HANDBOOK OF
Veterinary
Pain
Management

THIRD EDITION

HANDBOOK OF
Veterinary Pain Management

James S. Gaynor, DVM, MS, Dipl. ACVAA, Dipl. AAPM,
   IVAS, IVAPM
President and Medical Director
Animal Emergency Care Centers
Peak Performance Veterinary Group
HemoSolutions
Breckenridge and Colorado Springs, Colorado

William W. Muir III, DVM, PhD, Dipl. ACVAA, Dipl. ACVECC, VCPCS
Columbus, Ohio

ELSEVIER

ELSEVIER
MOSBY

3251 Riverport Lane
St. Louis, Missouri 63043

HANDBOOK OF VETERINARY PAIN
MANAGEMENT, Third edition   978-0-323-08935-7

> **Notices**
> Knowledge and best practice in this field are constantly changing. As new research and
> experience broaden our knowledge, changes in practice, treatment and drug therapy may
> become necessary or appropriate. Readers are advised to check the most current information
> provided (i) on procedures featured or (ii) by the manufacturer of each product to be
> administered, to verify the recommended dose or formula, the method and duration of
> administration, and contraindications. It is the responsibility of the practitioner, relying on
> their own experience and knowledge of the patient, to make diagnoses, to determine dosages
> and the best treatment for each individual patient, and to take all appropriate safety
> precautions. To the fullest extent of the law, neither the Publisher nor the Editor assumes
> any liability for any injury and/or damage to persons or property arising out of or related to
> any use of the material contained in this book.
>
>   The Publisher

Content Strategist: Penny Rudolph
Content Specialist: Katie Starke
Publishing Services Manager: Jeff Patterson
Senior Project Manager: Mary G. Stueck
Design Direction: Margaret Reid

Printed in India
Last digit is the print number: 9   8   7   6   5   4

CONTRIBUTORS

Leilani Alvarez, DVM, CVA, CCRT
Director
Integrative and Rehabilitative Medicine Service
Animal Medical Center
New York, New York
Chapter 18: Acupuncture

Steven C. Budsberg, DVM, MS, Dipl. ACVS
Professor
Department of Small Animal Medicine and Surgery
College of Veterinary Medicine
University of Georgia
Athens, Georgia
Chapter 8: Nonsteroidal Anti-inflammatory Drugs

Luis Campoy, LV, CertVA, Dipl. ECVAA, MRCVS
Associate Clinical Professor in Anesthesiology and Analgesia
Clinical Sciences
Cornell University College of Veterinary Medicine
Ithaca, New York
Chapter 11: Local Anesthetics
Chapter 12: Local and Regional Anesthetic Techniques

Robin Downing, DVM, CVA, CVPP, CCRP, Dipl. AAPM
Hospital Director
Downing Center for Animal Pain Management, LLC
Windsor, Colorado
Chapter 1: Pain Management and the Human-Animal Bond
Chapter 21: Therapeutic Goals
Chapter 23: Chronic Pain Cases

Mark E. Epstein, DVM, Dipl. ABVP (Canine/Feline),
Dipl. AAPM, CVPP
Senior Partner, Medical Director
TotalBond Veterinary Hospitals
Gastonia, North Carolina;
International Veterinary Academy of Pain Management
Past President
Nashville, Tennessee
Chapter 9: Opioids

James S. Gaynor, DVM, MS, Dipl. ACVAA, Dipl. AAPM, IVAS, IVAPM
President and Medical Director
Animal Emergency Care Centers
Peak Performance Veterinary Group
HemoSolutions
Breckenridge and Colorado Springs, Colorado

Michelle G. Hawkins, VMD, Dipl. ABVP (Avian)
Associate Professor, Companion Avian and Exotic Pets
Department of Medicine and Epidemiology
School of Veterinary Medicine
University of California–Davis
Davis, California

Matthew Johnston, VMD, Dipl. ABVP (Avian)
Associate Professor of Zoological Medicine
Clinical Sciences
Colorado State University
Fort Collins, Colorado

Darryl L. Millis, MS, DVM, Dipl. ACVS, CCRP, Dipl. ACVSMR
Professor of Orthopedic Surgery
Director, CARES Center for Veterinary Sports Medicine
Department of Small Animal Clinical Sciences
College of Veterinary Medicine
University of Tennessee
Knoxville, Tennessee

Craig Mosley, DVM, MSc, Dipl. ACVAA
Assistant Professor, Anesthesiology
College of Veterinary Medicine
Oregon State University
Coravallis, Oregon
Chapter 27: Reptile-Specific Considerations

William W. Muir III, DVM, PhD, Dipl. ACVAA, Dipl. ACVECC, VCPCS
Columbus, Ohio
Chapter 3: Pain and Stress: Stress-Induced Hyperalgesia and Hypoalgesia
Chapter 4: Definitions of Terms Describing Pain
Chapter 7: Overview of Drugs Administered to Treat Pain
Chapter 14: Alternative Drugs and Novel Therapies Used to Treat Pain
Chapter 15: Factors Influencing Analgesic Drug Selection, Dose, and Routes of Drug Administration
Chapter 16: Drug Interactions, Analgesic Protocols, and Their Consequences and Analgesic Drug Antagonism
Chapter 22: Acute Pain Management: A Case-Based Approach

Andrea Nolan, MVB, DVA, PhD, Dip ECVAA, Dipl. ECVPT, MRCVS
Professor
Edinburgh Napier University
Edinburgh, Scotland, United Kingdom
Chapter 6: Health-Related Quality of Life Measurement

Mark G. Papich, DVM, MS, Dip ACVCP
Professor of Clinical Pharmacology College of Veterinary Medicine North Carolina State University
Raleigh, North Carolina
Chapter 13: Glucocorticoids

Joanne Paul-Murphy, DVM, Dipl. ACZM, Dipl. ACAW
Professor
Department of Veterinary Medicine and Epidemiology
School of Veterinary Medicine
University of California–Davis
Davis, California
Chapter 26: Bird-Specific Considerations: Recognizing Pain Behavior in Pet Birds

Bruno H. Pypendop, DrMedVet, DrVetSci, Dipl. ACVAA
Professor
Department of Surgical and Radiological Sciences
School of Veterinary Medicine
University of California–Davis
Davis, California
Chapter 10: α₂-Agonists

Matt Read, DVM, MVSc, Dipl. ACVAA
Associate Professor (Anesthesiology and Therapeutics)
Department of Veterinary Clinical and Diagnostic Sciences (VCDS)
Faculty of Veterinary Medicine
University of Calgary
Calgary, Alberta, Canada
Chapter 11: Local Anesthetics
Chapter 12: Local and Regional Anesthetic Techniques

Jacqueline Reid, BVMS, PhD, Dipl. VA, Dipl. ECVAA
Professor
Honorary Senior Research Fellow
School of Veterinary Medicine
College of Medical, Veterinary and Life Sciences
University of Glasgow
Glasgow, Scotland, United Kingdom
Chapter 6: Health-Related Quality of Life Measurement

Sheilah A. Robertson, BVMS (Hons), PhD, Dipl. ECVAA, Dipl. ACVAA, Dipl. ECAWBM (WSEL) Specialist in Welfare Science, Ethics; Law, Dipl. ACAW, MRCVS
Associate Professor
Department of Small Animal Clinical Sciences
College of Veterinary Medicine
Michigan State University
East Lansing, Michigan
Chapter 24: Cat-Specific Considerations

E. Marian Scott, BSc, PhD, CStat
Professor
School of Mathematics and Statistics
College of Science and Engineering
University of Glasgow
Glasgow, Scotland, United Kingdom
Chapter 6: Health-Related Quality of Life Measurement

Andrea R. Slate, DVM
Assistant Director
Division of Comparative Medicine
Assistant Professor Department of Pathology and Cell Biology
University of South Florida
Tampa, Florida
Chapter 28: Regulations Regarding Pain and Distress in Laboratory Animals

Ashley J. Wiese, DVM, MS, Dipl. ACVAA
Staff Anesthesiologist
Department of Anesthesia
MedVet Medical and Cancer Center for Pets—Cincinnati, Dayton
Cincinnati, Ohio
Chapter 2: Nociception and Pain Mechanisms
Chapter 5: Assessing Pain: Pain Behaviors

M. Lesley Wiseman-Orr, BSc, PhD
Honorary Research Fellow
School of Mathematics and Statistics
College of Science and Engineering
University of Glasgow
Glasgow, Scotland, United Kingdom
Chapter 6: Health-Related Quality of Life Measurement

Tony L. Yaksh, PhD
Professor and Vice Chair for Research
Anesthesiology
Professor of Pharmacology
University of California–San Diego
La Jolla, California
Chapter 2: Nociception and Pain Mechanisms

This handbook is dedicated to all those animals who have needlessly suffered because of the lack of or inadequate treatment of pain and to all the individuals who have devoted their efforts to the alleviation of animal pain.

A COMPANION'S PAIN

Labored into the world
Vibrant life ripped from flesh
Flung towards days of wagging ease.
Comfort razed in an instant
A shrouded attack within
Writhe, recoil
Stifled whimper
Not too close! Trust growls distant
Flee, retreat, curl up close
Wrapped tight while hope tremors.
Pleading glance; lights wane and ebb
The tearless eye reveals nature's sting
On stoic souls;
Bearing it wisely
Grasping on instinct
Eased by the graciousness of man
Or Mercy.

— *Kristine J. McComis*†

---

†Deceased, 2010.

The third edition of *Handbook of Veterinary Pain Management* was developed after considering the suggestions and ideas of many practicing veterinarians, veterinary students, and individuals who have devoted their careers to the study of pain and its treatment. This edition contains updated information on drugs, dosages, and protocols, and incorporates a complete revision and expansion of several key areas of interest. We have included a new chapter on the pathophysiology of pain, particularly the mechanisms responsible for neuropathic pain and its treatment. We have also dedicated chapters to health-related quality of life (HQOL), physical rehabilitation in dogs and cats, therapeutic goals, regulatory issues and pain therapy considerations for laboratory animals used in biomedical research. This expansion provides more complete information for the alleviation of pain and suffering in animals.

This edition of the handbook is designed to deliver accurate and clinically useful information to practitioners and students interested in pain and pain therapy in animals. We have made every effort to ensure that the most recent information is presented.

As stated in our previous editions, the science of pain and its therapy continue to evolve, due in no small part to the exponential growth of scientific information regarding pain mechanisms and the ever-increasing number of therapeutic targets being discovered. Although all veterinarians take an oath to use their scientific knowledge and skills for "the relief of animal suffering," the treatment of pain has become a primary objective in a growing number of veterinary practices. Excellent textbooks describing the neuroanatomy, neurophysiology, and pathophysiology of pain are available to serve as the foundation of current understanding of main pathways and the mechanisms responsible for causing pain. The goal of this *Handbook* is to supplement this knowledge by providing a species-oriented, rapid, clinically applicable resource for use by all who diagnose and treat animal pain. The *Handbook* serves as a quick reference for pertinent physiologic and pharmacologic information, including drugs, drug dosages, and complementary therapeutic modalities used to treat pain. This *Handbook* also provides an extensive updated and detailed array of case examples of acute and chronic pain that can be used to provide a framework for discussion of pain therapy by practicing veterinarians, professional students, interns, residents, and veterinary technical support staff who are responsible for the day-to-day evaluation and care of animals. Similar to the previous edition, some information has been extrapolated from the human experience or is based on our collective clinical experience treating various animal species. Ideally, future basic and clinical investigations conducted in animals will provide guidance for therapeutic pain assessment and therapeutic modalities.

We thank all of the contributors for the time and effort they have dedicated to making this edition of the *Handbook* a reality. We also greatly appreciate the talented efforts of Tim Vojt, whose artwork has made written concepts visually understandable. Finally we would like to thank all those who have contributed their time, energy, and efforts toward improving the quality of life for all animals.

James S. Gaynor
William W. Muir III

Being admitted to the profession of veterinary medicine,

I solemnly swear to use my scientific knowledge and skills for the benefit of society through the protection of animal health, the relief of animal suffering, the conservation of livestock resources, the promotion of public health, and the advancement of medical knowledge.

I will practice my profession conscientiously, with dignity, and in keeping with the principles of veterinary medical ethics.

I accept as a lifelong obligation the continual improvement of my professional knowledge and competence.

Adopted by the American Veterinary Medical Association (AVMA) House of Delegates, July, 1969.

CONTENTS

PART ONE

Basic Concepts

CHAPTER 1

Pain Management and the Human-Animal Bond

Robin Downing

"Pain is a more terrible lord of mankind than even death itself."

Albert Schweitzer, MD

The Buddhists have a saying: "Pain is inevitable; suffering is optional." Those of us who work in veterinary medicine have pledged ourselves to recognize, relieve, and prevent pain and suffering in the animals entrusted to our care. The veterinarian's oath states in part, "I solemnly swear to use my scientific knowledge and skills for the . . . prevention and relief of animal suffering. . ." Ours is a sacred trust to advocate on behalf of beings who cannot advocate for themselves.

To review the history of veterinary pain management is to see the good, the bad, and the ugly. It was not so long ago that the "experts" believed that animals experience pain differently from humans. This was an easy conclusion to draw if we only *observed* animals. We could witness an animal with a known injury behaving much as it did before the injury had occurred. In dogs with advanced periodontal disease, for instance, it would be easy to conclude they must feel pain differently—or at least not as intensely—as we do, because they continue to eat and drink, whereas we would be immobilized by a similar issue. Cats are notorious for masking any weakness, including pain, until they are so ill or the pain so great that they can no longer function.

Humans have eschewed overt cruelty toward animals as far back as Biblical times. Charles Darwin (1872/1965) recognized that animals possess the fundamentals of consciousness. His reasoning was that "if animals show emotion through behavioral expression, then the behavioral expression of emotion in man must share a similar neurobiological evolution with the other animals capable of expressing similar emotions." It is only within the past several decades, however, that society has expanded its sensitivity to pain and suffering in animals. Our cultural norm now recognizes that *all* animal pain and suffering should be mitigated, whether we are considering the companion animals who share our homes and daily activities, the food and fiber animals who provide sustenance and substance, or the laboratory animals who provide opportunities for major medical breakthroughs. The veterinary profession is in the unique position to facilitate the ongoing expansion and sophistication of the pain relief available for and offered to all animals. For animals that are members of the family, the veterinary healthcare team has the opportunity to facilitate, enhance, lengthen, and strengthen the precious family-pet relationship. Relieving pain is one core competency through which to achieve that end.

Veterinary medicine has, throughout its history, emulated human medicine. Much of the current sophistication in veterinary care has been the result of reworking and reapplying human medical techniques in animals. Unfortunately, pain, pain relief, and pain medicine present challenges. The focus in both human and veterinary medicine has shifted away from the *art* of medicine to evidence based decisions or the *science* of medicine. Science is objective and can be measured. Pain, on the other hand, is a uniquely subjective experience—the antithesis of objective science. Regardless, veterinarians should employ techniques and therapies that represent best knowledge. Also, emulating a physician's focus on preserving life has caused veterinarians to emphasize life *quantity* in deference to life *quality*.

Richard D. Ryder, in his groundbreaking volume *Painism: A Modern Morality* (2001), coined several terms important to our consideration of animal pain. For Ryder, a being is "painient" if it has the capacity to feel pain, and "painience" is the principle that a moral code should be based on this capacity. Ryder goes on to state that the terms *pain* and *suffering* are interchangeable and that "what matters morally is the degree of pain and not who or what experiences it." In Ryder's worldview, pain is the common enemy all living beings face, and it is our common capacity for suffering that maps the similarity between humans and animals. The philosopher Jeremy Bentham, a contemporary of Rene Descartes, laid an important foundation for our current concerns when he wrote in 1780, "The question is not, can they reason? Nor, can they talk? But, can they suffer?"

It is useful to note that anesthesia for veterinary patients was actually developed *not* for pain relief, but for restraint. The idea was to provide chemical restraint in order to complete procedures on beings that could not simply be told to "hold still." Several types of drugs were employed for this. Barbiturates provide little to no analgesia once consciousness is regained. Dissociative drugs do not relieve pain or the effects of pain on the nervous system, but scramble cognitive function and pain *perception*. Paralytic drugs cause paralysis of the voluntary muscles, but do not blunt the pain experience in any way. An animal so affected feels every excruciating moment of its pain, but is trapped inside its own body, incapable of moving or escaping its pain. Sedative drugs affect mentation, but they do very little to mitigate the pain experience. A sedated animal may experience the full complement of its pain, but is too obtunded to react to it.

Likewise, there have been several persistent myths concerning animal pain that have influenced veterinary attitudes about administering pain medications perioperatively or after surgery or other trauma. It was thought that pain medication would suppress an animal's appetite, so withholding medication would encourage eating. Postoperative or post-trauma pain was considered to be a useful form of restraint that facilitated and prevented further tissue damage. If an animal's pain was relieved, it was thought, the animal would move around and "hurt itself." It was believed that animals do not feel pain, physiologically, in the same way as humans. It was thought that animals do not have the same subjective pain experience (suffering) as humans. Finally, it was thought that young animals feel less pain, or feel pain less intensely, than adult animals because the nervous systems of young animals are not as developed. This particular misconception also pervaded *human* medical opinions regarding infant pain as well. We now know that animals share very similar nervous system anatomy and physiology with humans. In fact, current research on the emotional lives of animals supports the notion that animals and humans share similar primal affective experiences. The implication being, to use a computer analogy, is that if they have the *hardware* (i.e., the nervous system), they can run the *program* (i.e., pain).

It is our moral imperative, as humans and as veterinarians, to recognize animals' capacity to feel pain. Consciousness is considered a core component of the pain experience—of painism, according to Ryder—but consciousness was once thought to reside in the neocortex of the brain, making it a uniquely human experience. The cognitive neuroscientists, neuropharmacologists, neurophysiologists, and computational neuroscientists who crafted the "Cambridge Declaration on Consciousness" (2012) drew quite a different conclusion. It appears that the neuroanatomy, neurochemistry, and other neurobiologic substrates of consciousness are not confined to cortical structures, and actually involve primitive subcortical structures activated by primitive emotions. Consequently, we must conclude that the neural elements needed to support consciousness are not uniquely human. In fact, there is a growing body of evidence to support the assertion that many animal species have nervous systems sophisticated enough to support complex cognitive processes as well as to experience stimuli as noxious. It is this noxiousness that is "fundamental to the cognitive emotional ... and hurtful nature of pain." Although the subcortical networks for processing pain may not be *homologous* across species, they most certainly are *analogous*.

Once we understand the painience of our patients—that is, their capacity to experience pain—(see Chapters 2 and 3) we can comprehend that uncontrolled pain and suffering inflict great harm, elevating prevention and control of pain to a moral imperative. Pain causes both physical *and* psychological damage. Pain delays healing, suppresses the immune system and increases blood viscosity, which can contribute to pathologic blood clot formation. It can increase the metastatic rate of some cancers. Pain inhibits normal behaviors and can precipitate abnormal behaviors (e.g. self-trauma, hiding, aggression). Although animals do not anticipate or fear death, they certainly do fear and try to avoid pain. We now understand that untreated pain can lead to death. Subjecting animals to unmitigated pain is surely the worst thing we as humans can do to them.

Companion animals have made a cultural migration of biblical proportion in our society. In addition, animals traditionally considered "production" species are playing new and different roles in our world. We have chickens in the back yard, goats are providing milk for personal family consumption, miniature pigs have become pets, and a variety of species including cats, dogs, birds and miniature horses now serve as therapy animals. Animals have moved from the back yard to the bedroom, and from the kennel to the couch. They have become members of the family. Many people now describe themselves as "pet parents." Animal life expectancies continue to lengthen, and the longer a pet lives, the deeper and more intimate the human-animal bond becomes. Pet owners' greatest fear is that their beloved animals will suffer. In fact, pain is often the key parameter by which the decision for humane euthanasia was determined.

Pain can put the human-animal bond in great jeopardy.

Buck was a 12-year-old Labrador retriever who was presented for euthanasia after he bit the family's 3-year-old son in the face. Buck's physical examination revealed a pain score of 7 out of 10 (0 = no pain; 10 = worst possible pain). His pain was especially intense in the lumbar and hip areas. It turned out that there were extenuating circumstances worth considering. The son, in whose life Buck had always played a prominent role, loved Buck so much that he wanted to show him by giving Buck a big hug around his midsection—in the precise area in which Buck had the greatest pain. That hug was so excruciatingly painful that Buck was overcome and responded to his pain the only way he knew how—by trying to escape and lashing out. Clearly, a biting dog presents an unacceptable risk to any 3-year-old child. In this case, however, it was Buck's pain that caused his dangerous behavior and threatened a rupture of the human-animal bond in that family. Fortunately for Buck, his pain was identified and treated successfully. Client education and a wellness program restored his place as a family member. He died from organ system failure 4 years later at the age of 16, secure in his place as a valued family member. Buck's situation is all too common for a dog with unrecognized pain who behaves unacceptably—straining, or even fracturing, the family-pet relationship.

Cats are not immune to similar situations.

Flower had become more and more reclusive, hiding behind furniture or under beds rather than interacting with her human family members. She became quite unkempt and developed a matted and dull hair coat, and anytime anyone attempted to groom her, she would become enraged and aggressive, scratching and biting to escape handling. The "last straw" for Flower's family came when she began darting out from her hiding places and biting the feet and ankles of family members and visitors to the home. These seemed to be unprovoked attacks, but a physical examination revealed an overall pain score of 8 out of 10 with generalized distribution over her torso. She had stopped grooming because it hurt her so much. She began biting feet and ankles as a "preemptive strike" to avoid being touched by the humans surrounding her. Avoiding any exacerbation of her pain became Flower's number one priority, and her avoidance and aggressive behaviors nearly fractured her relationship with her human family. After her pain was relieved, Flower's behavior transformed. She began grooming herself again and returned to the interactive, gregarious cat her family had loved and lost. Pain had compromised the human-animal bond between Flower and her human family members, threatening her very life.

The veterinary profession's sacred trust is to provide care for animals throughout the entire arc of their lives—from womb to tomb; from cradle to grave. This means supporting the human-animal bond through that entire arc. Pain interferes with the human-animal bond and interrupts the arc of life. Our animal patients do not deserve to hurt—rather, they need and deserve our best efforts to identify and relieve whatever pain they experience, no matter whether it is acute or chronic, mild or severe.

One implication of treating animal patients from the beginning to the end of their lives is that veterinary healthcare teams will inevitably face end-of-life issues with those patients. The implication for the family is that their bond of love with that animal is likely to be even stronger at 15 years of age than when that animal was 2. Even though animals do not fear death, humans certainly do. Speculation in the human pain management arena is that part of the reason people fear death is that they fear *pain* and death could be painful. It seems reasonable that our fear concerning the death of our pets is influenced by our fear that death will bring pain and suffering to them. Serious illness, chronic pain, approaching death were once managed primarily by humane euthanasia. The pet owner's worry was balancing comfort with the "escape" of humane euthanasia, trying to decide between euthanizing too soon and euthanizing too late.

Fortunately, we now have guidance for negotiating the minefield of animal pain and suffering. The late Dr. Lloyd Davis (1983), veterinary pharmacologist, once said of animal pain:

> "[O]ne of the psychologic curiosities of therapeutic decision-making is the withholding of analgesic drugs because the clinician is not absolutely certain that the animal is experiencing pain. Yet the same individual will administer antibiotics without documenting the presence of a bacterial infection. Pain and suffering constitute the only situation in which, I believe that, if in doubt, one should go ahead and treat."

Pain hurts. Our obligation as veterinarians is to advocate on behalf of animals who cannot advocate for themselves. That advocacy means actively preventing pain whenever we can, and relieving pain wherever we find it. The current state of the human-animal bond has influenced the evolution of pain prevention and wellness in veterinary medicine. Our culture and animal owners have demanded that the veterinary profession improve methods to treat pain in animals—in pets, in production animals, and in animal research subjects. The veterinary profession possesses the unique opportunity to support the human-animal bond for the entire arc of an animal's life—from cradle to grave. Anticipating and preventing pain, recognizing and relieving pain, and providing a humane and dignified exit from a painful existence are all important ways that veterinarians can facilitate, enhance, lengthen, and strengthen the human-animal bond. Managing pain is an individualized moving target and an ongoing process, and pain provides a moving target because the pathophysiologic processes responsible for pain change over time (see Chapter 2). Specialist in human pain management, James Giordano (2014) maintains that practicing pain medicine is an "ongoing clinical experiment with an N of one" (personal communication). We must be bold, yet work within (and generate) scientific evidence. We need to follow Albert Schweitzer's (1923) guidance: "[U]ntil we have drawn the animal into our circle of happiness, there can be no world peace." We need to take our obligation to our patients to heart.

SUGGESTED READING

AAHA/AAFP Pain Management Guidelines Task Force. AAHA/AAFP pain management guidelines for dogs and cats. J Am Anim Hosp Assoc. 43(5):235, 2007.

Bentham J. Introduction to the principles of morals and legislation. Oxford, UK, 1780, Clarendon Press.

Darwin C. The expression of the emotions in man and animals. Chicago, 1965, University of Chicago Press. (Original work published 1872.).

Davis LE. Species differences in drug disposition as factors in alleviation of pain. In: RL Kitchell, HH Erickson, E Carstens (Eds.): Animal pain: Perception and alleviation. Bethesda, Md., 1983, American Physiological Society.

Loveless SE, Giordano J. Neuroethics, panience, and neurocentric criteria for the moral treatment of animals. Camb Q Healthc Ethics. 23(2):163–172, 2014.

Mashour GA, Alkive MT. Evolution of consciousness: Phylogeny, ontogeny, and emergence from general anaesthesia. Proc Natl Acad Sci U S A. 110(Suppl 2):10359, 2013.

McCardle P, McCune S, Griffin JA, et al. (Eds.). Animals in our lives: Human-animal interaction in family, community, and therapeutic setting. Baltimore, 2011, Paul H Brookes Publishing.

Page G. Inside the animal mind: A groundbreaking exploration of animal intelligence. New York, 1999, Doubleday.

Panksepp J. Cross-species affective neuroscience decoding of the primal affective experiences of humans and related animals. PLoS One. 6(9):e21236, 2011.

Panskeep J, et al. (Eds.), Low P. Cambridge declaration on consciousness. Presented at the Francis Crick Memorial Conference on Consciousness in Human and non-Human Animals at Churchill College, University of Cambridge, Cambridge, UK, July 7, 2012.

Ryder RD. Animal revolution: Changing attitudes toward speciesism. Oxford, UK, 2000, Burg.

Ryder RD. Painism: A modern morality. London, 2001, Open Gate Press.

Schweitzer A. The philosophy of civilization, London, 1923, A & C Black.

Serpell J. In the company of animals: A study of human-animal relationships, Cambridge, UK, 1996, Cambridge University Press.

Shearer TS. Palliative medicine and hospice care protocols. Vet Clin North Am Small Anim Pract. 41(3):531–550, 2011.

Villalobos A, Kaplan L. Quality of life scale. In: Canine and feline geriatric oncology: Honoring the human animal bond, Table 10.1; p. 304, Ames, Iowa, 2007, Blackwell Publishing.

CHAPTER 2

Nociception and Pain Mechanisms

Ashley J. Wiese; Tony L. Yaksh

The International Association for the Study of Pain provides the broad definition of pain as "an unpleasant sensory and emotional experience associated with actual or potential tissue damage, or described in terms of such damage." Operationally, mechanical or thermal stimuli of sufficient intensity to result in tissue injury produce a hierarchy of responses including withdrawal of the affected body part (homotopic withdrawal reflexes), changes in autonomic outflow (increased heart rate and blood pressure, depending on the species), and activation of the hypothalamopituitary axis, yielding increased circulating concentrations of a variety of stress hormones (e.g., prolactin, adrenocorticotropic hormone [ACTH], cortisol). Sufficiently noxious stimuli yielding this hierarchy of observed effects result in a behavioral state manifested by complex escape activities and vocalization. The animal can become conditioned to undertake complex responses organized at the supraspinal level to avoid the environment in which that stimulus was applied—for example, the unconditioned application of the stimulus has intrinsic negatively reinforcing qualities. As will be reviewed later, these behavioral and physiologic effects will also occur after tissue or nerve injury.

The previous paragraph raises the issue of *anthropomorphism*, which means to attribute a human form or personality to an animal. Human nature is to project personal experiences and feelings onto animals because they cannot verbally describe how they feel. Although it is not really possible to know what are the thoughts of a nonverbal organism (be it a nonhuman species or a nonverbal human), the earlier commentary suggests that at the least for a given stimulus, (1) the attribute of the stimulus (potentially tissue injuring), (2) the physiologic response, and (3) the ability of the stimulus condition to sustain escape or avoidance are clear attributes of a nociceptive attribute. Mechanistic studies on the pharmacology and physiology of nociceptive states in human and nonhuman organisms frequently show a convergence suggesting that at least for mammals, nociceptive stimuli have a high degree of comparability. These parallels suggest that at the least it is ethically appropriate to adopt and use an anthropocentric viewpoint when assessing and treating pain in animals. The mechanisms believed to underlie nociception following acute high-intensity stimuli, tissue injury and inflammation, or nerve injury are reviewed.

THE PAIN PHENOTYPE

Peripheral nerves can be thought of as an extension of the central nervous system (CNS), consisting of sensory, motor, and autonomic nerve fibers. They are the links over which sensory and motor information are transmitted. The terminal ends of sensory nerve fibers recognize and transform (*transduce*) various environmental stimuli (thermal, chemical, mechanical) into electrical signals (*action potentials*) that are carried (*transmitted*) to the dorsal horn of the CNS, where they are encoded (*modulated*) and relayed (*projected*) to supraspinal sites within the brainstem (medulla, pons and mesencephalon, diencephalon and telencephalon) (Figure 2-1). Brainstem outflow drives various somatic and autonomic responses (e.g., activation of pathways leading to parasympathetic [vagal] and bulbospinal activation of preganglionic sympathetic outflow). Diencephalic afferent traffic drives hypothalamic circuits initiating hypothalamopituitary hormone release and in the thalamus provides the primary somatosensory terminations. Signals arising from the thalamofugal projections are integrated at the telencephalic

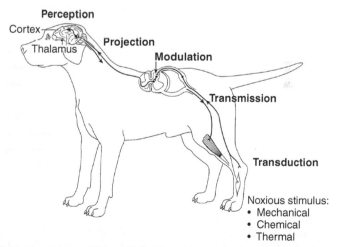

FIGURE 2-1   Pathways involved in nociception. Noxious stimuli (mechanical, chemical, thermal, electrical) are transduced (transduction) into electrical signals (action potentials) that are transmitted (transmission) to the spinal cord, where they are modulated (modulation) before being relayed (projection) to the brain for final processing and awareness (perception). Descending pathways from the brain modulate sensory input, and outputs from the spinal cord regulate skeletal muscle contraction.

level, identified (perceived), and transformed into appropriate self-preserving experiences and motor responses that are protective and remembered. Such input has a broad and pervasive effect on functionality of core systems and reflects on the imperative to appropriately and adequately manage pain states to maintain or reestablish homeostasis.

From an experiential point of view it is useful to discuss the origins of pain in terms of events initiated by the following:

- Acute high-intensity stimuli
- Tissue injury or inflammation
- Peripheral nerve injury

Acute Nociception

Pain reflects the interpretation of a nociceptive stimulus event as a *sensation* with highly aversive properties. Acute pain initiated by high-intensity stimuli is a psychophysical experience brought about by high-intensity, potentially tissue-damaging stimuli or peripheral nerve injury.

Nociception is the term used to describe the physiologic (*physiologic pain*) response (e.g., acute withdrawal; changes in autonomic outflow) generated by high-intensity stimuli.

- Such stimuli can sustain strongly motivating states.
- They can initiate and sustain avoidance behaviors cued by innocuous stimuli that have previously been paired with the nociceptive stimulus.

In the absence of prior conditioning or exposure, the manifestation of acute pain is accompanied by a constellation of observations:

- Withdrawal or guarding of the stimulated body part
- Activation of the autonomic nervous system
- A composite of behaviors that may include agitation and vocalization (see Chapter 5)

Somatotopic localization and classification of the acute nociceptive stimulus evoked response is characterized by the following:

- Restriction of the noxious sensation to the site of stimulation
- The magnitude of the evoked response (increased amplitude, increased strength, decreased latency) that co-varies with stimulus intensity (Figure 2-2)
- Termination of the response on removal of the acute stimulus, before development of tissue damage

Mechanical distortion, thermal stimuli (typically $>42°$ C [107.6° F]), or changes in the chemical milieu at the peripheral sensory nerve terminal evoke escape behavior in animals and the elicitation of activity in the adrenal-pituitary axis. The circuitry that serves in the transduction and encoding of this information includes the following:

- Primary sensory afferents
- Dorsal horn of the spinal cord

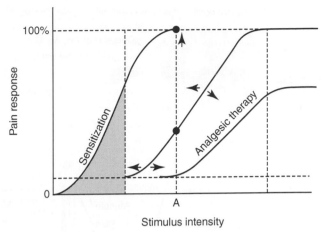

FIGURE 2-2   The pain threshold is the point at which stimulus intensity is just strong enough to be perceived as painful, e.g. a vocal report or of sufficient intensity to evoke an unconditioned escape response. Stronger stimuli elicit greater and longer pain responses until the maximum response possible is produced. The normal stimulus intensity-pain response curve is shown *(A)*. Increased responsiveness to a given stimulus that shifts the curve to the left is termed *hyperalgesia*. A decrease in the response to a given stimulus that shifts the curve to the right or decreases the slope of the curve is termed *analgesia* or *anesthesia*. A large left shift in the curve such that normally innocuous stimuli elicit a pain response is termed *allodynia*.

- Projection fibers to the brain
- Central pain processing centers

Primary Afferents and Dorsal Root Ganglia

The first-order neuron is the primary afferent. It is responsible for detecting and encoding the stimulus modality and intensity. The primary afferent nerve fiber is composed of populations of axons including large myelinated, small myelinated, and unmyelinated axons. Many of the Aδ and C sensory (afferent) nerve fibers innervating the viscera travel with sympathetic nerves (Figure 2-3). Axonal size and myelination dictate conduction velocity and are broadly associated with the encoding of different stimulus modalities (tactile, thermal, and/or chemical) (Table 2-1).

- Aβ (rapidly conducting) afferent nerve fibers typically respond to low-intensity mechanical (tactile, physical) stimuli (touch, pressure) and show rapid adaptation.
- Populations of Aδ fibers respond to low-intensity thermal or mechanical or high-intensity thermal or mechanical stimuli. The high-threshold Aδ nerve fibers are called *nociceptors*.
- C fibers typically respond to high-intensity thermal, mechanical, and chemical products and are called *polymodal nociceptors*.

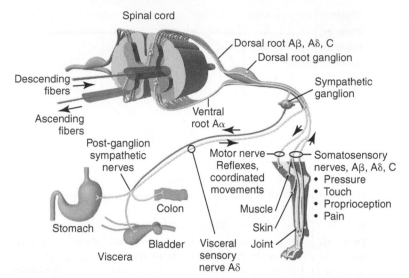

FIGURE 2-3   A simplified illustration of sensory (visceral and somatic) nerve fibers (Aβ, Aδ, C) that carry pressure, touch proprioception, and pain information as they travel to the dorsal root ganglia and then via the dorsal root nerve pathways to the brain. Many of the Aδ and C sensory (afferent) nerve fibers innervating the viscera travel with sympathetic nerves, passing through the sympathetic ganglia before reaching the dorsal root ganglia. Motor outflow innervating muscle is carried by nerve fibers (Aα).

TABLE 2-1	Primary Afferents Classed by Physical State, Size, Conduction Velocity, Effective Stimulus		
FIBER CLASS	**AXON DIAMETER**	**CONDUCTION VELOCITY**	**EFFECTIVE STIMULI**
Aβ (large myelinated)	12-20 μm	Group II (>40-50 m/sec)	Low-threshold mechanical (tactile or joint position)
Aδ (small myelinated)	1-4 μm	Group III ($10 < x < 40$ m/sec)	Low-threshold mechanical or thermal High-threshold mechanical or thermal (specialized nerve endings)
C (small unmyelinated)	0.5-1.5 μm	Group IV (<2 m/sec)	High-threshold thermal, mechanical, chemical (polymodal nociceptors)

- All afferents typically show two defining properties:
  - Minimal "spontaneous" activity in the absence of a stimulus
  - A monotonic increase in the frequency of firing with increasing stimulus intensities over the range of stimulus intensities to which they normally respond. For example, low-threshold Aδ thermal-sensitive

afferents respond with increasing frequency at temperatures ranging from 32° to 40° C, whereas high-threshold Aδ or C nociceptors respond with increasing stimulus intensity at temperatures ranging from 40° to 55° C.

Primary Afferents and Dorsal Root Ganglia Properties. The dorsal root ganglia (DRG) are cell bodies of afferent axons and thus provide the main trophic support for the afferent nerve. Proteins are transported centrally and peripherally to the terminals after synthesis in the DRG. Thus, primary afferent neurotransmitter synthesis occurs in the cell body of the DRG.

- The DRG neuron cell body is connected to the trunk of the axon by the glomerulus.
- The DRG demonstrates unique morphology for a neural structure situated outside the blood-brain barrier.
- The DRG display large *(type A)* and small *(type B)* neurons that give rise, respectively, to myelinated and unmyelinated afferent nerve fibers that project centrally (nerve roots) and peripherally (nerves).
- The DRG cells display *pericellular glial* cells that stain for glial fibrillary acidic protein *(GFAP)*. These are called *satellite cells* and invest the DRG neuron. Other cell types include Schwann cells and microglia.
- The DRG is well vascularized, and because it lies outside the blood-brain barrier, the vessels are innervated by *postganglionic sympathetic* efferents (as evidenced by dopamine β-hydroxylase–positive histochemistry).

Terminal Transduction and Action Potential Generation. Activation at the peripheral terminal generates an electrical (action) potential traveling locally in the peripheral terminal *(antidromic conduction)* and back to the spinal cord *(orthodromic conduction)*. Nerve terminals of the primary afferent neuron contain channels and receptors responsible for transduction of an external stimulus (thermal, mechanical, chemical). These channels vary in the modality to which they respond and the intensity of that preferred stimulus modality. The response properties of the different sensory and primary afferents thus reflect the constituencies of channels with which the different populations of afferents are endowed (Figure 2-4).

- Low-threshold transducers: Activated by events such as light touch (pacinian corpuscles) for mechanical stimuli or innocuous thermal intensities.
- High-threshold transducers: Activated only at extreme ranges of intensities, which may be noxious in character. Such transducers may be activated at different temperature ranges and by specific chemicals. Several examples are listed below.
  - Transient receptor potential cation channel subfamily V member 1 *(TRPV1)* is activated by temperatures higher than 52° C; known as *heat nociceptors*.
  - *TRPV8* is activated by temperatures lower than 19° C; known as *cold nociceptors*.

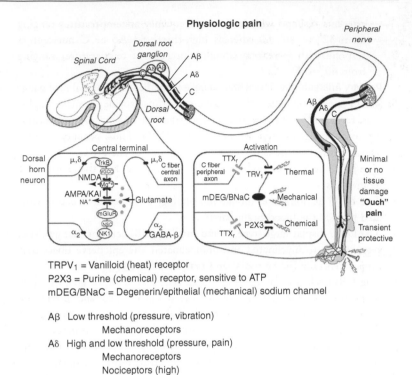

TRPV₁ = Vanilloid (heat) receptor

P2X3 = Purine (chemical) receptor, sensitive to ATP

mDEG/BNaC = Degenerin/epithelial (mechanical) sodium channel

Aβ Low threshold (pressure, vibration)
Mechanoreceptors
Aδ High and low threshold (pressure, pain)
Mechanoreceptors
Nociceptors (high)
C High threshold (pain)
Mechanoreceptors
Thermoreceptors
Nociceptors

FIGURE 2-4 Nociceptive (physiologic pain): Non–tissue-damaging stimuli activate peripheral pain receptors (nociceptors; *R*), which produce electrical signals that are transmitted by afferent Aδ and C sensory nerve fibers to the spinal cord and brain.

- It is important to note that these channels may also be activated by specific chemicals, for example, by *capsaicin* and *menthol*, which respectively initiate sensation of heat and cold when applied to the skin.
- Acid Sensing channels (ASIC) are a family of cation channels present on afferent nociceptors. They are typically activated by elevated hydrogen ion concentrations and a variety of chemicals including snake venoms.
- When activated, these channels increase cation currents, leading to a local depolarization of the terminal that in turn depolarizes local sodium channels to initiate a conducted action potential.

Transmission at the First-Order Synapse. The primary afferent synapse shows several specific characteristics and properties.

- Terminal depolarization leads to the opening of voltage-gated calcium channels (*CaV*) to activate synaptic proteins (soluble *N*-ethylmaleimide attachment proteins [*SNAREs*]), which mobilize synaptic vesicles to the terminal membrane. This mobilization leads to the *exocytosis* of the transmitter into the synaptic cleft.
- The released transmitters initiate postsynaptic excitation.
- Immunohistochemical analyses and pharmacologic studies show that the principal afferent transmitter contained within and released from small clear core synaptic vesicles is *glutamate*. The postsynaptic effect of glutamate is mediated by several eponymous *ionotropic* receptors:
  - α-Amino-3-hydroxy-5-methyl-4-isoxazolepropionic acid (AMPA) receptors mediate acute membrane activation through massive increase in sodium conductance.
  - *N*-Methyl-D-aspartate (NMDA) receptors, when activated, lead to a large increase in Ca^{2+} conductance and serve to mediate more persistent input, leading to more pronounced depolarization and activation.
- Populations of small nociceptive afferents may also contain and release from large dense core vesicles one or more peptides, such as substance P (sP), vasoactive intestinal peptide (VIP), somatostatin, the VIP homologue peptide histidine isoleucine (PHI), calcitonin gene-related peptide (CGRP), bombesin, and related peptides. The effects of each of the aforementioned peptides are mediated by specific eponymous receptors (e.g., neurokinin 1 for the neuropeptide sP).

Spinal Cord Dorsal Horn

The spinal cord second-order neurons in the dorsal horn relevant to nociceptive processing may be considered as being of several classes based on their anatomic location and response properties. These response properties are defined in large part by the input that they receive. The spinal cord is anatomically divided into several broad regions that are further subdivided into the so-called *Rexed laminae* (Figure 2-5), of which several play a key role in pain propagation.

Marginal Layer (Lamina I)

- Cells of the marginal layer contain neurons that respond to nociceptive and thermal input from Aδ and C fibers
- Because these cells receive largely nociceptive afferent input only, they are, broadly speaking, *nociceptive-specific neurons.*
- These cells project to the thalamus, periaqueductal gray matter (PAG), lateral parabrachial area, nucleus of the solitary tract, and medullary reticular formation (RF).

Substantia Gelatinosa (Lamina II)

- Lamina II primarily receives noxious or thermal stimuli from Aδ and nonpeptidergic C fibers.

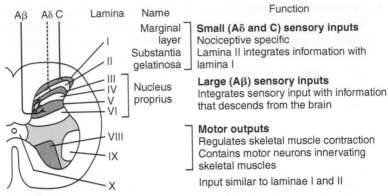

FIGURE 2-5   The gray matter of the spinal cord is divided into anatomically identified layers (Rexed laminae). The superficial and deep dorsal horn of the gray matter receives sensory input from Aβ, Aδ, and C nerve fibers. The ventral horn of the spinal cord contains motor neurons that innervate and regulate skeletal muscle contraction in response to afferent input. The white matter contains projection fibers that link the spinal cord with the brain.

- Lamina II is further subdivided into inner (IIi) and outer (IIo) regions based on the type of C-fiber input and cell morphology. Many of these cells are interneurons, employing either excitatory or inhibitory transmitters. Much regulation of dorsal horn input and output is regulated by the modulatory interneurons.

Nucleus Proprius (Laminae III Through VI)

- Neurons in laminae of the deep dorsal horn (so-called *lamina V neurons*) have their cell bodies deep, but send their dendrites dorsally toward the upper laminae. These neurons receive low-threshold sensory information (touch, innocuous temperature) from large Aβ fibers (which project deep into the dorsal horn). They also receive input on their distal dendrites from high-threshold Aδ and C fibers (located in the skin, muscle, and viscera) that project into laminae I and II and from excitatory interneurons.

- Because lamina V neurons receive convergent input from low-threshold afferents (and are thus activated by low-intensity input) and high-threshold input, they are referred to as *wide dynamic range (WDR)* neurons (Figure 2-6). Lamina V neurons respond to graded increases in stimuli (from light touch to modest pressure to nociceptive prick or pinch), a trait that is unique to these neurons and that likely plays an important role in both tissue and nerve injury states.

- Lamina VI is best developed in the cervical and lumbar enlargement (tumescence) areas.

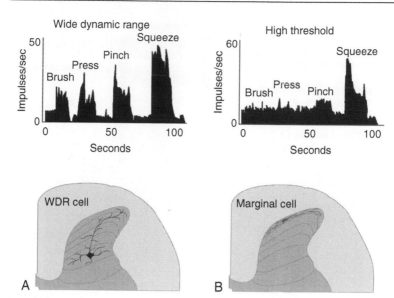

FIGURE 2-6   Firing pattern of second-order neurons. Firing pattern (impulses/sec) of a spinal dorsal horn wide dynamic range *(WDR)* neuron located primarily in lamina V **(A)** and a high-threshold (nociceptive-specific marginal) neuron **(B),** in response to graded intensities of mechanical stimulation (brush, pressure, pinch, squeeze) applied to the receptive fields of each cell. Note that response properties reflect their afferent connectivity within the spinal cord (see Figure 2-7).

Lamina X

- Lamina X is located around the central canal and is not physically part of the dorsal horn but receives nociceptive input that is more specific for visceral regions.

Projection Fibers to the Brain

Projection fibers consist of both afferent and efferent nerve fibers that couple the brain with the spinal cord. These projection fibers are myelinated nerves that are arranged in columns within the white matter surrounding the gray matter. The dorsal column relays somatic sensory information to the brain. The intermediate column contains sensory motor and autonomic nerve fibers descending from the brain and sensory pathways ascending to the brain.

Primary Afferent Projections

On entering the spinal cord, the central processes of the afferents collateralize (Figure 2-7).

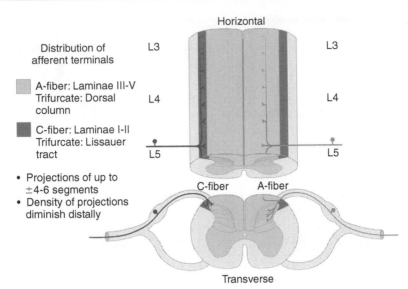

FIGURE 2-7 Spinal distribution of primary afferent nerve terminals in the dorsal horn. C fibers project into the dorsal horn at the segment of entry and collateralize to project rostrally and caudally in the lateral tract of Lissauer. Large A fibers project into the dorsal horn and send collaterals into the dorsal columns. For any given afferent axon, its densest terminations are within the segment of -fiber entry; but, there are also less dense collateralizations into the dorsal horn at more distal spinal segments. The density of collateralization corresponds to the strength of the excitatory drive into these distal segments. Thus, afferent input into one segment can provide some excitatory input into the dorsal horn at more distal segments.

- Small C-fiber afferents send projections in the segment of entry to ramify in the superficial dorsal horn (laminae I and II) and project rostrally and caudally several segments in the tract of Lissauer.
- Smaller Aδ myelinated fiber terminals are located in the marginal zone (lamina I), the ventral portion of lamina II (IIi) and throughout lamina III.
- Large Aβ-fiber afferents project into the deep dorsal horn (laminae III through VI) with ramifications into the superficial dorsal horn of the segment of entry and send collaterals rostrally and caudally in the *dorsal columns*, where they ramify in the deep dorsal horn.

It is important to emphasize that although the primary projection of afferent nerve fibers is in the dorsal horn at the segment of entry and it is in this segment that the afferent exerts its most potent excitatory effects, the collaterals spread excitatory nerve activity to adjacent segments. The farther away from the segment of entry, the smaller the excitatory influences become. For example, activation of a 3rd lumbar vertebral nerve root will activate neurons primarily in the lumbar 3 segment, but there may also be significant although less reliable activation of neurons several segments rostrally and caudally. The more distant the spinal cord segments are from the segment of entry (e.g., 12th thoracic vertebral nerve root), the less likely the neurons are to be activated, although some excitation in the form of small excitatory potentials may persist. If for any reason the more distant neurons become more excitable, then the subliminal excitatory input may be sufficient to activate a neuron that is normally activated only by a 12th thoracic vertebral nerve root. The size of the receptive field of that 12th thoracic vertebral nerve root neuron may now include areas of the body otherwise activated only by a 3rd lumbar vertebral nerve root input. This linkage is thought to be important in different forms of hyperalgesia observed after tissue and nerve injury.

Ascending Spinal Tracts

Output from the spinal cord arises from the superficial dorsal horn (laminae I and II) and lamina V. Second-order neurons project to supraspinal sites by several long and intersegmental tract systems that travel rostrally within the ventrolateral quadrant and are identified based on whether they cross or do not cross to the opposite side of the spinal cord and by their supraspinal projections. Classic studies have demonstrated that nociception and pain depend on a "crossed pathway," projecting contralaterally. Thus, unilateral injury or section of the ventrolateral quadrant will yield contralateral thermal or mechanical analgesia in dermatomes below the spinal level of the section.

- Spinoreticular fibers
  - Spinoreticular axons terminate ipsilaterally and contralaterally to their spinal site or origin. In the medulla, the fibers aggregate laterally, and collaterals of these fibers terminate in the more medially situated brainstem reticular nuclei. Reticulothalamic afferents excited by this input then project to the thalamus.
- Spinothalamic fibers
  - The cells of origin of the spinothalamic tract are the most extensively studied of the ventrolateral tract systems. Axons originating in the marginal layer and the neck of the nucleus proprius ascend predominantly in the contralateral ventral quadrant.
- Clinical experience suggests that the crossing may occur as much as several segments more rostrally. Thus, after spinal ventrolateral cordotomy the analgesic level may be several dermatomes caudal to the section.
- Although crossed fibers predominate, uncrossed fibers also represent an appreciable component of the spinothalamic population.

  Supraspinal Systems. The contralateral ventrolateral projection pathway may be divided into two principal projection motifs (Figure 2-8).
- Somatosensory pathway
  - The somatosensory pathway projects to the ventrobasal thalamus, and neurons in this region then project to the somatosensory cortex.
  - This projection pathway produces a precise somatotopic mapping of the body surface at each link.

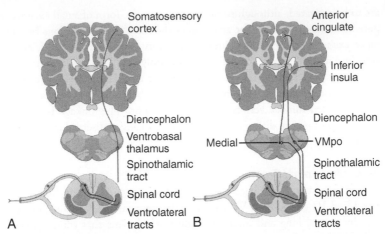

FIGURE 2-8   Summary of ascending pathways that originate from nociceptive specific (lamina I) and wide dynamic range (lamina V) neurons. **A,** The somatosensory pathway projects via the spinothalamic tract to the ventrobasal thalamus with projections to the somatosensory cortex. **B,** The affective-motivational pathway projects into the medial thalamus and posterior part of the ventral medial nucleus in the thalamus *(VMpo),* the pars oralis, and these project to the anterior cingulate and the inferior insula, respectively.

- Affective-motivational pathway
  - A second system projects into the more medial aspects of the thalamus, and these neurons project to a variety of sites including areas of the limbic forebrain, such as the anterior cingulate and the inferior insula. A poor somatotopic map characterizes this pathway.
- These pathways reflect the underlying dichotomy that pain may be considered to have.
  - The somatosensory pathway projecting though the somatosensory thalamus to the somatosensory cortex serves to encode stimulus localization and intensity (sensory-discriminative).
  - The medial system projecting though the medial thalamus and into regions such as the anterior cingulate and insula appears to encode information for regions that are classically associated with emotionality and affect (affective-motivational).
- In short, these events summarize the pathways and processes that are believed to underlie the primary functional motifs by which a high-intensity stimulus gives rise to higher-order processing, initiating an aversive state.

Central Pain Processing Centers

Perception.   The recognition and processing of sensory information (perception) occurs in multiple specific areas of the brain, which communicate via

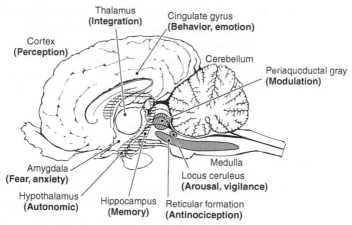

FIGURE 2-9   Regions of the brain associated with various functions and responses. The thalamus serves as the central integrating and transmission point for pain perception and subsequent responses.

interneurons to produce an integrated response that reflects the coordinated contributions of arousal, somatosensory input, and autonomic and motor output (Figure 2-9). Several neural pathways (redundancy) convey information from a specific body part (*parallel processing*) and help to ensure adequate input to the CNS. Neurons originating from laminae III, IV, and V ascend to synapse with neurons in the caudal medulla (brainstem) and relay information concerning tactile sensation, including touch, vibration, and limb proprioception.

The reticular activating system (RAS), located in the brainstem, is a critical center for the integration of these sensory experiences and the subsequent affective and motivational aspects of pain through projections to the medial thalamus and limbic system. The RAS mediates motor, autonomic, and endocrine responses. Neurons originating in laminae V and I synapse in the pons and medulla, midbrain, PAG, and thalamus. The PAG and thalamus serve as relay points for sensory information transfer; the former transfers information to the thalamus and hypothalamus, and the latter transfers information to the cerebral cortex. The three major pathways of the anterolateral system are the spinothalamic, spinoreticular, and spinomesencephalic tracts and are primarily involved in relaying painful and temperature-related sensations.

The thalamus relays information to the somatosensory cortex, which in turn projects the information to adjacent cortical association areas, including the limbic system. The limbic system includes the cingulate gyrus (behavior, emotion), amygdala (conditioned fear, anxiety), hippocampus (memory), hypothalamus (sympathetic autonomic activity), and locus ceruleus (arousal, vigilance, behavior) (see Figure 2-9). The caudal extension of the limbic system, the PAG, receives descending information from the cortex, amygdala, and hypothalamus and ascending projections from the medulla, medullary RF (including the locus ceruleus), and spinal cord.

The PAG is considered to be an important relay for descending facilitative and inhibitory (endogenous opioid) modulation of nociceptive input. The PAG connects with the rostral ventromedial medulla (RVM) and medullary RF, from which adrenergic and serotoninergic fibers descend to the dorsal horn of the spinal cord, inducing inhibitory or analgesic effects. Descending facilitation from the RVM is thought to be a critical component of many chronic pain states.

Collectively, these centers process sensory information that elicits fear, anxiety, and aggression and activate efferent pathways that mediate autonomic, neuroendocrine, and motor (skeletal and visceral) responses. Furthermore, all of these areas can be conditioned by visual, olfactory, auditory, and somatic or visceral stimuli that prepare the CNS for frightening or stressful events. The physiologic, biochemical, cellular, and molecular changes that occur in response to stressful or noxious events emphasize the tremendous plasticity of the CNS and highlight the importance of chronic stress in the development of pathologic pain (see Chapter 3).

Memory. The memory of pain is formed by several factors, including the animal's behavior pattern, the environment, the expectation of pain, and the intensity of painful events. The peak intensity of pain is the single most important factor in determining the memory of pain. *Neuroplasticity* refers to the ability of the nervous system to change or adapt its biochemical and physiologic functions in response to internal and external stimuli (including chronic drug use); the implication is that multiple minor sensory events or a single major sensory event can change the stimulus-response characteristics of the nervous system. Animals who have an inherent memory of pain or of a significant painful event are harder to treat, and animals in which pain has been allowed to persist for days to weeks are less responsive to analgesic therapy.

Tissue Injury and Inflammatory Pain States

The pain response generated by a stimulus that is severe enough to cause tissue injury differs in several important ways from the events evoked by a brief high-intensity noninjurious stimulus.

- The nociceptive pain state persists after termination of the injuring stimulus.
- The reported magnitude of the pain sensation associated with a given stimulus applied to the injured site is increased (*primary hyperalgesia*)—that is, a given stimulus applied to the injured site will evoke withdrawal or vocalization responses at shorter latencies and the magnitude (amplitude) of the responses will be enhanced; or, conversely, for a given

nociceptive response latency or amplitude, the stimulus intensity required to evoke that response will be reduced.

- Enhanced sensitivity to stimuli applied at sites *adjacent* to the injury site may develop (i.e., *secondary hyperalgesia*).
- The origins of these changes in response to tissue injury may reflect changes in peripheral terminal excitability (i.e., *peripheral sensitization*), and the ongoing activity in the pain-activated afferent sensory nerve results in an increased response within the spinal cord (i.e., *central sensitization*) (Figure 2-10).

Peripheral Origins of Tissue Injury Leading to Enhanced Pain States

Tissue injury elicits alterations in nociceptive afferent response characteristics that can be observed from any small afferent nerve innervating inflamed tissues (e.g., visceral afferents, musculoskeletal afferents, innervation of the cornea, tooth pulp, and meninges):

- An increase in ongoing (spontaneous) discharge of afferents innervating the site of injury or inflammation that is normally activated only by high-intensity stimulus (i.e., *silent nociceptors*—for example, a C fiber that normally fires at $50°$ C, may now start firing at $46°$ C).
- The monotonic increase (leftward shift) in the stimulus-response of afferents to stimulation reflects the fact that a given stimulus yields a yet greater afferent response. This left shift is consistent with the enhanced pain response produced by an otherwise mild aversive stimulus (e.g., severe stomatitis leads to an abnormal pain response to light touch in the oral cavity).
- The slope of the frequency-response curve is increased such that there is a greater increment in firing for any given increment in stimulus intensity (Figure 2-11).

Factors Leading to Altered Peripheral Afferent Response Properties. Altered response of small afferent nerves after local injury reflects changes in the local chemical milieu of the peripheral terminal that occur secondary to tissue damage and plasma extravasation resulting from enhanced capillary permeability. A variety of products are released from the following:

- Damaged tissue (e.g., K^+, H^+)
- Local inflammatory cells (e.g., histamine from mast cells; peptidase; prostaglandins [PGs] from macrophages; tumor necrosis factor [TNF])
- Blood products (5-hydroxytryptamine, or serotonin [5-HT] from platelets; bradykinin [BK] from endothelial cells)
- Transmitters released from local C-fiber primary afferents (e.g., sP, CGRP)

Collectively these many products are referred to as *inflammatory* or *sensitizing soup.*

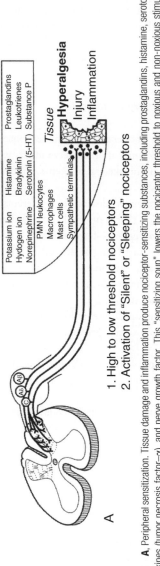

"Sensitizing soup"

Potassium ion	Histamine	Prostaglandins
Hydogen ion	Bradykinin	Leukotrienes
Norepinephrine	Serotonin (5-HT)	Substance P

PMN leukocytes
Macrophages
Mast cells
Sympathetic terminals

Tissue

Hyperalgesia
Injury
Inflammation

1. High to low threshold nociceptors
2. Activation of "Silent" or "Sleeping" nociceptors

FIGURE 2-10 A, Peripheral sensitization. Tissue damage and inflammation produce nociceptor-sensitizing substances, including prostaglandins, histamine, serotonin, bradykinin, proteases, cytokines (tumor necrosis factor—α), and nerve growth factor. This "sensitizing soup" lowers the nociceptor threshold to noxious and non-noxious stimuli and activates "silent" or "sleeping" nociceptors, resulting in hyperalgesia and allodynia.

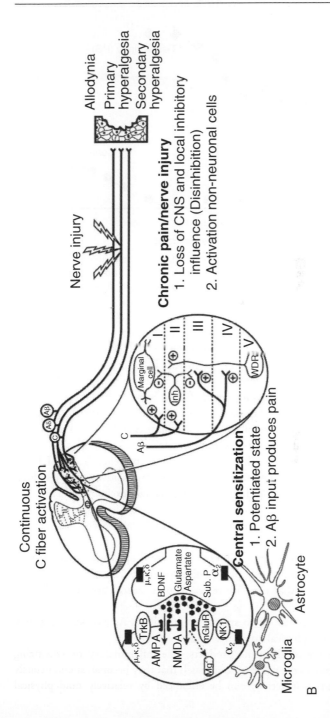

FIGURE 2-10—cont'd   **B,** Central sensitization. Strong (high-intensity) persistent stimuli activate C fibers, causing the release of a variety of transmitters, including glutamate, substance P (sP), and other factors such as brain-derived neurotrophic factor (BDNF) at central nerve terminals; this results in the activation of AMPA, NMDA, Neurokinin 1 and tyrosine receptor kinase B (Trk B) receptors, respectively, producing acute and long-lasting dull, aching, burning pain sensations. The activation of these receptors increases the activity of signaling molecules that alter gene expression and change the responsiveness (sensitize⁻ of the spinal cord to subsequent input. Chronic stimulation may result in neurochemical changes (neuroplasticity) in the spinal cord such that all stimuli produce pain. AMPA, a-amino-3-hydroxy-5-methyl-4-isoxazolepropionic acid; NMDA, N-Methyl-D-aspartate.

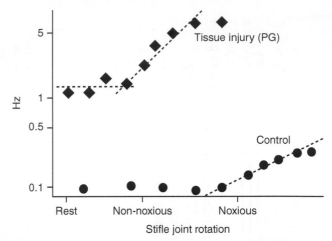

FIGURE 2-11 Increased slope and leftward shift of stimulus-response curve indicating a facilitated response to stimulus in an articular afferent nerve fiber after inflammation induced by prostaglandin I2 (PGI2) injection intra-articularly. After injection of PGI2 into the joint, joint manipulation even within a normal range of motion results in significant discharge.

These agents (*algogens*) released locally after injury typically activate eponymous receptors that are expressed on the peripheral terminal of the C fiber leading to activation of the C-fiber afferents (Table 2-2).

- Activation of these receptors leads to a persistent activation of C-fiber nerve terminals and ongoing small afferent nerve traffic—that is, a pain sensation. Activation of these receptors also serves to activate a variety of terminal protein kinases such as protein kinase A and C (PKA and PKC) as well as several mitogen-activated protein kinases (MAPKs).
  - These kinases phosphorylate transducer proteins (e.g., TRPV1) and local ion channels such as the voltage-sensitive (gated) sodium channels (NaVs), leading to their enhanced excitability. Thus any given stimulus will yield an enhanced afferent discharge.
- The degree of receptor activation reflects the local concentrations of the agents and the composite of products.

Silent Nociceptors. Many C fibers are activated only by intense physical stimuli. Articular and tooth pulp C-fiber afferents, as an example, have thresholds so high that they are referred to as "silent" or "sleeping" nociceptors.

- Afferents with little or no spontaneous activity. Activation occurs only with extreme physical stimuli.
- The presence of algogenic products (the inflammatory or sensitizing soup) sensitizes the nerve terminal such that they become "spontaneously active" and their activity can be enhanced by relatively mild physical stimuli.

TABLE 2-2	Activation and Sensitization of Nociceptors ("Inflammatory Soup")		
INFLAMMATORY MEDIATOR	**ORIGIN**	**TARGET RECEPTOR**	**NOCICEPTOR EFFECT**
Hydrogen ion	Damaged cells	Acid-sensing ion channels (ASICs) TRPV1	Activation
Potassium ion	Damaged cells	Two-pore potassium channels (K2P)	Activation
Prostaglandins (E2, I2)	Damaged cells	EP	Sensitization
Leukotrienes	Damaged cells		Sensitization
Bradykinin	Mast cells	Bradykinin (B1/B2)	Activation
Serotonin	Platelets, mast cells	Serotonin (5-HT)	Activation
Histamine	Mast cells		Activation
Substance P	Sensory nerve endings	Neurokinin 1 (NK1)	Sensitization
Calcitonin gene-related peptide (CGRP)	Sensory nerve endings		
Nerve growth factor	Sensory nerve endings, macrophages	Tyrosine kinase (TrkA)	Sensitization
Tumor necrosis factor–α	Macrophages	Tumor necrosis factor (TNF2)	Sensitization
Interleukins	Macrophages		Sensitization
ATP	Platelets		

ATP, Adenosine triphosphate *EP,* prostaglandin receptor; *TRPV1,* transient receptor potential cation channel sub family V member 1.

- Activation of silent nociceptors may contribute to the induction of hyperalgesia, central sensitization, and allodynia (see later).
- Many visceral nociceptors are silent nociceptors.
- Small innervating afferents with high threshold may display sprouting and develop neuromas during chronic inflammation of the joints. Neuromas are associated with nerve injuries and often display ongoing or ectopic activity. Accordingly this phenomenon may, in part, account for pain in osteoarthritis.

Spinal Origins of the Tissue Injury Enhanced Pain States

Acute activation of afferent nociceptors results in activation of the nociceptive pathways and a clearly defined pain behavior. The response of second-order dorsal horn neurons to such stimulation is related to the following:

- The afferent population activated (large vs. small afferents)
- The frequency of afferent activation, which is proportional to the magnitude of the stimulus

The nervous system's response to the acute stimulus is thus modeled in terms of a positive monotonic function of the activity in the afferent nerve and activity of supraspinally projecting neurons. Tissue injury or inflammation-induced enhanced activity initiates neurochemical cascades that lead to a *nonlinear* increase in the input-output function of the spinally projecting systems.

Central Facilitation. Dorsal horn WDR neurons exhibit a stimulus-dependent response to single C-fiber stimuli. Rapid, repetitive electrical stimulation of these C (but not A) fibers results in the phenomena of "wind-up": an increase in pain intensity over time caused by repeated stimulation of C fibers, leading to a progressively increasing electrical response in the corresponding spinal cord neurons. Wind-up reflects several important changes in response properties of these WDR cells:

- There is a progressively facilitated discharge in response to any given stimulus. This increase develops over intervals of seconds after the initiation of the stimulus train.
- This facilitation lasts for periods of seconds to minutes after termination of the stimulus.
- Low-threshold tactile (normally non-noxious) stimulation becomes increasingly effective in driving these afferent neurons and generating a noxious response (hyperalgesia).
- Conditioning input by the afferent nerve serves to enlarge the receptive field size of the neuron. Non-noxious afferent input from dermatomal areas adjacent to the un-injured region yields discomfort (allodynia).

Wind-up. Projection of WDR neurons supraspinally occurs through the ventrolateral quadrant of the spinal cord. The augmented response reflected by wind-up represents an important component of the encoding of the pain message and contributes to injury-induced hyperalgesia.

- A progressive and long-sustained partial depolarization of the cell, rendering the membrane increasingly susceptible to afferent C-fiber input
- A stimulus intensity reflective of the frequency of WDR discharge

Changes in Receptive Field Size That Occur With Tissue Injury. Changes in normal afferent input into collateral neurons located several spinal segments distal contribute to changes in receptive field size (see comments in preceding section on afferent dorsal horn collaterals):

- Distant collateral cell becomes sensitized during wind-up–induced spinal cord sensitization such that activation now occurs by input from the distal segment (dermatome).
- The receptive field now includes not only its original dermatomes, but dermatomes of the distant neurons, generating a referred pain state.

Dorsal Horn Circuitry. Nociceptive afferent nerve fibers release glutamate and peptides from their central terminals in the spinal cord (Figure 2-12). Additional peptides are released along with glutamate only when the afferent fibers fire action potentials at high frequencies (equivalent to severe injury).

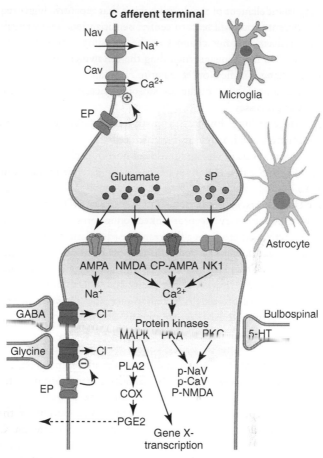

FIGURE 2-12   Primary afferent and second-order neuron synapse. Glutamate is the primary neurotransmitter released at the nerve terminal in the spinal cord (central terminals). Glutamate primarily activates α-amino-3-hydroxy-5-methyl-4-isoxazolepropionic acid *(AMPA)* and kainate (KA) receptors, producing transient or temporary ("ouch") pain. *CaV*, voltage-gated calcium channels; *COX*, cyclooxygenase; *CP-AMPA*, calcium-permeable AMPA; *EP*, prostaglandin receptor; *GABA*, γ-aminobutyric acid; *5-HT*, 5-hydroxytryptamine; *MAPK*, mitogen-activated protein kinase; *NaV*, voltage-sensitive (gated) sodium channel; *NK1*, neurokinin 1; *NMDA*, N-methyl-D-aspartate; *p*, permeable; *PGE2*, prostaglandin E2; *PKA*, protein kinase A; *PKC*, protein kinase C; *PLA2*, phospholipase A2; *sP*, substance P.

- Small nerve-fiber afferent input depolarizes terminals, opening voltage sensitive Ca^{2+} channels, leading to release of terminal neurotransmitters (glutamate and peptides).
- Neurotransmitters bind eponymous ionophores (AMPA, NMDA, calcium-permeable AMPA sites, and NK1 receptors) to activate second-order neurons.

- An important element of the dorsal horn is that repetitive high-frequency small afferent input will lead to central sensitization. The central sensitization reflects dynamic changes in the encoding process by a number of dorsal horn mechanisms, including the following:
  - Local changes in first-order synapse function
  - Increased excitability in the second-order neuron secondary to intracellular processes
  - A change in local inhibitory control leads to changes in bulbospinal modulation and finally non-neuronal cells
- These events result in changes in dorsal horn function that enhance the excitability of the dorsal horn systems over an extended time frame (seconds to days).

Acute-Onset Postsynaptic Events. Glutamate released from primary afferents activates two primary receptor-linked ionophores:

- *AMPA.* Activation produces a fast response (depolarization) that increases membrane permeability to sodium, yielding a prominent but transient depolarization. This likely accounts for the majority of the acute activation produced by brief activation of both low- and high-threshold afferents.
  - Some subtypes of AMPA receptors are able to gate calcium (e.g., calcium-permeable AMPA ionophores) and play a role in spinal facilitatory processes.
- *NMDA.* This ionophore does not appear to mediate acute excitation but is responsible for a slower-onset and longer-duration aching, burning pain response (slow response). Under normal resting membrane potentials, the NMDA receptor is in a state of magnesium block, preventing activation.
  - A modest depolarization of the membrane as produced during repetitive stimulation secondary to the activation of AMPA (glutamate), and the NK1 (sP) receptors remove the Mg^{2+} block, permitting glutamate to activate the NMDA receptor.
  - Activation of the NMDA channel permits the large-scale influx of Ca^{2+}.
  - Increases in intracellular calcium lead to activation of kinases (PKC, PKA, and tyrosine kinases), leading to increased sensitivity of NMDA receptors to glutamate.
  - Activation of the NMDA channel is responsible for central sensitization.
- Notably, blocking the spinal AMPA receptor can produce a virtual anesthetic-like state, whereas block of the spinal NMDA receptor (with agents such as ketamine) has no effect on acute nociception, but reduces facilitated states such as wind-up.

Delayed-Onset, Intermediate-Duration Postsynaptic Events. Persistence of C-fiber activity triggers other, more enduring intracellular biochemical cascades that also magnify and enhance the afferent response to yield a long-lasting spinal sensitization.

- Ca^{2+} *activation of phospholipase A2 (PLA2).* Arachidonic acid is released from plasma membranes, thus making it available as a substrate for cyclooxygenases (COX-1 and COX-2), resulting in production of PGs as well as other enzymes such as nitric oxide (NO) synthase producing NO.
  - The lipids act on specific PG receptors and NO on presynaptic second messengers to increase the amount of neurotransmitter released per action potential invading the terminal.
  - Glia are activated by PGs binding specific PG receptors, causing the release of additional neuroactive substances including proinflammatory cytokines and altering the activity of inhibitory interneurons (see the discussion of local regulatory interneurons).
- *Spinobulbospinal dorsal modulation.* The output of the local dorsal systems from lamina I neurons project into the medullary brainstem, activating bulbospinal serotonergic projections, which in turn project excitatory drive onto dorsal horn neurons, leading to a magnification of the response of the spinal projection neurons (see later discussion).
- *Changes in local inhibitory circuits.* Under normal circumstances, afferent input and large A low-threshold primary afferents are under inhibitory control by local γ-aminobutyric acid (GABA)–ergic and glycinergic interneurons. Some of the neurons are on the presynaptic terminal of the large (not small) afferents and on the second-order neuron. These inhibitory interneurons are often driven by large afferent input. This local circuit thus serves to regulate the excitation of the dorsal horn neurons otherwise initiated by afferent input (on the WDR neurons). Any process that reduces this GABAergic or glycinergic regulation will lead to an enhanced response of the second-order neuron otherwise evoked by the large afferent nerve fibers. It is interesting to note that the PG released by C-fiber input has been shown to suppress glycine receptor function, leading to an enhanced response evoked by the A-fiber input—for example, a substrate for tactile allodynia after tissue injury.

Slow-Onset, Long-Duration Postsynaptic Events. Increases in intracellular calcium lead to the activation of a variety of transcription factors that activate protein synthesis, resulting in the following:

- Increases in the activity of proinflammatory cascades—for example, increased expression of COX-2 and NO synthetase
- Upregulation of channel expression such as those for voltage gated calcium and sodium channels.
- These changes lead to long-term changes in sensitization of the dorsal horn as the result of a burst of high-frequency small afferent input.

Pharmacology of Central Facilitation—Non-Neuronal Cells. There are a variety of non-neuronal cells in the CNS. Among these are astrocytes and microglia. Microglia are resident macrophages that appear in the brain from the circulation during development (see Figure 2-12).

These astrocytes, microglia, and neurons form a complex in which each can influence the excitability of the other:

- Transmitters from primary afferents and intrinsic neurons (glutamate, adenosine triphosphate [ATP], sP) can overflow from the synaptic cleft to these adjacent non-neuronal cells and lead to their activation.
- Astrocytes may communicate over a distance by the spread of excitation through gap junctions (local nonsynaptic contacts).
- Astrocytes may communicate with microglia by the release of a number of products including glutamate or cytokines such as TNF and interleukin (IL)–1β.
- Neurons may activate microglia by the specific release of factors such as membrane chemokine (fractalkine), which can act on specific receptors found on microglia. This process is part of a complex cascade referred to broadly as *neuroinflammation*.
- Non-neuronal cells can influence synaptic transmission by their release of a variety of active products (such as ATP and cytokines). These glial cells regulate extracellular parenchymal glutamate by their glutamate transporters. This can serve to increase extracellular, activating neuronal glutamate receptors.
- Microglia (resident brain macrophages) are constitutively active. Microglia can also be upregulated after peripheral injury and inflammation.
- After tissue injury and inflammation, circulating cytokines (such as IL-1β, TNF-α) can activate perivascular astrocytes or microglia. Such activation provides a mechanism whereby circulating factors can alter neuronal excitability.

Local Regulatory Interneurons. WDR second-order dorsal horn neurons receive excitatory input from large afferents. This input is likely mediated by glutamate and by input into excitatory interneurons, which also release glutamate. The dorsal horn also has large populations of GABAergic and glycinergic interneurons that can interact with the GABA$_A$ and glycine chloride ionophores, respectively.

- These ionophores exert a potent inhibitory effect on pain that can varyingly have postsynaptic localization (second-order neurons) or presynaptic localization (primarily large afferents).
- WDR neurons receive convergent input from A and C nociceptive fibers. The presence of GABA or glycine ionophores on these terminals emphasizes that the input from large axons is under ongoing inhibitory control of a cell that is part of the nociceptive encoding pathway.
- Loss of inhibitory regulation *(disinhibition)*, as with blockade receptor antagonists (GABA$_A$, bicuculline; glycine, strychnine), will lead to a prominent state of tactile allodynia. Regulation of glycine receptor function by PGs provides an important mechanism whereby centrally acting COX inhibitors can alter inflammatory-induced hyperpathia.

Pharmacology of Central Facilitation—Spinobulbospinal Pathways. Bulbospinal pathways originating in nuclei in the medullary brainstem are activated by increases in high-intensity afferent input onto marginal (lamina I) cells that project into the periaqueductal gray, the parabrachial and the medulla. Whereas a component of descending inhibition mediates a local inhibition, the serotonergic pathway is facilitatory.

- Activation of subtypes of 5-HT receptors (5-HT3) contributes to spinal facilitation through excitation of dorsal horn neurons.
- Descending facilitation links higher-order function to spinal sensory processing.
- Emotions and conditioned memories can alter the nature of nociceptive input received by the brain—that is, aversive events may condition animals to show hyperalgesia.

Dorsal Root Ganglion Cells. Following tissue inflammation, a variety of changes may occur in the DRG:

- Increased presence of vascular adhesion factors cause migration of macrophages into the DRG (which lies outside the blood-brain barrier).
- Macrophages secrete proinflammatory products that lead to ectopic DRG activity.
- Similarly, there is activation of DRG satellite cells, glia, that surround DRG neurons.

These are considered to be potential sources of ongoing afferent traffic that would activate central neurons.

Summary

The post–tissue injury or inflammation pain state reflects several complex elements:

- Sensitization of the peripheral terminal in response to release of a variety of local factors that initiate spontaneous activity
- Facilitation of the response of the peripheral terminal to otherwise ineffective stimuli
- Potent central (spinal) sensitization that leads to enhanced responsiveness of dorsal horn neurons that receive ongoing small afferent traffic

These mechanisms lead to an enhanced response to input from the injured receptive field and an enlargement of the peripheral fields that can now activate those neurons originally unaffected by subliminal input. The augmentation reflects local synaptic circuitry, spinobulbospinal linkages, and products released from local non-neuronal cells.

NERVE INJURY

A variety of stimuli (mechanical trauma, chemicals, viral infections) can injure peripheral afferent nerves. Although there may be no evidence of tissue injury, the animal will exhibit behaviors that are aversive in nature and responds to otherwise innocuous stimuli that suggests pain or nociception. This state represents "neuropathic pain." Neuropathic pain has several properties that differentiate it from the events initiated by tissue injury.

After tissue injury and inflammation, pain subsides as the healing process takes place. The animal shows evidence of a different constellation of painful events following peripheral nerve injury:

- Ongoing incidences of sharp, shooting sensations referred to the peripheral distribution of the injured nerve.
- Abnormal painful sensations or responses evoked by light tactile stimulation of the peripheral body surface—that is, tactile allodynia (mediated by low-threshold mechanoreceptors [Aδ afferents]). This ability of light touch to evoke pain is evidence that the peripheral nerve injury has led to a reorganization of central processing—that is, it is not a simple case of a *peripheral sensitization* of otherwise high-threshold afferents.
- An ameliorating effect of sympathectomy of the afflicted limb and an attenuated responsiveness to analgesics such as opiates may be observed. This emphasizes the role of peripheral sympathetic nervous system activity in potentiating pain states (producing hyperalgesia).

These aberrant changes in sensory processing appear to arise from changes in the function of primary afferent function and in DRG and dorsal horn function secondary to responses to the peripheral injury.

Effects of Nerve Injury on Neuronal and Dorsal Root Ganglion Morphology

The peripheral afferent nerve initially dies back (*retrograde chromatolysis*) after an acute mechanical injury. This process proceeds for some interval after which the axon begins to sprout, sending growth cones forward.

- The growth cone frequently fails to make contact with the original target and displays significant proliferation. Collections of these proliferated growth cones form structures called *neuromas*.
- Examination of the neuroma reveals Schwann cell proliferation and increased invasion of postganglionic sympathetic efferents.
- In addition to changes in the peripheral axon, a variety of events indicate that the robust changes are also occurring in the dorsal root ganglion neurons of the injured axon.
- Examination of the DRG of the peripherally injured axon reveals a large number of events emphasizing the reactive changes in DRG function. It has been estimated that nerve injury can lead to changes in the expression levels of several thousands of genes.
- Examples of these reactive changes are noteworthy.
  - Marked increase in the expression of a variety of proteins, including those for channels (e.g., NaV and voltage-gated calcium channels, CaV)

- Transcription factors (e.g., activation transcription factor 3)
- Myriad membrane receptors (e.g., cytokine receptors [TNF receptors; IL-1β], α-adrenergic receptors; Toll-like receptors [TLRs]; protease-activated receptors [PARs])
- Glial (satellite cell) activation
- Increased innervation by postganglionic sympathetic afferents
- Appearance of inflammatory cells, for example, lymphocytes and macrophages

Spontaneous Pain State

The mechanism of changes in structure and function lead to a neuropathic pain phenotype after an injury to the nerve through afferent axonal changes.
- An initial burst of afferent firing secondary to the injury
- Silence for an interval of hours to days
- Development over time of persistent afferent traffic, which is noted in both myelinated and unmyelinated afferent axons

Ectopic activity is the origin of the ongoing pain state or dysesthetic sensation. Spontaneous activity in the afferent axon arises from the neuroma and from the DRG of the injured axon.

Recording from the afferent axon reveals that the afferent activity arises independently from two sources, the neuroma and the DRG neurons of the injured axon.

Mechanisms of Ectopic Afferent Activity

Changes in afferent terminal sensitivity and the presence of inflammatory products after nerve injury are responsible for ectopic activity.
- Sprouted afferent endings display increased sensitivity (receptor expression) to a number of humeral factors, such as prostanoids, catecholamines, and cytokines such as TNF. Sensitivity of the neuroma and DRG is of importance, given that after local nerve injury there is the release of a variety of cytokines, particularly TNF, that could directly activate the DRG and neuroma.
- After peripheral nerve injury, inflammatory cells appear in the DRG. As noted in the review of tissue injury, these macrophages can release products that can depolarize the DRG neurons.
- After nerve injury, sprouting of postganglionic sympathetic efferents occurs that can lead to the local release of catecholamines. This scenario is consistent with the observation that after nerve injury the postganglionic axons can initiate excitation in the injured axon.

Evoked Hyperpathia

Tactile sensitivity is mediated by low-threshold afferent (Aβ-fiber) stimulation. Several underlying mechanisms have been proposed to account for this seemingly anomalous linkage.

Dorsal Root Ganglion Cell Crosstalk

Single-unit recordings support the thesis that crosstalk develops between afferents in the DRG and in the neuromas.

- Depolarizing currents in one axon (e.g., an Aβ fiber) would generate a depolarizing voltage in an adjacent quiescent axon (e.g., a C fiber).
- This depolarization would allow activity arising in one axon to drive activity in a second.
- Accordingly, a large low-threshold afferent would drive activity in an adjacent high-threshold afferent. These events are thought to primarily occur in injured axons.

Dorsal Horn Reorganization

A variety of events occur in the dorsal horn after peripheral nerve injury, which suggests altered processing wherein the response to low-threshold afferent traffic can be exaggerated.

- *Increased spinal glutamate release.* Spinal glutamate release occurs in accord with increased spontaneous activity in the primary afferent and with the loss of intrinsic inhibition, which may serve to modulate resting glutamate secretion (see later discussion).
- *Non-neuronal cells and nerve injury.* Activation of spinal microglia and astrocytes occurs with nerve injury, leading to increased spinal expression of COX, nitric oxide synthetase (NOS), glutamate transporters, proteinases, and cytokines. Such biochemical components emphasize the *plasticity* of the nervous system and have been previously shown to play an important role in the facilitated state.
- *Loss of intrinsic GABAergic and glycinergic inhibitory control.* As noted earlier, a large number of small interneurons contain and release GABA and glycine. Animals undergoing antagonism of $GABA_A$ receptors or glycine receptors (i.e., bicuculline, strychnine) or animals genetically lacking glycine-binding sites often display a high level of tactile allodynia and spinal hyperexcitability. Loss of such inhibitory control may reflect the following:
  - Loss of GABAergic or glycinergic neurons.
  - Loss of $GABA_A$ or glycine receptors.
  - Change in inhibitory function of the GABA or glycine receptor. More recent work has suggested that after nerve injury, spinal neurons regress to a *neonatal phenotype* in which $GABA_A$ activation becomes *excitatory.* This change is secondary to reduced activity of a membrane Cl^- transporter, which changes the reversal current for the Cl^- conductance. Here, increasing membrane Cl^- conductance, as occurs with $GABA_A$ receptor activation, results in membrane depolarization that would make the inhibitory interneurons into a facilitatory component.

BOX 2-1	Mechanisms Responsible for Prolonged and Exaggerated Pain

- Peripheral sensitization (inflammatory soup)
- Wind-up (temporal summation of sensory inputs)
- Central sensitization
- Increased sympathetic innervation and excitation of dorsal root ganglia
- Disinhibition of inhibitory modulation of sensory inputs
- Redistribution of Aβ inputs from laminae III and IV to lamina II
- Abnormal patterns of spinal cord interneuronal communication
- Altered phenotype of damaged sensory nerve fibers (central nervous system plasticity)
- Abnormal patterns of peripheral nerve regeneration after trauma (neuroma)

- *Sympathetic sprouting.* After peripheral nerve injury, there is increased growth of postganglionic sympathetic terminals into the neuromas and into DRG of the injured axons.
  - These postganglionic fibers form baskets of terminals around DRG neurons.
  - Stimulation of preganglionic axons will produce activity in the sensory axon by an interaction both at the peripheral terminal at the site of injury and/or at the level of the DRG.

Summary

The mechanisms involved in pain after nerve injury include the following:
- Initiation of ectopic activity in the neuroma and in the DRG of the injured axon. This ectopic activity likely reflects the increased expression of receptors that are activated by inflammatory products at the site of the nerve injury and in the DRG and in ion channels such as those for NaV subtypes. Such products may arise in part from the post-ganglionic sympathetic nerves that invade the DRG.
- Prominent reorganization of dorsal horn processing as evidenced by the ability of low-threshold mechanoreceptors to initiate a pain state and enhanced dorsal horn activation. Components of this facilitation may reflect activation of non-neuronal cells and the change in the phenotype of the role played by otherwise inhibitory GABA$_A$ and glycine receptors.

The prolonged and exaggerated pain response observed after tissue or nerve injury arises as a result of this combination of events (Box 2-1).

CLINICAL PAIN

The preceding sections have heuristically discussed pain in terms of three discrete mechanisms: acute, tissue injury, and nerve injury and have emphasized the roles of peripheral, spinal and supraspinal mechanisms for producing pain.

The pain phenotype observed clinically results from one or more clinical pathologies and most likely results from more than one of these three mechanisms and produces multiple neuroendocrine responses (Table 2-3). This is illustrated in Table 2-4, using the example of an animal with pain from a metastatic disease. The importance of such interactions is the role played by multiple components when one considers pain therapeutics. The mechanism(s) whereby a drug alters the processing of pain information will ultimately depend on the role played by that target mechanism in the overall pain state. Moreover, in any given clinical condition the contributions of the various mechanisms may change throughout the day and over more extended periods of time.

TABLE 2-3   Pathophysiologic Consequences of Pain

SOURCE OF PAIN	SYMPTOMS
Cardiovascular	Tachycardia, hypertension, vasoconstriction, increased cardiac work and oxygen consumption
Pulmonary	Hypoxia, hypercarbia, atelectasis; decreased cough; ventilation/perfusion mismatch, predisposition to pulmonary infection
Gastrointestinal	Nausea, vomiting, ileus
Renal	Oliguria, urine retention
Extremities	Skeletal muscle pain, limited mobility, thromboembolism
Endocrine	Vagal inhibition; increased adrenergic activity, increased metabolism, increased oxygen consumption
Central nervous system	Anxiety, fear, sedation, fatigue, depression
Immunologic	Impairment, "sickness syndrome"

TABLE 2-4   Example of the Complex Nature of a Clinical Cancer Pain State Wherein Multiple Mechanisms are at Play

CANCER	ACUTE ACTIVITY (↑Aδ AND C SPINAL NEURONS ASCENDING ACTIVITY)	TISSUE INJURY (SENSITIZATION PERIPHERAL CENTRAL)	NERVE INJURY (ECTOPIC ACTIVITY SPINAL INHIBITION SPROUTING)
Tumor erosion (bone, tissue)	—	X	—
Tumor release of factors	X	X	—
Immune response (paraneoplastic)	—	—	X
Movement (incident pain)	X	X	—
Tumor compression	—	—	X
Radiation	—	—	X
Chemotherapy	—	—	X
Surgical section	—	X	X

SUGGESTED READING

Bueno L, Fioramonti J. Visceral perception: Inflammatory and non-inflammatory mediators. Gut. 2002; 51 Suppl 1: i19–23.

Craig AD. Interoception: The sense of the physiological condition of the body. Curr Opin Neurobiol. 2003; 13:500–505.

Dray A. Inflammatory mediators of pain. Br J Anaesth. 1995; 75:125–131.

Dubin AE, Patapoutian A. Nociceptors: The sensors of the pain pathway. J Clin Invest. 2010; 110:3760–3772.

Mashour GA, Alkire MT. Evolution of consciousness: Phylogeny, ontogeny, and emergence from general anesthesia. Proc Natl Acad Sci USA. 2013; 110:10357–10364.

Michaelis M, Häbler HJ, Jäenig W. Silent afferents: A separate class of primary afferents? Clin Exp Pharmacol Physiol. 1996; 23:99–105.

Milligan ED, Sloane EM, Watkins LR. Glia in pathological pain: A role for fractaline. J Neuroimmunol. 2008; 31:113–120.

Muir WW III, Woolf CJ. Mechanisms of pain and their therapeutic implications. J Am Vet Med Assoc. 200; 219:1346-1356.

Nickel FT, Seifert F, Lanz S, Maihöfner C. Mechanisms of neuropathic pain. Eur Neuropsychopharmacol. 2012; 22:81–91.

Ossipov MH, Dussor GO, Porreca F. Central modulation of pain. J Clin Invest. 2010; 120:3779–3787.

Petrenko AB, Yamakura T, Baba H, Shimoji K. The role of N-methyl-D-aspartate (NMDA) receptors in pain: A review. Anesth Analg. 2003; 97(4):1108–1116.

Raouf R, Quik K, Wood JN. Pain as a channelopathy. J Clin Invest. 2010; 120:3745–3752.

Rexed D. The cytoarchitectonic organization of the spinal cord in the cat. J Comp Neurol. 1952; 96:415–466.

Ru-Rong J, Woolf CJ. Neuronal plasticity and signal transduction in nociceptive neurons: Implications for the initiation and maintenance of pathological pain. Neurobiol Dis. 2001; 8:1–10.

Sandkuhler J. The organization and function of endogenous antinociceptive systems. Prog Neurobiol. 1996; 50:49–81.

Watkins LR, Milligan ED, Maier SF. Glial activation: A driving force for pathological pain. Trends Neurosci. 2001; 24:450–455.

Wieseler-Frank J, Maier SF, Watkins LR. Central proinflammatory cytokines and pain enhancement. Neurosignals. 2005; 14:166–174.

Willis AD, Westlund KN. Neuroanatomy of the pain system and of the pathways that modulate pain. J Clin Neurophysiol. 1997; 14:2–31.

Woolf CJ, Salter MW. Neuronal plasticity: Increasing the gain in pain. Science. 2000; 288:1765–1768.

Woolf CJ. What is this thing called pain? J Clin Invest. 2010; 120:3742–3744.

Xu Q, Yaksh TL. A brief comparison of the pathophysiology of inflammatory versus neuropathic pain. Curr Opin Anaesthesiol. 2011; 24:400–407.

Yaksh TL. Spinal systems and pain processing: Development of novel analgesic drugs with mechanistically defined models. Trends Pharmacol Sci. 1999; 20:329–337.

CHAPTER 3

Pain and Stress
Stress-Induced Hyperalgesia and Hypoalgesia

William W. Muir III

A nimal welfare, well-being, and contentment are all components of what is now collectively considered to be quality of life (QOL). QOL, for animals, has been defined as "a multidimensional, experiential continuum" that is composed exclusively of affect (i.e., to influence or produce change) (see Chapter 6). Most animals live in the present with little or no regard for the past or future; they live in "the now." Animals do not comprehend the meaning of pain or death, hence the importance of affect in determining the animal's interaction with its environment and its QOL. QOL for animals has been separated into two domains: comfort-discomfort and pleasure. The comfort-discomfort domain encompasses physical and emotional states and includes pain, thirst, hunger, disease, and responses to harsh environments, whereas emotional states include fear, anxiety, frustration, and depression. The pleasure domain includes physical and emotional states and activities such as physical contact, companionship, and mental stimulation. Quantitation of an animal's QOL may be the most noninvasive and promising method for determining the severity of an animal's condition. QOL, for animals, should always include the "five freedoms": (1) freedom from thirst, hunger, and malnutrition; (2) freedom from discomfort; (3) freedom to express normal behavior; (4) freedom from fear and distress; and (5) freedom from pain, injury, and disease (Box 3-1). Stress is the biologic response that animals exhibit when homeostasis (internal equilibrium) is threatened. Whether animals perceive pain and are stressed in the same way that human beings are is unlikely due to differences in their ability to comprehend the meaning of pain or its consequences. Regardless, pain produces stress and should be thought of in terms of the magnitude of the stress response that it produces, its potential to produce distress (stress that negatively affects biologic functions), and the degree of animal suffering incurred. In practical terms, the severity and duration of pain determine its consequences in terms of the continuum of stress–distress and suffering.

Stress occurs when animals experience disease, trauma, or surgery, or they perceive a threat such as unfamiliar environment or restraint. Conscious stressors (e.g., physical restraint, trauma) and unconscious stressors (e.g., anesthesia and surgery) can elicit stress. The role of the central nervous

> **BOX 3-1   The Five Freedoms**
>
> Freedom from thirst, hunger, and malnutrition
> - Access to food and fresh water
>
> Freedom from discomfort
> - Suitable environment, shelter, and a resting place
>
> Freedom to express normal behavior
> - Provision of space, facilities, and companionship
>
> Freedom from fear and distress
> - Environmental enrichment
>
> Freedom from pain, injury, and disease
> - Prevention of cruelty and illness

system (CNS) in modifying the body's response to various stressors (e.g., pain, surgery, restraint, confinement) varies among and within species and can be modified by domestication and training. Auditory and visual stimuli produce and potentiate somatosensory input to the CNS and elicits biologic responses identical to those produced by tissue damage. This input can modify the animal's memory and evoke predictable behavioral changes characterized by startle, fear, an attempt to escape, aggression (fight or flight), or submission. Dogs and cats, like all animals, respond to stressors by activating sensory, autonomic, endocrine, and immune responses that constitute a biologic defense mechanism targeted toward avoiding injury and maintaining homeostasis. Stress, then, serves a protective role by diverting the biologic resources of the body to cope with the stressor. This biologic defense mechanism functions to protect the animal and maintain homeostasis. Ineffective responses to stress, including the stress caused by pain, result in dysfunction, disability, depression and disease, and predispose to distress and suffering, collectively constituting a "sickness syndrome" that threatens life (Figure 3-1).

Stress does not cause pain, although it can change the pain experience. Acute and chronic pain, however, do produce stress and activate defensive biologic responses that result in profound physiologic and behavioral changes. Even without a painful stimulus, environmental factors (e.g., loud noise, restraint, predators) can produce a state of anxiety or fear in animals that sensitizes and amplifies the stress response and by doing so may aggravate or suppress pain. Stress has been demonstrated to either enhance pain (stress-induced hyperalgesia [SIH]) or suppress pain (stress-induced analgesia [SIA]) depending on the severity of pain and the animal's prior experience with stressful, painful, or environmental stimuli.

SICKNESS SYNDROME

"Sickness syndrome" occurs when animals are semi-continuously or continuously exposed to factors that activate the immune-inflammatory response

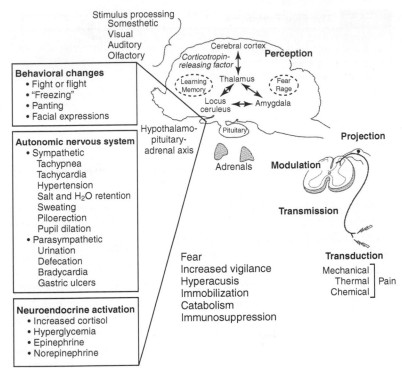

FIGURE 3-1 Stress response: Activation of the neural circuits (transduction, transmission, modulation, projection, perception) responsible for producing pain stimulates the thalamus, locus ceruleus, and amygdala, which induce fear, anxiety, and rage in animals, resulting in behavioral, autonomic, and neuroendocrine changes. Acute pain often produces fear, increased vigilance, and immobilization ("freezing" stance) in some animals, and chronic unrelenting pain can lead to loss of appetite, tissue catabolism, and immunosuppression and can alter learning patterns and memory.

(e.g., endotoxins, CNS trauma, reperfusion injury, chronic diseases). Proinflammatory cytokines "facilitate" or enhance pain in addition to producing malaise and fever. Animals generally exhibit clinical signs of hyperalgesia, depression, inappetence, somnolence, or may display signs of hypervigilence such as anxiety, restlessness, and hyperacusis, that can interfere with the animal's ability to rest or sleep. Cytokines activate glial cells in the CNS, contributing to the production and maintenance of a generalized central nervous system sensitized state (central sensitization). Sick animals may be more sensitive to external noxious stimuli and respond with signs of pain to nonnoxious stimuli. Therapeutic interventions to reduce this hyperalgesic state should include strategies to reverse glial cell activation and central sensitization. A decision to withhold analgesics in an apparently "sick" animal should take into account the potentially significant impact of "sickness syndrome," and the use of nonpharmacologic methods to manage pain, including a stress-free and protective environment (shelter, food, warmth, bedding).

DEFINING TERMS

Pain

Pain is defined as "an unpleasant sensory and emotional experience associated with actual or potential tissue damage or described in terms of such damage" (see Chapter 4). Pain produces biologic defense responses and physical or physiologic changes that are exhibited as behavioral aversion (dysphoria) or indifference to rewarding stimuli. Pain may be diffuse or localized and usually produces a desire to avoid, escape, or destroy the factors responsible for its production. Untreated or prolonged pain promotes an extended stress response, characterized by neuroendocrine dysregulation, fatigue, myalgia, abnormal behavior patterns, and altered physical performance.

Homeostasis

Homeostasis refers to the internal bodily adjustments that are made to maintain the "internal milieu"; these adjustments include but are not limited to changes in thermoregulation, metabolism, blood gases, acid base balance, hydration, and blood pressure.

Allostasis

Allostasis refers to the protective, coordinated, adaptive body reactions that ensure that the processes sustaining homeostasis stay within the normal range.

Stress

Stress is the animal's biologic (defense) response to factors that disrupt or threaten homeostasis. The stress response has three phases: detection (alarm reaction); resistance; and recovery or, if stressor is not removed, exhaustion. 'Surgical stress' is produced by surgical procedures and can be exaggerated by anesthesia and anesthetic technique. Surgical trauma causes activation of physiologic and immunologic processes designed to maintain or restore homeostasis and ensure survival. The surgical procedure, duration of surgery, surgeon, and magnitude of tissue damage produced during surgery determine the amount of trauma and the severity of surgical stress. Systemic cytokines (*interleukin [IL]–1, IL-6,* and *IL-8,* and *tumor necrosis factor–α [TNF-α]*) are indicative of a systemic inflammatory response (acute-phase response). Cytokines stimulate the release of acute-phase proteins (C-reactive protein, haptoglobin) from the liver and modulate both metabolic pathways and hormonal responses. Systemic increases in both C-reactive protein and haptoglobin are correlated with the severity of surgical stress. Anesthesia, particularly with inhalant anesthetics, opioids, and alpha-1 agonists modify and depress the surgical stress response.

Stressor

A *stressor* is any object or event that elicits a stress response—a physical, chemical, or emotional factor (e.g., trauma or fear) that causes physiologic tensions that can contribute to stress. The primary qualities of stressors are intensity, duration, and frequency.

Defense Response

The *defense response* refers to the adaptive psychophysiologic processes involved in the sensory detection, perception, and activation of autonomic, endocrine, and immune responses to tissue injury or threat of injury.

Distress

Distress is the state produced when the biologic cost of stress negatively affects biologic functions critical to homeostasis and the animal's well-being. Distress also means to cause pain or suffering or to make miserable.

Suffering

Suffering is defined as a perception or feeling of impending destruction or harm.

Sickness Response or Syndrome

The *sickness response* is cytokine-mediated and CNS dependent. Proinflammatory cytokines induce behavioral, neuroendocrine, and neurochemical changes characterized by dysphoria, anhedonia, indifference, depression, aggression, decreased appetite, poor health, and hyperalgesia.

BIOLOGIC COMPONENTS OF THE STRESS RESPONSE

The stress response is an adaptive pattern of behavioral, autonomic, endocrine, immune, hematologic, and metabolic changes directed toward the restoration of homeostasis (Box 3-2).

Most stress is short-lived because of the removal or short duration of exposure to the stressor. The nature, magnitude, and duration of the specific stimulus are important factors in determining the magnitude and extent of the adaptive defense responses elicited by the animal. Manipulation of a normal dog's hip joint or physical restraint of a cat, for example, generally elicits

BOX 3-2	Biologic Stress Response

- Behavioral
- Autonomic nervous system
- Neuroendocrine
- Immunologic
- Hematologic
- Metabolic
- Morphologic

only a temporary stress response. The response to stress prepares the animal for emergency situations and fosters survival in threatening circumstances (fight or flight). Acute and chronic pain are capable of producing a significant stress response in domesticated species. Pain induced by surgical or accidental trauma evokes responses characterized by activation of the sympathetic nervous system, secretion of glucocorticoids (primarily cortisol), hypermetabolism, sodium and water retention, and altered carbohydrate and protein metabolism (Box 3-3). Severe or relentless, stress can become maladaptive, producing distress and triggering self-sustaining neural endocrine, and immune cascades that overwhelm homeostatic mechanisms and can be responsible for self-mutilation, immune incompetence, and "sickness syndrome," culminating in death. Prior experience (memory) and current physical status (health, pain state) play an important role in determining the animal's adaptive and behavioral responses.

BOX 3-3	Systemic Effects of the Stress Response

Activation of central nervous system
- Hypothalamus, amygdala, locus ceruleus

Increases in autonomic activity
- Catecholamines

Endocrine response
- Pituitary hormone secretion
- Adrenal hormone secretion

Metabolic response
- Glucosemia
- Insulin resistance

Immune response
- Cytokine production
- Endogenous opioids and endocannabinoids
- Acute phase response
- Hematologic: neutrophil leukocytosis, lymphocyte proliferation

Morphologic response
- Failure to thrive, weight loss
- Accelerated aging

BEHAVIORAL INDICATORS OF STRESS AND PAIN

Pain is a stressor and can trigger changes in brain chemistry (neural plasticity) affecting the level of alertness, learning performance, and memory which lead to behavioral adjustments in addition to interdependent autonomic, endocrine, and immune alterations (Box 3-4). Intense stimulation of sensory (somatosensory, visual, acoustic) inputs to the brain activates the locus ceruleus (LC), limbic regions (e.g., hippocampus, amygdala, anterior thalamic nuclei), and cerebral cortex, which together produce adaptive responses. The stress induced when a cat is confronted by a dog, for example, amplifies both peripheral and central nervous system activity, leading to a defense response. Pain- and stress-induced increases in the concentration of corticotropin-releasing factor (CRF) in the hypothalamus, amygdala, and LC result in an increased startle response, anxiety, fear, and in some animals, rage. Therefore CRF serves as an excitatory neurotransmitter in the LC, releasing adrenocorticotropic hormone (ACTH), cortical norepinephrine (NE), dopamine, and 5-hydroxytryptamine (5-HT), which together result in hyper-responsiveness, hyperarousal, hypervigilance, and agitation. Prolonged stress impairs the animal's ability to learn and generally results in fear, periods of aggression, and avoidance behaviors.

CENTRAL NORADRENERGIC EFFECTS

The main neural substrates involved in the animal's response to aversive conditions including pain are the medial hypothalamus, amygdala, periaqueductal gray (PAG), and LC. Activation of the hypothalamus results in graded increases in CNS sympathetic output which leads to increases in heart rate and arterial blood pressure, sweating, piloerection, and pupil dilation. The PAG plays a central role in the descending modulation of *pain* and is

---

BOX 3-4	Behavioral Indicators of Stress and Pain

- Anxiety
- Fear
- Vocalization
- Aggression
- Disinterest
- Depression
- Poor appetite
- Facial expression
- Appearance
- Altered locomotion
- Abnormal posture
- Unsociable

important in the development of stress-induced hypoalgesia, discussed later. Noxious signaling increases activity in the LC noradrenergic neurons, and LC excitation appears to be a consistent response to nociception. The LC is the principal site for brain synthesis of NE. Any stimulus that threatens the biologic integrity of the animal increases the firing rate of the LC, and this in turn increases the release and turnover of NE in the brain, resulting in increases in vigilance, attention, and fear. The LC also responds to corticotropin-releasing hormone (CRH). LC neurons increase firing rates in response to CRF, and this increases NE levels throughout the CNS. Activation of the sympathetic nervous system is one of the principal effects initiated by stress.

NEUROENDOCRINE AXIS

The neuroendocrine axis and in particular the adrenal medulla, an endocrine organ, serve as a biologic interface for afferent sensory input and humoral communication between the CNS and the peripheral glands or organs (Figure 3-2). Auditory, visual, and somatosensory afferent sensory information

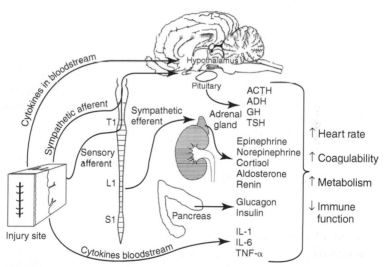

FIGURE 3-2 Acute surgical stimulation initiates the release of cytokines (interleukin [IL]-1, IL-6, tumor necrosis factor–α [TNF-α]) into the bloodstream and activation of the hypothalamic-pituitary-adrenal (HPA) system axis and the sympathetic nervous system. Activation of the hypothalamus and pituitary releases adrenocorticotropic hormone *(ACTH)*, vasopressin (or antidiuretic hormone *[ADH]*), growth hormone *(GH)*, and thyroid-stimulating hormone *(TSH)*. Sympathetic nervous system activation initiates the release of epinephrine, norepinephrine, cortisol, aldosterone, and renin. Together, these changes can alter hemodynamics, which elevates heart rate; increase blood coagulability predisposing to thrombosis; increase metabolism and caloric requirements; and when exaggerated, depress immune function.

TABLE **3-1**	Neurohumoral Response to Stress	
ENDOCRINE GLAND	**HORMONE**	**CHANGE**
Pituitary	Adrenocorticotropic hormone	Increase
	Growth hormone	Increase
	Vasopressin	Increase
	Thyroid-stimulating hormone	Increase or decrease
Adrenal cortex	Cortisol	Increase
	Aldosterone	Increase
	Catecholamines	Increase
Pancreas	Insulin	Often decreases
	Glucagon	Increase
Thyroid	Thyroxine	Decrease

is transmitted to the thalamus or directly to the amygdala, activating the hypothalamic-pituitary-adrenal (HPA) system (Table 3-1). This afferent information stimulates the secretion of CRF and vasoactive intestinal peptide (VIP), which in turn stimulates the pituitary gland to release ACTH, melanocortin, prolactin, vasopressin, thyroid-stimulating hormone (TSH), and growth hormone (GH). The metabolic consequences of these hormonal changes are increased catabolism, the mobilization of substrates to provide energy for tissue repair, and salt and water retention to maintain fluid volume and cardiovascular homeostasis. CRF, ACTH, and corticosterone are significant modulators of learning and memory processes. Acetylcholine (ACh) released from preganglionic descending sympathetic nerves during the stress response triggers secretion of NE, epinephrine (E), and neuropeptide Y (NPY; a vasoconstrictor) into systemic circulation. E and NE bind to adrenergic receptors, producing a general systemic arousal and prepares the animal for fight-or-flight. They increase heart rate and breathing, activate muscles, or dilate blood vessels (muscle, brain, lung, heart), and increase blood supply to organs involved in fight or flight.

Release of Corticotropin-Releasing Factor in the Brain

The release of CRF in the brain is one of the major components of the stress response, if not the most important. CRF acts synergistically with vasopressin to stimulate the production of ACTH and β-endorphin, thereby enhancing survival and producing analgesic effects, respectively. CRF also stimulates the adrenomedullary release of ACTH and catecholamines. CRF is an excitatory neurotransmitter in the brain, producing increased cortical NE release and excitation.

Adrenocorticotropic Hormone

ACTH release is stimulated by CRF, catecholamines, vasopressin, and VIP. The primary function of ACTH is to stimulate the adrenal cortex to secrete cortisol, corticosterone, aldosterone, and androgenic substances. ACTH also stimulates the adrenomedullary secretion of catecholamines. ACTH, cortisol, and NE and E levels are increased during emergence from anesthesia without surgery, suggesting that anesthesia alone produces a stress response in animals.

Cortisol

Serum cortisol concentration is an indicator of the severity of the stress response in most species. Mortality is increased in animals that are not able to increase serum cortisol concentrations. Etomidate, an injectable hypnotic recommended for anesthesia in high-risk cases, suppresses serum cortisol concentrations, an effect that is likely of little consequence when administered to normal healthy animals or when administered as a single bolus injection for induction to anesthesia. Etomidate may produce significant cardiorespiratory depression, however, when administered to catecholamine depleted or sympathetically exhausted animals. Cortisol stimulates gluconeogenesis, increases proteolysis and lipolysis, facilitates catecholamine effects, and produces anti inflammatory effects.

Catecholamines

Serum concentrations of NE, E, and dopamine are increased by CRF. Epinephrine causes glycogenolysis, gluconeogenesis, inhibition of insulin release, peripheral insulin resistance, and lipolysis. The increase of catecholamines into the systemic circulation is responsible for elevations in heart rate, respiratory rate, arterial blood pressure, and cardiac output. Increases in skeletal muscle blood flow prepare the animal for fight or flight.

Glucagon and Insulin

Endogenous endorphins, growth hormone, E, and glucocorticoids are capable of stimulating glucagon and insulin (β-adrenergic effect) secretion by the pancreas. More typically, however, surgical procedures cause an increase in glucagon secretion and a decrease in insulin secretion (α_2 effect), leading to hepatic glycogenolysis, gluconeogenesis from amino acids, glucosemia, and glucosuria.

Other Hormones

A variety of other hormones, including GH, TSH, and vasopressin, act together to protect cellular function and restore homeostasis.

Growth Hormone

GH stimulates protein synthesis and inhibits protein breakdown, promotes lipolysis, and produces anti-insulin effects. GH spares glucose for use by the nervous system.

Thyroid Hormones

Thyroxine and triiodothyronine are secreted into the systemic circulation from the thyroid gland during stimulation by TSH. Thyroid hormones stimulate carbohydrate metabolism and heat production and increase and sensitize β-adrenergic receptors in the heart, thereby enhancing the effects of circulating catecholamines.

Vasopressin

Vasopressin, also known as *antidiuretic hormone*, promotes water retention. Production and release of vasopressin into the systemic circulation in conjunction with increased concentrations of renin (sympathetic effect) increase the circulating blood volume, vascular tone, and vascular responsiveness to catecholamines, thereby supporting cardiovascular homeostasis.

METABOLISM

The net effect of the majority of the neurohumoral changes produced is to increase the secretion of catabolic hormones, promoting the production of metabolizable substrates from the breakdown of carbohydrates, fats, and proteins.

Carbohydrate Metabolism

Hyperglycemia is produced and may persist because of the stress induced production of glucagon and relative lack of insulin, although insulin levels may periodically increase. Pain can be responsible for increases in blood glucose, which is known to be associated with an increased incidence of wound infection, morbidity, and mortality.

Fat Metabolism

Lipolytic activity is stimulated by cortisol, catecholamines, and GH, resulting in an increase in circulating glycerol and free fatty acids. Glycerol in turn serves as a source for gluconeogenesis in the liver.

Protein Metabolism

Protein catabolism is a common consequence and a major concern after severe trauma or extensive surgical procedures. Cortisol increases protein catabolism, resulting in the release of amino acids. These amino acids can be used to form new proteins and to produce glucose and other substrates.

Protein supplementation (e.g., glutamine and arginine) during and after surgery results in fewer infections and shorter overall recovery time and may help to maintain body temperature (thermogenic effect). Prostaglandins (PGs; e.g., PGE_2) and cytokines may promote protein catabolism indirectly by increasing the energy expenditure of the body.

IMMUNE SYSTEM

Although the immune system is primarily considered in relation to the identification and destruction of foreign substances, it also functions as a diffusely distributed sense organ that communicates injury-related information to the brain. The immune system detects pain or injury in three ways: (1) through blood-borne immune messengers originating at the site of pain or injury; (2) through nociceptor-induced sympathetic activation and subsequent stimulation of immune tissues, and (3) through endocrine signaling that triggers the acute-phase reaction (Box 3-5). Pain intensity and duration are the key elements in determining the immune response (Box 3-6, Figure 3-3).

BOX 3-5   Immunologic and Hematologic Responses to Severe Stress

- Cytokine production
- Acute-phase response
- Neutrophil leukocytosis
- Lymphopenia
- Immune system depression

BOX 3-6   Neurotransmitters, Neuropeptides, Neurohormones, and Neuroendocrine Effector Molecules That Are Affected by Stress and Can Modulate Immune System Function* Neurotransmitters

- Acetylcholine
- Arginine vasopressin
- Cholecystokinin
- Corticosteroid
- Corticotropin
- Corticotropin-releasing factor
- Dopamine
- Epinephrine
- Growth hormone
- 5-Hydroxytryptamine (serotonin)
- Melatonin

- Neuroendocrine effector molecules
- Neurohormones
- Neuropeptides
- Norepinephrine
- Opiates
- Oxytocin
- Prolactin
- Sex steroids
- Substance P
- Thyroxine
- Vasoactive intestinal polypeptide

*These categories are not mutually exclusive. For example, the neuropeptides oxytocin and arginine vasopressin are also considered to be neurohormones.

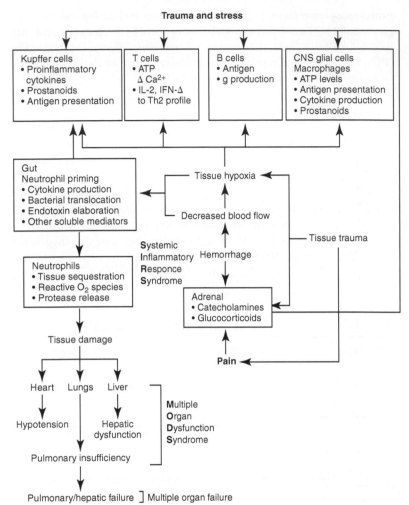

FIGURE 3-3   Schematic of the immune response to trauma and stress. Trauma-pain-stress results in a multitude of hematologic and immune-mediated responses that can provoke and support the systemic inflammatory response syndrome (*SIRS*) and lead to the development of multiple organ dysfunction syndrome (*MODS*). *ATP,* Adenosine triphosphate; *CNS,* central nervous system; *Ig,* immunoglobulin; *IFN,* interferon; *IL-2,* interleukin-2; *Th2,* T helper cells.

The messengers of the immune system are cytokines (e.g., IL-1, IL-6, TNF-α). Chronic pain also produces sustained increases in circulating concentrations of cortisol, NE, E, and glucagon, suppressing the humoral and cellular immune responses. The systemic release of endogenous opioids (endorphin and enkephalin) may contribute to immunosuppression.

Cytokines

A variety of low-molecular-weight proteins and cytokines (IL-1β, IL-2, IL-6, IL-8, IL-12, interferon-γ [IFN-γ], and TNF-α) are produced from activated leukocytes, fibroblasts, and endothelial cells in response to tissue injury. Cytokines help coordinate the nervous and immune systems. Their role is to protect the body by destroying and removing foreign invaders. When tissue trauma is severe, the excessive production of cytokines can lead to a systemic effect called the *systemic inflammatory response syndrome* (SIRS). Although pain has never been reported to cause SIRS, pain can contribute to the production of SIRS because it induces similar autonomic and endocrine effects. The major cytokines produced during stress are TNF-α, IL-1, and IL-6.

- IL-1 and IL-6 induce the release of acute-phase (inflammatory) reactants, cause fever, and initiate PG production (e.g., PGE_2). IL-1 and IL-6 can stimulate the secretion of ACTH from the pituitary gland and the subsequent release of cortisol.
- TNF-α can produce signs of shock, including hypotension, hemoconcentration, hyperglycemia, hyperkalemia, nonrespiratory acidosis, and activation of the complement cascade.

Peptides

Multiple peptides link the activities of the nervous and immune systems. CRF is a prominent peptide and functions as a neurotransmitter and a hormone. CRF produces both proinflammatory and anti-inflammatory effects. Other prominent proinflammatory and proalgesic neuropeptides include substance P (sP), calcitonin gene–related peptide (CGRP), and VIP. Somatostatin (SOM) is also released from peripheral C fibers and produces anti-inflammatory and analgesic effects, possibly acting as part of a negative feedback control system.

Acute-Phase Response

The acute-phase response can be triggered by severe stress from any cause. The main feature of the acute-phase response is the release of proteins from the liver, which act as inflammatory mediators and scavengers during tissue repair. These proteins include C-reactive protein, fibrinogen, macroglobulin, and antiproteinases. C-reactive protein is an excellent biomarker of physiologic stress, infection, and morbidity. Excessive production of these proteins can contribute to SIRS.

Endogenous Opioids

The immune system provides a rich source of endogenous opioid peptides (β-endorphin, enkephalin, dynorphin). The production of opioid peptides within immune cells located in inflamed tissue is enhanced by tissue trauma. Leukocytes secrete endogenous opioids in response to releasing factors such as CRF, NE, and proinflammatory cytokines. Endogenous opioids suppress peripheral C-terminal excitability and inflammatory mediator release, thus contributing anti-inflammatory effects in peripheral nociceptor activation. Brain opioid peptides are linked to emotion, vigilance, appetite and modify the response to stress and pain.

Endocannabinoids

Endocannabinoids are neuromodulatory lipids that activate cannabinoid receptors (CB_1, CB_2). Nerve, blood, and endothelial cells release endocannabinoids. CB_1 cannabinoid receptors occur principally in the brain, immune system, and other peripheral tissues. CB_2 receptors occur primarily in immune cells. Endogenous and exogenous cannabinoids produce anxiolytic, neuroprotective, and anti-inflammatory immune-suppressing effects and are involved in a variety of physiologic processes including appetite, pain sensation, mood, and memory. The endocannabinoid endogenous ligand anandamide activates both CB_1 and CB_2 receptors. Anandamide also binds to the vanilloid receptor TRPV1 (transient receptor potential cation channel subfamily V, member 1). TRPV1 receptors are present on C nociceptive terminals and the endings of primary sensory neurons (capsaicin-sensitive sensory neurons) in the dorsal horn of the spinal cord and brainstem. Peripheral nociceptor terminals express TRPV1 in response to tissue trauma. Anandamide modulates peripheral pain mechanisms through its dual agonist effects on TRPV1 and cannabinoid receptors. Low concentrations of anandamide induce CB_1 receptor–mediated inhibition of electrical impulses from neurons in the dorsal root ganglion. High concentrations of anandamide produce TRPV1 receptor–mediated neuropeptide release at central terminals of capsaicin-sensitive sensory neurons, thereby opposing peripheral CB-mediated inhibitory effects.

Hematology

The peripheral blood white cell count generally reflects a stress leukogram typified by an elevated number of mature and immature polymorphonuclear leukocytes (left shift) and reduced numbers of lymphocytes. Leukocytes are a rich source of cytokines, chemokines, peptides, and other signaling molecules that activate the stress response and modulate pain.

MORPHOLOGIC CHANGES

Morphologic changes associated with chronic stress or pain are typical of long-term aversive stimuli and include failure to thrive, hair loss or poor coat, weight loss, myopenia, and accelerated aging (see Chapters 5 and 6).

STRESS-INDUCED HYPOALGESIA AND HYPERALGESIA

Stress (anxiety, fear, pain) can produce either hypoalgesia or hyperalgesia. Clinically acute, severe pain is considered to be capable of producing a temporary loss of sensation, whereas chronic stressful or painful conditions generally increased pain sensitivity. Notably, supraspinal modulation of pain can either enhance nociception (descending facilitation) or reduce it (descending inhibition). Differences in the mechanisms for facilitation and inhibition of nociception have been linked to a variety of neurotransmitters. Neurotransmitters and neuropeptides that predominantly facilitate nociception include the excitatory amino acids glutamate, histamine, cholecystokinin, melanocortin, and the PGs. Neurotransmitters and neuropeptides that predominantly inhibit nociception include γ-aminobutyric acid (GABA), glycine, vasopressin, oxytocin, adenosine, endogenous opioids, and endocannabinoids. Neurotransmitters or neuropeptides that either facilitate or inhibit nociception include serotonin (5-hydroxytryptamine [5-HT]), NE, dopamine, dynorphin, ACh, and nitric oxide. It is important to note that, adding to the difficulty in unraveling the precise mechanisms responsible for pain facilitation or inhibition, the substrates and anatomic regions involved in pain modulation are often identical. Functional magnetic resonance imaging (fMRI) indicates that similar brain regions participate in modulating the response to stress and pain. Stress induced analgesia (SIA), placebo analgesia, diffuse noxious inhibitory control (DNIC), and fear-conditioned analgesia (FCA), for example, although differing with respect to the analgesia-inducing manipulation responsible for their production, activate similar brain regions including the insula, rostral anterior cingulate cortex, and PAG. The last is particularly important in descending pain modulation and in defensive behaviors.

Stress-Induced Analgesia

The ability of stress and pain to produce analgesia has been known for centuries. SIA is considered to be an innate suppression of pain during or after exposure to a stressful or fear-inducing stimulus. FCA is a survival response that occurs in response to noxious or aversive stimuli and can be produced by pavlovian conditioning. FCA is characterized by a decrease in nociception and has been demonstrated to suppress pain behaviors by more than 90%. This fact alone has important implications with regard to animal "conditioning," housing, restraint, and training techniques. The gate-control theory of Melzack and Wall in the mid-1960s provided a rudimentary understanding of pain modulation by theorizing that pain is modulated by the interaction between neurons at the spinal level and not by direct activation of pain receptors. The gate-control theory suggested that non-nociceptive firing from sensory Aβ fibers would "close the gate" to nociceptive signaling. Conversely, firing of nociceptive Aδ and C fibers would inhibit transmission of non-nociceptive signaling. Current evidence, however, suggests that both spinal pathways, through mechanisms described by the gate-control theory, and supraspinal descending opioid and nonopioid inhibitory pain pathways play a role in mediating SIA. When a painful stimulus serves as a stressor, there is an overlap of SIA and the phenomenon of DNIC. DNIC is observed when a strong sustained painful stimulus is applied at one site and subsequently decreases pain responsiveness to painful stimulation at multiple other sites. DNIC involves the endogenous opioid system. Placebo analgesia is mediated at the spinal level but also involves supraspinal brain structures. Opioid-mediated hypoalgesia is produced by activation of endogenous pain-inhibiting pathways from the PAG over the medulla to the spinal cord. It is interesting to note that although activation of all three major opioid receptor subtypes (μ, κ, δ) produces analgesia via inhibition of ascending pain fibers, central opioid receptor signaling produces opposing effects on mood: μ or δ receptor activation elevates mood, whereas activation of brain κ opioid receptors produces dysphoria and prodepressive-like behaviors (anhedonia, dysphoria, anxiety). Although κ signaling during acute stress produces analgesia and aversion, prolonged κ activation by the endogenous opioid agonist dynorphin in response to repeated stress or chronic painful conditions leads to persistent expression of behavioral signs characterized by indifference and depression, suggesting that κ-receptor agonists contribute to sensitization of stress-induced behaviors.

Stress-Induced Hyperalgesia

Stress induced hyperalgia (SIH), in contrast to SIA, is initiated by decreased GABA release and delayed $GABA_A$ receptor activation and is maintained or exaggerated by injury-induced increases in glutamate release and N-methyl-D-aspartate (NMDA) glutamate receptor activation at the spinal level. Inhibiting GABA and glycine in the spinal cord increases A fiber-mediated excitatory transmission in the superficial dorsal horn and produces tactile allodynia. Furthermore, immune-mediated increases in TNF-α reduce GABAergic interneuron activity and increase calcium levels in mitochondria, promoting the production of reactive oxygen species and reduced GABA release. Loss of local segmental inhibition in the dorsal horn is further accentuated by a loss of descending inhibitory control from the rostroventral medulla. In addition, increases in circulating concentrations of NE have been shown to exacerbate nociception after stress. Activation of sympathetic postganglionic nerves juxtaposed with peripheral sensory nerve fibers facilitates pain hypersensitivity via an α_1-adrenoceptor mechanism. Finally, the NE feedback inhibition at α_2-adrenergic receptors is likely reduced by stress. Central sensitization is considered to represent an injury-induced increase in excitatory activity in dorsal horn neurons. The synaptic changes underlying activity-dependent increases in dorsal horn neuron synaptic strength and excitability are mediated by NMDA; α-amino-3-hydroxy-5-methyl-4-isoxazolepropionic acid (AMPA); metabotropic glutamate receptors (mGluRs); sP neurokinin-1 (NK1) receptors; and brain-derived neurotrophic factor (BDNF) and its tyrosine kinase receptor–B (TrkB) (see Chapter 2). Loss of inhibitory modulation of dorsal horn neurons (disinhibition) produces deregulation of pain inhibitory mechanisms, whereas enhanced NE release from sympathetic postganglionic nerves results in significant sensitization of sensory afferents, resulting in SIH.

It is interesting to note that recent evidence suggests that endogenous opioids paradoxically trigger SIH by mechanisms located within the central nervous system. Notably, benzodiazepines (diazepam, midazolam) increase pain perception in humans, whereas the drugs propofol and dexmedetomidine produce analgesia. These observations have important implications for the selection and doses of drugs used to produce anesthesia in surgical candidates.

SUGGESTED READING

Butler RK, Finn DP. Stress-induced analgesia. Prog Neurobiol. 2009; 88:184–202.

Chapman CR, Tuckett RP, Song CW. Pain and stress in a systems perspective: Reciprocal neural, endocrine and immune interactions. J Pain. 2008; 9:122–145.

Carr DB, Goudes LC. Acute pain. Lancet. 1999; 353:2051–2058.

Carstens E, Moberg GP. Recognizing pain and distress in laboratory animals. ILAR J. 2000; 41(2)2:62–71.

Chapman CR, Gavrin J. Suffering: The contributions of persistent pain. Lancet. 1999; 353:2233–2237.

Charney DS, Grillon C, Bremner JD. The neurobiological basis of anxiety and fear: Circuits, mechanisms, and neurochemical interactions (part I). Neuroscientist. 1998; 4:35–44.

Charney DS, Grillon C, Bremner JD. The neurobiological basis of anxiety and fear: Circuits, mechanisms, and neurochemical interactions (part II). Neuroscientist. 1998; 4:122–132.

Clark JD, Rager DR, Calpin JP. Animal well-being. I. General considerations. Lab Anim Sci. 1997; 47:564–570.

Clark JD, Rager DR, Calpin JP. Animal well-being. II. Stress and distress. Lab Anim Sci. 1997; 47:571–585.

Curcio K, Bidwell LA, Bohart GV, et al. Evaluation of signs of postoperative pain and complications after forelimb onychectomy in cats receiving buprenorphine alone or with bupivacaine administered as a four-point regional nerve block. J Am Vet Med Assoc. 2006; 228:65–68.

Davis M. The role of the amygdala in fear-potentiated startle: Implications for animal models of anxiety. Trends Pharmacol Sci. 1992; 13:35–41.

Desborough JP. The stress response to trauma and surgery. Br J Anaesth. 2000; 85:109–117.

Dodam JR, Kurse-Elliott KT, Aucoin DP, et al. Duration of etomidate-induced adrenocortical suppression during surgery in dogs. Am J Vet Res. 1990; 51:786–788.

Donello JE, Guan Y, Tian M, et al. A peripheral adrenoceptor-mediated sympathetic mechanism can transform stress-induced analgesia into hyperalgesia. Anesthesiology. 2011; 114:1403–1416.

Erickson HH, Kitchell RL. Pain perception and alleviation in animals. Fed Proc. 1984; 43:1307–1312.

Foex BA. Systemic responses to trauma. Br Med Bull. 1999; 55:726–743.

Frolich MA, Zhang K, Ness TJ. Effect of sedation on pain perception. Anesthesiology. 2013; 118:611–621.

Giannoudis PV, Diopoulos H, Chalidis B, et al. Surgical stress response. Injury Int J Care Injured. 2006; 37S:S3–S9.

Imbe H, Iwai-Liao Y, Senba E. Stress-induced hyperalgesia: Animal models and putative mechanisms. Front Biosci. 2006; 11:2179–2192.

Khuseyinova N, Koenig W. Biomarkers of outcome from cardiovascular disease. Curr Opin Crit Care. 2006; 12:412–419.

Knoll AT, Carlezon WA Jr. Dynorphin, stress and depression. Brain Res. 2010; 1341:56–73.

Larauche M, Mulak A, Tache Y. Stress and visceral pain: From animal models to clinical therapies. Exp Neurol. 2012; 233:49–67.

Martenson MR, Cetas JS, Heinricher MM. A possible neural basis for stress-induced hyperalgesia. Pain. 2009; 142:236–244.

Michelsen J, Heller J, Wills F, et al. Effect of surgeon experience on the postoperative plasma cortisol and C-reactive protein concentrations after ovariohysterectomy in the dog: A randomized trial. Aust Vet J. 2012; 90:474–478.

McMillan FD. Quality of life in animals. J Am Vet Med Assoc. 2000; 216(12):1904–1910.

Nasraway SA Jr. Hyperglycemia during critical illness. JPEN J Parenter Enteral Nutr. 2006; 30:254–258.

Padgett DA, Marucha PT, Sheridan JF. Restraint stress slows cutaneous wound healing in mice. Brain Behav Immun. 1998; 12:64–73.

Quintero L, Cardenas R, Suarez-Roca H. Stress-induced hyperalgesia is associated with a reduced and delayed GABA inhibitory control that enhances post-synaptic NMDA receptor activation in the spinal cord. Pain. 2011; 152:1909–1922.

Richebe P, Rivat C, Cahana A. Stress-induced hyperalgesia: Any clinical relevance for the anesthesiologist. Anesthesiology. 2011; 114:1280–1281.

Rivat C, Becker C, Blugeot A, et al. Chronic stress induces transient spinal neuroinflammation, triggering sensory hypersensitivity and long-lasting anxiety-induced hyperalgesia. Pain. 2010; 150:358–368.

Rojas IG, Padgett DA, Sheridan JF, Marucha PT. Stress-induced susceptibility to bacterial infection during cutaneous wound healing. Brain Behav Immun. 2002; 16:74–84.

Stein C, Machelska H. Modulation of peripheral sensory neurons by the immune system: Implications for pain therapy. Pharmacol Rev. 2011; 63:860–881.

Suter MR, Wen YR, Decosterd I, et al. Do glial cells control pain. Neuron Glia Biol. 2007; 3:255–268.

Suzuki R, Rygh LJ, Dikenson AH. Bad news from the brain: Descending 5-HT pathways that control spinal pain processing. Trends Pharmacol Sci. 2004; 25:613–617.

Tang J, Gibson SJ. A psychophysical evaluation of the relationship between trait anxiety, pain perception, and induced state anxiety. J Pain. 2005; 6(9):612–619.

Weissman C. The metabolic response to stress: an overview and update. Anesthesia. 1999; 73:308–327.

Yates AR, Dyke PC II, Taeed R, et al. Hyperglycemia is a marker for poor outcome in the postoperative pediatric cardiac patient. Pediatr Crit Care Med. 2006; 7:351–355.

Yilmaz P, Diers M, Diener S, et al. Brain correlates of stress-induced analgesia. Pain. 2010; 151:522–529.

Zhang HJ, Huang YG. The immune system: A new look at pain. Chin Med J. 2006; 119:930–938.

CHAPTER 4

Definitions of Terms Describing Pain

James S. Gaynor; William W. Muir III

A working understanding of the terminology and definitions used to describe pain and analgesia is essential for clear and precise communication. By knowing the terminology, practitioners can speak intelligently and accurately to one another when discussing cases. The following terms and their definitions are arranged alphabetically and are used throughout this handbook.

DEFINITIONS

acupuncture The practice of inserting needles at certain points in the skin to achieve specific effects such as pain relief.

adjunctive Additional therapy used together with the primary treatment.

adjuvant A drug that is administered for a purpose other than analgesia but that has independent or additive pain-relieving effects. Treatment that is given in addition to the primary, main, or initial treatment.

agonist A drug that exerts its effect by binding to and activating specific receptors.

algogenic Pain inducing.

allodynia Pain caused by a stimulus that does not normally cause pain.

analgesia Loss of sensitivity to a stimulus that would normally produce pain (noxious stimulus).

analgesic ceiling effect The drug dosage beyond which no beneficial analgesic effect is observed. An analgesic ceiling effect is observed with both butorphanol and buprenorphine.

anesthesia Total or partial loss of sensation.

antagonist A drug that exerts its effect by competitively binding to receptors and preventing the effects of agonists.

central sensitization Sensitization of nerves in the spinal cord and brain due to amplification and facilitation of synaptic transfer from the peripheral nociceptor to dorsal horn neurons in the spinal cord. Central sensitization is triggered in central neurons by intense nociceptor input into the spinal cord (activity dependent) and is sustained beyond the initiating stimulus by changes in the molecular machinery of the cell (transcription dependent). Activation of N-methyl-D-aspartic acid (NMDA) receptors play a key role in the development of central sensitization.

distress Condition in which stress negatively affects biologic functions critical to the animal's well-being. Distress also means to cause pain or suffering or to make miserable.

dysesthesia Abnormal sense of touch.

epidural space The space above the dura mater. An injection into this area is commonly referred to as an *epidural*.

hyperalgesia An increased response to a stimulation that is normally painful (a heightened sense of pain) at the site of injury or in surrounding undamaged tissue. Stimulated nociceptors respond to noxious stimuli more vigorously and at a lower threshold.

Primary hyperalgesia—Increased sensitivity to a stimulus that is normally painful at the site localized to the area of tissue damage or inflammation.

Secondary hyperalgesia—Increased sensitivity to a stimulus that is normally painful in uninjured or inflamed tissues in areas around and beyond the site of primary site of tissue injury; caused by central sensitization.

hyperesthesia Increased sensitivity to touch.

hyperpathia A painful syndrome characterized by an increased reaction to a stimulus, especially if it is repetitive.

hypoalgesia Decreased sensitivity to a noxious stimulus.

hypoesthesia Decreased sensitivity to touch.

interventional pain management An invasive procedure to treat or manage pain through an injection of a drug or implantation of a drug delivery device.

local anesthesia The temporary loss of sensation in a defined part of the body without loss of consciousness.

multimodal analgesia The use of multiple drugs with different mechanisms of action, which may act at different levels of the nociceptive pathways, to produce enhanced (additive, superadditive) analgesic effects.

myofascial pain A syndrome of focal pain in a muscle or related tissues, stiffness, muscle spasm, and decreased range of motion.

nociception The neural processes for encoding pain: transduction, conduction, and central nervous system processing of nerve signals generated by the stimulation of nociceptors; the physiologic process that leads to the perception of pain.

noxious stimulus A stimulus (chemical, thermal, mechanical, electrical) that produces pain and damages or threatens to damage normal tissues.

opioid A drug that is related naturally or synthetically to morphine.

pain An unpleasant sensory and emotional experience associated with actual
or potential tissue damage or described in terms of such damage. The
inability to communicate verbally does not negate the need for appropriate pain-relieving treatment.

Acute pain—Pain that follows some bodily injury, disappears with healing, and tends to be self-limiting.

Adaptive pain—Pain that contributes to survival by limiting or preventing contact with or movement of the injured part until healing is
complete, thereby minimizing further damage. Inflammatory pain
is typically adaptive and decreases as the damage and inflammatory
response resolve.

Breakthrough pain—A transient flare-up of pain in the chronic pain setting that can occur even when chronic pain is under control.

Cancer pain—Pain that can be acute, chronic, or intermittent and is
related to the disease itself or to the treatment.

Central pain—Pain initiated or caused by dysfunction or a lesion in the
central nervous system.

Chronic pain—Pain that lasts several weeks to months and persists
beyond the expected healing time when nonmalignant in origin.

Clinical pain—Pain of inflammatory or neuropathic origin that is characterized by increased sensitivity to noxious (hyperalgesia) and non-
noxious stimuli and a spread of hypersensitivity to uninjured tissue
(secondary hyperalgesia). Differs from physiologic pain by the presence of pathologic hypersensitivity.

Deep pain—Pain that is present in "deep" anatomic structures (e.g., bone,
tendon, ligament, muscle).

Dysfunctional pain—Amplification of nociceptive signaling in the absence
of inflammation or neural lesions.

First pain—The initial well-localized and generally brief pain produced by
a noxious stimulus: produced by high-threshold nociceptors.

Inflammatory pain—Pain as a result of tissue damage and the release or
activation of local inflammatory mediators (e.g., prostaglandins,
hydrogen ion, histamine). Inflammatory pain typically decreases as
the damage and inflammatory response resolve.

Intractable pain—Intense, constant, usually chronic pain that does not
respond to any therapeutic medical intervention.

Maladaptive pain—Pain that is uncoupled from a noxious stimulus or
healing tissue and generally occurs in response to damage to the nervous system (neuropathic pain) or results from abnormal operation of
the nervous system (dysfunctional pain). Maladaptive pain is the
expression of abnormal sensory processing and usually is persistent
or recurrent; it is pain as disease.

Neuropathic pain—Pain that originates from injury or involvement of the peripheral or central nervous system and is described as burning or shooting, possibly associated with motor, sensory, or autonomic deficits.

Nociceptive pain—The sensation associated with the detection of potentially tissue-damaging noxious stimuli; this type of pain is protective.

Pathologic pain—A disease state that is caused by damage to the nervous system (neuropathic) or by its abnormal function (dysfunctional) and persists long after the healing process has occurred.

Perioperative pain—Pain that is present or occurs during the period extending from the time of hospitalization for surgery to the time of discharge.

Second pain—Delayed, diffuse and protracted, generally burning pain that persists after the termination of the noxious stimulus. Severe acute painful events (e.g., trauma) and chronic and visceral pain are almost always characterized by "second pain."

Superficial pain—Pain that originates in "superficial" tissues (e.g., skin, subcutis).

Visceral pain—Pain that originates from the body cavities (abdominal, thoracic) and the brain.

pain scales Visual, categoric, and numeric methods (instruments) used (by proxy) for diagnostic and therapeutic purposes to estimate the intensity of pain.

pain threshold The least amount of pain that an animal can recognize.

pain tolerance level The greatest level of pain that an individual can tolerate.

paresthesia A spontaneous or evoked abnormal sensation generally occurring in animals with neuropathic pain.

pathologic pain Pain that has an exaggerated response much beyond its protective usefulness. This is often associated with tissue injury incurred at the time of surgery or trauma.

peripheral sensitization Injury and inflammation of tissue result in alterations of the chemical environment of the peripheral nerve terminal of nociceptors. Injured or inflamed tissues release intracellular contents such as adenosine triphosphatase, K and hydrogen ions, cytokines, chemokines, growth factors, and prostaglandins. These factors act directly to activate (nociceptor activators) or to sensitize (nociceptor sensitizers) the terminal so that it becomes hypersensitive to subsequent stimuli.

physiologic pain Pain that acts as a protective mechanism and that is initiated by high threshold receptors. It is well localized and transient and incites individuals to move away from the cause of potential tissue damage or to avoid movement or contact with external stimuli during a reparative phase.

preemptive analgesia A pharmacologic intervention performed before a noxious event (e.g., surgery) that is intended to minimize the impact of the stimulus by preventing peripheral and/or central sensitization.

preventive analgesia Analgesic treatment that is initiated before a procedure to reduce the consequences of nociceptive transmission initiated by the procedure. The goal of preventative analgesia is to minimize sensitization induced by noxious perioperative stimuli including those arising before, during, and after the procedure. An analgesic therapy that is designed for the purpose of decreasing analgesic consumption relative to a placebo treatment or compared with no treatment and to produce an analgesic effect that extends for a period of time that outlasts the pharmacologic effects (more than 5.5 half-lives) for the drug in question.

radiculopathy Irritation of or injury (compression, inflammation, tissue damage) to a nerve root.

regional anesthesia The loss of sensation in part of the body caused by interruption of the sensory nerves conducting impulses from that region of the body.

sedation Central nervous system depression, mediated via the cerebral cortex, in which the individual is drowsy but arousable.

somatic pain Pain that originates from damage to bones, joints, muscle, or skin and is described in human beings as localized, constant, sharp, aching, and throbbing.

stress response Neuroendocrine-immune and behavioral response to actual or potential tissue damage ("fight-or-flight response").

subarachnoid space The space above the pia mater and below the arachnoid mater, in which cerebrospinal fluid can be found. A subarachnoid injection is also referred to as a "spinal."

suffering A state of emotional distress associated with events that threaten the biologic and/or psychosocial integrity of the individual. Suffering often accompanies severe pain but can occur in its absence; hence pain and suffering are phenomenologically distinct.

sympathetic mediated pain A syndrome in which there is abnormal sympathetic nervous system activity causing a severe debilitation that is often associated with tenderness to a light touch.

trigger zone or point Hypersensitive area on the body surface where touch or pressure elicits a painful response.

tolerance A shortened duration and decreased intensity of the analgesic, euphoric, sedative, and other central nervous system depressant effects, as well as considerable increase in the average dose required to achieve a given effect.

tranquilization A state of calmness, mediated through the reticular activating system, in which the individual is relaxed, awake, unaware of its surroundings, and potentially indifferent to minor pain.

visceral pain Pain that arises from stretching, distention, or inflammation of the viscera; is described as deep, cramping, aching, or gnawing, without good localization.

wind-up Sensitization of nociceptors and peripheral and central pain pathways in response to a barrage of afferent nociceptive impulses resulting in expanded receptive fields and an increased rate of discharge.

REFERENCE

International Association for the Study of Pain: IASP taxonomy. Retrieved from www.iasp-pain.org/AM/Template.cfm?Section=Pain_Definitions.

CHAPTER 5

Assessing Pain
Pain Behaviors

Ashley J. Wiese

Veterinarians must become familiar with characteristic behaviors for detecting and categorizing pain in animals. It is important to note that not all animals display pain-related behavior, and it should be emphasized that this does not mean the animal is not experiencing pain. Environmental factors, species, age, body condition, and concurrent disease can influence pain behavior and should be considered when one is evaluating animals. Spontaneous (unprovoked) and evoked responses should be recorded and quantified to categorize the severity of pain. Animal healthcare providers need to be familiar with placebo and nocebo influences they may evoke in animals. Learning produced by conditioning and expectancies plays an important role in placebo and nocebo effects. Both rely on a notion that conscious perception of sensory or social stimuli may act as a cue that triggers expectancy or a conditioned behavior.

Placebo: Inert substance that creates either a positive response or no response
Nocebo: A harmless substance that creates harmful effects in the subject

Objective, validated pain scoring systems should be employed to optimize the detection of painful animals and guide therapeutic intervention.

SPONTANEOUS PAIN BEHAVIORS

Attitude

Pain is almost always associated with changes in normal animal behavior (Box 5-1). Knowledge of the animal's normal behavior is required to optimally characterize subtle abnormalities. The history (e.g., activity, personality changes) and the owner's assessment are valuable aids. Common behaviors displayed by animals in pain include the following:

- Anxiety
- Depression
- Inappetence
- Reluctance to move
- Reclusive (noninteractive)
- Irritable-aggressive

BOX 5-1 | **Common Observational Indicators of Pain**

Dogs
- Decreased social interaction
- Anxious or glazed expression
- Submissive behavior
- Refusal to move
- Whimpering, whining, howling, growling
- Guarding behavior
- Aggression, biting
- Loss of appetite
- Self-mutilation

Rodents
- Reduced grooming
- Crouched stance, arched back
- Eye squinting
- Twitching
- Licking behavior

Cats
- Reduced activity
- Loss of appetite
- Does not interact or shows loss of curiosity
- Hiding
- Hissing, spitting, or growling
- Excessive licking or grooming
- Cessation of grooming
- Stiff posture or gait
- Guarding behavior
- Attempts to escape
- Tail flicking

Altered Facial Expressions and Appearance

Animals with chronic pain or stress often develop a dull, unkempt (ungroomed) appearance (Figure 5-1). Cats, a species known to groom regularly, that are experiencing chronic pain often stop grooming themselves, resulting in a dry, lusterless hair coat (Figure 5-2).

The FACES pain scale was originally developed for human pediatric patients to obtain self-reported assessments of pain. This pain scale has been adopted for use in human patients of all ages, given its simplicity and reliability as a pain assessment tool. Facial expressions are used to assess pain in laboratory animal species including mice, rats, and rabbits. Orbital tightening, cheek flattening, nares drawn vertically, whiskers extended horizontally or drawn toward the cheeks, and ear flattening are considered indicators of pain or discomfort in these species. A systematic analysis of changes in facial expression in animals in pain has not been conducted in companion animals.

Body Posture

Dogs and cats assume characteristic pain postures as pain intensity increases. The praying position, a stretched out stance (rocking horse appearance), or a hunched, base-wide stance are characteristic postures observed with abdominal pain (Figure 5-3). Despite being reluctant to move, animals in pain may become anxious, restless, and aggressive. Most important, there is a change in the routine pattern of behavior for the animal, which is best assessed by

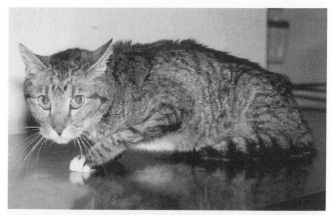

FIGURE 5-1   This cat with chronic pancreatitis attempted to hide or escape when approached. Note the dull, ungroomed hair coat.

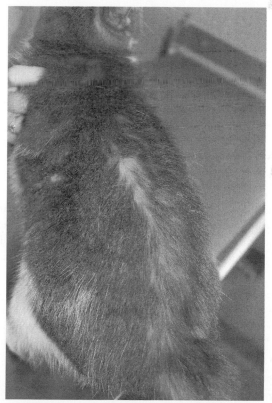

FIGURE 5-2   Some cats that have chronic pain and are stressed will lose their hair coat. This is particularly noticeable along the spine.

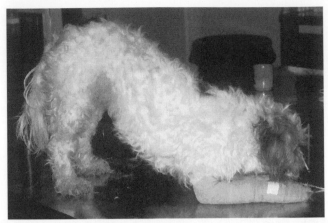

FIGURE 5-3 Reluctance to lie down. The so-called "praying" or "sphinx" position is characteristic of dogs and cats, respectively, with abdominal pain.

someone familiar with the animal's normal behavior. Characteristic positions indicative of pain or discomfort include the following:

- Curled position and reluctance to move
- Hunched, reluctant to lie down
- Tense or rigid
- Praying position (dogs); sphinx position (cats)
- Reduced weight bearing
- Licking or chewing at the site of pain

Activity Level

Reluctance to Move

Animals become reluctant to change position or move with increasing severity of pain (Figures 5-4 to 5-6). This minimizes movement-induced (incident) pain and facilitates healing. Even slight movement may evoke additional pain behaviors (e.g., limping or stilted gait), vocalization, or aggression.

Reluctance to Lie Down

Reluctance to lie down is often associated with acute abdominal or thoracic pain (Figure 5-7). Dogs or cats with abdominal pain may sit for hours or assume a "praying" position (see Figure 5-3). Animals may frequently attempt to sit or remain standing for hours (Figure 5-8).

Changing Positions

Restlessness and frequent changes in body position indicate that the animal is uncomfortable. Some dogs may shift from side to side, pace, or get up and lie

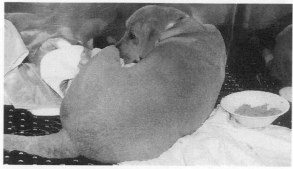

FIGURE 5-4 Reluctance to move and unresponsiveness. Abdominal pain caused this dog to lie facing the back of the cage for hours. Note the depressed facial expression.

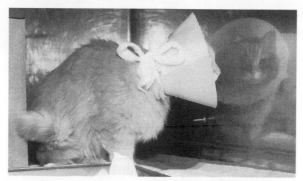

FIGURE 5-5 Reluctance to move. Abdominal (bladder) pain caused this cat to sit in the litter box facing the back of the cage.

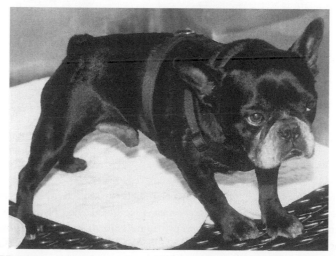

FIGURE 5-6 Reluctance to move. Pain caused by trauma to a cervical disk in a dog. Note the statue-like stance.

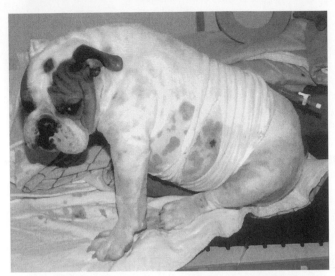

FIGURE 5-7 Reluctance to lie down. This dog with peritonitis would not lie down until exhausted.

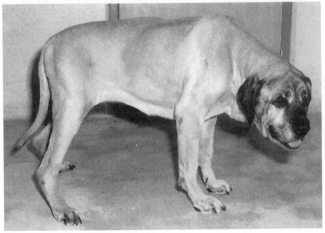

FIGURE 5-8 Reluctance to lie down. This dog with chronic bloat and abdominal pain remained standing in one spot until exhausted. Note the tense abdomen, open mouth breathing, and head-down, anxious expression.

down multiple times (Figure 5-9). Accelerometer-based activity counts in the home setting represent an objective means for quantifying restlessness and the animal's response to pain therapy. Some animals may change position frequently because of a full urinary bladder or the need to defecate. Good nursing practices, including manual bladder expression, are required when caring for animals in pain.

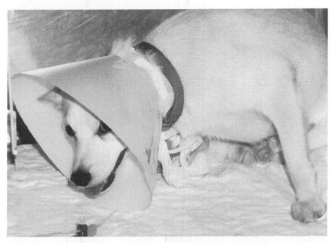

FIGURE 5-9 Shifting positions. This dog with abdominal pain would frequently get up and lie down. The dog was careful not to induce more pain, taking several minutes to lie down.

- Dogs and cats experiencing severe pain are often anxious and restless (getting up and lying down) and can become unmanageable or aggressive.
- Some animals become submissive or depressed (Figure 5-10). Depression is frequently associated with chronic pain. Many animals become reluctant to move or engage in physical activity.
- Some dogs and cats become increasingly protective and aggressive (Figure 5-11).

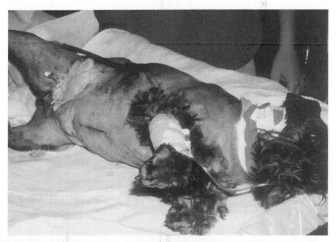

FIGURE 5-10 Submissive position. This dog with abdominal trauma demonstrated a submissive posture (on back, rear legs apart, ears flat) when approached.

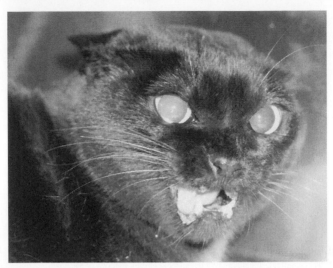

FIGURE 5-11   Aggression. Expression of aggression in a cat with a femoral fracture. Note the dilated pupils, flattened ears, and open mouth.

- Aggression usually occurs in response to acute-onset, severe pain. Often the slightest manipulation stimulates the animal to attempt to bite the handler.
- Small dogs usually become more vigilant, timid, and fearful.

Locomotor Activity

Musculoskeletal (long bone, joint) and associated soft-tissue pain often manifests as limping and guarding of the painful area (Figure 5-12). Limping helps to avoid further injury and increased pain associated with loading of the limb. Abnormal gaits including a stiff, stilted, or shifting weight carriage (i.e., stifle or coxofemoral osteoarthritis; elbow dysplasia, bone cancer) may be observed with increasing severity of pain (Figure 5-13). Unwillingness to rise or move and a slow, unstable transition from recumbency to standing represent additional signs of acute or chronic pain (see Figure 5-4). The aforementioned conditions are not likely to be observed in cats because of their natural propensity to hide signs of pain. Cats are much more likely to hide or attempt to escape (see Figure 5-1).

Focused Attention to Painful Area

Animals in pain tend to pay more attention to the area producing pain. Animals may rub painful areas of the body that they cannot tend to in other ways. Dogs and cats may begin to lick, bite, or chew at the site of pain. Self-mutilation, indicative of dysesthesia, is often indicative of peripheral nerve injury.

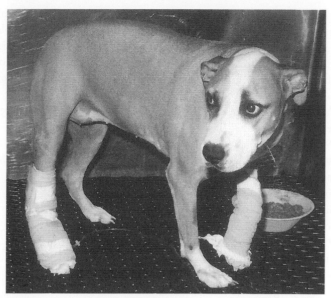

FIGURE 5-12 Acute pain. Left foreleg lameness in a dog. Pain causes the dog to lift its left foreleg and walk with a limp.

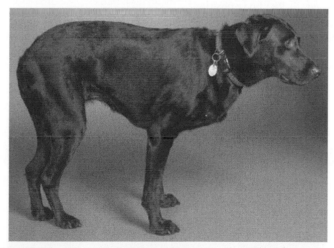

FIGURE 5-13 Chronic pain. Severe hip osteoarthritis in a dog. Note that the majority of the dog's weight is being carried on the front legs.

Vocalization

- Vocalization is associated with painful situations that are mild to severe, depending on the animal's personality and the environmental circumstances.
- Vocalization during recovery from anesthesia can suggest emergence delirium or pain. Delirious animals are often inconsolable and tend to react

equally to stimulation of painful and nonpainful areas. Animals vocalizing because of pain during recovery from anesthesia may be consolable but react to stimulation or manipulation of the painful area. Provision of analgesics with sedative properties such as opioids or α_2-agonists is advised when emergence delirium cannot be discerned from pain in postoperative animals.

- Vocalization is nonspecific. Animals may whine, whimper, cry, groan, howl, or scream.
- Vocalization may also be an example of increased anxiety.
- Whining may indicate a full bladder and the need to urinate or defecate.

Dogs. See Figure 5-14.

- Fixed glare, focused
- Glazed appearance
- Bulging, wide eyes
- Distant appearance
- Anxious appearance
- Depressed

Cats. See Figure 5-15.

- Furrowed brow
- Squinted eyes (Figure 5-16)
- Curled, tucked body position
- Poor hair coat, unkempt (see Figure 5-2)
- Disinterested; unresponsive

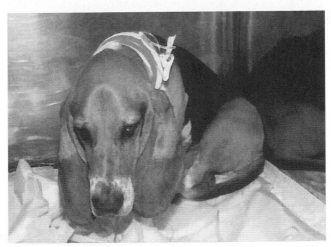

FIGURE 5-14   Dog facial expression. Note the head-down, fixed-gaze, and depressed expression. The dog was oblivious to its environment.

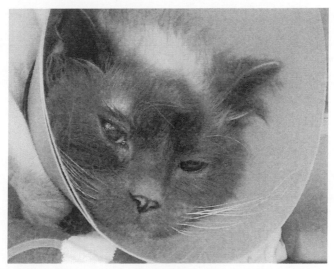

FIGURE 5-15   Facial expression in a cat with abdominal pain of unknown origin.

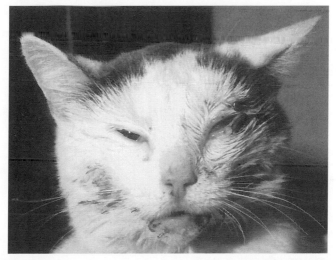

FIGURE 5-16   Cat facial expression. Note the squinted dull eyes and abnormal facial expression.

EVOKED PAIN BEHAVIORS

Physical interaction with animals is a necessary component of determining the presence and severity of pain. Assessment of evoked pain behaviors aids in determining an animal's pain condition and can help to confirm the evaluator's assumptions based on observation of the animal (Box 5-2). Physical

BOX 5-2 **Behavioral and Physiologic Signs Associated With Pain in Dogs and Cats**

Abnormal Posture
- Hunched-up guarding and tensing of abdomen
- "Praying" position for dogs (forequarters on the ground, hindquarters in the air), "sphinx" position for cats
- Sitting or lying in an abnormal position
- Not resting in a normal position (e.g., sternal or curled up)
- Statue-like appearance
- Abnormal body positioning (e.g., extended head and neck)

Abnormal Gait
- Stiff
- Partial or no weight bearing on injured limb
- Lameness, slight to obvious limp
- Reluctance to move

Abnormal Movement
- Thrashing
- Restlessness
- Circling
- Continuous activity

Vocalization
- Screaming, howling, barking, meowing
- Whining (intermittent, constant, or when touched)
- Crying (intermittent, constant, or when touched)

Miscellaneous
- Looking at, licking, or chewing the painful area
- Hyperesthesia or hyperalgesia
- Allodynia

Pain-Associated Characteristics That May Also Be Associated With Poor General Health (Medical Problems)
- Restlessness or agitation
- Trembling or shaking
- Tachypnea or panting
- Tucked tail (dogs) or tail flicking (cats)
- Depressed or poor response to caregiver
- Head hanging
- Not grooming
- Appetite decreased, picky, or absent
- Dull, depressed
- Lying quietly and not moving for hours
- Stuporous
- Urinates or defecates and makes no attempt to move
- Recumbent and unaware of surroundings
- Unwilling or unable to walk
- Bites or attempts to bite caregivers

BOX 5-2   Behavioral and Physiologic Signs Associated With Pain in Dogs and Cats—cont'd

Pain-Associated Characteristics That May Also Be Associated With Apprehension or Anxiety

- Restlessness or agitation
- Trembling or shaking
- Tachypnea or panting
- Low tail carriage
- Slow to rise
- Depressed (poor response to caregiver)
- Not grooming or excessive grooming
- Bites or attempts to bite caregiver
- Ears pulled back
- Restless
- Barking or growling (intermittent, constant, or when approached by caregiver)
- Growling or hissing (intermittent, constant, or when approached by caregiver)
- Sitting in the back of the cage or hiding (cat)

---

manipulation of suspected sources of pain and the surrounding area may identify areas of hyperalgesia, secondary hyperalgesia, or allodynia. The presence of hyperalgesia or allodynia is suggestive of a facilitated pain state (wind-up).

- Animals frequently respond with purposeful efforts to escape, and occasionally become aggressive (i.e., biting, scratching, kicking) in response to palpation of a painful area (Figures 5-11 and 5-17).

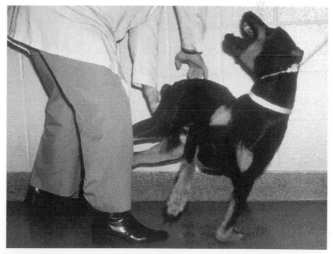

FIGURE 5-17   Response to manipulation. This dog became aggressive any time its pelvis was palpated.

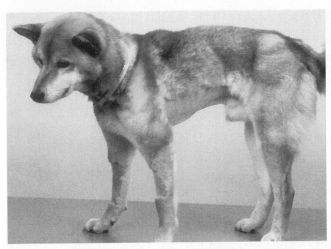

FIGURE 5-18 Abdominal pain. Abdominal splinting ("tucked up") or tenseness in response to abdominal palpation as a result of abdominal pain.

- Abdominal splinting or tenseness in response to abdominal palpation may cause abdominal pain or referred spinal pain (Figure 5-18).
- Animals may exhibit defensive behavior or withdraw to avoid being touched (see Figure 5-17).
- Stoic animals may simply freeze or look at the area in question (Figures 5-19 and 5-20).

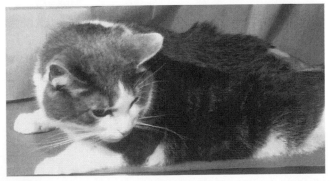

FIGURE 5-19 Looking at the painful area. This cat would sit and stare at its rear end. Its tail had been traumatized in an automobile accident.

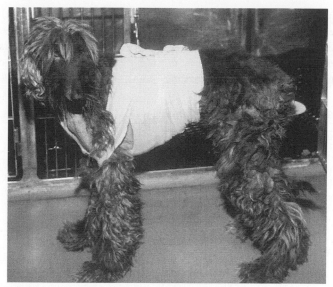

FIGURE 5-20 Looking at the painful area. This dog would stare at its left chest wall after a thoracotomy.

PHYSIOLOGIC INDICATORS OF PAIN

Physiologic manifestations of pain are largely related to activation of the sympathetic nervous system. The fight-or-flight response to actual or perceived stressors (i.e., pain) will activate the sympathetic nervous system, leading to release of cortisol from the adrenal cortex and catecholamines from the adrenal medulla. Physiologic indicators of acute pain in awake animals are generally transient and tend to be episodic in animals with chronic painful conditions. Noxious stimuli during lighter stages of general anesthesia will generate autonomic responses such as tachycardia, hypertension, and hyperventilation (or breath holding in some species). Deep anesthesia generally abolishes all physiologic responses to noxious (surgical) stimulation. Despite their potential value as indicators of pain, physiologic parameters should not be the only method used to identify or assess pain because the sympathetic nervous system and the stress response can be activated by nonpainful conditions (e.g., fear, disease).

- Non-noxious stressors (i.e., "white coat syndrome" or presence of a potential predator producing anxiety or fear responses) and metabolic derangements (i.e., hyperthermia) can generate physiologic responses similar to those elicited in response to noxious stimuli.
- Maximally stressed animals (i.e., septic peritonitis, polytrauma) may exhaust their sympathetic reserves, which may preclude the expected physiologic responses to pain.

- Autonomic responses (tachycardia, hypertension, hyperventilation) may be markedly depressed by general anesthesia.
- Anesthesia in the absence of a noxious stimulus can trigger a mild stress response that becomes apparent in the early postanesthetic period, creating physiologic conditions that may mimic pain.

Physiologic Indicators of Pain

- Hyperventilation or tachypnea
- Tachycardia (mild, moderate, or severe)
- Pupil dilation
- Hypertension
- Hyperthermia
- Increased serum cortisol and catecholamines (epinephrine)

Appetite

Anorexia is common in dogs or cats with significant acute or chronic pain. The animal may be misdiagnosed as having some other systemic problem. Concurrent causes of anorexia (e.g., gastrointestinal disorders) must be excluded. Various responses to food that may be exhibited by animals in pain include the following:

- Disinterest
- Poor appetite
- Food hiding

Elimination Habits

Urination and bowel habits may be affected by pain.

- Dogs and cats experiencing pain may lose their house-training habits because of the discomfort associated with ambulation, posturing, and reluctance or inability to move without pain.
- Dogs and cats may urinate frequently because of painful distention of the bladder or irritation (inflammation) of the bladder or urethra.
- Urine retention and constipation may occur in animals in pain that are administered opioids (e.g., morphine or hydromorphone).

FACTORS INFLUENCING THE ASSESSMENT OF PAIN BEHAVIORS

- Species, environmental factors, and concurrent diseases are the most influential factors that affect how likely and in what fashion an animal demonstrates pain. Consider the fight-or-flight response to stressors and the total submissive behavior of various species when threatened.

- Environmental factors (e.g., hospital setting, presence of perceived predators, confinement) may alter the likelihood of an animal to display characteristic pain behaviors, thereby confounding the evaluator's assessment.
- Evaluators of pain must be familiar with the species, and when possible the individual animal's normal behavior and its response to aversive or noxious stimuli, to accurately evaluate pain.
- Subjective, semi-objective, and objective pain assessment tools have been developed to standardize pain evaluative methods. A validated questionnaire using owner-perceived pain assessment, the Canine Brief Pain Inventory (CBPI), has been developed to better characterize chronic pain in dogs with osteoarthritis and bone cancer.
- Some animals appear more stoic and less inclined to display normal behavioral characteristics of pain than others. Giant breed dogs, for example, generally are very passive and may not demonstrate pain behaviors even when experiencing severe pain. The caregiver should consider breed and owner-reported pet behavior when assessing pain.
- The impact of age on pain perception has garnered mixed results, with studies reporting increased, decreased, or no change in pain sensitivity with increasing age. Degeneration of descending inhibitory mechanisms and neuronal cell death, autonomic dysfunction, and dysregulation of the hypothalamic-pituitary-adrenal axis occur with increasing age. All of these factors will affect pain processing and perception. Neonates have poor sensory discrimination because of incomplete axonal myelination and lower pain thresholds resulting from incompletely developed inhibitory systems and cortical processing center.

Behavioral and Categorical Methods for Assessing Pain in Animals

Subjective Verbal Pain Scale

Subjective verbal pain scales aimed at determining the severity of pain can aid in developing appropriate therapeutic analgesic regimens (Box 5-3).

- Subjective verbal scoring systems use a simple approach of assigning words to qualify pain, such as no pain; mild, moderate, or severe pain; or a number based on the degree of presumed pain the animal is experiencing.

BOX **5-3**	**Simple Subjective Verbal Pain Scale**

This is a simple descriptive scale used to estimate an animal's current pain status.

0 = No pain
1 = Mild pain
2 = Moderate pain
3 = Severe pain

- Advantages of this system are that it is simple to use and it aids in the planning of perioperative pain management. Inherent in this approach is that severe pain involving tissue and nerve damage is best managed by a multimodal analgesic approach.
- Subjective verbal scoring systems do not objectively quantitate the severity of pain (e.g., whether moderate pain is twice as severe as mild pain), making it difficult to compare individual animals and their response to analgesic therapy.

Visual Analogue Scale

The visual analogue scale (VAS) is one of the most extensively used subjective pain scoring systems in human and veterinary medicine. There are both numeric and non-numeric versions. The scale consists of a horizontal line measuring 100 mm in length with a vertical line border at both ends. Identifiers such as "no pain (0)" and "worst possible pain (10 or 100)" are usually present at the left and right borders, respectively (Figure 5-21). Occasionally VASs may have descriptors preplaced along the horizontal line to segmentalize the scale; however, this practice is not recommend because of the introduction of bias.

Behavioral Categories and Physiologic Parameters

- Demeanor: anxious, depressed, distressed, quiet
- Response to people: aggressive, fearful, indifferent
- Response to food: disinterested, eating hungrily, picking
- Posture: curled, hunched, rigid, tense
- Mobility: lame, slow or reluctant, stiff, unwilling to rise
- Activity: restless, still, sleeping
- Response to touch: crying, flinching, growling, guarding
- Attention to painful area: biting, chewing, licking, looking
- Vocalization: crying, groaning, howling, screaming

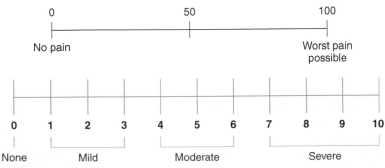

FIGURE 5-21 A typical visual analogue scale (VAS) used to estimate *(top)* and verbally categorize *(bottom)* pain intensity in animals.

- Physiologic and behavioral signs: tachycardia, panting, tachypnea, pyrexia, salivating, trembling, guarding, muscle spasm, dilated pupils, and so on

The care provider places a vertical line along the horizontal scale believed to represent the severity of the animal's pain. The line can be dated and time stamped, making it possible to use the same template for multiple evaluations. Annotations, such as before (B) and after (A) therapy, can be noted below the dates and times placed on the scale.

Advantages of the VAS are its simplicity of use as a semiquantitative means for assessing pain, the ability to trend pain over time, and its usefulness as a record of the animal's response to therapy. The VAS may be more discriminatory than subjective numeric scoring systems because it provides a greater range of scoring options (0 to 10).

Similar to subjective verbal scoring systems, the VAS does not provide an objective quantitation of pain (i.e., a score of 4 does not represent twice the pain as a score of 2), making it difficult to compare the severity of pain and response to therapy among animals. The VAS may appear to be, but erroneously, more statistically sensitive for evaluating pain compared with subjective numeric or verbal scoring systems, leading to overconfidence in the results. Interobserver variability with either method is quite high, limiting the accuracy of subjective numeric and verbal or VAS scoring systems, especially with multiple observers and/or when untrained co-workers are assessing the animal's pain. "Number bias" (preference for select numbers) is significant.

Simple Descriptive Pain Scale

The simple descriptive pain scale (SDPS) is analogous to the verbal rating scale used in human medicine. This scale assigns descriptors to the varying severities of pain, thereby providing greater objectivity to pain assessment (e.g., none, mild, moderate, severe). The descriptors are often assigned a number that is used for calculating the animal's pain score. Numerous versions of this scoring system have been developed for investigational studies, with descriptors ranging from basic (e.g., none, mild, moderate, or severe) to more detailed versions using brief definitions to describe each descriptor (e.g., anxious, depressed, aggressive, uncontrollable).

- Advantages of the SDPSs include their simplicity and the minimal training required for use. Most behavioral characteristics are identified and defined, and many apply across species.
- Like verbal scoring systems and the VAS, most SDPSs demonstrate poor sensitivity, leading to the potential for overestimation or underestimation of pain severity. There is also a high potential for significant interobserver variability. "User bias" (personal opinion) resulting from the observer's personal experience or opinion influences the pain score.

Numeric Rating Scale

The numeric rating scale (NRS) is another type of ordinal scale that attempts to remove evaluator subjectivity by assigning numeric values to indicate severity of pain. The NRS consists of multiple categories (e.g., 1 to 4, 1 to 6, 1 to 10) that list various descriptors (no pain, mild pain, moderate pain, severe pain, very severe pain) about each category in an attempt to quantify a gradual increase in pain intensity (Figure 5-22). The descriptors are assigned a numeric value analogous to increasing intensity; however, the individual categories are not weighted by importance. Scores from each category are summed to yield an overall pain score. Multiple categories such as physiologic (e.g., heart rate, respiratory rate, blood pressure), behavioral, and grooming changes are included in an attempt to make the score more objective.

- NRSs are more systematic and detailed and less subject to bias than most other pain assessment instruments. The inclusion of multiple categories permits a more critical assessment of the severity of the animal's pain. Most are easy to complete and ultimately assign a numeric value to the animal's pain level.
- Disadvantages include difficulty in applying this scale to multiple species because of species-specific behavioral and physiologic categories. Many NRS instruments are not weighted (i.e., each descriptor is treated equally) or robust (i.e., they do not apply to all circumstances) and are specifically directed toward animals with acute, chronic, orthopedic, or visceral pain. Others are designed for evaluation of a specific species (e.g., cats).
- The ability of NRSs to distinguish among delirium, dysphoria, and pain, particularly during the postanesthetic period, is poor.

Categorical Scoring Systems

Variations of the NRS include categoric NRSs (C-NRSs), wherein observations are grouped and weighted by assignment of a numeric score (e.g., 0 to 3). Scores are assigned within each category and summed to yield a "pain score." This type of system attempts to improve on the inadequacies of the standard NRS by applying more importance to key behavioral and physiologic variables; however, this method is still limited by the different and somewhat arbitrary definitions derived by different

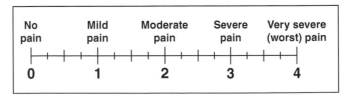

FIGURE 5-22 Numeric pain rating scale.

authors and how the instrument is applied. This predicament was illustrated by application of a C-NRS to a postoperative animal from which analgesics were withheld. The animal was lying quietly in its cage; was unwilling to move, eat, or drink; and appeared depressed. The University of Melbourne Pain Scale (UMPS) suggested a pain score of 4/27; however, a more thorough physical examination produced a pain score of 18/27. Several C-NRS instruments are listed here and can be obtained from various websites.

Owner assessment may be equally as effective as purely objective (force plate) pain scoring systems. Lameness assessment with force plate gait analysis (FPGA) and owner assessment of chronic pain with the CBPI are valid and reliable methods of evaluating canine orthopedic pain, particularly pain caused by osteoarthritis.

- **UMPS** (Box 5-4). The UMPS incorporates physiologic and behavioral parameters into six categories to assess postoperative pain in dogs. The assessor assigns a descriptor that approximates the animal's behavior in each category. The value for the descriptor is added to the animal's total

---

BOX 5-4   University of Melbourne Pain Scale (UMPS)

CATEGORY	DESCRIPTOR	SCORE
1. Physiologic data		
a.	Physiologic data within reference range	0
b.	Dilated pupils	2
c. Choose only one	Percentage increase in heart rate relative to preprocedural rate	
	>20%	1
	>50%	2
	>100%	3
d. Choose only one	Percentage increase in respiratory rate relative to preprocedural rate	
	>20%	1
	>50%	2
	>100%	3
e.	Rectal temperature exceeds reference range	1
f.	Salivation	2
2. Response to palpation (choose only one)	No change from preprocedural behavior	0
	Guards/reacts* when touched	2
	Guards/reacts* before touched	3
3. Activity (choose only one)	At rest: sleeping	0
	At rest: semiconscious	0
	At rest: awake	1
	Eating	0
	Restless (pacing continuously, getting up and down)	2
	Rolling, thrashing	3

Continued

BOX 5-4	University of Melbourne Pain Scale (UMPS)—cont'd	

CATEGORY	DESCRIPTOR	SCORE
4. Mental status (choose only one)	Submissive	0
	Overtly friendly	1
	Wary	2
	Aggressive	3
5. Posture		
a.	Guarding or protecting affected area (includes fetal position)	2
b. Choose only one	Lateral recumbency	0
	Sternal recumbency	1
	Sitting or standing, head up	1
	Standing, head hanging down	2
	Moving	1
	Abnormal posture (e.g., prayer position or hunched back)	2
6. Vocalization† (choose only one)	Not vocalizing	0
	Vocalizing when touched	2
	Intermittent vocalization	2
	Continuous vocalization	3

Modified from Firth AM, Haldane SL: Development of a scale to evaluate postoperative pain in dogs. J Am Vet Med Assoc 1999; 214: 651-659.

*Includes turning head toward affected area; biting, licking, or scratching at the wound; snapping at the handler; or tense muscle and a protective (guarding) posture.

†Does not include alert barking.

The pain scale includes six categories. Each category contains descriptors of various behaviors that are assigned numeric values. The assessor examines the descriptors in each category and decides whether a descriptor approximates the dog's behavior. If so, the value for that descriptor is added to the animal's pain score. Certain descriptors are mutually exclusive (e.g., a dog cannot be in sternal recumbency and standing at the same time). These mutually exclusive descriptors are grouped together with the notation "choose only one." For the fourth category, mental status, the assessor must have completed a preprocedural assessment of the dog's dominant or aggressive behavior to establish a baseline score. The mental status score is the absolute difference between preprocedural and postprocedural scores. The minimum possible total pain score is 0 points; the maximum possible pain score is 27 points.

pain score. Prior knowledge of the animal's behavior is necessary for determining mental status and change associated with the procedure. Possible pain scores are a low of 0 to a high of 27.

- **Glasgow Composite Measure Pain Score** (GCMPS). The GCMPS is a composite pain scale comprising seven behavioral categories with associated descriptors. The specific descriptors identified for each category comprise 47 words selected from a collection of 279 words to describe pain behaviors. The short form of the GCMPS (GCMPS-SF) (Box 5-5) was developed specifically for clinical application. It includes six behavioral categories with associated descriptors with a possible pain score of 0 for the lowest score or a high of 24.

BOX 5-5	**Short Form of the Glasgow Composite Measure Pain Scale**

Dog's name _____ Date / / Time

Hospital Number _____

Procedure or Condition _____

_____

In the sections below please circle the appropriate score in each list and sum these to give the total score

A. Look at dog in Kennel
Is the dog
(i)

Quiet	0
Crying or whimpering	1
Groaning	2
Screaming	3

(ii)

Ignoring any wound or painful area	0
Looking at wound or painful area	1
Licking wound or painful area	2
Rubbing wound or painful area	3
Chewing wound or painful area.	4

In the case of spinal, pelvic or multiple limb fractures, or where assistance is required to aid locomotion do not carry out section **B** and proceed to **C**
Please tick if this is the case ☐ then proceed to C

B. Put lead on dog and lead out of the kennel
When the dog rises/walks is it?
(iii)

Normal	0
Lame	1
Slow or reluctant	2
Stiff	3
It refuses to move	4

C. If it has a wound or painful area including abdomen, apply gentle pressure 5 inches round the site
Does it?
(iv)

Do nothing	0
Look round	1
Flinch	2
Growl or guard area	3
Snap	4
Cry	5

D. Overall
Is the dog?
(v)

Happy and content or happy and bouncy	0
Quiet	1
Indifferent or non-responsive to surroundings	2
Nervous or anxious or fearful	3
Depressed or non-responsive to stimulation	4

Is the dog?
(vi)

Comfortable	0
Unsettled	1
Restless	2
Hunched or tense	3
Rigid	4

Total Score (i+ii+iii+iv+v+vi) = _____

Reid J, Nolan AM, Hughes JML, Lascelles D, Pawson P, Scott EM: Development of the short-form Glasgow Composite Measure Pain Scale (CMPS-SF) and derivation of an analgesic intervention score, *Animal Welfare* 2007, 16(S):97-104.

- **Colorado State University Acute** (canine and feline) **and Chronic** (canine) **Pain Scales** (Figures 5-23, 5-24, and 5-25). These are numeric and categoric, convenient pain scales that are easy to use in a clinical setting.
- **CBPI** (Figure 5-26). The CBPI is an owner-applied questionnaire designed to quantitate the severity and impact of chronic pain in dogs with osteoarthritis. Originally modeled off the Brief Pain Inventory developed

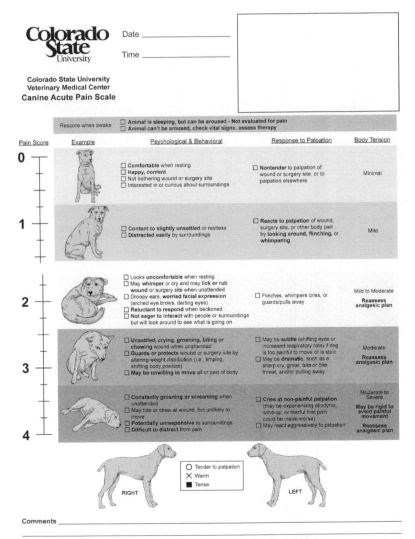

© 2006/PW Hellyer, SR Uhrig, NG Robinson

Supported by an Unrestricted Educational Grant from Pfizer Animal Health

FIGURE 5-23 Colorado State University Medical Center Canine Acute Pain Scale. (Courtesy Peter Hellyer, Samantha Uhrig, Narda Robinson.)

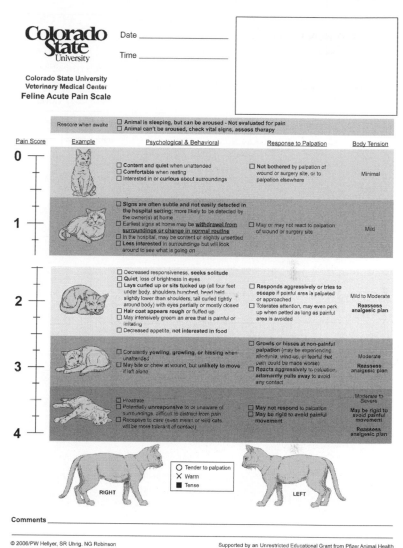

FIGURE 5-24 Colorado State University Medical Center Feline Acute Pain Scale. (Courtesy Peter Hellyer, Samantha Uhrig, Narda Robinson.)

for self-reporting pain in humans, the CBPI has been validated for use in dogs with osteoarthritis and bone cancer pain. Averaging the response to four questions that are scored from 0 to 10 generates a pain severity score. Interference of the animal's pain with its daily function is measured by averaging the score of six questions scaled from 0 to 10. Individual scores for pain and interference questions may also be used individually.

Colorado State University

Colorado State University
Veterinary Medical Center
Canine Chronic Pain Scale

Date _____

Time _____

Many signs of chronic pain are non-specific; rule out anxiety, poor general health, and systemic disease as part of a full workup.

Pain Score	Example	Psychological & Behavioral	Postural	Response to Palpation
0		☐ Happy, energetic ☐ Interested in or curious about surroundings ☐ Responsive; seeks attention	☐ Comfortable when resting ☐ Stands and walks normally ☐ Normal weight bearing on all limbs	☐ Minimal body tension ☐ Does not mind touch ☐ No reaction to palpation of joint
1		☐ Subdued to slightly unsettled or restless ☐ Distracted easily by surroundings ☐ Responsive; may not initiate interaction	☐ Stands normally, may occasionally shift weight ☐ Slight lameness when walking	☐ Mild body tension ☐ Does not mind touch except painful area ☐ Turns head in recognition of joint palpation
2		☐ Anxious, uncomfortable ☐ Not eager to interact with people or surroundings but will look around to see what is going on ☐ Loss of brightness in eyes ☐ Reluctant to respond when beckoned	☐ Abnormal weight distribution when standing ☐ Moderate lameness when walking ☐ May be uncomfortable at rest	☐ Mild to moderate body tension ☐ Doesn't mind touch far away from painful area ☐ Pulls limb away during palpation of affected joint **Reassess analgesic plan**
3		☐ Fearful, agitated, or aggressive ☐ Avoids interaction with people and surroundings ☐ May lick or otherwise attend to painful area	☐ Abnormal posture when standing ☐ Does not bear weight on affected limb when walking ☐ Guards painful area by shifting body position	☐ Moderate body tension ☐ Tolerates touch far away from affected limb ☐ Vocalizes or responds aggressively to palpation of affected joint **Reassess analgesic plan**
4		☐ Stuporous, depressed ☐ Potentially unresponsive to surroundings ☐ Difficult to distract from pain	☐ Reluctant to rise and will not walk more than 5 strides ☐ Does not bear weight on limb ☐ Appears uncomfortable at rest	☐ Moderate to severe body tension ☐ Dislikes or barely tolerates any touch (may be experiencing allodynia, wind-up, or fearful that pain could be made worse) ☐ Will not allow palpation of joint **Reassess analgesic plan**

Additional Comments:

© 2008/ NG Robinson, SL Shaver   Supported by an Unrestricted Educational Grant from Pfizer Animal Health

FIGURE 5-25   Colorado State University Medical Center Canine Chronic Pain Scale. (Courtesy Peter Hellyer, Samantha Uhrig, Narda Robinson.)

Today's Date: ☐☐ / ☐☐ / ☐☐
Month   Day   Year

Patient/Study ID# _____

Canine Brief Pain Inventory (CBPI)

Description of Pain:

Rate your dog's pain.

1. Fill in the oval next to the <u>one number</u> that best describes the pain at its **worst** in the last 7 days.

   ○ 0   ○ 1   ○ 2   ○ 3   ○ 4   ○ 5   ○ 6   ○ 7   ○ 8   ○ 9   ○ 10
   No Pain   Extreme Pain

2. Fill in the oval next to the <u>one number</u> that best describes the pain at its **least** in the last 7 days.

   ○ 0   ○ 1   ○ 2   ○ 3   ○ 4   ○ 5   ○ 6   ○ 7   ○ 8   ○ 9   ○ 10
   No Pain   Extreme Pain

3. Fill in the oval next to the <u>one number</u> that best describes the pain at its **average** in the last 7 days.

   ○ 0   ○ 1   ○ 2   ○ 3   ○ 4   ○ 5   ○ 6   ○ 7   ○ 8   ○ 9   ○ 10
   No Pain   Extreme Pain

4. Fill in the oval next to the <u>one number</u> that best describes the pain as it is **right now**.

   ○ 0   ○ 1   ○ 2   ○ 3   ○ 4   ○ 5   ○ 6   ○ 7   ○ 8   ○ 9   ○ 10
   No Pain   Extreme Pain

Description of Function:

Fill in the oval next to the **one number** that describes how during the past 7 days **pain has interfered** with your dog's:

5. **General Activity**

   ○ 0   ○ 1   ○ 2   ○ 3   ○ 4   ○ 5   ○ 6   ○ 7   ○ 8   ○ 9   ○ 10
   Does not   Completely
   Interfere   Interferes

6. **Enjoyment of Life**

   ○ 0   ○ 1   ○ 2   ○ 3   ○ 4   ○ 5   ○ 6   ○ 7   ○ 8   ○ 9   ○ 10
   Does not   Completely
   Interfere   Interferes

FIGURE 5-26   University of Pennsylvania Canine Brief Pain Inventory. (Courtesy Dorothy D. Brown.)

Continued

Today's Date: ☐☐ / ☐☐ / ☐☐
                Month   Day   Year

Patient/Study ID# _____

Description of Function (continued):

Fill in the oval next to the one number that describes how during the past 7 days **pain has interfered** with your dog's:

7. **Ability to Rise to Standing From Lying Down**

○ 0   ○ 1   ○ 2   ○ 3   ○ 4   ○ 5   ○ 6   ○ 7   ○ 8   ○ 9   ○ 10
Does not   Completely
Interfere   Interferes

8. **Ability to Walk**

○ 0   ○ 1   ○ 2   ○ 3   ○ 4   ○ 5   ○ 6   ○ 7   ○ 8   ○ 9   ○ 10
Does not   Completely
Interfere   Interferes

9. **Ability to Run**

○ 0   ○ 1   ○ 2   ○ 3   ○ 4   ○ 5   ○ 6   ○ 7   ○ 8   ○ 9   ○ 10
Does not   Completely
Interfere   Interferes

10. **Ability to Climb Up (for example Stairs or Curbs)**

○ 0   ○ 1   ○ 2   ○ 3   ○ 4   ○ 5   ○ 6   ○ 7   ○ 8   ○ 9   ○ 10
Does not   Completely
Interfere   Interferes

Overall Impression:

11. Fill in the oval next to the one response best describes your dog's overall quality of life over **the last 7 days**?

○ Poor   ○ Fair   ○ Good   ○ Very Good   ○ Excellent

FIGURE 5-26, cont'd University of Pennsylvania Canine Brief Pain Inventory. (Courtesy Dorothy D. Brown.)

Novel Pain Scoring Systems

Mouse Grimace Scale. The Mouse Grimace Scale (MGS) was developed based on the premise that animals are capable of demonstrating facial expressions suggestive of pain or discomfort (Figure 5-27). Such scoring systems are being developed for all domesticated species and provide a unique, validated adjunct to behavior-based and reflex response systems for assessing pain in mice that is applicable to clinical and laboratory research settings. The MGS is particularly useful in the laboratory setting, where researchers and animal care staff may have limited knowledge of behavioral signs of pain in animals. Since the advent of the MGS, similar facial expression scales intended to detect pain in rats and rabbits have been developed but have yet to be developed and validated for dogs and cats.

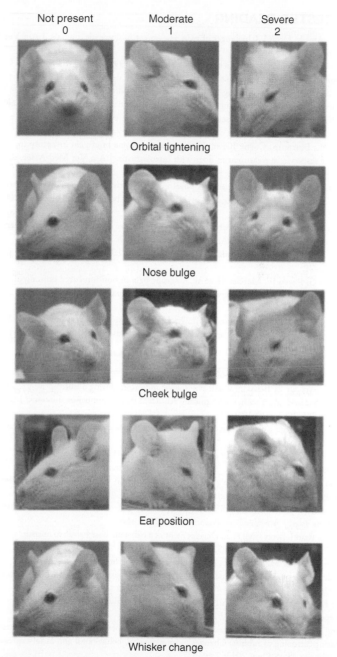

FIGURE 5-27   The Mouse Grimace Scale. Differences in facial expression. (From Langford DJ, et al. Coding of facial expressions of pain in the laboratory mouse. Nature Methods. 2010; 7:447-449.)

SUGGESTED READING

Anil SS, Anil L, Deen J. Challenges of pain assessment in domestic animals. J Am Vet Med Assoc. 2002; 220:313–319.

Bateson P. Assessment of pain in animals. Anim Behav. 1991; 42:827–839.

Bergeron N, Dubois MJ, Dumont M, et al. Intensive care delirium screening checklist: Evaluation of a new screening tool. Intensive Care Med. 2001; 27:859–864.

Brondani JT, Luna SPL, Padovani CR. Refinement and initial validation of a multidimensional composite scale for use in assessing acute postoperative pain in cats. Am J Vet Res. 2011; 72:174–183.

Brown DC, Boston R, Coyne JC, et al. Ability of the canine brief pain inventory to detect response to treatment in dogs with osteoarthritis. J Am Vet Med Assoc. 2008; 233:1278–1283.

Brown DC, Boston R, Coyne JC, et al. A novel approach to the use of animals in studies of pain: Validation of the canine brief pain inventory in canine bone cancer. Pain Med. 2009; 10:133–142.

Cambridge AJ, Tobias KM, Newberry RC, et al. Subjective and objective measurements of postoperative pain in cats. J Am Vet Med Assoc. 2000; 217:785–790.

Carstens E, Moberg GP. Recognizing pain and distress in laboratory animals. ILAR J. 2000; 41:62–71.

Chanques G, Payen JF, Mercier G, et al. Assessing pain in non-intubated critically ill patients unable to self report: An adaptation of the behavioral pain scale. Int Care Med. 2009; 35:2060–2067.

Conzemius MG, Hill CM, Sammarco JL, et al. Correlation between subjective and objective measures used to determine severity of postoperative pain in dogs. J Am Vet Med Assoc. 1997; 210:1619–1622.

Firth AM, Haldane SL. Development of a scale to evaluate postoperative pain in dogs. J Am Vet Med Assoc. 1999; 214:651–659.

Gelina C, Arbour C. Behavioral and physiologic indicators during a nociceptive procedure in conscious and unconscious mechanically ventilated adults: Similar or different? J Crit Care. 2009; 24:628e7–628e17.

Hansen B. Through a glass darkly: Using behavior to assess pain. Semin Vet Med Surg Small Anim. 1997; 12:61–74.

Hansen B. Assessment of pain in dogs. ILAR Journal. 2003; 44:197–205.

Hielm-Bjorkman AK, Hannu R, Tulamo RM. Psychometric testing of the Helsinki chronic pain index by completion of a questionnaire in Finnish by owners of dogs with chronic signs of pain caused by osteoarthritis. Am J Vet Res. 2009; 70:727–734.

Holton LL, Scott EM, Nolan AM, et al. Comparison of three methods used for assessment of pain in dogs. J Am Vet Med Assoc. 1998; 212:61–66.

Holton L, Reid J, Scott EM, et al. Development of a behavior-based scale to measure acute pain in dogs. Vet Rec. 2001; 148:525–531.

Hudson JT, Slater MR, Taylor L, et al. Assessing repeatability and validity of a visual analogue scale questionnaire for use in assessing pain and lameness in dogs. Am J Vet Res. 2004; 65:1634–1643.

Jensen KB, Kaptchuk TJ, Kirsch I, et al. Nonconscious activation of placebo and nocebo pain responses. PNAS. 2012; 109:15959–15964.

Keating SCJ, Thomas AA, Flecknell PA, et al. Evaluation of EMLA cream for preventing pain during tattooing of rabbits: Changes in physiological, behavioural and facial expression responses. PLoS One. 2012; 7:e44437.

Langford DJ, Bailey AL, Chanda ML, et al. Coding of facial expressions of pain in the laboratory mouse. Nat Methods. 2010; 7:447–449.

Lascelles BD, Hansen BD, Roe S, et al. Evaluation of client-specific outcome measures and activity monitoring to measure pain relief in cats with osteoarthritis. J Vet Intern Med. 2007; 21:410–416.

Mathews KA. Pain assessment and general approach to management. Vet Clin North Am Small Anim Pract. 2000; 30:729–752.

Morton CM, Reid J, Scott M, et al. Application of a scaling model to establish and validate an interval level pain scale for assessment of acute pain in dogs. Am J Vet Res. 2005; 66:2153–2166.

Reid J, Nolan AM, Hughes JML, et al. Development of the short-form Glasgow Composite Measure Pain Scale (CMPS-SF) and derivation of an analgesic intervention score. Animal Welfare. 2007; 16:97–104.

Sotocinal SG, Sorge RE, Zaloum A, et al. The rat grimace scale: A partially automated method for quantifying pain in the laboratory rat via facial expressions. Molecular Pain. 2011; 7:55–65.

Wiseman-Orr ML, Nolan AM, Reid J, et al. Development of a questionnaire to measure the effects of chronic pain on health-related quality of life in dogs. Am J Vet Res. 2004; 65:1077–1084.

Wiseman-Orr ML, Scott EM, Reid J, et al. Validation of a structured questionnaire as an instrument to measure chronic pain in dogs on the basis of effects on health-related quality of life. Am J Vet Res. 2006; 67:1826–1836.

Yazbek KVB, Fantoni DT. Validity of a health-related quality-of-life scale for dogs with signs of pain secondary to cancer. J Am Vet Med Assoc. 2005; 226:1354–1358.

Zamprogno H, Hansen BE, Bondell HD, et al. Item generation and design testing of a questionnaire to assess degenerative joint disease-associated pain in cats. Am J Vet Res. 2010; 71:1417–1424.

Health-Related Quality of Life Measurement

Jacqueline Reid; M. Lesley Wiseman-Orr; Andrea Nolan; E. Marian Scott

Quality of life (QOL) is a general term used in a variety of disciplines in which it is accepted that QOL is, like pain, a multidimensional construct that is subjectively experienced by and is uniquely personal to the individual. Previously in formal veterinary or scientific contexts the focus was on welfare and its measurement, but more recently the application of the term *quality of life* to animals has been more common. Some use these terms interchangeably, but we believe there to be a distinction between the two, as follows. *Welfare* can be conceptualized as a complex construct that combines both subjective and objective aspects of the conditions of life for animals—for example, as described in the Five Freedoms of the Farm Animal Welfare Council. Although the importance to its welfare of how the animal feels is now widely recognized, practical welfare measurement is still most usually concerned with ensuring that minimum standards of care are provided—that is, it is focused on the avoidance of suffering rather than the promotion of the best possible welfare. If we adopt for animals a conceptualization and definition of QOL that is similar to that for people, then consideration of QOL in veterinary and animal science offers the opportunity to make explicit the importance of the individual's perspective, and to significantly shift the focus in animal welfare from the avoidance of poor QOL to the attainment of good and even excellent QOL.

Health-related quality of life (HRQL) is concerned with those aspects of QOL that change as a result of ill health and medical interventions. We have proposed the following definition of QOL:

> Quality of life is the subjective and dynamic evaluation by the individual of its circumstances (internal and external) and the extent to which these meet its expectations (which may be innate or learned and which may or may not include anticipation of future events), which results in, or includes, an affective (emotional) response to those circumstances (Wiseman-Orr, Scott, Reid, et al., 2006).

Consequently, HRQL is the subjective evaluation of circumstances that include an altered health state and related interventions.

The incidence of chronic disease in companion animals is increasing. In the past two decades small animal practitioners have seen a marked change in the demographics of the pet population with an increase in the geriatric population of dogs and cats, resulting in more frequent presentations of chronic conditions, many of which are painful, such as osteoarthritis and painful tumors. Pain is defined by the International Association for the Study of Pain as a sensory and emotional experience, and it is the emotional component of this complex experience that makes pain something that is suffered. In the case of persistent pain, the emotional component can come to dominate the sufferer. Human chronic pain is often associated with fear, anger, anxiety, or depression, all of which may be caused by and may in turn exacerbate a patient's pain. Chronic pain therefore can have a widespread impact on patients' social and psychological as well as physical well-being, resulting in significantly reduced QOL. Recognition of the effects of chronic pain on QOL in humans has led to the development of instruments to measure chronic pain through such impacts, and many of the instruments now used in people are concerned primarily with the way in which the chronic condition disrupts activities of daily living and alters QOL. Irrespective of whether or not pain is a feature, chronic disease frequently has a deleterious impact on QOL. For example although lymphoma is generally recognized to be nonpainful, it can cause depression and lethargy as well as weight loss and weakness, and although chemotherapy increases life expectancy, owners often report side effects that might affect QOL.

Pain and QOL are uniquely personal subjective experiences that render impossible any scientific certainty about their perception—even about how they are perceived by another person. However, most scientists now consider that, unless proven otherwise, the ethically correct stance is to assume that many nonhuman animal species may suffer pain and be affected by a range of other circumstances in a similar way to humans. Accordingly, certainly in the case of chronic pain, we should assume that this may have a negative effect on an animal's QOL as it does on our own, and anecdotal evidence and recent studies have provided some evidence for this.

THE IMPORTANCE OF MEASURING THE IMPACT OF CHRONIC DISEASE ON HRQL IN ANIMALS

The assessment of pain is not an isolated element, but rather is an ongoing and integral part of total pain management. The current trend in managing chronic osteoarthritis in dogs is toward using combinations of therapeutic agents accompanied by lifestyle and dietary management, and in oncology clinicians must choose from a range of therapeutic options. To assess clinical change, gauge treatment efficacy, and guide treatment decisions, including decisions regarding the appropriateness of euthanasia, many clinicians and their clients would find it helpful to have access to valid, reliable and responsive measures of pain and HRQL as they attempt to identify the best course of action for the treatment of an animal that cannot speak for itself.

With greater choice of treatment options and increased affordability has come increasingly demanding ethical decision making in general as well as in specialist veterinary practice. This is particularly evident in the field of oncology, where increased survival is often achieved by the aggressive use of potentially aversive treatment protocols that may reduce HRQL both during and after treatment. In palliative care, too, treatments can have negative as well as positive impacts on QOL that must be weighed against each other and against valuations of *quantity* of life. An instrument that can be used with confidence to measure QOL and to monitor clinical change in an individual, as well as to provide data that would facilitate the development and selection of treatments with known effectiveness and impact, should reliably inform such difficult decision making, potentially reducing animal suffering as well as lessening the moral distress often felt by those involved in such decisions, whether veterinary practitioner or client.

The current emphasis on evidence-based veterinary medicine, in which decisions on adopting, modifying, or abandoning treatment methodologies are made according to peer-reviewed evidence, requires that robust measures of clinical impact be developed. It is the unpleasant feelings associated with pain—pain's emotional component—that cause an animal to suffer. Measuring that emotional component of an animal's pain or HRQL represents a huge challenge. In the past two decades the medical profession has recognized the importance of the valid and reliable measurement, however difficult to achieve, of how people are feeling, but until relatively recently there have been no such instruments for veterinary use. Measurement of an animal's pain and QOL has used indirect clinical measures and the subjective judgment of the veterinarian and/or client: an assessment approach of questionable validity, reliability, and sensitivity, and one that is at risk of positive and negative bias.

THE CHALLENGES FACING VETERINARY MEDICINE

Animals are incapable of verbal self-report and so must rely on an observer to assess their subjective experiences. Although self-reports, often using structured questionnaire instruments designed for the purpose, are currently regarded as the gold standard in assessing a person's pain and QOL, there are human sufferers who lack the necessary language skills or cognitive abilities to make such a report—for example, infants and those who are cognitively impaired. In such cases, caregivers and parents have been used as observers and reporters of behavioral indicators associated with pain and QOL, with some success. In the case of chronic pain in dogs, recent studies have highlighted the importance of using the owner as such an observer because subtle behavioral disturbances may be apparent only outside of a clinical setting (within which they may be masked by fear, excitement, or anxiety associated with being in an unfamiliar environment), and changes in behavior may be so gradual that they are apparent only to someone very familiar with the individual animal.

Behavioral disturbances have long been recognized as potential indicators of the presence of pain in animals. These include changes in demeanor, aggressiveness, submissiveness, fearfulness, restlessness, lethargy, activity, inquisitiveness, vocalization, self-mutilation, appetite, drinking, urination, grooming, and social behavior. However, it is important to bear in mind that each species may manifest unique pain-related behaviors or behavioral disturbances, often rooted in the evolutionary process (e.g., selection pressures may have ensured that prey species do not "advertise" an increased vulnerability to predators). Even within a species, such as the dog, it is possible that breed differences will result in differences in the impact of chronic pain on QOL. For example, poor QOL may be more quickly reflected in reduced appetite for some breeds of dog than for others that have a tendency to obesity and therefore may be expected to be highly motivated to eat.

Developing an instrument that is scientifically robust, and fit for its intended purpose, is undoubtedly the greatest challenge of all, irrespective of whether the instrument is designed for humans or for nonhuman species. Our medical colleagues have addressed this challenge over the last two decades by using psychometric methods that were first established by psychologists and psychiatrists to measure intangible constructs, such as anxiety and depression, through formally assessed structured questionnaires. These methods have been adopted increasingly in the measurement of human pain and HRQL and are well established; the creation of such assessment tools can be summarized as follows:

- Specify measurement goals (and hence the ideal measurement scale): What is to be measured, in which population, and for what purpose.
- Develop a pool of potential items for the instrument.
- Select suitable items from the pool and subject to expert validation.
- Incorporate selected items into an instrument, with consideration given to layout, response options, instructions to respondent, and administration.
- Pretest the instrument to ensure that the target respondent can use the instrument correctly.
- Field test the instrument to evaluate its psychometric properties (e.g., validity and reliability).

Instrument development is an iterative process, in which instruments are continuously refined and retested with new populations, in new contexts, and for new purposes.

HEALTH-RELATED QUALITY OF LIFE INSTRUMENTS

Properties

HRQL instruments are designed to assess the wide-ranging impacts of chronic disease and also treatment effects and side effects. They are increasingly valued as outcome measures in human medicine and are likely to become so in veterinary medicine as suitable instruments become available. Instruments to measure pain and HRQL can be used to measure differences between animals at a point in time (discriminative purposes) or differences within an animal over time (evaluative purposes). They can be disease specific, focusing on particular conditions, or they can be generic, designed to be used in a variety of contexts. Disease-specific instruments can be more responsive to clinical change, but generic instruments can be valuable indicators of a range of impacts associated with disease and its treatment, and may be the only option when an animal is suffering from more than one condition.

To be scientifically sound, a measurement instrument must possess the fundamental properties of validity and reliability and, in the case of evaluative instruments, responsiveness to clinical change.

- Validity (criterion, content, and construct) is the most fundamental attribute of an instrument because it provides evidence that the instrument is able to measure what it was designed to measure. Validity is not determined by a single statistic, but by a body of research that supports the claim that the instrument is valid. There are three types of validity.
  - Content validity focuses on the relevance and adequacy of the items within the instrument. The simplest form of content validity is face validity, which uses expert opinion to establish whether, "on the face of it," the items appear relevant to and encompassing of the attribute(s) to be measured.
  - Criterion validity is a measure of how well an instrument relates to other measures or outcomes (the criteria) already established for the attribute being measured.
  - Construct validity is demonstrated when hypotheses that are based on the construct being measured are devised and tested. A number of approaches exist to examine the construct validity of a new questionnaire instrument; these include factorial validity and known-groups validity. Factorial validity requires the analysis of relationships between questionnaire item responses with a multivariate statistical technique called *factor analysis*. Known groups (also known as extreme groups) validity is demonstrated when the instrument correctly distinguishes between groups that would be expected to have quite different scores.
- Reliability is a measure of whether an instrument can measure accurately and repeatedly what it is intended to measure, so that measurements of individuals on different occasions, or by different observers, or by similar or parallel tests, produce the same or similar results. If an instrument is to be used by an independent observer, then inter-rater reliability—the degree to which two or more observers who concurrently apply the instrument to the same subject arrive at similar scores—is a good indicator of the reliability of an instrument. Alternatively, test-retest reliability is

demonstrated when the scores provided by a single observer applying the instrument on two separate occasions to an unchanging subject are in agreement.

- Responsiveness in a clinical instrument is the property that ensures that the instrument is sensitive enough to detect differences in health status that not only are statistically significant, but are also important to the clinician or to the animal.

- To be useful in the busy clinical environment, an instrument must also have utility that encompasses the following:
  - Acceptability: The instrument is easy and rapid to complete.
  - Feasibility: The instrument is easy to administer and process.
  - Interpretability: The instrument provides a useful reference point. For example, an acute pain scale might supply the user with an intervention level for analgesic administration, or an HRQL instrument might supply the user with normative values for comparative purposes.

QUESTIONNAIRE DESIGN

Response Options

Each item in a structured questionnaire instrument is accompanied by a response option or options. These may be dichotomous (yes or no), categoric, and/or ordinal (e.g., mild, moderate, severe; numeric Likert-type scale) or even more complex. If responses are likely to lie on a continuum, it is important that respondents have the opportunity to answer in this way to ensure minimum loss of information and to minimize error. For example, for a question about anxiety, more and better information will be captured by offering the opportunity to indicate an amount of anxiety than would be captured by simply asking if the subject is or is not anxious.

Respondent Bias

Any questionnaire instrument is subject to the risk of respondent bias. Respondent bias can be reduced with comparative methods that use expert judgment to scale the value of each item response during instrument development. The result of this is that when the questionnaire instrument is used, the extent to which each response option represents the "right" or "wrong" answer is to some extent hidden from the respondent, thus making biased responding more difficult. A range of established comparative methods can be used for this purpose. In addition, a range of design features can be used to minimize the risk of respondent bias, such as considerations of number, type and arrangement of items, delivery methods, and even titling of the instrument.

Status Quo

A number of tools intended to measure pain and HRQL in animals have been developed in recent years. Veterinary practitioners who want to improve the management of pain in their animals are faced with a range of instruments to choose from. Instruments should be chosen for a particular purpose and population. The key questions to consider when selecting an instrument for a particular purpose are as follows:

- What does the instrument intend to measure, and what is its validity for this purpose? (For example, consider how measurement goals were defined, how items were generated and selected, and with what population(s) and in what contexts the instrument has been tested.)
- Do the response options seem appropriate, and is the method of generating instrument scores from item responses fully explained and justified?
- What evidence has testing of the instrument provided for its:
  - Criterion or construct validity?
  - Reliability?
  - Responsiveness (for evaluative instruments)?
  - Utility?

To assist the reader, Tables 6-1, 6-2, and 6-3 summarize the general and psychometric properties of generic and disease-specific instruments, available at the time of writing, that have some published evidence of validity. Please note that the information is presented as published by the instrument developers and does not represent any judgment of individual instruments by us.

CONCLUSION

Increasingly, measurement of companion animal QOL or HRQL is becoming more and more necessary in clinical practice as medical advances lead to animals living longer with painful chronic disease, and evidence-based medicine requires that robust measures of clinical impact be developed. The development of valid, reliable, and responsive measurement instruments for QOL and HRQL in animals is both time-consuming and challenging as well as costly, but in our view the resourcing and carrying out of such research is mandatory if we are to maintain rigorous scientific standards in modern veterinary medicine and improve the well-being of animals under our care.

TABLE 6-1	General Properties of Generic Health-Related Quality of Life (HRQL) Instruments Using the Owner as Respondent						
INSTRUMENT	**PURPOSE OR USE**	**DELIVERY**	**ITEMS**	**OUTPUT**	**CONSTRUCTION**	**AVAILABILITY**	**COMMENTS**
Karnofsky's score modified for cats (Hartmann and Kuffer, 1998)	Measures ability to carry on normal activities in life; uses a scale of 0 to 100%	Paper	22	Unclear but assumed to be single score from 0 to 100	Modified from Karnofsky's score for human patients	Published in reference	Score is composite of owner responses and clinician general condition scores
Preliminary discriminative questionnaire for assessment of nonphysical aspects of QOL of dogs (Wojciechowska et al., 2005, 2005)	Provides a framework for further development of an HRQL instrument	Telephone	27	Calculated single QOL score	Based on objective list theory	From corresponding author on request	Questionnaire did not discriminate sick from healthy dogs
VetMetrica (Reid et al., 2013)	1. General health and wellness measure 2. Monitoring the effectiveness of therapeutic interventions in any disorder affecting the QOL of dogs	Online	46	Profile of HRQL made up of scores in vitality, pain, distress, and anxiety	Psychometric methodology using dog owners as key informants	*www.vetmetrica.com* Password protected; for access, contact jacky.reid@newmetrica.com	Online delivery minimizes respondent bias HRQL profile generated automatically and instantaneously at server

QOL, Quality of life.

TABLE 6-2 General Properties of Disease-Specific Health-Related Quality of Life (HRQL) Instruments Using the Owner as Respondent

INSTRUMENT	ITEMS	OUTPUT	CONSTRUCTION	AVAILABILITY	COMMENTS
Helsinki Chronic Pain Index (HCPI) Indication: Osteoarthritis in dogs (Hielm-Björkman et al., 2003, 2009)	11	Single aggregate score of 1 to 44	Psychometric methodology	Contact anna.hielm-bjorkman@helsinki.fi	Created in Finnish English version available
Canine Brief Pain Inventory (CBPI) Indication: Osteoarthritis in dogs (Brown et al., 2007, 2008)	11	Two scores for pain: severity and interference One score for global QOL	Psychometric methodology	Download from *www.CanineBPI.com*	Modeled closely on the human self-report Brief Pain Inventory (BPI)
Liverpool Osteoarthritis in Dogs (LOAD) Indication: Elbow arthritis in dogs (Hercock et al., 2009; Walton et al., 2013)	31 reduced to 14 for analysis	Single aggregate score	Items generated by veterinary practitioners and specialists	*www.liv.ac.uk/sath/services/LOAD.pdf*	
Weighted QOL assessments for dogs with spinal cord injuries (Budke et al., 2008; Levine et al., 2008)	Five domains of QOL	Weighted quality of life score 0 to 100	Adapted from the schedule for the evaluation of individual quality of life–direct weighting for people	Contact authors	Specifically designed for individual dogs

QOL, Quality of life.

TABLE 6-3   Other Disease-Specific Instruments

INSTRUMENT	ITEMS	OUTPUT	CONSTRUCTION	AVAILABILITY	COMMENTS
Questionnaire on the QOL of dogs with atopic skin disease and their owners (Favrot et al., 2010)	Dog QOL: 14 Impact on family: 13 Overall assessment: 2	Not specified	Modeled on a number of instruments validated for the evaluation of QOL of children affected by atopic dermatitis and their parents	From authors on request	
Questionnaire on the QOL of dogs with skin diseases and their owners (Noli et al., 2011, 2011)	15	Single aggregate score for dog and owner separately	Psychometric methodology using dog owners as key informants	From authors on request	Measures impact of atopic dermatitis and other painful skin diseases
Functional evaluation of cardiac health (FETCH) in dogs (Freeman et al., 2005)	18	Single aggregate score	Modeled on the Minnesota Living with Heart Failure Questionnaire for people	Questionnaire items published in paper, but full questionnaire available from authors	
HRQL scale for dogs with pain secondary to cancer (Yazbek and Fantoni, 2005)	12	Single aggregate score	Not reported	Published in reference	
HRQL diabetic cats and dogs (DIAQoL-pet) (Niessen et al., cats, 2010; dogs, 2012)	29	Single average weighted impact score (AWIS)	Literature and focus groups—health professionals and owners	Available online at *www.rvc.ac. uk/diabetes*	

QOL, Quality of life.

SUGGESTED READING

Brearly JC, Brearly MJ. Chronic pain in animals. In: PA Flecknell, A Waterman-Pearson (Eds): Pain management in animals. London, 2000, Saunders.

Brown DC, Boston RC, Coyne JC, et al. Development and psychometric testing of an instrument designed to measure chronic pain in dogs with osteoarthritis. Am J Vet Res. 2007; 68:631–637.

Brown DC, Boston RC, Coyne JC, Farrar JT. Ability of the Canine Brief Pain Inventory to detect response to treatment in dogs with osteoarthritis. J Am Vet Med Assoc. 2008; 233:1278–1283.

Budke CM, Levine JM, Kerwin SC, et al. Evaluation of a questionnaire for obtaining owner-perceived, weighted quality-of-life assessments for dogs with spinal cord injuries. J Am Vet Med Assoc. 2008; 233:925–930.

Costello AB, Osborne JW. Best practices in exploratory factor analysis: Four recommendations for getting the most from your analysis. Pract Assess Res Eval. 2005; 10:1–9.

Dawkins MS. (2004) Using behaviour to assess animal welfare. Anim Welfare. 2004; 13:S3–S7.

Duncan IJH, Fraser D. Understanding animal welfare. In: MC Appleby, BO Hughes (Eds): Animal welfare. Wallingford, 1997, CAB International.

Favrot C, Linek M, Mueller R, Zini E. Development of a questionnaire to assess the impact of atopic dermatitis on health-related quality of life of affected dogs and their owners. Vet Dermatol. 2010; 21:64–70.

Freeman LM, Rush JE, Farabaugh AE, Must A. Development and evaluation of a questionnaire for assessing health-related quality of life in dogs with cardiac disease. J Am Vet Med Assoc. 2005; 226(11):1864–1868.

Gingerich DA, Strobel JD (2003) Use of client-specific outcome measures to assess treatment effects in geriatric, arthritic dogs: controlled clinical evaluation of a nutraceutical. Vet Ther. 4(4):376–386.

Hare B, Brown M, Williamson C, Tomasello M. The domestication of social cognition in dogs. Science. 2002; 298(5598):1634–1636.

Hartmann K, Kuffer M. Karnofsky's score modified for cats. Eur J Med Res. 1998; 3:95–98.

Hercock C, Pinchbeck G, Giejda A, et al. Validation of a client-based clinical metrology instrument for the evaluation of canine elbow osteoarthritis. J Small Anim Pract. 2009; 50:266–271.

Hielm-Björkman AK, Kuusela E, Liman A, et al. Evaluation of methods for assessment of pain associated with chronic osteoarthritis in dogs. J Am Vet Med Assoc. 2003; 222:1552–1558.

Hielm-Björkman AK, Rita H, Tulamo RM. Psychometric testing of the Helsinki chronic pain index by completion of a questionnaire in Finnish by owners of dogs with chronic signs of pain caused by osteoarthritis. Am J Vet Res. 2009; 70:727–734.

Holton L, Scott EM, Nolan AM, et al. The development of a composite measure scale to assess pain in dogs. J Vet PharmTher. 1997; 20(Suppl1):167–168.

Hudson JT, Slater MR, Taylor L, et al. Assessing repeatability and validity of a visual analogue scale questionnaire for use in assessing pain and lameness in dogs. Am J Vet Res. 2004; 65 (12):1634–1643.

Juniper EF, Guyatt GH, Jaeschke R. How to develop and validate a new health-related quality of life instrument. In: B Spilker: Quality of life and pharmacoeconomics in clinical trials, ed 2, Philadelphia, 1996, Lippincott-Raven Publishers.

Levine JM, Budke CM, Levine GJ, et al. (2008) Owner-perceived, weighted quality-of-life assessments in dogs with spinal cord injuries. J Am Vet Med Assoc. 2008; 233 (6):931–935.

Lynch S, Savary-Bataille K, Leeuw B, et al. Development of a questionnaire assessing health-related quality-of-life in dogs and cats with cancer. Vet Compar Oncol. 2011; 9:172–182.

Maria A, Iliopoulou BE, Kitchell V, et al. (2013) Development of a survey instrument to assess health-related quality of life in small animal cancer patients treated with chemotherapy. J Am Vet Med Assoc. 2013; 242:1679–1687.

McMillan FD. Maximising quality of life in ill animals. J Am Anim Hosp Assoc. 2003; 39:227–235.

Niessen SJ, Powney S, Guitian J, et al. Evaluation of a quality of life tool for cats with diabetes mellitus. J Vet Int Med. 2010; 24:1098–1105.

Niessen SJ, Powney S, Guitian J, et al. Evaluation of a quality of life tool for dogs with diabetes mellitus. J Vet Int Med. 2012; 26:953–961.

Noli C, Minafo G, Galzerano M. Quality of life of dogs with skin diseases and their owners. Part 1: Development and validation of a questionnaire. Vet Dermatol. 2011; 22:335–343.

Noli C, Minato G, Galzenaro M. Quality of life of dogs with skin diseases and their owners. Part 2: Administration of a questionnaire in various skin diseases and correlation to efficacy of therapy. Vet Dermatol. 2011; 22:344–351.

Reid J, Wiseman-Orr ML, Scott EM, Nolan AM. Development, validation and reliability of a web-based questionnaire instrument to measure health-related quality of life in dogs. J Small Anim Pract. 2013; 54:227–233.

Rutherford KMD. Assessing pain in animals. Animal Welfare. 2002; 11:31–53.

Scott EM, Fitzpatrick JL, Nolan AM, et al. Evaluation of welfare state based on interpretation of multiple indices. Animal Welfare. 2003; 12:457–468.

Skevington SM. Investigating the relationship between pain and discomfort and quality of life, using the WHOQOL. Pain 1998; 76:395–406.

Streiner DL. (1993) Research methods in psychiatry. A checklist for evaluating the usefulness of rating scales. Can J Psych. 1993; 38:140–148.

Streiner DL, Norman GR. Health measurement scales. A practical guide to their development and use, ed 2, New York, 1995, Oxford University Press.

Walton MB, Cowderoy E, Lascelles D, Innes JF. Evaluation of construct and criterion validity for the 'Liverpool Osteoarthritis in Dogs' (LOAD) clinical metrology instrument and comparison to two other instruments. PLoS One. 2013; 8(3):e58125.

Ware JE, Sherbourne CD. The MOS 36-item short-form health survey (SF-36): I. Conceptual framework and item selection. Med Care. 1992; 30:473–483.

Wemelsfelder F, Hunter EA, Mendl MT, Lawrence AB. The spontaneous qualitative assessment of behavioural expressions in pigs: first explorations of a novel methodology for integrative animal welfare measurement. Appl Anim Behav Sci. 2000; 67 (3):193–215.

Wiseman-Orr ML, Nolan AM, Reid J, et al. Development of a questionnaire to measure the effects of chronic pain on health-related quality of life in dogs. Am J Vet Res. 2004; 65:1077–1084.

Wiseman-Orr ML, Scott EM, Reid J, et al. Validation of a structured questionnaire as an instrument to measure chronic pain in dogs on the basis of effects on health-related quality of life. Am J Vet Res. 2006; 67:1826–1836.

Wojciechowska JI, Hewson CJ. Quality-of-life assessment in pet dogs. J Am Vet Med Assoc. 2005; 226(5):722–728.

Wojciechowska JI, Hewson CJ, Stryhn H, et al. Development of a discriminative questionnaire to assess nonphysical aspects of quality of life of dogs. Am J Vet Res. 2005; 66 (8):1453–1460.

Wojciechowska JI, Hewson CJ, Stryhn H, et al. Evaluation of a questionnaire regarding nonphysical aspects of quality of life in sick dogs. Am J Vet Res. 2005; 66 (8):1461–1467.

Yazbek KV, Fantoni DT. Validity of a health-related quality-of-life scale for dogs with signs of pain secondary to cancer. J Am Vet Med Assoc. 2005; 226:1354–1358.

Yeates J, Main D. Assessment of companion animal quality of life in veterinary practice and research. J Small Anim Pract. 2009; 50:274–281.

PART TWO

Pain Therapy

Pain Therapy

CHAPTER 7

Overview of Drugs Administered to Treat Pain

William W. Muir III

SEROTONIN SYNDROME

A drug is any chemical substance introduced into the body that produces a physiologic effect or is used in the treatment, cure, prevention, or diagnosis of disease. Ideally, drug treatment of pain is directed at the mechanism(s) responsible for pain and should be tailored to the cause, severity, and duration (acute or chronic) of pain. Few if any drugs can be considered to produce excellent or even good analgesia for extended periods without the risk of side effects or toxicity. Inadequate evidence, limited formulations, and an astonishing absence of controlled clinical trials limit the chronic administration of many drugs in dogs and cats. Drugs that have demonstrated efficacy in the treatment of pain fall into one of six broad categories: opioids, nonsteroidal anti-inflammatory drugs (NSAIDs), α_2-agonists, local anesthetics, corticosteroids, and others. Many "other" and "adjunctive" (added to) medications are known to alter central or peripheral neuronal activity (e.g., neuroleptics [tranquilizers], anticonvulsants, antidepressants, and topical preparations) or to produce anti-inflammatory effects, thereby enhancing the analgesic effect of known analgesics. This chapter provides a general overview of the drugs administered for the treatment of pain, emphasizing the most clinically relevant aspects of each drug group (Table 7-1) and how these drugs act to produce analgesia (Figure 7-1). Subsequent chapters describe specific representatives of each drug group, emphasizing mechanism of action, relevant pharmacology and pharmacokinetics, side effects, toxicity, and potential drug interactions.

NONSTEROIDAL ANTI-INFLAMMATORY DRUGS

See Chapter 8 for more information on NSAIDs.

NSAIDs represent a diverse group of chemical compounds that produce *analgesia, anti-inflammatory* and *antipyretic* effects. They are currently the most popular analgesic drugs used for the treatment of acute and chronic pain in dogs and cats (Box 7-1). NSAIDs act by inhibiting the various isoforms of cyclooxygenase (COX) synthase or, in the case of the "dual"

TABLE 7-1	Principal Analgesic Drug Classes		
	RELATIVE EFFICACY		
DRUG	**CHRONIC USE**	**ACUTE USE**	**PRACTICAL ISSUES**
Opioids	+/−	++	Bradycardia, tolerance
NSAIDs	++	+/−	Analgesic efficacy; renal, liver toxicity
α_2-Agonists	−	+	Sedation, bradycardia, respiratory depression
Local anesthetics	−	+++	Loss of motor control; CNS toxicity
Adjunct and adjuvant therapies	++	+/−	Depression, somnambulant, drug interactions, drug-specific effects

Key: +, Efficacious; −, minimal efficacy; *CNS*, central nervous system; *NSAIDs*, nonsteroidal anti-inflammatory drugs.

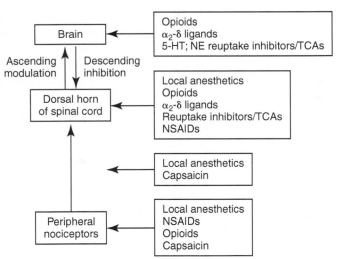

FIGURE 7-1   Principal sites of drug action. *5-HT*, 5-Hydroxytryptamine; *NE*, norepinephrine; *NSAIDs*, nonsteroidal anti-inflammatory drugs; *TCAs*, tricyclic antidepressants.

inhibitors, COX and 5-lipoxygenase (LOX) (LOX-COX inhibitors; no longer available in the United States). COX and LOX are responsible for prostaglandin (e.g., prostaglandin E_2) and leukotriene (e.g., leukotriene B_4 [LTB_4]) production, respectively. Prostaglandins produce their algesic, proinflammatory, and pyretic effects by activating prostaglandin receptors (e.g., eicosanoid receptors [EP receptors]) throughout the body. Leukotrienes stimulate chemotaxis and are associated with increased neutrophil activation and subsequent neutrophil adhesion and degranulation. Leukotrienes

BOX 7-1	Nonsteroidal Anti-inflammatory Drugs

Salicylic Acid
- Aspirin

Para-**aminophenol**
- Acetaminophen

Fenamic Acid
- Flunixin meglumine

Pyrazolones
- Dipyrone
- Phenylbutazone

Propionic Acids
- Carprofen
- Ketoprofen
- Naproxen
- Ibuprofen

Oxicams
- Piroxicam
- Meloxicam

Acetic Acids
- Ketorolac
- Etodolac

Coxibs
- Deracoxib
- Robenacoxib
- Firocoxib

Lipoxygenase or Cyclooxygenase Inhibitor
- Not available in the United States

play an important role in mediating inflammation, promoting tissue and in particular gastrointestinal mucosal damage and pain. At least two types of COX exist: COX-1 and COX-2. Although COX-1 is considered to be a constitutive or "housekeeping" enzyme and to be involved in cell signaling and maintenance of tissue homeostasis, both COX-1 and COX-2 have been demonstrated to have housekeeping roles in select tissues. COX-1 inhibition is believed to be responsible for the majority of acute and chronic toxicities of NSAIDs, especially gastrointestinal ulceration, although one theory contends that inhibition of COX-1 or both of the COX enzymes shunts substrate toward the production of leukotrienes, increasing the production of LTB_4 and thereby exacerbating mucosal damage. COX-2 is often but inappropriately referred to as *inducible COX* and is the principal enzyme responsible for the overproduction of prostaglandins after acute injury or infection. Most NSAIDS that are currently available inhibit COX-1 and COX-2 isoenzymes, although several are relatively selective (deracoxib, robenacoxib), if not specific (firocoxib) for COX-2. The availability of COX-2-selective NSAIDs (firocoxib, deracoxib, robenacoxib) offers the potential to provide improved analgesic and anti-inflammatory effects with minimal interference of gastrointestinal physiology. The nonsedating, analgesic, and low-toxicity profile of newer NSAIDs (e.g., deracoxib, firocoxib, robenacoxib) has helped to decrease traditional concerns regarding gastrointestinal toxicity, although the potential for renal toxicity and blood clotting abnormalities remains.

Pharmacologic Considerations

Regardless of their diverse chemical structure and selectivity for COX-1, COX-2, or LOX, most NSAIDs produce dose- and individual animal–dependent analgesic effects. It is noteworthy that COX-1 selective NSAIDs (e.g., aspirin and ibuprofen [weakly]) inhibit platelet aggregation. Although efforts have been made to match a specific NSAID to the dependence of inflammation on COX-1 or COX-2 activation, this goal has not been and is unlikely to be achieved. As stated earlier, the majority of proinflammatory prostaglandins induced by acute tissue damage or trauma are produced by upregulation of COX-2, suggesting that drugs that inhibit COX-2 should be more effective analgesic, anti-inflammatory, and antipyretic drugs. This conjecture remains clinically unproven in veterinary species. Similarly, NSAIDs that interfere with normal homeostatic activity (COX-1 effects) should be more likely to produce toxicity. Clinically, the last conclusion is generally true because drugs that produce COX-2 inhibitory effects exhibit a lower tendency to produce gastrointestinal toxicity or interfere with clotting than COX-1 inhibitors. Nevertheless, given the potential for serious side effects, veterinarians should consider analgesic adjuncts (tramadol, gabapentin, amantadine) if standard NSAID therapy does not produce the desired analgesic effects. It is important to note that all currently available NSAIDs can produce renal toxicity.

Central Nervous System

NSAIDs do not alter the animal's level of consciousness or behavior. Analgesia, although primarily resulting from the local inhibition of prostaglandins, may also be caused by the inhibition of prostaglandin generation in the central nervous system (CNS). The activation of glial cells and microglia within the CNS by proinflammatory cytokines and lymphokines is suspected to be responsible for the production of prostaglandins including tumor necrosis factor–α (TNF-α) that contribute to central sensitization and amplification of pain-associated chronic pain states. The use of NSAIDS that target CNS sites may have special advantage in providing analgesia for chronic pain. NSAIDs are synergistic with opioids for producing analgesia and reduce the amount of opioid required to produce effective analgesia.

Neurons within the hypothalamus that are responsible for regulating body temperature are affected by prostaglandins, resulting in an increase in the thermoregulatory set point and onset of fever. NSAIDs return the set point to normal by inhibiting prostaglandin production.

Respiratory System

NSAIDs do not produce clinically relevant effects on the respiratory system. NSAIDs may, however, improve respiratory function in animals with inflammatory-mediated bronchoconstrictive diseases. On rare occasions, NSAIDs have been incriminated in the production of acute asthma-like signs. The mechanism for this response is unclear, but it has been suggested that leukotrienes (e.g., LTC_4 and LTD_4) may increase when arachidonate metabolism is diverted from the COX pathway to the LOX pathway. Increased production of LTC_4 and LTD_4 causes airway hyperreactivity and bronchial contractions.

Cardiovascular System

NSAIDs do not produce significant cardiovascular effects. Inhibition of prostaglandin production after infection, trauma, or a generalized systemic inflammatory response can help prevent vasodilation, edema, and platelet aggregation. Some NSAIDs, particularly those that are more COX-1 selective (e.g., aspirin), are noted for their inhibitory effect on platelet aggregation and are routinely used in humans to limit the possibility of stroke and heart attack (one baby aspirin daily). NSAIDs, particularly COX-1 selective, can produce prolonged bleeding times and the development of edema at sites of tissue injury. NSAIDs occasionally cause fluid retention in animals with heart failure.

Other Organ Systems

Gastrointestinal System

Prostaglandins play an important role in the development of a protective gastric barrier to intraluminal acidity by stimulating mucous production and bicarbonate secretion and promoting blood flow. Prostaglandins also sustain cell turnover and repair and maintain normal gut motility. The use of NSAIDs predisposes animals to gastric erosions and ulceration, often requiring treatment (Box 7-2).

Renal and Genitourinary Systems

Various prostaglandins, produced by both COX-1 and COX-2, are involved in the regulation of renal blood flow, glomerular filtration rate (GFR), the release of renin, reabsorption of water, and excretion of sodium and potassium. Young and older animals are at increased risk of NSAID-associated renal toxicity. NSAIDs may cause hyperkalemia because of inhibition of aldosterone. This effect will be greater in animals with heart failure or those administered potassium-sparing diuretics or angiotensin-converting enzyme (ACE) inhibitors (e.g., enalapril). The release of the prostaglandins

BOX 7-2	Treatment of Gastrointestinal Side Effects of Nonsteroidal Anti-inflammatory Drugs

- Discontinue nonsteroidal anti-inflammatory drug
- Initiate antibiotic therapy
- Sucralfate, 0.5 to 1.0 g PO
- Ranitidine, 2.5 mg/kg IV q12h
- Famotidine, 0.5 to 1 mg/kg IV q12h
- Misoprostol, 0.7 to 5 µg/kg PO q8h

(e.g., prostacyclin and prostaglandin E_2) is increased by volume depletion, glomerular disease, renal insufficiency, hypercalcemia, and the vasoconstrictors angiotensin II and norepinephrine. Prostaglandins antagonize the vasoconstrictor effects of angiotensin II and norepinephrine, thereby maintaining GFR. Inhibition of prostaglandin synthesis by NSAIDs can lead to reversible renal ischemia, a decline in glomerular hydraulic pressure (the major driving force for glomerular filtration), and acute kidney injury. The rise in the plasma creatinine concentration usually occurs within the first 3 to 7 days after initiating NSAID therapy.

Liver Function and Hemostasis

Hepatopathies are relatively uncommon in animals receiving NSAIDs. NSAID administration can produce mild hepatic changes characterized primarily by increases in liver enzymes without clinical signs or hepatic dysfunction. Idiosyncratic reactions are rare, resulting in hepatic dysfunction or failure, but have been reported in dogs (acetaminophen, carprofen, etodolac, ibuprofen) and cats (acetaminophen). Acetaminophen undergoes minor metabolism by P-450 mixed function oxidase to a highly reactive metabolite, N-acetyl-para-benzoquinoneimine (NAPQI), which is inactivated through glucuronidation with glutathione, in the liver. Saturation of glucuronidation and sulfation pathways and depletion of glutathione stores cause NAPQI metabolite to bind to hepatic cell membranes, causing hepatocyte injury and potentially cell death. Cytopathic injury (hepatocellular injury, necrosis) and cholestasis may occur, suggesting caution in animals with preexisting hepatic disease. NAPQI also causes severe oxidative stress to red blood cells. The oxidant damage to heme ions results in methemoglobin, a form of hemoglobin which does not carry oxygen. Ferrous iron is oxidized to ferric iron, converting hemoglobin to methemoglobin. Oxidation of hemoglobin may also cause Heinz body formation. In addition, aspirin and other COX-1 inhibitors inhibit platelet COX, thereby blocking the formation of thromboxane A_2, impairing thromboxane-dependent platelet aggregation and consequently predisposing to a prolonged bleeding time.

Clinical Issues

NSAIDs are effective for the treatment of mild to moderate pain associated with osteoarthritis and are frequently administered as part of a multimodal pain therapy program. NSAIDs act synergistically with opioids. The routine perioperative and, in particular, preoperative administration is controversial. All NSAIDs are potentially toxic to the kidneys, especially in animals with evidence for preexisting renal disease, which are dehydrated, hypovolemic, anemic (Hct <24%) or aged. If an NSAID is administered before anesthesia and surgery, the Hct and mean arterial blood pressure (MAP >60 mm Hg) should be monitored. Although most effective for treating pain caused by tissue damage (e.g., hypersensitivity), NSAIDs rarely eliminate all pain and are relatively ineffective for treating severe pain. Gastrointestinal, renal, or hepatic toxicity, and excessive bleeding are potential problems associated with the clinical use of NSAIDs. These issues are particularly important in very young or old animals and in animals that are immunocompromised or have preexisting cardiovascular, renal, or liver disease. The potential for altered platelet function and blood dyscrasias should be considered if NSAIDs are to be administered chronically. Significant differences among drugs and their metabolism by different species (dogs versus cats) emphasize the importance of strict adherence to dose recommendations and administration schedules if toxicity is to be prevented. Potential drug interactions include hypocoagulability when combined with other drugs that interfere with platelet function, and interference with the effects ACE inhibitors. The exact mechanisms of this latter interaction remain unresolved.

OPIOIDS

See Chapter 9 for more information on opioids.

The term *opioid* is preferred to the older name *narcotic* because by definition narcotics include any drug that induces sleep, and most opioid analgesics do not induce sleep—at least not in animals. Simply stated, opioids include any one of a growing number of natural and synthetic compounds that produce morphine-like effects by acting on one of multiple opioid receptors (e.g., OP_3 [μ; MOP], OP_2 [κ; KOP], and OP_1 [δ; DOP]) (Table 7-2). The principle desired effect of opioid administration is analgesia, although mild sedation is frequently observed and desired, at least in animals. Opioids are categorized as opioid agonists, partial agonists, agonist-antagonists, and antagonists (Table 7-3). Partial agonists (e.g., buprenorphine: mixed-action μ opioid partial agonist/κ opioid antagonist) bind to and activate opioid receptors but produce only partial efficacy relative to full agonists. Opioid partial agonists produce morphine-like effects, can act as antagonists, and are generally less toxic (although often less effective) than opioid agonists. Opioid agonist-antagonists produce opioid effects and lower dosages are additive with full opioid agonists. Larger doses of opioid agonist-antagonists and partial agonists can act as antagonists of full opioid agonists because of their relatively high affinity for opioid receptors. Opioid antagonists (e.g., naloxone and naltrexone) are devoid of agonist activity and are used clinically to antagonize or reverse opioid effects (see Table 7-3).

Opioids vary in their receptor specificity, potency, and affinity for the different opioid receptors (μ, κ, δ), resulting in a wide variety of clinical effects depending on the dosage and the species (e.g., dog, cat) they are administered to. Most opioid agonists have a relatively high affinity for μ receptors and are noted for their ability to produce analgesia and mild sedation (e.g., morphine, meperidine, and hydromorphone).

TABLE 7-2   Opioid Receptor Classification

OPIOID RECEPTOR SUBTYPES	CLASSIFICATION*	DISTRIBUTION	LIGAND	FUNCTION
μ_1 μ_2 μ_3	MOP (OP$_1$)	Brain, spinal cord, periphery sensory neurons Immune cells, amygdala, endothelial cells	Morphine	Analgesia, euphoria, depression, dysphoria Respiratory depression Dysregulated gut and bladder motility ↓ Temperature
κ_{1a} κ_{1b} κ_{2a} κ_{2b} κ_3	KOP (OP$_2$)	Brain, spinal cord, peripheral sensory neurons (gut)	Dynorphin	Analgesia Minimal sedation Dysphoria
δ_1 δ_2	DOP (OP$_3$)	Brain, peripheral sensory neurons	Leu-enkephalin Met-enkephalin	Analgesia, euphoria CNS depression, dysphoria Respiratory depression
Nociceptin	NOP? (OP$_4$)	Brain, spinal cord		Anxiety, depression Appetite stimulation

*International Union of Basic and Clinical Pharmacology.

TABLE 7-3   Selectivity of Opioid Receptor Subtypes

DRUG	μ	κ	δ
Agonists			
Codeine	+	+	+
Fentanyl	++++	−	+
Hydromorphone and oxymorphone	+++	+	+
Meperidine	++	+	++
Methadone	+++	+	++
Morphine	+++	++	++
Partial and Mixed Agonists			
Buprenorphine	(+++)	−	−
Butorphanol	++	(++)	−
Dezocine*†	+		
Nalbuphine†	+	(+++)	(++)
Pentazocine	+	(++)	+
Antagonists			
Naloxone	+++	++	+++
Naltrexone	+++	++	++
Atypical Opioids			
Tramadol*	+	?	?
Tapentadol*	+	?	?

Key: +, Mild effect; ++, moderate effect; +++, pronounced effect; ++++, very pronounced effect; () partial agonist effects; ?, unknown; −, little or no effect.
*In addition to suggested norepinephrine reuptake inhibition and α_2 receptor agonist.
†Not controlled.

Pharmacologic Considerations

As suggested in Table 7-2, different opioids produce varied pharmacologic effects based on their ability to combine with and activate opioid receptors located in the CNS and peripherally. The prevalence, location (central or peripheral), and density of the opioid receptors in different species, the opioid receptor selectivity, the severity of pain, and the influence of various diseases ultimately determine the pharmacologic effects of the opioid in any given animal. Methadone, for example, is known to act primarily at μ opioid receptors but it also inhibits N-methyl-D-aspartate (NMDA) receptors in the spinal cord, potentially increasing its efficacy for the treatment of severe acute and chronic pain syndromes. Although the CNS-associated analgesic effects of opioids have been emphasized, their effects on peripheral opioid receptors should not be underestimated and are the basis for their administration intra-articularly.

Central Nervous System

Opioids relieve or reduce pain by combining with opioid receptors in the CNS and periphery. Opioids are generally considered to be the most effective of all analgesic medications but vary widely in their analgesic efficacy when used to treat naturally occurring pain (e.g., superficial, visceral, or deep). Fentanyl, for example, is at least 100 times more potent than morphine and produces excellent analgesia when administered at what would be considered extremely small doses (micrograms per kilogram) compared with most opioid analgesics (e.g., morphine, oxymorphone, and butorphanol [milligrams per kilogram]).

Most opioid agonists produce species-dependent minimal to moderate CNS effects that generally result in sedation. Opioid agonists almost always produce CNS and respiratory depression or arrest when administered with tranquilizers (neuroleptanalgesia) or with injectable or inhalant anesthetics, especially when administered to animals that are already depressed, have suffered head trauma, or are clinically debilitated or demented. Cats may become disoriented and display signs of delirium and excitability when larger doses of opioids are administered, and some dogs may react wildly and aggressively. Both dogs and cats become sensitive to loud or high-pitched noises (i.e., hyperacusis). Increased doses of opioids can produce nervousness, agitation, increased locomotor activity, dysphoria, and potentially hyperthermia (cats). MOP and KOP receptors are thought to be in balance, with μ and κ receptor activation producing hyperthermia and hypothermia, respectively. Cats are particularly susceptible to the neuroexcitatory effects of opioids and μ opioid agonists are more likely to produce opioid-induced neurotoxicity (OIN) and hyperthermia than partial agonists or agonist-antagonists. Morphine can produce excitement and mania ("morphine mania") in cats. This response is now known to be species and dose dependent. Myoclonus and seizures can be triggered on rare occasions and have been attributed to drug metabolites, solution preservatives, and preexisting CNS disorders. Aged animals may be particularly susceptible to the CNS and behavioral effects of opioids, with some animals demonstrating indifference, malaise, disorientation, hyperalgesia, agitation, and aggressive behavior. Some animals may become timid and attempt to escape when approached. Dogs may exhibit a "release of suppressed behavior" manifesting as aggression when any drug that alters CNS cognitive activity is administered. Changes in behavior and aggression and the development of opioid-induced hyperalgesia (OIH) have been attributed to central neurochemical mechanisms.

Nausea and vomiting (dogs and cats) and panting (dogs) are acute phenomena that are most commonly observed after intramuscular opioid administration. Opioids are known to stimulate the chemoreceptor trigger zone (CTZ) and reset thermoregulatory centers in the hypothalamus, resulting in a slight fall in body temperature in dogs. Vomiting (less common in cats) may be considered an advantage in animals that have recently eaten and are scheduled for surgery. Vomiting and retching, however, are problematic if the animal is believed to have a pharyngeal, esophageal, or gastric foreign body. Panting is a common clinical sign after the administration of most opioid agonists to dogs and may not provide adequate ventilation because of increases in dead space ventilation. Dogs and cats that have been administered opioids as preanesthetic medication may require manual or mechanical ventilation to achieve adequate ventilation, maintain adequate oxygenation, and avoid respiratory acidosis. Shivering is common after anesthesia because body temperature may be decreased. Shivering increases postoperative oxygen and caloric requirements, which could become important in older, very young, and small animals. Shivering may also be a sign of inadequate analgesia. Some opioids (e.g., meperidine) decrease the incidence of shivering by lowering the shivering thermal threshold.

Most opioids depress the cough reflex by a central mechanism. Cough suppression is produced at subanalgesic doses and is prominent with less potent opioids (e.g., codeine) and opioid agonist-antagonists (e.g., butorphanol). Cough suppression may lead to the accumulation of mucous secretions in the airways of animals recovering from anesthesia, predisposing to upper airway obstruction.

Opioids generally produce pinpoint pupils (miosis) in dogs as a result of CNS stimulation of parasympathetic segments of the oculomotor nerve. This response can be inhibited by prior administration of anticholinergic drugs (e.g., atropine and glycopyrrolate). The pupil dilates (mydriasis) in cats as a result of stimulation of CNS sympathetic pathways.

Respiratory System

Opioid administration may exaggerate the respiratory depressant effects of adjunctive drugs that produce CNS depression and/or anesthesia. Opioids increase the concentration of carbon dioxide necessary to stimulate the rate and depth of breathing (increase respiratory threshold) and depress the ventilatory drive to increases in inspired concentrations of carbon dioxide (decrease respiratory sensitivity). Clinically, both effects predispose animals to hypoventilation and the development of respiratory acidosis. Respiratory depression is not frequently reported in conscious dogs or cats administered opioids compared with humans. The best explanation for this difference is that most opioids do not produce the same degree of euphoria and CNS depression in dogs or cats as they do in humans. In other words, the degree of opioid-induced respiratory depression in dogs and cats is related to the amount of preexisting CNS depression. As long as the animal remains conscious, it is unlikely to develop significant respiratory depression. Respiratory depression in animals administered tranquilizers or sedatives in conjunction with opioids, before or during anesthesia, is of greater concern. These animals may require assisted or controlled ventilation.

Chest wall rigidity, or "woody chest syndrome," can occur in dogs or cats administered large or repeated doses of opioids (e.g., fentanyl). Increased chest wall muscle rigidity resulting in increased thoracic and abdominal efforts to breathe may be related to the CNS excitation.

Cardiovascular System

Opioids produce relatively few if any clinically significant cardiovascular side effects in dogs and cats when administered at recommended doses. Sinus bradycardia and first-degree (prolonged PR interval), second-degree (P wave not followed by a QRS interval), and, rarely, third-degree (no relationship between P wave and QRS complexes) atrioventricular block can occur because due to vagally mediated increases in parasympathetic tone; these conditions are almost always responsive to anticholinergic therapy (atropine, glycopyrrolate).

Opioids can produce clinically significant decreases in the force of cardiac contraction (inotropy), arterial blood pressure, and cardiac output when administered rapidly intravenously or in large doses. Some opioids (e.g., morphine and meperidine) are noted for causing histamine release and the splanchnic sequestration of blood (dogs), which could exacerbate hypotension. The clinical impact of these effects, at the currently prescribed dosages of opioids, remains to be demonstrated. Histamine release in cats is signaled by increased redness of the ears and paws.

Other Organ Systems

Gastrointestinal System

The precise mechanisms responsible for opioid-induced nausea and vomiting are incompletely understood and involve both central and peripheral sites including the vomiting center, CTZs, the cerebral cortex, and the vestibular apparatus of the brain. Nausea and vomiting are treated by administering opioid receptor antagonists (e.g., naloxone, naltrexone). Regardless, a specific role for other opioid receptors such as the κ opioid receptor (KOR) or δ opioid receptor (DOR) in contributing to or modulating opioid-induced nausea and vomiting (OINV) cannot be ruled out. The emetic effects of some opioids seem to be dependent on activation of DOR. In clinical settings, multiple receptors may play a role in contributing to nausea and vomiting. Some of the emetogenic receptors that have been proposed are dopamine-2 (D_2) receptor; histamine-1 (H_1) receptor; DOR; 5-hydroxytryptamine (serotonin) ($5\text{-}HT_3$) receptor; acetylcholine (ACh) receptor; neurokinin-1 (NK1) receptor; and cannabinoid receptor 1 (CB_1). Receptors that are antagonized by antimemetics include D_2 (haloperidol); H_1 (promethazine); DOR (naloxone); $5\text{-}HT_3$ (ondansetron, tropisetron, dolasetron, granisetron); ACh (scopolamine); NK1 (maropitant); and CB_1 (dronabinol).

Opioids, particularly μ-receptor agonists, delay gastric emptying and prolong intestinal transit time. Gastric and intestinal smooth muscle tone are increased, producing "ropy guts" that are particularly evident after the administration of an opioid to puppies or kittens. Increases in intestinal smooth muscle tone are caused by centrally mediated increases in vagal tone and activation of opioid receptors throughout the gastrointestinal tract. The onset of opioid-induced gastrointestinal effects may result in defecation and a period of diarrhea in dogs. This is followed by a decrease in propulsive peristaltic activity and absorption of water from the intestinal tract, predisposing the animal to constipation, a condition that becomes more prominent when opioids are administered chronically. Opioids increase esophageal, biliary, duodenal, and anal sphincter tone, making it difficult to perform endoscopic examinations, particularly of the duodenum. Opioids should be avoided in animals believed to have an obstructed biliary tract or biliary neoplasm. Butorphanol or butorphanol drug combinations are generally preferred for endoscopic procedures involving the gastrointestinal system because of lesser effects on gastrointestinal motility and sphincter activity.

Genitourinary System

Opioids inhibit the voiding reflex and increase external urethral sphincter tone, resulting in urine retention. Urine retention can be an important postsurgical consideration in dogs and cats that have undergone prolonged orthopedic surgical procedures or abdominal surgery or in animals with pre-existing bladder dysfunction.

Although popular because of their analgesic and sedative effects, most opioids decrease uterine contractions, thereby prolonging labor. This issue may be of little consequence if a cesarean section is performed. Respiratory depression of the fetus is of potential concern, however, and can be treated by administration of an opioid antagonist or doxapram.

Clinical Issues

Opioids are controlled substances, making their clinical use potentially problematic because of strict ordering, storage, and record-keeping requirements (see Definition of Controlled Substance Schedules: *www.deadiversion.usdoj.gov/ schedules*). These bureaucratic issues aside, opioids are the most effective therapy for pain from all causes and are critical components of multimodal therapeutic pain regimens. Opioids are less effective, however, in the treatment of pain caused by nerve injury and other forms of neuropathic pain (e.g., spinal cord compression). The routine clinical use of opioids for analgesia or as preanesthetic medication must be considered within the framework of the animal's medical problems, the severity of pain, and the potential for additive effects or synergism with anesthesia. Low doses of opioid agonist-antagonists (e.g., butorphanol), for example, can be additive with full opioid agonists (e.g., hydromorphone and oxymorphone). Opioid antagonist effects, however, are to be expected when larger or repeated doses of an opioid agonist-antagonist (e.g., butorphanol or pentazocine) or partial agonist (e.g., buprenorphine) are administered. Furthermore, not all opioid effects can be antagonized. The administration of the partial agonist buprenorphine, for example, after administration of an opioid agonist (e.g., meperidine or hydromorphone) may lead to increased respiratory depression in some animals. As noted, low doses of opioids may produce excitatory effects in some species, especially cats. It has been suggested that the administration of low doses of an opioid antagonist (naltrexone) before administration of a full opioid agonist (morphine, hydromorphone) may help to prevent opioid-related side effects, enhance opioid-related analgesia, and attenuate the development of tolerance associated with chronic opioid use. The clinical usefulness and relevance of this suggestion remains to be validated in clinical veterinary practice. Finally, diseases (liver, renal, CNS) and drugs (anesthetics) that prolong opioid metabolism and elimination may be responsible for prolonged drug effects, resulting in extended periods of depression and unconsciousness.

α_2-AGONISTS

See Chapter 10 for more information on α_2-agonists.

α_2-Agonists produce sedative, muscle relaxant, and analgesic effects in animals (Box 7-3). Mild to moderate analgesia can be produced, but are

BOX 7-3 α_2-Agonists

- Clonidine
- Detomidine
- Dexmedetomidine
- Medetomidine
- Romifidine
- Xylazine

associated with moderate to profound degrees of sedation. It is important to note that α_2-agonists act synergistically with opioids to produce analgesia. α_2-Agonists produce clinically relevant pharmacologic effects by activating a variety of α_2-receptor subtypes (e.g., α_{2A}, α_{2B}, α_{2C}, and α_{2D}) in the CNS and periphery. The discovery of a receptor-based mechanism has led to the identification and synthesis of α_2-receptor antagonists (e.g., yohimbine, tolazoline, and atipamezole). Based on differences in chemical structure, some α_2-agonists are capable of activating imidazoline receptors (I_1, I_2) and producing direct vascular effects (e.g., xylazine). The diversity in chemical structure coupled with α_2 receptor specificity, density, and location are responsible for considerable differences in drug dosages and the effects of α_2-agonists among and within species. α_2-Agonists are notorious for the frequency, scope, and severity of their cardiovascular-respiratory side effects, particularly the production of sinus bradycardia and bradyarrhythmias. α_2-Antagonists must be administered with caution to very young, aged, or debilitated animals and are contraindicated in most (not all) animals with cardiovascular disease.

Pharmacologic Considerations

More than with any other group of drugs that produce analgesia, the clinical use of α_2-agonists is dependent upon their dose-dependent CNS (sedative), cardiovascular, and respiratory effects. Consideration must be given to the potential for profound sedation, unexpected or startle-behavior, bradycardia, and respiratory depression. The potential for drug interactions (anticholinergic drugs and α_2-agonists) and amplification of cardiorespiratory depression is considerable.

Central Nervous System

α_2-Agonists activate presynaptic and postsynaptic α_2 receptors in the CNS, producing anxiolysis, sedation, and analgesia. Sedation in dogs and cats is attributed to activation of CNS α_{2A} receptors in areas of the brain that are responsible for awareness, arousal, and vigilance. Activation of α_1 and imidazoline receptors (regulate CNS norepinephrine release) may play some part in the pharmacology of most α_2-receptor agonists because most α_2 receptors activate both types of receptors. Large doses of relatively non-selective α_2-agonists (xylazine, romifidine) produce an initial period of reduced or poor sedation attributed to the activation of CNS α_1 receptors. Lower doses of α_2-agonists are capable of eliciting a release of "suppressed behavior" and increase the potential for a "startle response" to loud noises. Dogs or cats that appear sedated can become suddenly aroused and may attempt to bite if disturbed. Many dogs, cats, and especially horses seem to demonstrate increased sensitivity to sound and initial tactile contact. Microdoses (<1 $\mu g/kg$) of α_2-agonist produce minimal cardiorespiratory effects and can be administered to enhance the analgesic effects of opioids.

Activation of α_2 receptors in the brain and spinal cord decreases pain-related neurotransmitter release and interferes with sensory transmission. α_2-Agonists also act peripherally at α_2 receptors to produce analgesia, and some α_2-agonists (e.g., xylazine) are known to produce local anesthetic effects. Activation of presynaptic α_2 receptors inhibits the release of excitatory neuropeptides and substance P, centrally. Activation of postsynaptic α_2 receptors hyperpolarize neurons, thereby decreasing the activity of nociceptive neurons. α_2-Adrenergic and opioidergic systems have common effector mechanisms in the *locus ceruleus*, probably via a common transduction mechanism, representing a supraspinal site of action. In the spinal cord the analgesic action of α_2-agonists is likely related to activation of the descending medullospinal noradrenergic pathways or to the reduction of spinal sympathetic outflow at presynaptic ganglionic sites.

Activation of α_2 receptors within the CTZ is responsible for nausea and vomiting, common side effects of α_2-receptor drugs after administration to dogs and cats.

All α_2-agonists impair the control of body temperature through CNS-mediated dose-dependent effects on temperature thresholds for sweating, vasoconstriction, and shivering. These effects predispose dogs and cats to hypothermia both intraoperatively and postoperatively. α_2-Agonists help to prevent shivering. The administration of an α_2-agonist can cause intense peripheral vasoconstriction and an inability to dissipate heat and may trigger hyperthermia in some animals. Hyperthermia is more likely to occur in hot, humid environments.

Respiratory System

α_2-Agonists produce dose-dependent decreases in respiratory rate and volume that parallel the degree of CNS depression. Pronounced CNS depression is associated with an increase in the threshold to P_{CO_2} (i.e., higher P_{CO_2} required to stimulate breathing) resulting in significant respiratory acidosis and hypoxemia in older or sick animals. α_2-Agonists may also decrease Pa_{O_2} independent of increases in Pa_{CO_2} most likely due to a decrease in pulmonary blood flow and ventilation-perfusion abnormalities. Clinical doses generally produce mild respiratory depression and respiratory acidosis ($\uparrow$ P_{CO_2}).

α_2-Agonists cause considerable relaxation of upper airway muscles in the pharynx and larynx, which can result in irregular breathing patterns, inspiratory dyspnea, and upper airway obstruction, particularly in brachycephalic breeds or animals with upper airway disease (e.g., neoplasms, collapsing trachea).

Cardiovascular System

α_2-Agonists produce multiple and at times profound cardiovascular effects. Chief among their effects are decreases in heart rate (sinus bradycardia) and cardiac output. Sinus bradycardia and bradyarrhythmias are common occurrences after the administration of an α_2-agonist. First- and second-degree atrioventricular block occur commonly. Third-degree atrioventricular block and sinus arrest with ventricular escape beats are occasionally observed. Atrioventricular block and decreases in heart rate are caused by decreases in CNS sympathetic output and increases in vagally mediated parasympathetic tone, suggesting that the administration of an anticholinergic (e.g., atropine or glycopyrrolate) may be effective therapy. The coadministration of an anticholinergic to dogs or cats that have been administered an α_2-agonist predisposes them to the development of cardiac arrhythmias, including ventricular tachycardia and, rarely, ventricular fibrillation. Therefore anticholinergics and α_2-agonists should not be coadministered or administered to animals with preexisting ventricular arrhythmias, myocardial contusion, heart failure, or any other cause of ventricular electrical instability. Some α_2-agonists (e.g., xylazine) transiently sensitize the heart to catecholamine-induced arrhythmias.

Arterial blood pressure usually increases briefly (5 to 10 minutes) and then decreases from baseline values after the administration of an α_2-agonist. The early period of vasoconstriction and hypertension is initiated by stimulation of peripheral vascular α_1 and α_2 receptors and is responsible for increases in baroreceptor reflex activity and vagal tone and the development of bradyarrhythmias. The long-term decrease in arterial blood pressure parallels decreases in CNS sympathetic output and heart rate.

Cardiac output decreases almost immediately after the administration of an α_2-agonist, primarily because of a decrease in heart rate ($CO = HR \times$ Stroke volume, where CO is cardiac output and HR is heart rate). The short-term and long-term decrease in cardiac output has also been attributed to vasoconstriction (increased afterload) and decreases in central nervous system sympathetic output.

Other Organ Systems

Gastrointestinal System

Vomiting and retching are common consequences of α_2-agonist administration to dogs and cats. Lower doses (microdoses) and subcutaneous administration help decrease the occurrence of this side effect, which is mediated by

α_2-receptor effects in the CTZ in the CNS. α_2-Agonists produce immediate and pronounced decreases in gastrointestinal motility in dogs and cats that can last for several hours. Gastrointestinal stasis is caused by stimulation of α_2 receptors in the gut and increases in serum gastrin concentration. This effect is dose dependent but is believed to be responsible for postoperative ileus, gas accumulation, and potentially the development of bloat in dogs.

Endocrine System

α_2 Receptors modulate the release of insulin by the pancreas, causing a transient decrease in serum insulin concentration and an increase in serum glucose, resulting in glycosuria. This effect is mediated by α_2-receptor modulation of insulin secretion by beta cells in the pancreas.

Renal and Genitourinary Systems

α_2-Agonists promote diuresis due to their glucosuric effects and direct actions on the renal tubules to decrease renal tubular salt and water absorption. Labor can be delayed and prolonged as a result of sedative and muscle relaxant effects.

Clinical Issues

Microdoses (≤ 1 µg/kg) and infusions (≤ 1.0 µg/kg/hr) of α_2-agonists produce anxiolytic, mild-moderate sedative, and opioid- and anesthetic-sparing effects. α_2-Agonists are potentially useful as analgesics for minor medical or surgical procedures or as preanesthetic medication before general anesthesia. The administration of an anticholinergic for the treatment of bradycardia, although indicated, may precipitate ventricular arrhythmias. The best approach to the treatment of severe bradycardia with hypotension may be the administration of an α_2-antagonist (atipamezole). α_2-Agonists are excellent anxiolytics, however, and the administration of low doses (microdoses of ≤ 1 µg/kg) or infusions (0.2 to 1.0 µg/kg/hr) with opioids or NSAIDs as part of a multimodal treatment approach for procedural or postoperative pain can be very effective. α_2-Agonists may have considerable benefit as analgesics when administered into the epidural or subarachnoid space.

LOCAL ANESTHETICS

See Chapters 11 and 12 for more information on local anesthetics.

All local anesthetics block the initiation and conduction of electrical impulses (action potentials) in nerves (Box 7-4). Small-diameter, unmyelinated (Aδ, C) nerve fibers are blocked first in preference to large myelinated

BOX 7-4	Local Anesthetic Drugs

ESTER-LINKED DRUGS	AMIDE-LINKED DRUGS
• Benzocaine	• Articaine
• Chloroprocaine	• Bupivacaine
• Cocaine	• Etidocaine
• Procaine	• Lidocaine
• Proparacaine	• Mepivacaine
• Tetracaine	• Prilocaine
	• Ropivacaine

Mexiletine is an oral antiarrhythmic drug with lidocaine-like activity.

fibers $(A\beta)$, thereby producing a loss of sensation (analgesia) and varying degrees of paralysis (i.e., loss of motor function). More specifically, local anesthetics block sodium ion channels in neuronal cells and other tissues, thereby preventing an influx of sodium ions, membrane depolarization, and a decrease in propagated action potentials. The intensity of the local anesthetic drug effect is determined by local pH, temperature, and blood flow. Tissue acidosis reduces local anesthetic effect. Nonspecific membrane effects similar to those produced by inhalant anesthetics may be partially responsible for CNS-mediated analgesic activity. Analgesia is a direct result of sodium ion channel blockade and membrane stabilization. Local anesthetics are most frequently administered at specific sites (topical, local) or on nerves (regional) to produce analgesia but can also be infused perioperatively to reduce anesthetic and opioid requirements.

Pharmacologic Considerations

Although noted for their analgesic effects after topical, local, or regional administration, most local anesthetic drugs produce mild CNS depressant (anesthetic-sparing), antiarrhythmic, anti-inflammatory, antishock, and gastrointestinal promotility effects. Significant differences exist among local anesthetics regarding their metabolism, elimination, and potential for toxicity. Cats are much more susceptible to the neurotoxic side effects of local anesthetics than dogs.

Central Nervous System

Local anesthetics produce analgesia by suppressing or blocking electrical activity in sensory nerves. The preferential blockade of small unmyelinated nerves suggests that smaller doses should limit motor dysfunction, although some degree of motor impairment is usually observed at clinically relevant drug doses.

Low doses of local anesthetics produce negligible effects on the CNS, mild sedation, a generalized decrease in neuronal activity, and a centrally mediated decrease in sympathetic activity. Most local anesthetics potentiate the effects of injectable anesthetics (e.g., thiopental, propofol) and inhalant anesthetics (e.g., isoflurane, sevoflurane), resulting in a decrease in the amount of anesthetic required (anesthetic sparing) to produce unconsciousness and surgical anesthesia.

Large doses of local anesthetics are capable of producing CNS stimulation typified by nervousness, disorientation, nystagmus, nausea, excitement, agitation, and seizures. These effects are believed to be caused by the inhibition of inhibitory neurons within the CNS and, when severe, can result in respiratory paralysis and death.

Respiratory System

Clinically recommended doses of local anesthetics produce minimal if any significant effects on the respiratory system other than those associated with their CNS effects.

Solutions containing local anesthetic drugs have the potential to produce hypotension secondary to sympathetic blockade and resultant vasodilatation. The cranial migration of the local anesthetic to the C5-C6 nerve roots after epidural or spinal (subarachnoidal) administration can paralyze the diaphragm, resulting in hypoventilation and apnea.

Cardiovascular System

Therapeutic doses of lidocaine produce minimal cardiovascular effects in otherwise healthy dogs and cats. Heart rate may increase as a result of sympathetic suppression, vasodilatation, and mild decreases in arterial blood pressure.

A large dose or the rapid intravenous administration of a local anesthetic drug can decrease cardiac output, arterial blood pressure, and heart rate. The decrease in cardiac output is caused by decreases in CNS sympathetic output, myocardial contractile force, and venous return. These effects are dependent on dose and rate of drug administration and are more prominent in stressed or sick animals that depend on sympathetic tone for maintenance of homeostasis.

All local anesthetics produce antiarrhythmic effects but have the potential to produce sinus bradycardia, bradyarrhythmias, and hypotension when administered too rapidly by the intravenous route. Blockade of sodium channels throughout the heart decreases conduction of electrical impulses, leading to conduction disturbances and ventricular dysrhythmias due to a reentry. This effect is particularly notable when excessive doses of bupivacaine are administered. Local anesthetics should not be administered to dogs or cats with high-grade (two or more blocked P waves) second-degree or third-degree atrioventricular block because they can cause further depression of conduction and suppress ventricular escape beats, leading to cardiac arrest.

Other Organ Systems

Gastrointestinal System

High sympathetic tone can cause complete gut stasis and may be responsible for the development of ileus after surgery. Local anesthetics promote gastro-intestinal motility by suppressing sympathetic tone.

Hematopoietic System

Some local anesthetics (e.g., Cetacaine [benzocaine, butamben, and tetra-caine hydrochloride], benzocaine, and dibucaine) can produce methemoglo-binemia (ferric [Fe^{3+}]; reduced ability to release oxygen) and tissue hypoxia. This is particularly important in puppies and cats of all ages.

Clinical Issues

Currently available local anesthetic drugs lack selectivity (i.e., they block both sensory and motor nerves) and can produce motor paralysis. Local anes-thetics produce good to excellent analgesia when administered topically, locally, and for regional anesthesia, but at the expense of motor impairment, which can become problematic in some animals. The systemic infusion of lidocaine produces clinically relevant analgesia and anesthetic-sparing effects when administered as adjunctive therapy with inhalant (e.g., isoflurane, sevo-flurane) or injectable (e.g., ketamine, propofol) anesthetics, opioids, or α_2-agonists. Mexiletine ("oral lidocaine") has been administered as an alternative to injectable lidocaine for this purpose, although clinically relevant analgesic effects have not been validated in dogs or cats. Toxicity (CNS, cardiovascu-lar) is most likely to occur after accidental intra-arterial injection or overdose or when multiple bolus injections of smaller doses are administered over a short period (Box 7-5). Cats are more susceptible to the CNS side effects of local anesthetics than dogs, mandating a reduction in intravenous bolus administration (<0.5 mg/kg IV). Cimetidine and other drugs that impair liver metabolism can prolong the elimination of local anesthetics and increase the potential for toxicity.

ADJUNCT AND ADJUVANT ANALGESICS FOR THE TREATMENT OF PAIN

A growing number of chemicals representing widely diverse drug classes are being increasingly prescribed as adjunctive or adjuvant therapy for the treat-ment of acute and, more commonly, chronic (neuropathic, cancer, muscle, bone) pain (see Chapter 14) (Tables 7-4 and 7-5). The ultimate goal is to eliminate or suppress pain and thereby improve the animal's quality of life (see Chapter 6). Adjunct drugs are drugs that are administered to supple-ment the effects of the primary drug rather than as the primary drug.

BOX 7-5	Local Anesthetic Drug Toxicity

Central Nervous System
- Excitation
- Disorientation
- Shivering
- Licking, nausea, vomiting
- Convulsion
- Depression
- Hypoventilation
- Loss of consciousness
- Coma
- Respiratory depression or arrest

Cardiovascular System
- Tachycardia
- Hypotension
- Sinus bradycardia
- Arrhythmia
- Cardiac arrest

TABLE 7-4	Drugs Administered as Adjuvant or Adjunctive Therapy

DRUG CATEGORY	POSSIBLE SIDE EFFECTS
Corticosteroids	
Dexamethasone Prednisolone Prednisone	Tissue edema, immune suppression
Local Anesthetics	
Lidocaine Mexiletine	Central nervous system toxicity, cardiovascular depression
Tranquilizers and Muscle Relaxants	
Acepromazine Chlorpromazine Diazepam Midazolam	Central nervous system depression, hypotension
Anticonvulsants	
Carbamazepine Gabapentin Pregabalin Phenytoin	Disorientation, depression, somnambulance
Antidepressants	
Amitriptyline Clomipramine	Depression, disorientation, agitation, anticholinergic effects
Antianxiety Drugs	
Buspirone Duloxetine Fluoxetine Trazodone	Seizures, somnolence, vomiting, serotonin syndrome

Continued

TABLE 7-4	Drugs Administered as Adjuvant or Adjunctive Therapy—cont'd
DRUG CATEGORY	**POSSIBLE SIDE EFFECTS**
Bisphosphonates	
Alendronate	
Pamidronate	
Tiludronate	
Zoledronate	
Cannabinoid	
Dronabinol	Depression, disorientation
Calcium Channel Blocker	
Diltiazem	
Ziconotide (N-type)	
Sympatholytics	
Atenolol	Bradycardia, hypotension
Prazosin	
Propranolol	
Miscellaneous Drugs	
Amantadine	Depression, disorientation, agitation, seizures
Baclofen	
Capsaicin*	
Clonidine	
Codeine	
Dextromethorphan	
Dezocine	
Ketamine	
Magnesium salts ($Mg^{2-}SO_4^{2-}$)	
Tapentadol	
Tramadol	

*Topical.

Adjuvant drugs modify the effect of the primary drug and may have an indication other than pain. Corticosteroids, anticonvulsants, antidepressants, antiviral medications (NMDA receptor antagonists), immunosuppressants, anticancer agents, bisphosphonates, herbal remedies, and a variety of nutritional supplements are all capable of modifying the pain experience. Many of these drugs produce analgesia by multiple mechanisms. Some produce NMDA receptor blocking activity (amantadine, dextromethorphan, methadone) and are administered in conjunction with NSAIDs and opioids to control chronic pain. Tramadol and tapentadol act at opioid receptors, inhibit the reuptake of serotonin and norepinephrine, and are administered alone or as adjunct therapy with NSAIDs to control chronic pain. Tapentadol

TABLE 7-5	Adjuvant and Analgesic Drug Dosages	
DRUG	**DOSAGE IN DOGS**	**DOSAGE IN CATS**
Corticosteroids		
Dexamethasone	0.10-0.15 mg/kg SC, PO	0.10-0.15 mg/kg SC, PO
Prednisolone	1.0-2.2 mg/kg PO	1-2 mg/kg PO
Prednisone	1.0-2.2 mg/kg PO	1-2 mg/kg PO
Local Anesthetics		
Lidocaine	2-4 mg/kg IV bolus and then 25-75 µg/kg IV infusion	0.25-1.0 mg/kg IV bolus and then 10-40 µg/kg IV infusion
Mexiletine	4-10 mg/kg PO	—
Tranquilizers and Muscle Relaxants		
Acepromazine	0.025-1.13 mg/kg IV, SC, IM	0.05-2.25 mg/kg IM, SC, IV, PO
Chlorpromazine	0.05-0.50 mg/kg SC, IM; 0.8-4.4 mg/kg PO	0.5 mg/kg IM, IV; 2-4 mg/kg PO
Diazepam	0.1-0.5 mg/kg IV; 0.5-2.2 mg/kg PO	0.1-0.5 mg/kg IV; 0.5-2.2 mg/kg PO
Midazolam	0.066-0.22 mg/kg IV, IM	0.066-0.22 mg/kg IV, IM
Anticonvulsants		
Carbamazepine	Not recommended	—
Gabapentin*	1-5 mg/kg PO, initial dose	—
Pregabalin*	1-5 mg/kg PO, initial dose	
Phenytoin	20-35 mg/kg PO	2-3 mg/kg PO
Antidepressants		
Amitriptyline	1-2 mg/kg PO	1-2 mg/kg PO
Clomipramine	1-3 mg/kg PO	1-5 mg/kg PO
Antianxiety Drugs		
Fluoxetine	0.5-2.0 mg/kg PO?	—
Duloxetine	1.0 mg/kg PO?	—
Buspirone	1.0 mg/kg PO?	—
Trazodone	2 mg/kg PO?	—
Bisphosphonates		
Alendronate	1 mg/kg PO	—
Tiludronate	2 mg/kg SC, four treatments	
Calcium Channel Blocker		
Diltiazem	0.5-1.5 mg/kg PO	1.75-2.5 mg/kg PO
Ziconotide?		
Sympatholytics		
Atenolol	0.25-1.0 mg/kg PO	1-2 mg/kg
Prazosin	1 mg/15 kg PO	—
Propranolol	0.125-1.10 mg/kg PO	0.4-1.2 mg/kg PO

Continued

TABLE 7-5	Adjuvant and Analgesic Drug Dosages—cont'd	
DRUG	**DOSAGE IN DOGS**	**DOSAGE IN CATS**
Miscellaneous Drugs		
Amantadine	2-5 mg/kg PO	3-5 mg/kg PO
Baclofen	1 mg/kg PO?	—
Clonidine	10 μg/kg IV	10 μg/kg IV
Codeine	1-2 mg/kg PO	—
Dextromethorphan	0.5-2 mg/kg PO, SC, IV	—
Ketamine	0.5 mg/kg SC 20 μg/kg/min IV	0.5 mg/kg SC 5-10 μg/kg/min IV
Magnesium salts ($Mg^{2-}SO_4^{2-}$)	0.3-0.5 mg/kg/day IV	0.3-0.5 mg/kg/day mg/kg IV
Tramadol	2-5 mg/kg PO, bid-tid	1-3 mg/kg PO, sid-bid
Tapentadol	1-2 mg/kg PO, bid	—

Key: ?, Dose not substantiated (to effect).
*Titrated to effect.

(see Chapter 14) is a centrally acting analgesic having both μ-opioid receptor agonist and norepinephrine reuptake inhibition activity with minimal serotonin reuptake inhibition. This dual mode of action may make tapentadol, like tramadol, useful as an adjunct for the treatment of chronic and neuropathic pain. The gabapentanoids (gabapentin, pregabalin), originally developed for the treatment of epilepsy, have become popular for the treatment of neuropathic pain. Recent evidence, however, suggests that they are also effective as adjunctive therapy for the treatment of inflammatory pain caused by accidental and surgical trauma. Gabapentin and pregabalin bind to the α_2-δ subunit of voltage-gated P/Q-type calcium channels, thereby inhibiting calcium influx and the consequent release of pain producing neurotransmitters. Gabapentin and pregabalin exert an analgesic effect by activating descending inhibitory noradrenergic pathways that regulate neurotransmission of pain signals in the dorsal horn of the spinal cord. The mechanism of action of gabapentin and pregabalin has also been linked to modulation of AMPA, NMDA receptors, and ATP-sensitive potassium channels, although conclusive evidence for their analgesic effects at these targets has been contradictory.

Capsaicin is an odorless fat-soluble naturally occurring alkaloid derived from chili peppers and responsible for their hot taste. It is rapidly absorbed through the skin and activates transient receptor potential variant 1 (TRPV1) receptors in sensory nerves, causing a hot or burning sensation. Subsequently, analgesia results from the local depletion of substance P, leading to a desensitization of small sensory nerves. Sensory nerves become insensitive to noxious heat and chemical stimuli and lose their ability to release mediators involved in neurotransmission and inflammation. Topically applied capsaicin is administered to alleviate pain associated with neuropathic and chronic musculoskeletal pain and to treat pruritus. Capsaicin has also been infused into the bladder to reduce incontinence in animals with bladder hyperactivity. Drugs administered to produce anxiolysis and muscle relaxation (e.g., acepromazine, diazepam) induce adjunctive analgesic effects when combined with inhalant (e.g., isoflurane, sevoflurane) or injectable (e.g., ketamine, propofol) anesthetics, opioids, or α_2-agonists. The potential to produce significant drug interactions, side effects (lethargy, muscle weakness, somnolence), and toxicity must always be considered. The co-administration of acepromazine and opioids, for example, may improve over-all analgesic efficacy but also increases the potential for lethargy, muscle weakness, and respiratory depression. To date, there are no controlled clinical trials demonstrating the efficacy or safety for most if not all of the drugs considered to be useful for producing adjuvant analgesia.

An increasing number of drugs developed as anticonvulsants, antidepressants, or behavior modifiers have demonstrated efficacy either alone or as adjuncts for the treatment of chronic and neuropathic pain. These drugs encompass a diverse group of chemicals that include but are not limited to tricyclic antidepressants, selective and nonselective amine (serotonin [5-HT]; norepinephrine) reuptake inhibitors, and antiepileptics. The precise mechanism(s) responsible for their analgesic effects likely involve multiple modalities (Table 7-6). Serotonin and norepinephrine are both involved in the regulation of nociception at different levels of the nervous system, particularly in their regulation of descending inhibitory pathways. Central inhibitory pathways are compromised (disinhibition) in chronic and neuropathic

TABLE 7-6	Proposed Analgesic Mechanisms of Antidepressant and Antiepileptic Drugs				
MECHANISM OF ACTION	**SITE OF ACTION**	**TCAs**	**SNRIs**	**SRIs**	**AEs**
Reuptake inhibition of	Serotonin	+	+	+	—
monoamine	Noradrenaline	+	+	—	—
Receptor antagonism	α_2-Agonist	+	—	—	—
	NMDA	+	(+)	—	—
Blocker or activator of ion	Na^+ channel blocker	+	(+)	(?)	+
channels	Ca^{2+} channel blocker (α_2-δ ligands)	+	?	(+)	+
	K^+ channel activator	+	?	—	?
GABA$_B$ receptor	γ-receptor function	+	?	+	+
Opioid receptor binding and mediating effect	μ and δ opioid	(+)	(+)	(+)	—
Inflammation	PGE$_2$ production TNF production	+	?	+	—

Key: +, Positive effect; (+), questionable effect; ?, uncertain; —, no effect; *AEs,* Antiepileptics (e.g., gabapentin); *GABA,* γ-aminobutyric acid; NMDA, *N*-methyl-D-aspartate; PGE$_2$, prostaglandin E$_2$; *SNRIs,* serotonin-norepinephrine reuptake inhibitors (e.g., duloxetine); *SRIs,* serotonin reuptake inhibitors (e.g., fluoxetine); *TCAs,* tricyclic antidepressants (e.g., amitriptyline); *TNF,* tumor necrosis factor.

pain conditions (neuroplasticity), leading to an exaggerated response to nociceptive input (see Chapter 2). Their efficacy for the treatment of chronic and
neuropathic pain in animals with naturally occurring disease is rational based
on experimental evidence but speculative based on the absence of prospective,
randomized, blinded, and controlled clinical trials.

SEROTONIN SYNDROME

The CNS production of serotonin modifies behavior, attention, cardiorespiratory function, pain perception, aggression, motor function, temperature
regulation, sleep, appetite, and sexual activity. Excessive amounts of serotonin in the CNS can result in the development of "serotonin syndrome" and
may develop when two or more drugs and/or supplements that are capable of
increasing CNS serotonin concentrations are administered together. Serotonin syndrome usually occurs early during treatment but may develop at any

---

BOX 7-6   Drugs Associated With Serotonin Syndrome

Medications That Increase Presynaptic Release of Serotonin
- Amphetamine
- Methylphenidate
- 3,4-Methylenedioxymethamphetamine (MDMA, ecstasy)

Medications That Inhibit the Reuptake of Serotonin into the Presynaptic Neuron
- Amitriptyline
- Bupropion
- Chlorpheniramine
- Clomipramine (Clomicalm)
- Duloxetine
- Fluoxetine (Reconcile)
- Paroxetine
- Sertraline
- Trazodone
- Venlafaxine
- Fentanyl
- Demerol
- Tramadol
- Tapentadol

Medications That Inhibit the Metabolism of Serotonin
- Amitraz (Mitaban, Preventic collar)
- Linezolid
- Selegiline (Anipryl)

Medications That Act as Serotonin Agonists at the Postsynaptic Membrane
- Buspirone
- Lithium
- Lysergic acid diethylamide (LSD)

time during drug therapy. Excessive amounts of serotonin in the CNS can produce diarrhea, mydriasis, tachycardia, tachypnea, hypertension, and fever. Some animals develop hyperreflexia, myoclonus, and tremors. Disorientation, agitation, and seizures may occur. Serotonin syndrome can be facilitated by foods that increase the synthesis of serotonin (L-tryptophan, cheese) and by medications that promote serotonin synthesis, increase the presynaptic release of serotonin, or inhibit the reuptake of serotonin by presynaptic neurons. Some medications inhibit the metabolism of serotonin and facilitate the action of serotonin at the presynaptic neuron. The most common drug combinations that cause serotonin syndrome are monoamine oxidase inhibitors (MAOIs: selegiline [Anipryl]) and serotonin selective reuptake inhibitors (SSRIs), MAOIs and tricyclic antidepressants, MAOIs and tryptophan, and MAOIs and tramadol (Box 7-6).

SUGGESTED READING

Al-Hasani R, Bruchas MR. Molecular mechanisms of opioid receptor-dependent signaling and behavior. Anesthesiology. 2011; 115:1363–1381.

Angst MS, Clark JD. Opioid-induced hyperalgesia. Anesthesiology. 2006; 104:570–587.

Argoff C. Mechanisms of pain transmission and pharmacologic management. Curr Med Res Opin. 2011; 27:2019–2031.

Autefage A, Palissier FM, Asimus E, et al. Long-term efficacy and safety of firocoxib in the treatment of dogs with osteoarthritis. Vet Rec. 2011; 168:617–622.

Bennett WM, Henrich WL, Stoff JS. The renal effects on nonsteroidal anti-inflammatory drugs: Summary and recommendations. Am J Kidney Dis. 1996; 28(S1):S56–S62.

Benyamin R, Trescot AM, Datta S, et al. Opioid complications and side effects. Pain Physician. 2008; 11:S105–S120.

Buvanendran A, Kroin JS. Useful adjuvants for postoperative pain management. Best Pract Res Clin Anaesthesiol. 2007; 21:31–49.

Carroll GL, Simonson SM. Recent developments in nonsteroidal anti-inflammatory drugs in cats. J Am Anim Hosp Assoc. 2005; 41:347–354.

Cashmore RG, Harcourt-Brown TR, Freeman PM, Granger N. Clinical diagnosis and treatment of suspected neuropathic pain in three dogs. Australian Vet J. 2009; 87:45–50.

Costa L, Major PP. Effect of bisphosphonates on pain and quality of life in patients with bone metastases. Nature Clin Prac Oncol. 2009; 6:163–174.

Dahl JB, Moiniche S. Pre-emptive analgesia. Br Med Bull. 2004; 71:13–27.

Ejaz P, Bhojani K, Joshi VR. NSAIDs and kidney. J Assoc Phys India. 2004; 52:632–640.

Gilron I, Flatters SL. Gabapentin and pregabalin for the treatment of neuropathic pain: A review of laboratory and clinical evidence. Pain Res Manag. 2006; 11(Suppl A):16A–29A.

Giovannoni MP, Ghelardini C, Vergelli C, et al. α-Agonists as analgesic agents. Med Res Rev 2009; 29:339–368.

Hamza M, Dionne RA. Mechanisms of non-opioid analgesics beyond cyclooxygenase enzyme inhibition. Curr Mol Pharmacol. 2009; 2:1–14.

Hartrick CT, Hernandez JRR. Tapentadol for pain: A treatment evaluation. Ex Opin Pharmacother. 2012; 13:283–286.

Hayman M, Kam PCA. Capsaicin: A review of its pharmacology and clinical applications. Curr Anaesth Crit Care. 2008; 19:338–343.

Hoskin PJ, Hanks GW. Opioid agonist-antagonist drugs in acute and chronic pain states. Drugs. 1991; 41:326–344.

Innes JF, Clayton J, Lascelles BDX. Review of the safety and efficacy of long-term NSAID use in the treatment of canine osteoarthritis. Vet Rec. 2010; 166:226–230.

Kaufman E, Epstien JB, Gorsky M, et al. Preemptive analgesia and local anesthesia as a supplement to general anesthesia. A review. Anesth Prog. 2005; 52:29–38.

Ko JC, Raffe MR, Knesl O, et al. Analgesia, sedation and anesthesia: Making the switch from medetomidine to dexmedetomidine. Compendium Cont Ed Vet. 2009; 31 (Suppl 1A):1–16.

Koppert W. The impact of opioid-induced hyperalgesia for postoperative pain. Best Pract Res Clin Anaesth. 2007; 21:65–83.

KuKanich B, Bidgood T, Knesl O. Clinical pharmacology of nonsteroidal anti-inflammatory drugs in dogs. Vet Anaesth Analg. 2012; 39:69–90.

Kurz A, Ikeda T, Sessler DI, et al. Meperidine decreases the shivering threshold twice as much as the vasoconstriction threshold. Anesthesiology. 1997; 86:1046–1054.

Lascelles BDX, Court MH, Hardie EM. Nonsteroidal anti-inflammatory drugs in cats: A review. Vet Anaesth Analg. 2007; 34:228–250.

Lee M, Silverman S, Hansen H, et al. A comprehensive review of opioid-induced hyperalgesia. Pain Physician. 2011; 14:145–161.

Lemke KA. Perioperative use of selective alpha-2 agonists and antagonists in small animals. Can Vet J. 2004; 456:475–480.

Lesnial A, Lipkowski AW. Opioid peptides in peripheral pain control. Acta Neurobiol Exp. 2001; 71:129–138.

Lussier D, Huskey AG, Portenoy RJ. Adjuvant analgesics in cancer pain management. The Oncologist. 2004; 9:571–591.

Maizles M, McCarberg B. Antidepressants and antiepileptic drugs for chronic non-cancer pain. Am Fam Physician. 2005; 71:483–490.

Manzanares J, Julian MD, Carroscosa A. Role of the cannabinoid system in pain control and therapeutic implications for the management of acute and chronic pain episodes. Curr Neuropharmacol. 2006; 4:239–257.

Martel-Pelletier J, Lajeunesse D, Reboul P, et al. Therapeutic role of dual inhibitors of 5-LOX and COX, selective and non-selective nonsteroidal anti-inflammatory drugs. Ann Rheum Dis. 2003; 62:501–509.

McEwen BS, Kalia M. The role of corticosteroids and stress in chronic pain conditions. Metabol Clin Exp. 2010; 59(S1):S9–S15.

McLure HA, Rubin AP. Review of local anaesthetic agents. Minerva Anesthesiol. 2005; 71:59–74.

Mico JA, Ardid D, Berrocoso E, et al. Antidepressants and pain. Trend Pharmacol Sci. 2006; 27:348–354.

Mohammad-Zadeh LF, Moses L, Gwaltney-Brant SM. Serotonin: A review. J vet Pharmacol Ther. 2008; 31:187–199.

Moreau M, Rialland P, Pelletier JP, et al. Tiludronate treatment improves structural changes and symptoms of osteoarthritic in the canine anterior cruciate ligament model. Arthritis Res Ther. 2011; 13:1–13.

Muir WW. Pain. In: WW Muir, JAE Hubbell, R Bednarski et al. (Eds.) Handbook of veterinary anesthesia, ed 5, St Louis, 2013, Mosby.

Nimmrich V, Gross G. P/Q-type calcium channel modulators. Br J Pharm. 2012; 167:741–759.

O'Connor N, Dargan PI, Jones AL. Hepatocellular damage from nonsteroidal anti-inflammatory drugs. Q J Med. 2003; 96:787–791.

Paronis CA, Bergman J. Buprenorphine and opioid antagonism, tolerance and naltrexone-precipitated withdrawal. J Pharmacol Exp Ther. 2011; 336:488–495.

Posner LP, Pavuk AA, Rokshar JL, et al. Effects of opioids and anesthetic drugs on body temperature in cats. Vet Anaesth Analg. 2010; 37:35–43.

Power I. An update on analgesics. Br J Anaesth. 2011; 107:19–24.

Ren K, Dubner R. Interactions between the immune and nervous systems in pain. Nature Med. 2010; 16:1267–1276.

Renyu L, Huang Z-P, Yeliseev A, et al. Novel molecular targets of dezocine and their clinical implications. Anesthesiology. 2014; 120:714–723.

Salerno A, Hermann R. Efficacy and safety of steroid use for postoperative pain relief. J Bone Joint Surg. 2006; 88:1361–1372.

Schafer AI. Effects of nonsteroidal anti-inflammatory drugs on platelet function and systemic hemostasis. J Clin Pharmacol. 1995; 35:209–219.

Schmidt PC, Ruchelli G, Mackey SC, Carroll IR. Perioperative gabapentinoids. Anesthesiology. 2013; 119:1215–1221.

Simpson BS, Papich MG. Pharmacologic management in veterinary behavioral medicine. Vet Clin Small Anim. 2003; 33:365–404.

Sinclair MD. A review of the physiological effects of α_2-agonists related to the clinical use of medetomidine in small animal practice. Can Vet J. 2003; 44:885–897.

Sindrup SH, Jensen TS. Efficacy of pharmacological treatments of neuropathic pain: An update and effect related to mechanism of drug action. Pain. 1999; 83:389–400.

Thomas DE, Lee JA, Hovda LR. Retrospective evaluation of toxicosis from selective serotonin reuptake inhibitor antidepressants. J Vet Emerg Crit Care. 2012; 22:674–681.

Trescot AM, Datta S, Lee M, et al. Opioid pharmacology. Pain Physician. 2008; 11: S133–S153.

Ungpraser P, Kittanamongkolehai W, Price C, et al. What is the "safest" nonsteroidal anti-inflammatory drugs. Am Med J. 2012; 3:115–123.

Vallejo R, Barkin RL, Wang VC. Pharmacology of opioids in the treatment of chronic pain syndromes. Pain Physician. 2011; 11:E343–E360.

Verdu B, Decosterd I, Buclin T, et al. Antidepressants for the treatment of chronic pain. Drugs. 2008; 68:2611–2632.

Wieseler-Frank J, Maier SF, Watkins LR. Central proinflammatory cytokines and pain enhancement. Neurosignals. 2005; 14:166–174.

Young A, Buvanendran A. Recent advances in multimodal analgesia. Anesthesiology Clin. 2012; 30:91–100.

CHAPTER 8

Nonsteroidal Anti-inflammatory Drugs

Steven C. Budsberg

Nonsteroidal anti-inflammatory drugs (NSAIDs) share therapeutic actions including analgesia and anti-inflammatory and antipyretic capabilities despite differences in chemical structure. Although chemically related, these compounds vary widely in their structure, and their classification based on chemical structure still engenders some controversy. NSAIDs have a unifying action biochemically in the inhibition of the cyclooxygenase (COX) enzymes. Historically, NSAIDs are one of the most commonly used classes of drugs in humans. The same statement is now made about NSAIDs in small animal clinical practice. There are several reasons for the dramatic increase in NSAID use in companion animals. There is now a better understanding of the need to manage acute and chronic pain in small animal medicine. Pain control is a very important mission for the practicing veterinarian. NSAIDs provide an effective means to accomplish this goal. Furthermore, there is now the availability of NSAIDs with improved safety and efficacy targeted for small animals (primarily dogs). For the most part, currently prescribed NSAIDs are very safe drugs, with only a small percentage of animals experiencing serious complications. However, these problems have achieved significant proportions based on the fact that so many animals are taking these agents each year—thus a small percentage becomes a very large number. Because these drugs are remarkably effective yet carry a significant risk potential, one must closely evaluate and monitor their use in each animal.

MECHANISM OF ACTION

Prostaglandin Inhibition

The mechanism of actions of NSAIDs is a continually evolving story that started in the early 1970s with the publication of two manuscripts that examined the ability of aspirin to inhibit prostaglandin production. Eicosanoids, which include the compounds known as prostaglandins, are derived from arachidonic acid (AA). It is the ability of NSAIDs to interfere with eicosanoid synthesis and the subsequent alteration of different physiologic systems that explains the numerous effects seen in the body with NSAID administration. Significant portions of the analgesic and anti-inflammatory clinical effects seen with NSAID administration are related to the inhibition of the COX enzyme isoforms.

The last 20 years have seen the discovery, identification, and considerable elucidation of a group of COX enzymes. Two isoforms, COX-1 and COX-2, are well established, with the presence of a third isoform, COX-3 (which is an alternative splice variant of COX-1) identified but with unclear activity and physiologic effects. Discovery of the first two isoforms generated a hypothesis that their functions were mutually exclusive, with COX-1 involved with normal physiologic functions of various systems and COX-2 involved in pathologic processes. Current data about these enzymes has shown that this initial paradigm was an oversimplification. COX-1 is now primarily considered the constitutive isoform of COX and is responsible for basal prostaglandin production for homeostasis in many tissues. It exists in many tissues of the body including the stomach, kidney, platelets, and reproductive tract, where it catalyzes the synthesis of prostaglandins involved in the daily "housekeeping" functions. COX-1 is expressed at sites of inflammation, but this is likely a function of basal rather than induced expression. COX-2 is usually thought of as the induced isoform and is found in sites of inflammation, yet it is expressed constitutively in several tissues including the brain, kidney, reproductive system, and eye. Cells that express COX-2 include endothelial cells, smooth muscle cells, chondrocytes, fibroblasts, monocytes, macrophages, and synovial cells. Various cytokines and growth factors rapidly induce the expression of COX-2.

The COX enzymes initiate a complex cascade that results in the conversion of polyunsaturated acids to prostaglandins and thromboxane (Figure 8-1). Briefly, AA is transformed into prostaglandin G_2 (PGG_2) and then PGH_2 by COX. Further enzymatic conversion of PGH_2 leads to the functionally important prostaglandins (types D, E, F, and I) and thromboxane. With regard to pain, prostaglandins, primarily PGE_2, contribute to the inflammatory response by causing vasodilation and enhancing the effects of other cytokines and inflammatory mediators. The production of PGE_2 at various sites of inflammation appears to be mediated primarily by COX-2. Thus, when an inflammatory event occurs within the tissue, COX-2 enzyme production is induced, followed by an increase in prostaglandin concentrations. The selective inhibition of certain prostaglandins primarily produced by COX-2 should allow for the therapeutic analgesic and anti-inflammatory effects while greatly diminishing the unwanted side effects caused by COX-1 inhibition. However, complete COX-2 inhibition is detrimental to many normal physiologic functions including the healing of gastric ulcers. Therefore it is important to accurately assess COX-2 selectivity, and current methods to make such assessments are not clear-cut. COX selectivity is a measure of the relative concentrations of a drug required to inhibit

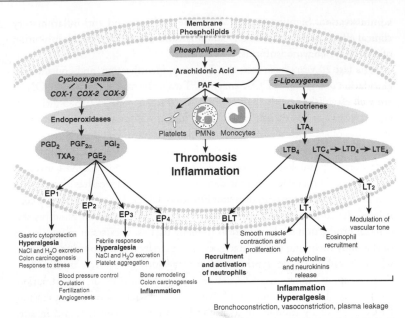

FIGURE 8-1   The breakdown of membrane phospholipids and arachidonic acid cascade as influenced by cyclooxygenase and lipoxygenase leads to the production of prostaglandins and leukotrienes, which activate membrane receptors to produce myriad effects including pain and inflammation. See text for details.

each COX isoenzyme and usually is determined by in vitro studies. Current ex vivo and limited in vivo data have confirmed COX-2 selectivity or COX-1 sparing effects of certain compounds. In addition, recent studies have provided a model to show the physiologic effects of COX selectivity in target tissues in dogs with osteoarthritis (OA). It is interesting to note that comparison of prostaglandin production in the stomach and duodenum has shown much lower concentrations in the duodenum. A dual COX and 5-lipoxygenase (5-LOX) inhibitor (tepoxalin) has been available on the veterinary market (currently not available). This drug blocks both the COX and the 5-LOX metabolic pathways (see Figure 8-1). Although this drug is a nonspecific inhibitor of the COX enzymes, it appears to have the same gastrointestinal (GI) toxicity as the COX-1 selective agents and less than the nonselective COX inhibitors. The exact mechanism of why this dual inhibition limits the GI toxicity is not well described.

Site of Action

Data now support the concept that NSAIDs act on both the peripheral tissue injury site as well as at the level of the central nervous system (CNS). They inhibit the peripheral COX-2 enzyme to block the formation of

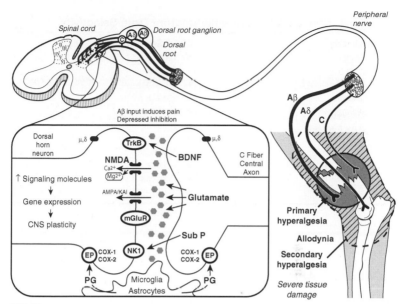

FIGURE 8-2 The release of prostaglandins *(PGs)* from activated microglia and astrocytes within the central nervous system *(CNS)* and spinal cord results in the exaggerated release of substance P and other excitatory amino acids from presynaptic terminals, promoting the development of central sensitization, pain facilitation, and hyperalgesia.

prostaglandins such as PGE_2 and PGI_2, which function to dilate arterioles and sensitize peripheral nociceptors to the actions of mediators (e.g., histamine and bradykinin), which produce localized pain and hypersensitivity. PGE_2 produced by COX-2 plays a pivotal role in sustaining acute pain sensation by increasing nociceptor cyclic AMP, which decreases the nociceptor threshold of activation. Centrally, COX-2-mediated prostaglandins such as PGE_2 are involved in spinal nociception and central sensitization (Figure 8-2). COX-2 is expressed in the brain and spinal cord and is upregulated in response to traumatic injury and peripheral inflammation. COX-2–activated PGE_2 lowers the threshold for neuronal depolarization, increasing the number of action potentials and repetitive spiking. The actions of COX-2 are thought to contribute to neuronal plasticity and central sensitization. These insights do provide information into the potential value of developing centrally acting agents that alter receptor-mediated actions of prostanoids or enzyme inhibitors that can target specific sites in the prostaglandin cascade. However, these data should not lead directly to the conclusion that spinally delivered NSAIDs will be more effective than systemic delivery (Box 8-1).

BOX 8-1	Nonsteroidal Anti-inflammatory Drug Selectivity

Nonselective
- Aspirin
- Etodolac?
- Ketoprofen
- Ketorolac
- Naproxen

COX-LOX Inhibitor
- Tepoxalin

COX-2 Selective (COX-1 Sparing)
- Carprofen
- Cimicoxib
- Deracoxib
- Etodolac?
- Firocoxib
- Flunixin meglumine
- Mavacoxib
- Meloxicam
- Robenacoxib
- Piroxicam
- Tolfenamic acid

CLINICAL APPLICATIONS

Indications

NSAIDs can be used to relieve pain in a variety of clinical settings. Efficacy of NSAIDs is comparable to that of opioids in many instances of musculoskeletal and visceral pain. However, for major pain such as fractures, data are not available to substantiate this claim. NSAIDs can be used for cases of acute pain, either traumatic or surgically induced, and for chronic pain such as OA. Efficacy and toxicity are often individualized, and individual monitoring is mandatory. There are numerous initiating pathways that produce pain that are not fully understood, and it would be naïve to think that all pathways will react in the same manner to different drugs. In addition, the heterogeneity of the animal's response to a given NSAID in terms of efficacy and toxicity may be accounted for by slight variations in genetic expression or gene polymorphism of the COX enzymes known as the "COX continuum." It must also be remembered that in humans, NSAID therapy has a modest effect (20% to 30%) in pain reduction, and thus to optimize treatment programs, nonpharmacologic modalities are needed and have been emphasized (see Chapters 17, 18, 19).

Choosing and Monitoring the Use of Nonsteroidal Anti-inflammatory Drugs

- Use products with history of clinical experience and good safety profiles.
- Use only one NSAID at a time, and ensure adequate dosage.
- Adapt therapy to suit individual requirements. Begin with the recommended dose for an extended period of time (at least 10 to 14 days) in animals with chronic pain, and if this is efficacious, attempt to reduce

the administered dose at regular intervals (e.g., weekly) until the lowest dose providing the maximum benefit has been achieved.
- Review therapy frequently, and change to alternative NSAIDs if there is a poor response to therapy.
- Avoid NSAIDs in animals with known contraindications to their use.
- Observe for potential toxicity. Increased vigilance and monitoring are required for at-risk individuals. If indicated, establish renal and hepatic status of the animal before NSAID administration.

Contraindications

The following recommendations are general guidelines, and the type of NSAID (e.g., COX-1 sparing [COX-2 specific]) may alter these recommendations as more data become available.

Contraindications to NSAID use are as follows:
- Animals receiving any type of systemic corticosteroids.
- Animals receiving concurrent NSAIDs.
- Animals with documented renal or hepatic insufficiency or dysfunction.
- Animals with any clinical syndrome that creates a decrease in the circulating blood volume (e.g., shock, dehydration, hypotension, or ascites).
- Animals with active GI disease.
- Animals that have experienced trauma with known or suspected significant active hemorrhage or blood loss.
- Pregnant animals or in females in which pregnancy is being attempted.
- Animals with significant pulmonary disease. (This may be less important with COX-2–specific drugs.)
- Animals with any type of confirmed or suspected coagulopathies. (This may be less important with COX-2–specific drugs.)

Specific Compounds

Approved Compounds

The approved NSAIDs available to the clinician vary considerably around the world. It is very important for practitioners to remember that the clinical response to a particular drug is quite individualized. Dogs may respond favorably to one product and not another, so if an NSAID is indicated in a case and the first product used does not achieve a positive clinical response, do not forsake NSAIDs, but try a different product (Table 8-1).

Carprofen. Carprofen is a member of the arylpropionic acid class of NSAIDs. Carprofen has been shown to be COX-1 sparing (COX-2 selective) both in vitro and in vivo. Carprofen is approved, both in oral and injectable formulations, to treat pain and inflammation associated with OA and postoperative pain in dogs. Carprofen has been shown to improve limb function in clinical trials of dogs with naturally occurring OA. Three long-term

TABLE 8-1	Doses of Nonsteroidal Anti-inflammatory Drugs (NSAIDs) in Dogs and Cats		
DRUG	**DOSAGE IN DOGS**	**DOSAGE IN CATS**	**COMMENTS**
Nonselective			
Aspirin	10-25 mg/kg q8-12h PO with food	5-20 mg/kg, q48-72h, PO with food	Not for chronic use or osteoarthritis Cats: antithrombotic
Etodolac	10-15 mg/kg q24h PO		
Ketoprofen	NR	2 mg/kg, once PO or SC, then 1 mg/kg q24h for 3-5 days	
Selective			
Carprofen	2.2 mg/kg q12h or 4.4 mg/kg q24h PO Perioperative: 4.4 mg/kg once SC	Perioperative: 4 mg/kg once SC	Not for chronic use in cats
Cimicoxib	2 mg/kg q24h PO	Not established	
Deracoxib	1-2 mg/kg q24h PO	Not established	
Firocoxib	5 mg/kg q24h PO	Not established	
Mavacoxib	2 mg/kg on days 1, 14, and 30, then once a month	Not established	Do exceed 6 months of continuous administration
Meloxicam	0.2 mg/kg day 1 SC or PO followed by 0.1 mg/kg q24h PO	Perioperative: 0.1-0.3 mg/kg SC once 0.05 mg/kg PO q24h	
Piroxicam	0.3 mg/kg q24-48h PO	Not established, although 0.3 mg/kg q24h is used	
Robenacoxib	1 mg/kg q24h PO Perioperative: 2 mg/kg SC once	1 mg/kg q24h PO Perioperative: 2 mg/kg SC once	Cats: 3-11 days of administration
Tolfenamic acid	4 mg/kg q24h PO or SC for 3-5 days	4 mg/kg q24h PO or SC for 3-5 days	
COX-LOX Inhibitor			
Tepoxalin	10 mg/kg q24h PO	Not established	

studies (84 days and 120 days) found that carprofen was well tolerated, and subjectively dogs appeared to improve over the treatment period. Carprofen is also effective in providing postoperative analgesia in both orthopedic and soft tissue procedures. Carprofen does not appear to affect platelet function or cause excessive bleeding in surgical procedures, although more recent data demonstrate some changes in platelet function with uncertain clinical significance. Adverse effects associated with carprofen are very limited, with the majority being GI in nature. Furthermore, administration of carprofen to healthy dogs undergoing anesthesia has not shown alterations in renal function or hemostasis. Association of carprofen with liver dysfunction deserves special attention (see potential side effects), but the reported incidence of liver dysfunction is less than 0.06% of all dogs treated. In certain countries, a single injectable dose in cats is approved for pain. Although there are ample data to support single-dose use for perioperative pain, repetitive administration in cats *is not recommended* until additional safety and efficacy data have been produced with multiple dosage protocols.

Cimicoxib. Cimicoxib is a member of the coxib class of NSAIDs. Cimicoxib has been approved by the European Union as an oral formulation in dogs for treatment of pain and inflammation associated with OA and postoperative pain. Limited data are available on Cimicoxib; one study documented noninferiority compared with carprofen in managing postoperative pain in dogs undergoing either orthopedic or soft-tissue surgery. No peer-reviewed published pharmacologic data are available currently on this drug. Some data are available as part of cimicoxib's approval process in Europe.

Deracoxib. Deracoxib is a member of the coxib class of NSAIDs. Deracoxib has been shown to be COX-1 sparing (COX-2 selective) in vitro and in vivo. Deracoxib is approved in an oral formulation in dogs for treatment of pain and inflammation associated with OA and postoperative pain associated with orthopedic surgery. Deracoxib has been demonstrated to provide effective analgesia for acute postoperative pain involving cruciate ligament stabilization. It has also been demonstrated to provide effective relief of pain in clinical OA trials in dogs. Deracoxib is also effective in providing postoperative analgesia in both dental and soft-tissue procedures. In these studies, reported adverse effects were few; however, a recent report does document serious GI complications. Adverse events seemed to be related to higher (3 to 4 mg/kg) dosages or concurrent use of corticosteroids or other NSAIDs in most cases. An additional laboratory study was done to evaluate safety in long-term administration of deracoxib. At recommended doses, deracoxib was well tolerated; dose-dependent renal injury occurred, but at dosages three times above the label recommendation. Deracoxib does not appear to significantly alter platelet function in dogs without preexisting coagulopathies. Although limited data on pharmacokinetics are available in cats, safety and efficacy have not been studied, and use in cats is not advised.

Etodolac. Etodolac is a member of the pyranocarboxylic acid class of NSAIDs. In vitro data suggest that etodolac is not COX-2 selective in dogs. However in vivo data are conflicting, with evidence suggesting that platelet thromboxane and gastric prostaglandin PGE_1 were not inhibited by etodolac in dogs at recommended therapeutic doses. Thus it is difficult to definitively state whether or not etodolac is COX-1 sparing in vivo. Etodolac is approved as an oral formulation for use in managing pain and inflammation associated with canine OA. Clinically it has been shown to improve rear limb function in dogs with chronic OA. Adverse events are primarily seen in the GI tract; however, keratoconjunctivitis sicca has also been associated with etodolac administration.

Firocoxib. Firocoxib is a member of the coxib class of NSAIDs. In vitro and in vivo data support firocoxib as a COX-1–sparing (COX-2–selective) drug. Firocoxib is approved as an oral formulation with an indication for the management of pain and inflammation associated with OA in dogs. Clinically it has been shown to improve limb function in dogs with OA. Clinical trials suggest that firocoxib may have some superiority in owner and veterinarian subjective evaluations with regard to lameness resolution when compared with carprofen and etodolac in dogs with lameness associated with OA. Long-term administration of firocoxib showed continued improvements over the year of treatment. Firocoxib is also effective in providing postoperative analgesia. Clinical data suggest a low rate of adverse events, limited primarily to the GI tract. Two additional studies that evaluated long-term therapy (90 days) with firocoxib in dogs (including geriatric animals) described minimal adverse events.

Ketoprofen. Ketoprofen is a member of the arylpropionic acid class of NSAIDs. Ketoprofen inhibits both COX isoenzymes without selectivity in dogs. Because of this inhibition of both COX enzymes, ketoprofen is expected to have significant antithromboxane activity. Although ketoprofen can be used to effectively manage postoperative pain, there may be a propensity for postoperative hemorrhage. Ketoprofen is approved for use in dogs and cats in Europe and Canada in oral and parenteral formulations. The only data available to the clinician regarding clinical use of this product is in an acute pain model and perioperative pain management. Adverse events are the aforementioned excessive bleeding and GI effects (primarily vomiting).

Mavacoxib. Mavacoxib is a member of the coxib class of NSAIDs. Mavacoxib is approved by the European Union as an oral formulation in dogs for treatment of pain and inflammation associated with OA. Mavacoxib has published pharmacologic data but no clinical data beyond what are available in the application for approval in Europe and one abstract from a meeting in 2009. Mavacoxib is a long-acting agent with an approved administration regimen consisting of a loading dose repeated at 14 days and thereafter at an administration interval of 1 month.

Meloxicam. Meloxicam is a member of the oxicam family of NSAIDs. Recent in vivo and in vitro data have shown meloxicam to be COX-1 sparing (COX-2 selective). It is approved for use in dogs for the control of pain and inflammation associated with OA and is available in oral, transmucosal oral mist, and parenteral formulations. Published efficacy data are available for chronic and perioperative pain management. A recent study documents preferential accumulation of meloxicam in experimentally inflamed joints. Meloxicam administration to euvolemic dogs undergoing anesthesia has not resulted in alterations in renal function or hemostasis. Evaluation of platelet function indicates that meloxicam does not significantly alter platelet function in normal animals. The incidence of adverse events with meloxicam is low, and they are primarily GI effects.

Meloxicam is approved for use in cats, but that approval is limited to a single dose to control pain and inflammation associated with orthopedic surgery, ovariohysterectomy, and castration in the United States. Several studies support the use of meloxicam for postoperative pain. Chronic use of meloxicam is approved in several countries. Use in cats from 5 days to indefinite administration to provide analgesia for locomotor disorders including OA has been described at several different dosage levels (0.01 to 0.05 mg/kg orally [PO]) daily. Although these data exist, clinical efficacy is supported by data generated from studies using the 0.05 mg/kg dose PO every 24 hours. At lower dosage regimens (0.01 to 0.03 mg/kg PO q24h), meloxicam has been shown to be well tolerated and safe in cats including cats with chronic renal dysfunction. Recent data suggest that meloxicam has no effect on platelet function in healthy cats.

Robenacoxib. Robenacoxib is a member of the coxib class of NSAIDs. In vitro and in vivo data support robenacoxib as a COX-1–sparing (COX-2–selective) drug in both dogs and cats. Robenacoxib is approved for only dogs or both dogs and cats depending on the country. Indications in the dog are for treatment of pain and inflammation associated with orthopedic or soft-tissue surgery as well as the treatment of pain and inflammation associated with chronic OA (depending on the country). Robenacoxib has been shown to maintain elevated concentrations in inflamed joints (either experimentally induced or with chronic OA) when compared with the serum concentrations over time. In the cat, approved indications (depending on the country) may include treatment of postoperative pain and inflammation associated with orthopedic and soft tissue surgeries as well as the acute pain and inflammation associated with musculoskeletal disorders. Length of approved treatment times in the cat varies from 3 to 11 days. Robenacoxib was shown to have a very good safety profile with daily administration in studies of 28 and 42 days in healthy young cats (5 to 8.5 months of age).

Tepoxalin. Tepoxalin is a dual COX-LOX inhibitor, inhibiting both COX isoenzymes and LOX. This dual inhibitor drug offers an alternative method of blocking the metabolic pathways responsible for pain and inflammation. Tepoxalin has been approved for use in dogs to control pain and inflammation associated with OA and is available in an oral formulation. Both in vitro and in vivo data support its ability for dual COX-LOX inhibition. Unfortunately, there are no published reports available to support clinical efficacy and safety beyond data submitted for government approval in the dog. Tepoxalin administration did not alter renal function in healthy dogs receiving an angiotensin-converting enzyme inhibitor. Available data suggest that tepoxalin used chronically did not alter renal function in dogs with chronic renal disease and OA. Adverse events with tepoxalin are low, primarily GI effects in the dog. There is one report of successful off-label use of tepoxalin in cats.

Tolfenamic Acid. Tolfenamic acid is an anthranilic acid derivative and a member of the fenamate class of NSAIDs. It is approved in Canada and Europe in both an oral and a parenteral formulation for dogs and cats. In vitro data support COX-1–sparing (COX-2–selective) activity. However, in vivo data to confirm these actions is not available. Some clinical data support the use of tolfenamic acid in dogs and cats. Strict recommendations on limiting the use of this product are apparently related to its relatively narrow therapeutic range. The most common adverse events are GI related (diarrhea and vomiting) and perioperative bleeding.

Compounds Used Off-Label

Nonapproved NSAIDs that have been recommended for use off-label include aspirin, piroxicam, and a plethora of human products. The vast majority of the human products have limited to no data for dogs or cats regarding correct dosage for efficacy or safety.

Aspirin. Aspirin is historically the most commonly used NSAID in dogs and cats. It is relatively effective, inexpensive, and readily available. Aspirin is not COX-1 sparing (COX-2 selective). However, with the introduction of more effective and safer products, aspirin use has declined. Adverse events are primarily GI related and are not uncommon. The frequency of GI toxicity increases as the dose increases. Buffered aspirin has been demonstrated to cause less GI irritation than plain aspirin when administered to dogs. Aspirin also has antithromboxane effects and is used as an antiplatelet drug in humans and veterinary species. A final possible area of concern is the use of one of the COX-1–sparing NSAIDs concurrently or immediately after administration of aspirin. Recently, lipoxin A_4 and its epimeric counterpart, aspirin-triggered lipoxin (ATL), have been shown to exert protective effects in the stomach. ATLs diminish gastric injury most likely via release of nitric oxide from the vascular endothelium. However, concurrent administration of COX-1–sparing (COX-2–selective) drugs (see Box 8-1) with aspirin results in the complete inhibition of ATLs and causes significant exacerbation of gastric mucosal injuries. Therefore clinicians should make sure that dogs are not on aspirin when prescribing COX-1–sparing NSAIDs, and owners must be informed of the potential risks of such concurrent therapy. It is important to remember that the formation of ATLs has yet to be proven in the dog. However, it would be surprising to find that they are not formed since they have been found in other species.

Piroxicam. Piroxicam is a member of the oxicam family of NSAIDs. In vitro data suggest that piroxicam is COX-2 selective in dogs. However, in vivo data are not available to confirm these results. Piroxicam has an elimination half-life of approximately 40 hours in the dog and 12 hours in the cat. Piroxicam has long been used as an antineoplastic agent to treat transitional cell carcinoma, and it is now also being used as an adjunct therapy in other chemotherapy regimens to treat squamous cell carcinoma and mammary carcinoma. Although antineoplastic activity has been linked to COX-2 inhibitory activity, other factors may also play a role in piroxicam's antineoplastic activity. Based on clinical response and the long elimination half-life, once-daily or once-every-other-day administration has been successfully used in the dog. Piroxicam has been administered at a dose of 0.3 mg/kg orally once daily for many months for the treatment of canine transitional cell carcinoma. Approximately 18% of the dogs demonstrated adverse GI signs. Clinical reports are vague regarding exact adverse events, but these events seem to be limited. Gastroendoscopic evaluation of healthy dogs given piroxicam at a dose of 0.3 mg/kg orally once daily for 28 days failed to demonstrate a difference in gastroduodenal lesion development between treated and control dogs. Additional data are needed before sweeping recommendations on use in pain management can be made.

POTENTIAL SIDE EFFECTS

See Box 8-2.

Adverse Effects

Gastrointestinal Effects

See Boxes 8-3 and 8-4. The most common problems associated with NSAID use in dogs and cats involve the GI tract. Some GI toxicities associated with NSAID use may be caused by inhibition of endogenous prostaglandins. Signs range from vomiting and diarrhea, including hematemesis and melena, to a silent ulcer that results in perforation. The true overall incidence of GI toxicity in dogs or cats treated with NSAIDs is unknown

---

BOX 8-2   Key Points to Minimize Adverse Reactions

- Every effort should be made to prevent rather than treat the adverse reactions associated with nonsteroidal anti-inflammatory drug (NSAID) use.
- Chronic use is often necessary; the goal should be to use the minimum amount of drugs to maintain the animal's now improved function.
- Concurrent use of other NSAIDs or corticosteroids provides no additional therapeutic benefit but does increase the potential for adverse reactions.
- As the animal ages or the addition of medications for unrelated problems increases, so should the monitoring for potential problems.

BOX 8-3 Toxicity of Nonsteroidal Anti-inflammatory Drugs

CLINICAL SIGNS	LABORATORY FINDINGS

Gastrointestinal (GI) Toxicity

- Vomiting
- Diarrhea
- Nausea
- Darkened stools (melena)
- Inappetence or anorexia
- Lethargy
- Hematochezia
- Depression
- Abdominal tensing

Decreased hematocrit and total protein
Increased blood urea nitrogen (BUN) because of GI hemorrhage
Elevated leukocyte count

Nephrotoxicity

- Polyuria and polydipsia
- Vomiting and anorexia (as a result of uremic toxin production)
- Oliguria or anuria
- Other signs of chronic or acute renal failure

Increased BUN, creatinine
Decreased urine specific gravity (best to review serial urine specific gravity values)
Cast formation
Proteinuria

Hepatotoxicity

- Icterus
- Lethargy
- Vomiting
- Weight loss
- Hepatic encephalopathy

Increased alanine aminotransferase (ALT)
Increased aspartate aminotransferase (AST)
Increased alkaline phosphatase (ALP)
+/− hyperbilirubinemia
+/− hypoalbuminemia

Gastrointestinal Bleeding

Consequences of Bleeding

- Pale mucous membranes
- Lethargy
- Dyspnea
- Prolonged bleeding at venipuncture sites
- Excessive bleeding during minor surgical procedures

BOX 8-4 Gastrointestinal Effects of PGD$_2$, PGE$_2$, PGF$_{2\alpha}$ Drugs

- ↓ Mucin
- ↓ Neutral mucosal pH
- ↓ Bicarbonate
- ↓ Blood flow
- ↑ Leukocyte adherence
- ↑ Intestinal permeability

- Gastric hypermotility
- Uncoupling of enterocyte mitochondrial oxidative phosphorylation
- Gastrointestinal erosions and ulcers
- Bleeding and perforation

PG, Prostaglandin.

because unfortunately, many reports include the use of inappropriate doses of NSAIDs or *concurrent administration of other medications (especially other NSAIDs or corticosteroids)*. Previous GI bleeding or the presence of other systemic diseases may contribute to adverse reactions. The effect of aging on an individual's ability to metabolize NSAIDs is likely to be quite variable. Various gastroprotectant strategies should be considered when NSAIDs are prescribed for chronic use (Table 8-2).

Hepatic Effects

See Box 8-3. Hepatotoxicosis caused by NSAIDs is generally considered to be idiosyncratic. Carprofen has been associated with an idiosyncratic cytotoxic hepatocellular reaction. Anorexia, vomiting, and icterus along with increased hepatic enzyme levels have been seen. The onset of signs were seen by 21 days in the vast majority of dogs. Most dogs recovered with cessation of treatment and with supportive care. Other NSAIDs can induce the same problems, and liver function must be monitored with use of all NSAIDs.

TABLE **8-2**	Doses of Drugs Used for Treatment of Nonsteroidal Anti-inflammatory Drug (NSAID) Toxicity in Dogs and Cats	
DRUG	**DOSAGE**	**RECOMMENDATIONS**
H₂-Receptor Blockers		
Famotidine	0.5 mg/kg q12-24h PO, SC, IM, IV	Decrease dosage in renal failure.
Nizatidine	2.5-5.0 mg/kg q24h PO	
Mucosal Protectant		
Sucralfate	Dogs: 0.5-1.0 g/dog q8-12h PO	If co-administering oral antibiotics, separate administration by at least 2 hr.
	Cats: 0.25 g/cat q8-12h PO	If co-administering antacids, administer at least 30 min after sucralfate administration.
		Use cautiously in renal failure.
		Side effect: constipation.
Proton Pump Inhibitors		
Omeprazole	Dogs: 0.5-1.0 mg/kg q24h PO	Do not administer partial tablet or capsule unless dissolved in HCO_3^-.*
	Cats: 0.7 mg/kg q24h PO	
Pantoprazole	0.7-1.0 mg/kg, q24h, PO, IV	
Prostaglandin Analogue		
Misoprostol	Dogs: 3-5 µg/kg q6h PO	Side effects: diarrhea, abortion.
	Cats: Not established	

Continued

TABLE 8-2	Doses of Drugs Used for Treatment of Nonsteroidal Anti-inflammatory Drug (NSAID) Toxicity in Dogs and Cats—cont'd	
DRUG	**DOSAGE**	**RECOMMENDATIONS**
Promotility Agent		
Metoclopramide	0.2-0.4 mg/kg q8h 30 min before eating, PO, IM, SC; or 1-2 mg/kg/ 24 hr, given in fluids continuous rate infusion	Not for use in animals with mechanical gastric outflow obstruction. Should not be used in combination with phenothiazines, butyrophenones, or narcotics. Physically incompatible when mixed with cephalothin sodium, sodium bicarbonate, chloramphenicol sodium succinate, or tetracycline. Side effects: anxiety, agitation, tremors, twitching.
Fluid Therapy		
Administer IV fluids to enhance NSAID excretion at a diuretic rate for at least 48 hr if potentially renally toxic dose has been ingested.		
Hepatotherapy		
Discontinue NSAID and begin IV fluids; administer vitamin K_1 (1-2 mg/kg PO or SC) and control vomiting with metoclopramide, maropitant, or dolasetron or ondansetron (serotonin [5-HT$_3$] receptor antagonists). Consider SAMe, N-acetylcysteine, ursodiol.		

*To prepare an oral suspension, dissolve 20-mg capsule or tablet in 10 mL of 8.4% HCO_3^- to make a 2-mg/mL solution; good for 7 days.

BOX 8-5	Risk Factors for Nonsteroidal Anti-inflammatory Drugs

- Age
- Anemia
- Anesthesia
- Heart failure
- Hypotension
- Hypovolemia
- Pre-existing renal disease
- Renal toxicity

Renal Effects

See Boxes 8-3 and 8-5.

Renal dysfunction may occur with NSAID administration as a consequence of prostaglandin inhibition (Figure 8-3). Renal prostaglandin synthesis is very low under normovolemic conditions. When normovolemia is challenged, prostaglandin synthesis is increased and important to maintaining renal perfusion (see Figure 8-3). NSAID use must be considered very carefully in hypovolemic animals. This is especially important to remember with the increasing use of NSAIDs perioperatively for pain management. It must be noted that the COX-1–sparing NSAIDs do not infer greater safety in

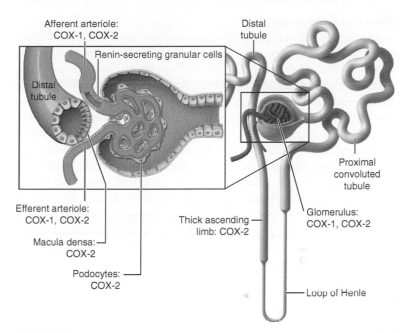

FIGURE 8-3   Cyclooxygenase enzymes *(COX-1, COX-2)* are important regulators of renal blood flow and renal tubular function. Their inhibition by all currently available NSAIDs can result in vasoconstriction of afferent and efferent blood vessels, glomerular dysfunction, and abnormal tubuloglomerular feedback, resulting in renal failure.

the kidney. There are some data to suggest that NSAIDs can be used safely in dogs and cats with chronic renal disease in which hydration can be maintained.

Effects on Cartilage

NSAIDs are used frequently and often chronically in animals with osteoarthritis. Studies have demonstrated a variety of effects on proteoglycan synthesis when chondrocytes or cartilage explants are incubated with an NSAID in vitro. The most pronounced effects have been seen in chondrocytes from osteoarthritic joints, although a lesser effect has been demonstrated on normal cartilage. Aspirin is uniformly reported to cause inhibition of proteoglycan synthesis; conflicting data exist for other NSAIDs, such as etodolac, showing both potential negative and positive effects; and there is a final group, including meloxicam, piroxicam, tepoxalin, and carprofen, in which no effect or even some increased synthesis of proteoglycan has been noted. The significance of these in vitro findings remains unclear, and there are now experimental data suggesting that NSAIDs and dual inhibitors can slow the progression of OA in vivo; however, the clinical significance of these data in the clinical setting with naturally occurring disease is unknown.

Effects on Bone Healing

Pain management is an important component of the care of animals with fractures. It is interesting to note that prostaglandins also play an important role in bone repair and normal bone homeostasis. Experimental studies support the hypothesis that both nonspecific and specific COX inhibitors (COX-1 sparing) do impair bone healing. With the nonspecific NSAIDs, the effects appear to be both time and dose dependent. Whether COX-1–sparing drugs have the same effects on fracture healing, spinal fusions, and bone ingrowth remains controversial, but recent data support that the effects of COX-1–sparing drugs are dose and time dependent and are reversible. These statements are based on rabbit, rat, and mouse induced fracture models that show that COX-1–sparing agents do alter bone healing. However, the most recent data confirm that after cessation of NSAIDs, fracture healing returns to its normal rate, and therefore judicious use of postoperative NSAIDs can be recommended. Stated another way, any potential adverse effects must be weighed against potential benefits that include but are not limited to improved analgesia and earlier return to function (both mobilization of the limb and the individual and weight bearing), and data support use of NSAIDs in the immediate postoperative period as long as the administration is not continuous for several weeks.

Cardiovascular Effects

Nonselective NSAIDs inhibit the platelet COX-1 enzyme and cause a significant decrease in the amount of thromboxane A_2 (TXA_2) produced by activated platelets. Thromboxane is an important promoter of platelet aggregation in most dogs and is released by activated platelets to recruit additional platelets to the site of vessel injury. Thromboxane is also a potent vasoconstrictor. A decrease in thromboxane release can result in prolongations of primary hemostasis. COX-1–sparing (COX-2–selective inhibitor) drugs do not have this effect on thromboxane production and likely do not clinically affect primary hemostasis, depending on the study methodology. The actions of thromboxane are balanced at the vessel level by the presence of prostacyclin (PGI_2), which is produced by COX enzymes in the vascular endothelial cells. PGI_2 is a strong inhibitor of platelet aggregation and also results in vasodilation. In the presence of endothelial inflammation (such as that caused by atherosclerotic plaques), the expression of COX-2 in the endothelial cells increases and may produce the majority of prostacyclin in that area. When COX nonselective NSAIDs are administered, the expression of both thromboxane from platelets and PGI_2 from endothelial cells is decreased, preserving the balance. In certain circumstances of endothelial inflammation (e.g., with atherosclerosis), specific COX-2 inhibitors may decrease the endothelial production of PGI_2 (mainly from COX-2) without a concomitant decrease in platelet thromboxane (produced only by COX-1), and consequently may result in the development of a hypercoagulable state.

SUGGESTED READING

Agnello KA, Reynolds LR, Budsberg SC. In vivo effects of tepoxalin, a dual COX/LOX inhibitor, on prostanoid and leukotriene production in dogs with osteoarthritis. Am J Vet Res. 2005; 66:966–972.

Aragon CL, Hofmeister EH, Budsberg SC. Systematic review of clinical trials of treatments for osteoarthritis in dogs. J Am Vet Med Assoc. 2007; 230:514–521.

Autefage A, Gossellin J. Efficacy and safety of the long-term oral administration of carprofen in the treatment of osteoarthritis in dogs. Revue De Medicine Veterinaire. 2007; 158:119–127.

Barry S. Non-steroidal anti-inflammatory drugs inhibit bone healing: A review. Vet Comp Orthop Traumatol. 2010; 6:385–392.

Bennett D, Zainal Ariffin SM, Johnston P. Osteoarthritis in the cat: 2. How should it be managed and treated? J Feline Med Surg. 2012; 14:76–84.

Bergh MS, Budsberg SC. The coxib NSAIDs: Potential clinical and pharmacological importance in veterinary medicine. J Vet Intern Med. 2005; 19:633–643.

Bienhoff SE, Smith ES, Roycroft LM, Roberts ES. Efficacy and safety of deracoxib for control of postoperative pain and inflammation associated with soft tissue surgery in dogs. Vet Surg. 2012; 41:336–344.

Blois SL, Allen DG, Wood RD, Conlon PD. Effects of aspirin, carprofen, deracoxib, and meloxicam on platelet function and systemic prostaglandin concentrations in healthy dogs. Am J Vet Res. 2010; 71:349–358.

Brainard BM, Meredith CP, Callan MB, et al. Changes in platelet function, hemostasis, and prostaglandin expression after treatment with nonsteroidal anti-inflammatory drugs with various cyclooxygenase selectivity's in dogs. Am J Vet Res. 2007; 68:251–257.

Carmichael S. Clinical use of non-steroidal anti-inflammatory agents (NSAIDs); the current position. Euro J Companion Anim Pract. 2011; 21:171–177.

Davila D, Keeshen TP, Evans RB, Conzemius MG. Comparison of the analgesic efficacy of perioperative firocoxib and tramadol administration in dogs undergoing tibial plateau leveling osteotomy. J Am Vet Med Assoc. 2013; 243:225–231.

Edamura K, King JN, Seewald W, et al. Comparison of oral robenacoxib and carprofen for the treatment of osteoarthritis in dogs: A randomized clinical trial. J Vet Med Sci. 2012; 74:1121–1131.

Fiorucci S, Antonelli E. NO-NSAIDs: From inflammatory mediators to clinical readouts. Inflamm Allergy Drug Targets. 2006; 5:121–131.

Gowan RA, Lingard AE, Johnston L, et al. Retrospective case-control study of the effects of long-term dosing with meloxicam on renal function in aged cats with degenerative joint disease. J Feline Med Surg. 2012; 13:752–761.

Grosser T, Fries S, FitzGerald GA. Biological basis for the cardiovascular consequences of COX-2 inhibition: Therapeutic challenges and opportunities. J Clin Invest. 2006; 116:4–15.

Gruet P, Seewald W, King JN. Robenacoxib versus meloxicam for the management of pain and inflammation associated with soft tissue surgery in dogs: A randomized, non-inferiority clinical trial. BMC Vet Res. 2013; 2:9:12.

Gunew MN, Menrath VH, Marshall RD. Long-term safety, efficacy and palatability of oral meloxicam at 0.01-0.03 mg/kg for treatment of osteoarthritic pain in cats. J Feline Med Surg. 2008; 10:235–241.

Humber LG. On the classification of NSAIDs. Drug News Perspect. 1992; 102–103.

Innes JF, Clayton J, Lascelles BDX. Review of the safety and efficacy of long-term NSAID use in the treatment of canine osteoarthritis. Vet Rec. 2010; 166:226–230.

ISFM and AAFP Consensus Guidelines. Long-term use of NSAIDs in cats. J Feline Med Surg. 2012; 12:521–538.

Jones CJ, Budsberg SC. Physiologic characteristics and clinical importance of the cyclooxygenase isoforms in dogs and cats. J Am Vet Med Assoc. 2000; 217:721–729.

Jones CJ, Streppa HK, Budsberg SC. In vivo effect of a COX-2 selective and nonselective nonsteroidal anti-inflammatory drug (NSAID) on gastric mucosal and synovial fluid prostaglandin synthesis in dogs. J Vet Internal Med. 2001; 15:273.

Kamata M, King JN, Seewald W, et al. Comparison of injectable robenacoxib versus meloxicam for peri-operative use in cats: results of a randomised clinical trial. Vet J. 2012; 193:114–118.

Khan SA, McLean MK. Toxicology of frequently encountered nonsteroidal anti-inflammatory drugs in dogs and cats. Vet Clin Small Anim. 2012; 42:289–306.

Knapp DW, Richardson RC, Chan TC, et al. Piroxicam therapy in 34 dogs with transitional cell carcinoma of the urinary bladder. J Vet Intern Med. 1994; 8:273–276.

KuKanich B, Bidgood T, Knesl O. Clinical pharmacology of nonsteroidal anti-inflammatory drugs in dogs. Vet Anaesth Analg. 2012; 39:69–90.

Luna SP, Basílio AC, Steagall PV, et al. Evaluation of adverse effects of long-term oral administration of carprofen, etodolac, flunixin meglumine, ketoprofen, and meloxicam in dogs. Am J Vet Res. 2007; 68:258–264.

Monteiro-Steagall BP, Steagall PVM, Lascelles BDX. Systematic review of nonsteroidal anti-inflammatory drug induced adverse effects in dogs. J Vet Intern Med. 2013; 27 (5):1011–1019.

Punke JP, Speas AL, Reynolds LR, Budsberg SC. Effects of firocoxib, meloxicam, and tepoxalin on prostanoid and leukotriene production by duodenal mucosa and other tissues of osteoarthritic dogs. Am J Vet Res. 2008; 69:1203–1209.

Reymond N, Speranza C, Gruet P, et al. Robenacoxib vs. carprofen for the treatment of canine osteoarthritis; a randomized, noninferiority clinical trial. J Vet Pharmacol Ther. 2012; 35:175–183.

Slingsby LS, Waterman-Pearson AE. Postoperative analgesia in the cat after ovariohysterectomy by use of carprofen, ketoprofen, meloxicam or tolfenamic acid. J Small Anim Pract. 2000; 41:447–450.

Staffieri F, Centonze P, Gigante G, et al. Comparison of the analgesic effects of robenacoxib, buprenorphine and their combination in cats after ovariohysterectomy. Vet J. 2013; 197:363–367.

Streppa HK, Jones CJ, Budsberg SC. Differential biochemical inhibition of specific cyclooxygenases by various non-steroidal anti-inflammatory agents in canine whole blood. Am J Vet Res. 2002; 63:91–94.

Surdyk KK, Brown CA, Brown SA. Evaluation of glomerular filtration rate in cats with reduced renal mass and administered meloxicam and acetylsalicylic acid. Am J Vet Res. 2013; 74:648–651.

Surdyk KK, Sloan DL, Brown SA. Renal effects of carprofen and etodolac in euvolemic and volume-depleted dogs. Am J Vet Res. 2012; 73:1485–1489.

Vane JR, Bakhle YS, Botting RM. Cyclooxygenases 1 and 2. Ann Rev Pharmacol Toxicol. 1998; 38:97–120.

Vanegas H, Schaible HG. Prostaglandins and cyclooxygenases in the spinal cord. Prog Neurobiol. 2001; 64:327–363.

Wallace JL, Zamuner SR, McKnight W, et al. Aspirin, but not NO-releasing aspirin (NCX-4016), interacts with selective COX-2 inhibitors to aggravate gastric damage and inflammation. Am J Physiol Gastrointest Liver Physiol. 2004; 286:G76–G81.

Watkins LR, Hutchinson MR, Ledeboer A, et al. Glia as the "bad guys": Implications for improving clinical pain control and the clinical utility of opioids. Brain Behav Immun. 2007; 21:131–146.

Wooten JG, Blikslager AT, Marks SL, et al. Effect of nonsteroidal anti-inflammatory drugs with varied cyclooxygenase-2 selectivity on cyclooxygenase protein and prostanoid concentrations in pyloric and duodenal mucosa of dogs. Am J Vet Res. 2009; 70:1243–1249.

CHAPTER 9

Opioids

Mark E. Epstein

O pioids have been used to modify pain since the beginning of recorded history, and the reason is simple: Receptors for naturally occurring opioids (endorphins, enkephalins, dynorphins) are distributed ubiquitously throughout the body and can be found in both central (spinal cord and brain) and peripheral tissues, with natural and synthetic compounds being capable of binding to these receptors as well. The term *opioid* is preferred to the term *narcotic* because drugs in this class can be defined as any natural or synthetic compound that exerts its effects by interacting with cell membrane opiate receptors. Opioids remain the most efficacious systemic means of controlling acute or postoperative pain, and can play a role in the management of chronic pain, as well. *The choice of opioid, route, dose, and duration of administration is dependent on clinical preferences and individual patient needs.*

OPIOID NEUROBIOLOGY

The opioid receptor is a serpentine molecule embedded in the cell membrane with one terminal ending that is exposed to the extracellular environment (binding site for drugs); the other terminus is intracellular. Several different opioid receptor types and subtypes have been isolated, each with a variant effect. The historic categorization of mu (μ), kappa (κ), delta (δ), and sigma (σ) opioid receptor types is simplistic in that it requires only minor amino acid changes to modify an opioid receptor from one type to another, and many hybrid subtypes have been identified in recent years. Furthermore opioid expression is an extremely plastic endeavor, dependent on intrinsic and extrinsic factors that modify a given individual's subsequent receptor expression. These factors include, but are not limited to, locus in the body, type of tissue injury, duration of tissue injury, comorbidities, species, and individual biologic variations. Efforts have been made to reclassify opioid receptors according to a rubric aligned with gene expression; however, convention allows the continued use of the familiar and traditional Greek letter categories, and in particular μ and κ receptors as the two that are most commonly manipulated in animals to modify pain (Table 9-1).

TABLE 9-1	Classification of Opiate Receptors and Their Effects
CLASS	**EFFECTS**
μ-1	Supraspinal analgesia
μ-2	Respiratory depression
	Bradycardia
	Physical dependence
	Euphoria
μ-3	Hyperpolarization of peripheral nerves induced by inflammation or immune response
κ	Analgesia
	Sedation
	Miosis
δ	Modulation of μ receptor activity

Mu Receptor

- Activation of a μ opioid receptor inhibits presynaptic release (especially in the dorsal horn of the spinal cord) of and postsynaptic response (especially in the dorsal root ganglion) to excitatory neurotransmitters. The proposed mechanism includes opioid receptor coupling with the G proteins coupling at the opioid intracellular C-terminus adjacent to the cell membrane. This leads to decreased intracellular formation of cyclic adenosine monophosphate (cAMP), which diminishes cell-membrane calcium channel phosphorylation (closing off the voltage-gated calcium channel, impeding calcium influx) and opens potassium channels, enhancing potassium influx. The resulting effect is hyperpolarization of the neuron and blockade of substance P release. Nociceptive transmission is thus greatly impeded.[1]

- Recent investigations have established that there are several subunits of intracellular G protein (G_1 to G_5, G_{stim}), and their variability plays a role in the specific action of different opioids.

- Some drugs fully bind and activate the μ receptor, and others do so only partially; and some drugs bind more tightly to the receptor (i.e., they have a higher affinity) than others. For example, buprenorphine binds only partially to the μ receptor, but in some circumstances may have a higher affinity for it than a pure μ-agonist (Box 9-1) such as morphine; given the presence of both drugs, the buprenorphine may thus preferentially bind even though it does so only partially.

- Other drugs bind tightly to the μ receptor with an affinity greater than μ-agonists but elicit no pharmacologic action; these are termed μ-*antagonists*, and examples include butorphanol and naloxone.

Kappa Receptors

Activation of κ receptors (especially in the spinal cord) induces an inhibitory neurotransmitter effect by increasing phosphodiesterase activity; this induces

---

BOX 9-1 | **Definitions**

- A pure opioid *agonist* binds to one or more types of receptor and causes certain effects, such as analgesia or respiratory depression (e.g., morphine).
- An opioid is considered a *partial agonist* if its binding at a given receptor causes an effect that is less pronounced than that of a pure agonist (e.g., buprenorphine).
- An opioid *antagonist* binds to one or more types of receptor but causes no effect at those receptors. By competitively displacing an agonist from a receptor, the antagonist effectively "reverses" the effect of the agonist (e.g., naloxone).
- An opioid *agonist-antagonist* binds to more than one type of receptor, causing an effect at one but no effect or a less pronounced effect at another (e.g., butorphanol).

---

catabolism of intracellular cAMP, which hyperpolarizes interneurons and increases their firing threshold. The pain-modifying effect of κ-receptor activation is relatively minor and short-lived compared with μ-receptor activation.

Delta and Sigma Receptors

The δ and σ receptors are less understood and currently are not targets for pain modification. They appear to be localized in higher centers (brain) and are considered responsible for some of the more profound psychomimetic and dysphoric properties of opioids and other drugs. The σ receptors, in fact, are no longer considered opioid receptors at all, because they are activated by nonopioid compounds such as phencyclidines.

Opioid Receptor Tropism: Which to Target?

- A therapeutic goal of systemic opioid is to maximize the mechanisms of opioid analgesia in the dorsal horn of the spinal cord (laminae I to V, the substantia gelatinosa, and dorsal root ganglia) while minimizing effects in the brain.
- Mu receptors are found in the various higher centers such as the mesencephalic periaqueductal gray matter, reticular formation, medulla, substantia nigra, ventral forebrain, and amygdala. Activation of μ receptors in these centers contributes to many of the undesirable adverse effects (AEs) of opioids, such as sedation, agitation, dysphoria, nausea, and respiratory depression. In the ventral tegmental area, opioids inhibit release of the neurotransmitter γ-aminobutyric acid (GABA), which induces dopamine release in the nucleus accumbens and creates the euphoria attributable to opioids but also becomes a prime mechanism for creating dependence in humans.
- Activation of μ receptors in peripheral tissue can be of great benefit when the opioid is applied locally or regionally (e.g., epidurally, intraarticularly) and can decrease the systemic requirements for opioid and other analgesic medications.

Opioids, Immunomodulation, and Spinal Cord Glia

- Opioids and their interaction with inflammation have received significant attention in recent years. Inflammatory cells contribute to hyperalgesia by releasing cytokines and other nerve-sensitizing products; however, they also have opioid receptors that can suppress this activity, and furthermore, these cells can also release endogenous opioids.
- Mu opioid activity can activate the hypothalamic-pituitary-adrenal axis, leading to hypercortisolemia with resultant suppression of lymphocyte and natural killer (NK) cell activity.
- It is interesting to note that not all opioids have the same effects; for example, morphine and fentanyl exhibit far more immunomodulatory activity than do buprenorphine and hydromorphone.[2]
- Glial cells in the spinal cord were once thought to merely perform non-neuronal supporting roles in the spinal cord, including scaffolding (astrocytes), immune-regulating and macrophage activity (microglia), and production of myelin (oligodendrocytes). They are now known to be highly interactive with nociceptors and pain processing.
- Glia are immunocompetent and have receptors for opioids, viruses, bacteria, tissue breakdown–products such as thrombin, and inflammatory cytokines. Once activated, glial cells contribute to exaggerated and sustained pain states as well as opioid dysregulation. Glial cells may in fact be a significant contributor to neuropathic pain, opioid tolerance, and opioid-induced hyperalgesia (OIH).

SIDE EFFECTS AND TOXICITY

Possible side effects of opioid administration are many and varied, although rarely problematic enough to prevent its use. In fact, one of the major advantages of opioids in pain management is their safety when used responsibly.

- In the veterinary acute care setting, opioid AEs generally are more likely to occur with intravenous administration and to animals not in pain (i.e., when opioids are used as a premedicant, because with preexisting pain, μ receptors are upregulated and the opioid distributes to these first).
- Although opioids are considered to be quite safe, the multimodal approach to pain management is designed, among other things, to be opioid sparing, to help minimize the potential for opioid-related AEs.
- Because wide biologic variation exists in animal response to disease, trauma, surgery, pain, and drug intervention, the clinician must attempt to prevent where possible and otherwise be prepared to encounter, recognize, and treat opioid AEs if and when they occur.
- In humans, the top seven opioid AEs are constipation; persistent nausea; dizziness and vertigo; somnolence and drowsiness; vomiting; dry skin and pruritus; and myoclonus and urinary retention.

- Data are not available in animals, but in an anecdotal, informal poll, the most frequently perceived AEs were reported to be dysphoria (41%); persistent inappetence with or without nausea (15%); ileus or constipation (13%); ineffectiveness (7%); and respiratory depression (3%). Twenty percent of veterinarians reported not having observed AEs.[3]

Sedation and Central Nervous System Depression

- Sedation and central nervous system (CNS) depression are more commonly observed in dogs than in cats.
- Sedation is generally considered an advantage when an opioid is used as a preanesthetic or in the immediate postoperative period when rest is desirable. This effect is often knowingly enhanced when an opioid is combined with other presurgical or postsurgical medications such as a phenothiazine (acepromazine), benzodiazepine (midazolam), or α_2-agonist (dexmedetomidine) to create a profoundly relaxed, stress-free, comfortable, and anesthetic-sparing state. However, sedation may be undesirable in the postoperative period if it interferes with return to normal behaviors such as eating and drinking. The degree of sedation is considered dose dependent.
- Options for treating excessive sedation are as follows:
  1. Reduce the dosage of opioid or, if necessary, withdraw altogether.
  2. Administer a low dose of an agonist-antagonist such as butorphanol or nalbuphine in conjunction with a pure agonist such as morphine.
  3. Administer a low dose of a pure antagonist such as naloxone in conjunction with a pure agonist such as morphine.

Excitement or Dysphoria

- Significant species and individual variation exists, with cats, horses, and northern breeds of dogs (e.g., Alaskan Malamutes and Siberian Huskies) apparently more susceptible to dysphoria of pure μ-agonists, and Labrador Retrievers to butorphanol-induced dysphoria.
- Determination of whether an agitated animal is dysphoric or in pain is important because the treatment for each situation may be different. A rough rule of thumb is that animals in pain will generally respond to human interaction, whereas animals with dysphoria will not. (See Chapters 3 and 4 for more information on assessing pain and analgesia.)
- The recommended dosages (in milligrams per kilogram) for most opioids in cats are as low as one tenth those recommended for dogs.
- Options for treatment of dysphoria or agitation include the following:
  1. Administration of a tranquilizer such as acepromazine (0.01 to 0.03 mg/kg) or a sedative such as dexmedetomidine (microdoses as low as 0.5 μg/kg intravenously [IV]) should help to calm the animal.
  2. Administration of an agonist-antagonist such as butorphanol antagonizes the excitatory effects of a pure agonist such as morphine, without

antagonizing analgesia. A study in cats demonstrated that 0.1 mg/kg each of oxymorphone and butorphanol provided synergistic analgesia without excitement.[4]

Cardiovascular Effects

- Bradycardia occurs as a result of opioid-induced medullary vagal stimulation; however, cardiac output is maintained because of compensatory mechanisms that increase stroke volume, and bradycardia is not considered clinically significant.
- Rarely, animals may develop second-degree atrioventricular block.
- Prevention and treatment: atropine (0.02 to 0.04 mg/kg) or glycopyrrolate (0.005 to 0.02 mg/kg), administered subcutaneously (SC), intramuscularly (IM), or IV, will increase the heart rate, but the clinical importance and wisdom of this in most animals is controversial.
- With the exception of meperidine, opioids generally cause little to no direct depression of myocardial contractility.

Respiratory Depression

- Respiratory depression results from an opioid-induced decrease in responsiveness of the brainstem respiratory center to $Paco_2$.
- In humans, opioid-induced respiratory depression can be profound, but in animals, clinically useful analgesic dosages and routes of opioids *alone* are unlikely to produce clinically significant respiratory depression.
- However, when opioids are used IV and/or in high dosages to provide surgical analgesia (such as fentanyl infusions at 20 µg/kg/hr or higher) or when they are used in conjunction with other respiratory depressant drugs (such as thiopental, propofol, or the inhaled anesthetics), the respiratory depression can be clinically significant even to the extent that assisted or controlled ventilation may be required.

Panting

- Panting may occur in some dogs after opioid administration, particularly after oxymorphone administration, because of resetting of the thermoregulatory center in the thalamus (the normothermic dog perceives it is hot, eliciting the panting to cool).
- Panting animals do not necessarily hyperventilate; in fact, they may hypoventilate because of low tidal volume and become hypercapnic.
- Panting can range from the merely inconvenient (e.g., motion artifact during radiography) to causing interference with rewarming of a hypothermic animal (e.g., in postoperative recovery).

Cough Suppression or Depression of Laryngeal Reflexes

- Opioid-induced cough suppression can be desirable or undesirable, depending on circumstances.

- Many dogs can be intubated after receiving IV administration of an opioid and benzodiazepine, and an opioid and dexmedetomidine, even though they remain conscious. This technique can be used to induce profound neuroleptanalgesia in critically ill animals, thus avoiding the use of more depressant anesthesia-induction drugs.
- Depression of laryngeal reflexes might be desirable when a brachycephalic (or other airway-challenged) dog is recovering from anesthesia, because it will allow the animal to tolerate the endotracheal tube for a longer time, during which inhaled anesthetic can be eliminated. However, insensitivity to the endotracheal tube can lead to undesirably protracted extubation times; in those cases a small dose of an agonist-antagonist such as nalbuphine or butorphanol (0.05 mg/kg IV) or a very small dose of an antagonist such as naloxone (1 to 10 μg/kg IV) may restore laryngeal reflexes and allow safe extubation.

Histamine Release

- Histamine release can occur with administration of certain opioids (particularly morphine and meperidine administered IV), resulting in sequelae of vasodilation and hypotension and, if extreme, gastrointestinal (GI) ulceration. Histamine release is the source of pruritus and allergic hypersensitivity in humans.
- Morphine may thus not be the ideal opioid to administer in animals with hypovolemic or hypotensive shock (e.g., after trauma, with gastric dilatation-volvulus [GDV]), IV during anesthesia, or before mast cell tumor resection.
- Morphine should be given by the IV route only if given cautiously and slowly and in low doses. It is recommended to avoid IV administration of meperidine altogether.
- No significant histamine release occurs after administration of oxymorphone, hydromorphone, fentanyl, or methadone, so these opioids are considered safer for IV use and in cases of existing hypotension.

Nausea and Vomiting

- Transient vomiting commonly follows administration of opioids as a result of μ-receptor binding in the chemoreceptor trigger zone in the medulla and the adjacent emetic center.[5] Vomiting is quite common when opioids are administered as a preanesthetic to animals not in pain, especially dogs; conversely, these effects are less common when opioids are administered to animals with preexisting pain (e.g., after trauma or surgery).[6]
- Some clinicians view preoperative vomiting as an advantage, ensuring that the stomach is empty; other clinicians wish to choose an opioid that minimizes nausea. The effect is most predictable with morphine, oxymorphone, and hydromorphone and is less commonly noted with methadone, buprenorphine, and butorphanol.

- Persistent postoperative opioid-induced nausea is a frequent complaint in humans, resulting from effects on both central and peripheral sites including the vomiting center, chemoreceptor trigger zones, the cerebral cortex, and the vestibular apparatus of the brain, as well as the GI tract itself.[7] It is less often appreciated in dogs and cats but can be suspected if animals are inappetent.
- Defecation may result from an initial increase in GI tone.

Constipation

- Opioids can cause increased GI sphincter tone and reduced peristalsis, leading to the common complaint in humans of constipation with long-term use of (often oral) opioids. In humans, a lack of bowel movement postoperatively is a major reason to delay discharge from the hospital. However, in dogs and cats it is not reported to be a significant clinical problem in short-term pain management, although it is unknown whether this is a dose-dependent and/or time-dependent factor versus a species difference (e.g., receptor distribution and expression).
- Peripherally acting µ opioid receptor antagonists (PAMORs) are now available. These agents permit the central analgesic effect of the opioid while blocking its effect on GI motility.
  1. Alvimopan (Entereg) is administered orally (PO) to prevent postoperative opioid-induced ileus
  2. Methylnaltrexone (Relistor) is administered SC to prevent constipation during long-term opioid administration

Urinary Retention

Urinary retention is caused by increased detrusor muscle tone and increased vesical sphincter tone. In animals it is most commonly associated with epidural morphine administration. In extreme cases the bladder may require temporary catheterization or manual expression.

Effect on Biliary Smooth Muscle

- In humans, morphine and fentanyl (and, less commonly used in veterinary medicine, meperidine and pentazocine) constrict the sphincter of Oddi, causing pain from increased pressure within the common bile duct and making use of these opioids suboptimal to treat pancreatitis or biliary disease. Partial- and agonist-antagonist opioids do not appear to have this effect in humans.
- Dogs generally have separate bile and pancreatic ducts, and there are no reports that use of any opioid worsens or prolongs pancreatitis or biliary disease. Most cats, however, do have a common pancreatic and bile duct, so butorphanol, nalbuphine, or buprenorphine may be the best choice for pain management in cats with pancreatitis.

Decreased Lower Esophageal Tone, Reflux, Esophagitis

- Studies have described opioid-induced gastroesophageal reflux from decreased lower gastroesophageal tone,[8] and there are case reports of clinically relevant postoperative esophagitis and esophageal dysfunction in both dogs and cats.[9] However, the prevalence and overall clinical relevance remain unknown.
- Some clinicians minimize this AE by coadministering histamine-antagonists or proton pump inhibitors preoperatively, and having the animal maintain an elevated head-chest orientation intraoperatively and during recovery.

Hyperthermia

- Cats may develop hyperthermia (103° to 105 ° F) several hours after the administration of μ-opioid agonists (morphine, oxymorphone, and, most implicated, hydromorphone[10]). Animals usually respond to antipyretics and other supportive care. Hyperthermia is not generally seen in cats given buprenorphine.

Pupil Size

- Humans and dogs experience miosis with opioids; cats experience mydriasis.[11]

SPECIAL ISSUES

Comprehensive Drug Abuse Prevention and Control Act (United States)

- Drugs are classified according to potential for abuse.
  1. Most opioid agonists have a high potential for abuse and are listed in Schedule II: morphine, hydromorphone, methadone, meperidine, and others.
  2. Butorphanol, an opioid agonist-antagonist with moderate abuse potential, is listed in Schedule IV.
- Prescribing of controlled substances is regulated in the United States.
  1. Veterinarian must register with the Drug Enforcement Administration (DEA) (registration to be renewed every 2 years).
  2. Veterinarian must keep inventory of controlled substances.
  3. Controlled substances must be ordered by using special forms.

Tolerance and Physical Dependence

- Definition of opioid tolerance: decreased response to escalating doses of opioid, resulting from signaling cascades that force calcium channels to remain open despite the presence of opioid.
- Clinically, occurrence of tolerance in animals is anecdotal and apparently rare.

- Tolerance can develop quite rapidly, or slowly over time.
  - Acute (minutes to hours) mechanism: receptor phosphorylation (which allows calcium channels to remain open and maintains the neuron in a hypopolarized state), uncoupling of opioid receptors from G protein, and opioid receptor downregulation (internalization of receptor from cell membrane to cytoplasm). This phenomenon appears to occur with high doses of immediate-release opioids—that is, high opioid plasma levels even though over a short period of time.
  - Chronic (days to weeks) mechanism: increased intracellular cAMP (receptor phosphorylation allowing calcium channels to remain open and maintaining the neuron in a hypopolarized state) and opioid activation of spinal glial cells.
- Nociceptive stimulation reportedly antagonizes or prevents development of tolerance to fentanyl. Therefore, tolerance is less likely to occur during pain management.
- Definition of dependence: the inability to withdraw use of opioids when there is no objective indication for the drug.
  - Mechanism: production of neurotropic compounds in higher CNS centers, including dopamine (nucleus accumbens) and brain-derived neurotrophic factor (BDNF; in the ventral tegmental area);[12] and downregulation of endogenous opioid production.
  - In humans, dependence involves a combination of biological, psychological, and social factors.
  - Dependence considered rare in animals.

Opioid-Induced Hyperalgesia

- Opioid-induced hyperalgesia (OIH) is described as the paradoxical potentiation of pain by the use of opioid.
- Reports indicate that OIH may occur in 20% or more of humans receiving long-term opioids, but it is also reported postsurgically and may be both dose and time dependent.[13]
- The mechanism is not well understood but appears to be an imbalance of pronociceptive and antinociceptive systems, whereby antinociceptive systems are less responsive to opioids and pronociceptive systems are activated.[14] This may include the following:
  - N-methyl-D-aspartate (NMDA)–mediated activation of central glutaminergic system.
  - Preferential binding of opioid to excitatory G_{stim}-protein.
  - Upregulation of central μ receptors.
  - Activation of opioid receptors on spinal glial cells, which then promote depolarization of second-order neurons without a nociceptive stimulus from the primary afferent neuron.

- Increased cholecystokinin in the rostroventral medulla (RVM), leading to increased nociceptive output to the spinal cord through descending pathways.
- Release of excitatory neuropeptides such as substance P.
- OIH may be difficult to distinguish from opioid tolerance.

Gene Expression and Opioid Metabolism

- Select genes have been identified in humans that regulate the speed and completeness of opioid metabolism (e.g., *OPRM1* for morphine and *CYP2D6* for codeine and tramadol) and tendency to cause AEs.
- Some animals may be very rapid or much slower metabolizers of various opioids and may be less or more sensitive to opioids and susceptible to their AEs, based on their specific gene expression directing receptor trafficking and pattern of G-protein formation.
- Currently there is no translational effect from gene mapping to clinical medicine; the totality of opioid metabolism and individual effect is dependent on multiple alleles rather than the few individual genes presently known.
- Future developments of opioid use include genotype-based diagnostics and custom designing of opioid protocols that maximize individual safety and analgesic effect.

Limitations of Clinical Research

- Universal certitude about the efficacy of various opioids in animals, and even simpler matters such as duration of drug effect, is almost impossible to achieve.
- Conclusions are confounded not only by species and aforementioned individual gene expression differences, but by the wide variety of methodology and outcome measurements reported throughout the literature.
- Therefore the clinician is cautioned to rely more heavily on individual animal assessment than published pharmacokinetic or pharmacodynamic data.

INJECTABLE OPIOID CLASSES AND MEMBERS

Pure or Full Mu Agonists

Morphine*

DESCRIPTION: Morphine is the principal alkaloid derived from opium and the prototypical opioid agonist with which all others are compared (Table 9-2). For many reasons, morphine is generally considered a primary analgesic in small animal practice.

Continued

---

*Morphine, morphine sulfate injection; Roxane Laboratories, Inc.

TABLE 9-2	Comparative Potencies, Suggested Doses, and Administration Frequencies of Common Opioid Analgesics			
OPIOID ANALGESIC	**RELATIVE POTENCY**	**DOG DOSE**	**CAT DOSE**	**COMMENTS**
Morphine	1 mg/kg	0.5-2.0 mg/kg q2-4h	0.2-0.5 mg/kg q3-4h	Oral tablets and suspension also available Use caution when given IV (histamine release)
Morphine, sustained release (oral)		2-5 mg/kg q12h		Bioavailability is poor when morphine is given PO
Oxymorphone	10 mg/kg	0.05-0.4 mg/kg q2-4h	0.02-0.1 mg/kg q3-4h	Minimal to no histamine release
Hydromorphone	10-15 mg/kg	0.05-0.2 mg/kg q1-4h	0.05-0.1 mg/kg q2-6h	Minimal to no histamine release
Methadone	1-1.5 mg/kg	0.5-1 mg/kg	0.1-0.5 mg/kg	Single dose recommended Oral suspension also available
Meperidine	0.1 mg/kg	3-5 q1-2h mg/kg	3-5 q1-2h mg/kg	Not recommended for intravenous use (histamine release)
Fentanyl	100 mg/kg	*Loading:* 2-5 µg/kg *CRI:* 2-5 µg/kg/hr (pain management); 10-45 µg/kg/hr (surgical analgesia and minimum alveolar concentration reduction)	*Loading:* 1-3 µg/kg *CRI:* 1-4 µg/kg/hr (pain management); 10-30 µg/kg/hr (surgical analgesia)	CRI required for sustained effect
		Recuvyra transdermal injectable: 2.7 mg/kg	N/A	One dose only, provides analgesia for 4 days

TABLE 9-2	Comparative Potencies, Suggested Doses, and Administration Frequencies of Common Opioid Analgesics—cont'd			
OPIOID ANALGESIC	**RELATIVE POTENCY**	**DOG DOSE**	**CAT DOSE**	**COMMENTS**
Sufentanil	1000	5 µg/kg loading; 0.1 µg/kg/min	?	Unpredictable sedation; may require tranquilizer
Alfentanil	10	?	?	Rapid onset, short duration (10 min?)
Remifentanil	50 mg/kg	*Loading:* 4-10 µg/kg *CRI:* 4-10 µg/kg/hr (pain management); 20-60 µg/kg/hr (surgical analgesia)	?	Extremely rapid elimination
Butorphanol	3-5 mg/kg	0.1-0.4 mg/kg q1-4h	0.1-0.4 mg/kg q2-6h	
Butorphanol, oral		0.5-2 mg/kg q6-8h	0.5-1 mg/kg q6-8h	
Buprenorphine	25 mg/kg	0.005-0.02 mg/kg q8-12h	0.005-0.02 mg/kg q8-12h; 0.01-0.02 mg/kg PO, tid, qid	May be difficult to antagonize *Cats:* Instill in cheek pouch for oral transmucosal absorption
Nalbuphine	1 mg/kg	0.5-1 mg/kg q1-4h	0.2-0.4 mg/kg q1-4h	
Pentazocine	0.25-0.5 mg/kg	1-3 mg/kg q2-4h	1-3 mg/kg q2-4h	

Drugs may be administered intravenously, intramuscularly, and subcutaneously unless otherwise stated. Doses are in milligrams per kilogram unless otherwise stated. Required doses and duration of analgesia vary from individual to individual; these are guidelines only.
Key: *CRI,* Constant rate infusion; *N/A,* not applicable.

ANALGESIC EFFICACY: Potency is not the same thing as efficacy. Although other opioids may be more potent, currently none is more effective than morphine at relieving pain. Cats lack glucuronate metabolism, resulting in minimal production of the analgesic M6G metabolite (none after IM administration, and only 50% of cats produce it after IV morphine administration).[15] However, some studies have demonstrated a pain-modifying effect for morphine in cats.[16]

UNIQUE FEATURES AND EFFECTS

1. No ceiling effect. Higher doses will escalate not only the analgesic effect but the likelihood of AEs such as respiratory depression, decreased minute volume, and increased arterial carbon dioxide tension.
2. Histamine release occurs especially with IV administration, and can occur within 1 minute and persist for at least 60 minutes in dogs. This may make morphine, especially IV morphine, less ideal during hypotension (shock, anesthesia) and before mast cell tumor excision. If administered IV, use a conservative dose and administer slowly.
3. Vomiting can be expected after subcutaneous administration even after low doses in animals without pain (e.g., as a presurgical medication); less commonly, defecation may be noted. Less common if administered IV, chronically, or in animals with pain.
4. Cardiovascular effects: Morphine generally causes minimal depression of cardiac contractility but can cause bradycardia, which is generally responsive to anticholinergic agents. Histamine release, if it occurs, may result in hypotension.
5. Depression of the cough center and therefore protracted time to extubation postsurgically.
6. Increased antidiuretic hormone, with urine production decreased by up to 90%.
7. Excitement or dysphoria: dose and species dependent (cats, horses more susceptible).

DURATION: Analgesic effects of systemically administered morphine appear to be longest among the pure-μ agonists, 2 to 4 hours after IV administration[17,18] and 4 or more hours after IM or SC administration.[19] This may be considered an advantage in the management of acute pain associated with trauma or surgery.

COST: Morphine is inexpensive enough that cost should not be an excuse for inadequate treatment of pain.

Hydromorphone* (Dilaudid)

DESCRIPTION: A semisynthetic opioid.
ANALGESIC EFFICACY: Hydromorphone has the same efficacy as morphine in dogs.[20] Hydromorphone may produce better analgesia than morphine in cats.
DURATION: Duration is shorter than morphine in dogs, perhaps 1 to 2 hours after IV administration and up to 2 hours after IM or SC administration.[20,21] In cats, hydromorphone may have a longer duration of action (longer than 7 hours in a thermal threshold model)[22] but may be dose-dependent.[23]

---

*Hydromorphone, hydromorphone HCl (Dilaudid); Purdue Pharma LP.

COST: Currently, hydromorphone is more expensive than morphine but less expensive than oxymorphone.

OTHER COMMENTS: Although hydromorphone can induce some histamine release, the effect is mild compared with that of morphine[24] and hydromorphone may be preferred, especially IV, during hypotension (dehydration, shock, anesthesia) and before mast cell tumor excision. Hydromorphone appears to produce less sedation than morphine or oxymorphone in dogs and cats. These features and the relatively short duration of action make hydromorphone arguably the most versatile of parenteral μ-agonist opioids. Nausea appears somewhat less pronounced than with morphine when given in dogs without pain, but transient vomiting can still be expected. In cats, hydromorphone is implicated more than other opioids in episodes of hyperthermia.[10]

Oxymorphone (Opana and Opana ER)*

DESCRIPTION: A semisynthetic opioid.

ANALGESIC EFFICACY: Similar to other pure agonists morphine and hydromorphone.

DURATION: Based on the plasma half-life of approximately 1 hour in dogs, duration is longer than that of hydromorphone and approaches that of morphine, approximately 3 to 4 hours after both IV and SC administration in dogs;[25] in cats the plasma half-life is somewhat longer (approximately 90 minutes versus 30 to 40 minutes in dogs) after IV administration.[26]

OTHER EFFECTS

1. Oxymorphone does not cause histamine release;[27] therefore, it is safer than morphine for IV administration during hypotension (dehydration, shock, anesthesia), and before mast cell tumor excision.
2. Clinical impression suggests that oxymorphone may be less likely to produce excitement than morphine, but more likely to induce panting than morphine.

COST: Oxymorphone is approved for use in dogs and cats but is considerably more expensive than morphine.

Methadone†

DESCRIPTION: A synthetic opioid.

ANALGESIC EFFICACY: Similar to morphine.

DURATION: Based on pharmacokinetics, 5 to 6 hours' duration can be expected after IV administration in dogs. After SC administration, the plasma half-life is more variable and far longer, ranging from 6 to 14 hours, but pharmacodynamics have not been assessed.[28] In cats, efficacy can be expected to last at least 2 hours after IV administration and at least 4 hours after oral transmucosal (OTM) administration.[29]

OTHER COMMENTS: Methadone administered IV is the least likely of the μ-agonist opioids to cause vomiting or elicit histamine release. It may also be an attractive opioid alternative in animals[30] because of mild to moderate NMDA receptor antagonist activity and evidence of effectiveness in rodent models of

Continued

---

*Oxymorphone (Opana), oxymorphone HCl injection; Endo Pharmaceuticals, Inc.
†Methadone (Dolophine); Roxane Laboratories, Inc.

neuropathic pain,[30] adding another pain-modifying effect and possibly helping to prevent opioid tolerance. Methadone has significant sedative properties, and several studies have demonstrated potential usefulness of the parenteral formulation in both dogs[31] and cats.[32] An oral methadone hydrochloride solution is commercially available; however, pharmacokinetic data in dogs and cats is lacking, and anecdotally appears to be bitter leading to excessive salivation after administration in dogs and cats.

Meperidine* (Demerol)

DESCRIPTION: Meperidine is a weak synthetic opioid one fourth to one tenth as potent as morphine. Because of its short duration and possible cardiovascular effects, meperidine has found limited use in veterinary medicine.

ANALGESIC EFFICACY: Similar to morphine.

DURATION: Less than 1 hour in the dog.[33]

OTHER COMMENTS

1. Negative inotropy: Unlike other opioids, meperidine reportedly may have significant negative inotropic effects.
2. Histamine release: Like morphine, meperidine can induce histamine release. For this reason intravenous use is discouraged, and meperidine is not the ideal opioid in animals experiencing hypotension or undergoing mast cell excision.

Fentanyl[†]

DESCRIPTION: A short-acting synthetic opioid with a potency 80 to 100 times that of morphine.

ANALGESIC EFFICACY: Similar to morphine. Fentanyl can decrease the minimum alveolar concentration (MAC) requirement for inhaled anesthetics by up to 63%.

DURATION: The half-life of fentanyl is very short, with clinical effects lasting only about 30 minutes after a single injection. For clinical application, the duration of fentanyl is commonly extended by administering it as a constant rate infusion— intraoperatively to augment surgical analgesia and to reduce the requirement for inhalation anesthetics (10 to 45 µg/kg/hr) and postoperatively for pain management (2 to 5 µg/kg/hr). Despite the supposed short duration of action of fentanyl, there is a great deal of individual variation in recovery time after infusions.

OTHER COMMENTS

1. The use of fentanyl intraoperatively may be especially advantageous in animals with compromised cardiac function because (unlike inhaled anesthetics) it causes minimal cardiovascular depression or hypotension while contributing to significant reduction in the MAC requirement.
2. Experimental findings and clinical impression suggest that tolerance to fentanyl can occur, perhaps as soon as 3 hours after administration is begun.

---

*Meperidine, meperidine HCl; Roxane Laboratories, Inc.

†Fentanyl, fentanyl citrate injection; Baxter Healthcare Corp.

‡Sufentanil; Taylor Pharmaceuticals.

Sufentanil[‡]

> **DESCRIPTION:** A synthetic opioid about 1000 times as potent as morphine.
> **DURATION:** About half as long as that of fentanyl.
> **OTHER COMMENTS:** Currently, sufentanil is not commonly used for pain management in animals.

Alfentanil*

> **DESCRIPTION:** A synthetic opioid about 25 times as potent as morphine.
> **DURATION:** Shorter in duration than fentanyl.
> **OTHER COMMENTS:** Currently, alfentanil is not commonly used for pain management in animals.

Remifentanil[†]

> **DESCRIPTION:** Remifentanil is another synthetic opioid that is about half as potent as fentanyl and is unique among opioids in that it is metabolized by nonspecific esterases that occur in blood and tissues throughout the body (mainly in skeletal muscle). This gives remifentanil the clinical advantage of extremely rapid clearance that does not depend on liver or kidney function.
> **DURATION:** Because of remifentanil's rapid clearance, constant rate infusion is required for sustained analgesia. Recovery is generally expected to occur within 3 to 7 minutes after termination of an infusion.
> **OTHER COMMENTS:** Remifentanil may be useful in situations in which intense analgesia is needed for a short or variable period.

Carfentanil[‡]

> **DESCRIPTION:** Synthetic opioid approximately 10,000 times more potent than morphine.
> **OTHER COMMENTS:** Used mainly for capture of wild and feral animals; not normally used in pain management.

Partial Mu Agonist

Buprenorphine[§] (Buprenex)

> **DESCRIPTION:** Buprenorphine is different from other opioids in that it is considered a partial agonist and binds more slowly at μ receptors although with greater affinity than morphine (and will displace it if the two are given together, although this effect may be clinically significant only at higher doses). Also, in contradistinction to pure μ-agonists, buprenorphine does exhibit a ceiling effect, meaning neither AEs nor
> *Continued*

[‡]Sufentanil; Taylor Pharmaceuticals.

*Alfentanil; Akorn.

[†]Remifentanil (Ultiva); Abbott Laboratories.

[‡]Carfentanil (Wildnil); Wildlife Pharmaceuticals.

[§]Buprenorphine (Buprenex Injectable); Reckitt Benckiser Pharmaceuticals, Inc.

analgesia becomes more pronounced at higher doses.[34] In fact, the analgesic effect may actually diminish at higher doses as it displaces endogenous opioids off μ receptors and elicits an apparent κ-antagonist effect.

ANALGESIC EFFICACY: Buprenorphine's partial, rather than full, binding at the μ receptor and its bell-shaped response curve suggest that this opioid may not provide adequate analgesia for moderate to severe pain, and escalating doses may detract from, rather than enhance, its analgesic effect.

ONSET: Buprenorphine has a slower onset of action than many other opioids, with its peak effect delayed up to an hour even after IV administration. Some studies have demonstrated negligible serum levels after subcutaneous administration.[35]

DURATION: Although a purported advantage of buprenorphine is its long duration of analgesia (up to 12 hours), its clinical analgesic effect in animals often seems to wane by 6 hours. The literature reflects wide individual variability in degree and duration of plasma levels and analgesic effect, which may not be related to plasma levels and may be in part dose dependent.[36] Some recent work by Gaynor suggests that buprenorphine administered subcutaneously to cats at much higher than customary doses (0.24 mg/kg) is safe and allows for an analgesic duration of up to 24 hours.

OTHER COMMENTS

1. Once bound to μ receptors, buprenorphine is reportedly difficult to displace, meaning that its effects may be difficult to antagonize.
2. A great benefit of the drug in veterinary medicine is that its pK_a (8.4) closely matches the pH of the feline oral mucosa (9.0), which allows for nearly complete absorption when the drug is given buccally (OTM route) in that species,[37] with kinetics nearly identical to those after IV and IM administration,[38] and very little sedation. However, one study in cats undergoing ovariohysterectomy found that IV and IM administration provided superior analgesia to OTM and SC administration.[39]
3. OTM absorption in the dog appears to be much lower than in cats (approximately 40%),[40] and large doses (volumes) are required for a clinical effect to be achieved;[41] therefore the usefulness of OTM buprenorphine is limited in this species, albeit present and similar to that in humans.

COST: Buprenorphine is considerably more expensive than morphine.

Agonist-Antagonists

Butorphanol*

DESCRIPTION: Butorphanol is a synthetic opioid believed to exert its effects mainly at κ receptors; it produces varying degrees of analgesia and sedation with minimal cardiopulmonary depression. Butorphanol binds to, but has minimal effect at, μ receptors and consequently is labeled a μ-receptor antagonist. At low doses the analgesic potency of butorphanol is about three times that of morphine; doses greater than about 0.8 to 1 mg/kg are associated with a ceiling effect, such that no further enhancement of analgesia (or AEs) occurs. The potency cannot be

---

*Butorphanol; Pfizer and West-ward Pharmaceutical Corp.

compared with that of morphine because of different maximal analgesic effects. Potency is defined as the relative dose to achieve a 50% maximal effect.

ANALGESIC EFFICACY: Butorphanol appears to be a less effective analgesic than morphine and other pure μ-agonist opioids. It demonstrates poor analgesia in a canine tail-clamp model;[42] therefore it appears to be more appropriate for mild to moderate and for visceral pain than for severe or somatic pain.

DURATION: The duration of analgesia from butorphanol is debatable and probably varies depending on the species, degree of pain, and route of administration. Some studies suggest a duration of visceral analgesia of less than an hour in dogs,[43] whereas others indicate a longer duration of up to 3 to 7 hours, particularly in cats.[44,45]

OTHER COMMENTS

1. Interaction of butorphanol with pure agonists:
   - Traditionally, it was thought that simultaneous or sequential administration of an agonist-antagonist such as butorphanol and a pure agonist such as oxymorphone or morphine would be counterproductive in that the agonist-antagonist may inhibit or even reverse the analgesic effects of the agonist.
   - However, studies examining the actual clinical effect reveal a variety of outcomes: no change in analgesia but a reduction in opioid AEs, reduction in analgesia and reduction in AEs, and improvement in analgesia with a reduction in AEs.
   - For example, in a feline study combining butorphanol with oxymorphone (0.05 to 0.1 mg/kg of each) in which a colonic balloon model was used for visceral pain, results included synergistic analgesia, minimal cardiopulmonary effects, and decreased excitement or dysphoria compared with oxymorphone alone.[4] This result suggested that a combination of an agonist-antagonist and a pure agonist may have advantages, particularly in species or individuals prone to opioid-induced dysphoria. However, in another feline study in which butorphanol was combined with hydromorphone, although duration of analgesia was enhanced, the intensity of analgesia was reduced.[46]

2. Butorphanol may partially antagonize the sedative or respiratory depressant effects of a pure μ-agonist such as morphine or oxymorphone, without completely removing analgesia. This technique is particularly useful for reversal of excessive sedation and restoration of laryngeal reflexes so that the animal can be extubated in recovery. For this purpose, butorphanol, 0.05 mg/kg, administered IV is generally safe and effective.

3. Butorphanol has been effectively used in combination with other drugs such as α$_2$-agonists and ketamine.

Nalbuphine*

DESCRIPTION: A κ-agonist and partial μ-antagonist, nalbuphine produces effects similar to those of butorphanol.

Continued

---

*Nalbuphine, nalbuphine HCl injection; Hospira, Inc.

OTHER COMMENTS

1. Cost: nalbuphine was once substantially less expensive than butorphanol, but more recently the cost differential has become less significant.
2. Nalbuphine is not on the DEA scheduled substance list because of its low abuse potential.
3. Partial antagonism of pure agonists: Nalbuphine, like butorphanol, may also be effective in partially antagonizing the sedative effects of a μ-agonist, at a dose of 0.1 to 0.5 mg/kg administered IV.
4. One recent study in humans reports success with repeated weekly injections in relieving animals previously suffering from refractory chronic pain.[47]

Pentazocine*

DESCRIPTION: Pentazocine is another κ-agonist and μ-antagonist similar to butorphanol and nalbuphine, producing mild analgesia of uncertain duration.

OTHER COMMENTS: Pentazocine appears to be less reliable than butorphanol or nalbuphine as a partial antagonist for other opioids. It is currently not in common veterinary use.

Antagonists

Opioid antagonists are often used to arouse animals that have sustained opioid overdose or are excessively sedated or obtunded from opioid administration. One should remember that use of opioid antagonists at customary doses will reverse both adverse and analgesic effects; for an animal that is potentially in pain, the result may be intense acute pain with accompanying and detrimental sympathetic stimulation. Therefore, opioid antagonists should be used conservatively and only with good reason in animals experiencing pain, and clinicians will have to decide if a partial μ-agonist (e.g., buprenorphine) or μ-antagonist/κ-agonist (e.g., butorphanol) might better provide the reversal of opioid AEs while maintaining some degree of analgesia. If bradycardia is the main opioid AE of concern, an anticholinergic such as atropine or glycopyrrolate should be used instead of an opioid antagonist to restore a normal heart rate without affecting individual comfort. Naloxone does not induce any effects when administered alone.

Naloxone[†] (Narcan)

DESCRIPTION: The prototypical μ-antagonist, naloxone effectively reverses the effects of an opioid agonist, causing increased alertness, responsiveness, and coordination, as well as increased awareness of pain if present.

DURATION: The duration of naloxone is shorter than that of many opioid agonists; an IV injection of naloxone, 0.01 mg/kg, lasts 20 to 40 minutes, whereas 0.04 mg/kg,

---

*Pentazocine (Talwin); Hospira, Inc.

[†]Naloxone, naloxone HCl injection; Hospira, Inc.

administered IM, lasts 40 to 70 minutes.[48] Therefore, animals should be watched for recurrence of opioid effects, including resedation, after a dose of naloxone.

OTHER COMMENTS

1. Excitement or anxiety may accompany naloxone reversal of the effects of an opioid agonist.
2. Although not common, cardiac dysrhythmias such as ventricular premature contractions can occur after naloxone reversal of the effects of an opioid, particularly if conditions favor high levels of circulating catecholamines.
3. In potentially painful situations (such as after surgery), the dose of naloxone should be greatly reduced and given in small increments—just to the point of arousal—to avoid precipitating a painful recovery. For this purpose, a total dose of 0.001 to 0.01 mg/kg IV may be sufficient.
4. Microdoses (0.004 mg/kg) of the μ-antagonist naloxone added to patient-controlled analgesia (PCA) have diminished opioid-associated adverse events.[49] In humans, microdoses as low as 0.01 to 0.05 μg/kg (0.00001 to 0.00005 mg/kg) of naloxone IV have been used to improve the analgesia provided by buprenorphine.[50]
   - Such medications hold great promise in minimizing constipation and other peripheral AEs, which commonly force the withholding of opioids.[51]
   - The mechanism appears to be preferential binding to stimulatory G protein (G_{stim}), while not binding to G_1 protein. This permits the standard opioid analgesic activity while inhibiting any neural excitatory activity.

Nalmefene*

DESCRIPTION: An opioid antagonist approximately four times as potent as naloxone.

DURATION: Nalmefene works as quickly as naloxone but its duration of action is approximately 1 to 2 hours[52] (about twice that of naloxone). In one study, it more completely returned dogs to a normal (nonsedated) state after oxymorphone administration.[53] Therefore, nalmefene may be advantageous in preventing recurrence of undesirable opioid effects when it is used to antagonize a long-acting opioid.

OTHER COMMENTS: Dosages for animals have not been well established, but in humans, dosages may vary from 0.25 to 30 μg/kg. Nalmefene is not currently available in United States.

Naltrexone†

DESCRIPTION: Another pure opioid antagonist, about four times more potent than naloxone.

Continued

---

*Nalmefene (Revex).

†Naltrexone (Revia); Teva Women's Health, Inc.

DURATION: In humans the duration is about twice that of naloxone, but in dogs, pharmacokinetic studies suggest that naltrexone is not much longer-acting than naloxone.[54]

OTHER COMMENTS

1. Based on these findings, a dose of 0.0025 mg/kg IV should effectively antagonize a pure agonist for approximately 2 hours.

2. Methylnaltrexone appears to have the ability to reverse peripheral opioid AEs while allowing the central pain-modifying effect of μ-agonists to remain. In humans, the SC-administered Relistor (Salix Pharmaceuticals, Inc.) is labeled for the prevention and treatment of opioid-induced constipation.

CLINICAL USE OF OPIOIDS

Systemic

Acute Pain

- *Perioperatively:* Opioids are administered systemically preoperatively, intraoperatively, and postoperatively. Preoperatively in animals without preexisting pain, opioids may be administered on the low end of the dosage range.

- *Post-trauma:* Early and aggressive intervention for pain, including the use of systemic opioids, is increasingly recognized as a critical component to reducing morbidity, mortality, and the incidence or severity of chronic, exaggerated pain states after severe trauma. In animals with preexisting pain, opioids may be administered on the mid to higher end of the dosage range.

Chronic Pain

Systemic (generally orally administered) opioids may play a selective but important role in the management of chronic pain conditions in animals. Indications may include the following:

- Cancer (especially osteosarcoma or other bone metastasis)
- Palliative end-of-life care
- Breakthrough acute-on-chronic pain conditions such as intervertebral disk disease and a variety of maladaptive pain states (e.g., complex regional pain syndrome)

Regional or Local Administration

Epidural

- Epidural administration of morphine is widely practiced in a variety of species, including dogs, cats, and horses.

- Morphine, 0.1 mg/kg, administered epidurally provides analgesia with fewer side effects than systemically administered morphine.
  1. Onset: Approximately 30 to 60 minutes in small animals; longer in horses.
  2. Duration: Approximately 18 to 24 hours.
- Preservative-free morphine is recommended because preservatives may be neurotoxic. However, in horses and other large animals, preservative-containing morphine is typically used but is diluted with sterile physiologic saline.

Intra-articular

- Trauma or inflammation up-regulates opioid receptors on synovial nociceptive nerve terminals and/or inflammatory cells (possibly μ_3 receptors).
- Morphine instilled into joints at the end of surgery reportedly provides up to 6 to 18 hours of analgesia, with doses of 0.1 mg/kg diluted with saline to a volume of 0.1 to 0.5 mL/kg.[55,56]
- Based on human studies, application of a tourniquet proximal to the joint is recommended for 10 minutes after injection but is rarely done in veterinary practice.
- Intra-articular morphine administration may be combined with a local anesthetic such as bupivacaine for enhanced analgesia.

Topical Application on Cornea

- Results are conflicting regarding efficacy of topical opioids on corneal pain in dogs, and these agents have not been evaluated in other animal species.
- In one study a specially prepared, pH-controlled 1% morphine sulfate solution was applied to experimentally induced corneal ulcers in dogs and was associated with decreased pain behaviors (reduced blepharospasm and lower esthesiometer readings) without affecting healing.[57]
- Other studies with topical morphine[58] and nalbuphine[59] have demonstrated disappointing analgesic effects on corneal pain in dogs.

Adjunct to Local Anesthetics

- Studies in humans reveal that adding small amounts of opioids can double or triple the duration of local anesthetics.
- Reported doses of opioids added to local anesthetics to extend duration vary but include morphine, 0.075 mg/kg,[60] and buprenorphine, 0.003 mg/kg[61] to 0.04 mg/kg.[62]

SUSTAINED-RELEASE AND EXTENDED-DURATION PARENTERAL OPIOIDS

There is increasing interest in sustained-release and/or long-acting parenteral opioid formulations and technologies for use in humans and animals,

---

BOX 9-2 **Parenteral Opioid Sustained-Release Technologies**

Transdermal
- Patches
  - Reservoir gel
    - Fentanyl (Duragesic, generic)
  - Non–gel matrix systems
    - Buprenorphine (Butrans, Transtec, Buprederm)
    - Fentanyl (generic, Mylan, Sandoz)
  - Iontophoretic
    - Fentanyl (IONOSYS)
- Transdermal solution: Recuvyra (not injectable)

Injectable Subcutaneous
- Liposome encapsulated
  - Oxymorphone, hydromorphone, morphine
  - No commercial products at this time
- Sustained-release polymer
  - Buprenorphine

---

one of which has recently received U.S. Food and Drug Administration (FDA) approval in dogs; others are under current investigation (Box 9-2). The technologies are generally divided between transdermal (reservoir and non–gel matrix) patches and injectable applications (liposome-encapsulated [LE] agents and sustained-released polymers). A third technology, iontophoresis, uses electrical current to deliver drugs transdermally; the only FDA-approved product in humans (IONSYS, for fentanyl administration as a patient-controlled delivery system) has been plagued by technical problems and has been withdrawn from the market. A fourth, novel transdermal technology has recently been added to the veterinary market.

Reservoir Patches

Reservoir patch technology places the opioid in a gel that transverses a semipermeable membrane via concentration gradient into the stratum corneum of the skin.

Fentanyl

Fentanyl has been available in the United States as a transdermal reservoir gel patch delivery system* since 2005, labeled in humans for breakthrough cancer pain, and has been studied (and used off-label) in dogs, cats, and rabbits. Results have demonstrated usefulness in these species[63,64] but also wide variability in serum concentrations.[65–67] Variability is probably further enhanced by body location on which applied, body condition, body or ambient temperature,

---

*Duragesic patch; Ortho-McNeil-Janssen Pharmaceuticals, Inc.

quality of adhesiveness, and more. An additional concern with this technology is human exposure to the reservoir, which is not only easily divertible for illicit use, but also potentially dangerous, possibly causing death when ingested (and to which children have been susceptible). Furthermore, the far off-label use in veterinary medicine raises concerns with regards to practitioner liability in the event of an adverse event or human exposure.

DOSAGE: 2 to 4 µg/kg/hr.
1. Patch sizes: 25, 50, 75, or 100 µg/hr.
2. For very small animals, remove the backing from only a portion of the patch that represents an appropriate dose (e.g., for a 4-kg cat, use a 25-µg/hr patch with only half the backing removed, resulting in a dose of 12.5 µg/hr, or 3.125 µg/kg/hr).

APPLICATION
1. Site is the back of the neck or shoulders, lateral thorax, or metatarsus.
2. Clip hair; clean skin with water only.
3. Apply patch and hold firmly in place for at least 2 minutes.
4. Apply a bandage over the patch.
5. Because this product is not labeled for use in veterinary medicine, it does not come with warnings against human exposure, and it can be argued that historical use by veterinarians and staff has been cavalier in this regard. Customary safety measures against human precautions should be taken including wearing of personal protective equipment when handling, segregating the pet from children during and after the pet wears the patch, proper disposal as hazardous waste, and so on.
6. Use of Duragesic patches in dogs and cats may now be supplanted by other long-acting opioid preparations (see Recuvyra and buprenorphine SR, respectively, below).

ONSET: 12 hours (cats), 24 hours (dogs).
DURATION: 72 to 104 hours.

Non–Gel Matrix Patches

Non–gel matrix patch technology embeds the opioid into the adhesive itself; the drug is then continually released into the skin.

Fentanyl in a generic matrix patch was approved for administration in humans in 2005 (Mylan Pharmaceuticals, Technologies). The use, safety, pharmacokinetics, and pharmacodynamics have not been studied in dogs and cats.

Buprenorphine as a matrix transdermal patch has been available in Europe since 2001 (Transtec, Grünenthal), and was approved by the FDA (Butrans, Purdue Pharma) in 2010. Rabbits and rodents achieved rapid plasma levels (1 to 24 hours), with peak analgesic activity with the tail-flick and writhing model at 3 to 4 hours and sustained for 72 hours of the study.[68] However, in one feline study using a 35-µg/hr patch, plasma levels were negligible and there were no changes in thermal thresholds.[69] The experience in dogs is somewhat better. In one canine study, use of a 70-μg/hr patch resulted in sustained plasma concentrations of 0.7 to 1.8 ng/mL within 36 hours of application.[70] Another canine study that used a 52.5-μg/hr patch found peak plasma levels of 1.54 ng/mL; analgesic efficacy was found to be noninferior to that of intravenous buprenorphine in mechanical and thermal thresholds within 36 hours of application, and analgesic effects lasted until the patch was removed. However, there was some inconsistency because 3 of the 10 dogs had recorded negligible plasma levels.[71] An additional clinical canine study found the 70-μg/kg patch to be noninferior to subcutaneous buprenorphine after ovariohysterectomy.[72]

Topical Transdermal Solution

Transdermal technology combines the opioid with a solvent and penetration enhancer, driving drug into the skin and allowing slow release into circulation from that site.

Fentanyl

In 2012 the FDA approved a novel transdermal fentanyl product for perioperative soft-tissue and orthopedic surgical pain in dogs. Recuvyra uses a liquefied drying agent and solvent (isopropyl alcohol) and a penetration enhancer (octyl salicylate, also used in sunscreen). When the solution is applied to the skin via a patented device, the fentanyl is delivered into the stratum corneum. There it forms a depot for slow release by passive diffusion into circulation; 99% penetration from the surface of the skin occurs within 2 to 4 minutes. The time to maximum concentration (T_{max}) is 13.6 hours. From there this product exhibits "flip-flop" kinetics: the rate of absorption is slower than the rate of elimination. Studies demonstrate analgesic plasma levels and effects for 2 hours to 4 days, and a large study found it noninferior to buprenorphine administered IM every 6 hours.[73] Administration instructions are very specific because of the highly concentrated nature of the product (50 mg/mL; 1000 times more concentrated than current commercial product). The product overcomes some of the disadvantages or limitations of other forms of sustained opioid administration, including Duragesic patch, constant rate IV infusions, and repeat parenteral dosing.

> **DOSAGE:** 2.7 mg/kg; dogs only.
> **APPLICATION**
> 1. Site is the back, between shoulder blades.
> 2. Special applicator tip comes as unit with syringe, must be in contact with skin.
> 3. To be administered only in hospital; administrator should wear personal protective equipment.

4. Maximum of 0.5 mL/site; if dose requires additional sites, they should be 1 inch apart until entire dose administered.
5. Administrator should restrain animal for 2 minutes; contact with administration site should be avoided for 72 hours, including isolation from children, and hands washed if occurs.

ONSET: 2 to 3 hours.
DURATION: 4 days.
COMMENTS

1. Sedation or inappetance may be seen as with other opioids at standard doses, but for longer periods of time. Dose attenuation may help minimize frequency and severity of such events, but efficacy and duration have not yet been established for below-label dosing.
2. Reversal, if required (as in the case of accidental overdose), is accomplished with naloxone 40 µg/kg (0.04 mg/kg) IM administered PRN (usually every 1 to 2 hours) until AEs resolve (will also reverse analgesic effects). Off-label, some clinicians may use naltrexone every 3 to 4 hours, nalmefene, or butorphanol to reverse the µ-agonism.
3. Transdermal absorption does not occur in humans, so contact with the application site is not known to be problematic after the initial application period; however, skin-to–mucous membrane (e.g., licking fingers after contact, as might occur with children) may lead to systemic absorption of fentanyl, and consultation with a physician is recommended in this instance.
4. Contraindications: on sites other than between shoulder blades, other species besides dogs, on abnormal skin, dogs with paralytic ileus, repeat doses, hypovolemic or debilitated dogs, and dogs with known hypersensitivity to fentanyl.

Sustained-Release Polymers

Opioids and other drugs can be combined with water-insoluble polymers; when injected SC, this mixture precipitates as a reservoir that degrades while slowly releasing the active drug. Buprenorphine is available in a compounded (non–FDA approved) sustained-release formulation. Unpublished pharmacokinetic (PK) data in dogs report plasma levels adequate for analgesia for over 72 hours,[74] but there are anecdotal reports of prolonged and in some cases dramatic sedation, especially at the higher end of the dosage range in larger dogs.[75] Unpublished PK data in cats report superior maintenance of plasma levels adequate for analgesia over 3 days when compared with repeated OTM administration.[76,77] One published pharmacodynamic (PD) study in cats found SR buprenorphine to be noninferior to every 12 hours OTM administration for 3 days after ovariohysterectomy, with minimal AEs.[78] Similar positive outcomes have been observed in unpublished studies with non-human primates[79] and rodents,[80] and in one published rat study.[81]

Liposome-Encapsulated Formulations

LE opioids are injected SC; they are sequestered in the liver and slowly released into circulation as the lipid is metabolized.

In animals, the efficacy, durability, and tolerability of LE hydromorphone have been demonstrated in dogs, with adequate serum levels up to 4 days[82] and superior analgesic effect 12 hours after ovariohysterectomy compared with subcutaneous morphine.[83] This same formulation, route, and dose demonstrated favorable pharmacokinetics and tolerability in rhesus macaques when compared with subcutaneous or intravenous hydromorphone.[84] Similar studies with LE oxymorphone and hydromorphone have been performed in laboratory animals, demonstrating durability, tolerability, and effectiveness (rhesus macaques[85] and rodents[86-88]). No commercial subcutaneous LE opioid product is available on the market; current formulations are expensive to manufacture and have poor shelf-lives, but efforts are under way to overcome these shortcomings. However, a stable, preservative-free multivesicular LE morphine product has been approved by the FDA for epidural use in humans (DepoDur) and is designed to provide analgesia for 48 hours.

ORAL OPIOIDS

Commercial oral opioid preparations are widely available, and although dogs exhibit a robust first-pass effect limiting bioavailability,[17] these drugs are not without usefulness. Hydrocodone, codeine (both alone and in combination with acetaminophen), hydromorphone (Dilaudid), and sustained-released forms of oral opioids including morphine (MS Contin), oxycodone (Oxy-Contin), and oxymorphone (Opana ER)[89] are all available by prescription. PK data exist for some of these formulations,[90-94] but PD (efficacy) data are currently lacking in dogs and cats.

- Oral morphine is less than 20% bioavailable in the dog, and the per-rectal route appears to offer no advantage over the oral route.[95] However, one study investigating oral morphine incorporated into a polymer granule formulation to protect from gastric acidity revealed high bioavailability in dogs.[96]
- Oral hydrocodone in dogs has approximately 50% of the bioavailability found in humans.[94] Oral codeine in dogs does not significantly metabolize to morphine as it does in humans; however, dogs do produce another μ-agonist metabolite, codeine-6-glucoronide, in significant quantities,[93] and this metabolite is thought to render an analgesic effect in this species.[97]
- Oral hydrocodone doses are reported at 0.22 to 0.5 mg/kg, and codeine at approximately 1 mg/kg.[98] When used in combination with commercially available generic acetaminophen products (in *dogs only*), however, these opioid doses would result in very high doses of the acetaminophen; thus acetaminophen-opioid combinations are usually calculated on the basis of the acetaminophen dose (10 to 15 mg/kg PO bid or tid).[98]

- The usefulness of highly potent oral opioids such as oxycodone and oxymorphone in veterinary medicine is not established, and their use might be discouraged because of high human abuse potential and risks of diversion.
- Oral methadone appears to have low oral bioavailability (<20%, compared with >70% in humans) and rapid clearance in dogs.[99] In humans, the sedative effect is far more prolonged than the analgesic effect, and this, in addition to the cardiac irregularities attributed to methadone, have contributed to many accidental deaths.[100] At this time, until more is understood about the pharmacokinetics and pharmacodynamics of oral methadone in dogs, its use cannot be recommended in veterinary medicine.
- Tramadol has also become a popular adjunct to pain management in humans because of its effectiveness as a weak synthetic opioid and as a norepinephrine and serotonin (inhibitory neurotransmitters) agonist. It is increasingly popular in veterinary medicine as well.
  - However, conversion to the active μ-agonist M1 metabolite appears to be minimal in the dog (with per-rectal administration offering no advantage in this regard),[101-103] indicating that most of its activity and increasingly established usefulness in this species are likely derived from its serotoninergic and noradrenergic, rather than opioid, activity.
  - In contradistinction, cats do appear to manufacture the M1 metabolite with a sustained half-life,[104] qualifying this agent as an opioid in this species, and the clinical usefulness as an adjunct to nonsteroidal anti-inflammatory drugs (NSAIDs) during ovariohysterectomy has been established.[105]
  - Tapentadol (Nucytna) is a new centrally acting analgesic with a dual mode of action similar to that of tramadol: μ-opioid receptor agonism and inhibition of norepinephrine reuptake. Unlike tramadol, however, it is the parent compound, not a metabolite, that provides both of these effects, and thus this agent may offer an alternative superior to tramadol in dogs. Unfortunately, recent data from the United States reveal that in dogs this drug has low oral bioavailability,[106] and one evaluation revealed poor performance on a tail-flick model of evaluation of analgesic effect.[107] Its future usefulness in veterinary medicine is unknown.
  - Tramadol (and tapentadol) should be used only cautiously in combination with other serotoninergic or monoaminergic medications such as tricyclic antidepressants, serotonin-norepinephrine reuptake inhibitors (SNRIs), amitraz-containing compounds, and selegiline.

ORAL TRANSMUCOSAL OPIOIDS

Commercial opioid OTM preparations are FDA approved in humans for breakthrough (cancer) pain and addiction, but pharmacokinetics and pharmacodynamics in dogs and cats are not established, and the usefulness of many agents in animals is limited by the drugs' delivery systems.

- Examples include fentanyl buccal tablets and suckers (Actiq, Fentora) for breakthrough (cancer) pain and buprenorphine for addiction (Suboxone, in a 4:1 buprenorphine:naloxone combination, and Subutex). Fentanyl is also available as an OTM sublingual spray (Subsys) and intranasal spray (Lazanda), although there are no data in the literature to validate either PK or PD of these preparations in dogs or cats.
- Clinical usefulness of OTM administration of injectable buprenorphine is established in cats. Analgesic effects of OTM buprenorphine can also be achieved in dogs, but the doses and volumes are so high that it may preclude practical usefulness. (See earlier discussion of buprenorphine.)
- In cats, one study does illustrate favorable bioavailability of OTM-administered injectable methadone.[108]

REFERENCES

1. Barkin RL, Iusco M, Barkin SJ. Opioids used in primary care for the management of pain: A pharmacologic, pharmacotherapeutic, and pharmacodynamics overview.
   In: Boswell MV, Cole BE (Eds.). Weiner's pain management: A practical guide for clinicians, ed. 7. Boca Raton, Fla., 2006, Taylor & Francis.
2. Sacerdote P. Opioids and the immune system. Palliat Med. 2006; 20 Suppl 1:s9–15.
3. Epstein ME. Opioids: A practical guide and new developments. North American Veterinary Conference, 2012.
4. Briggs SL, Sneed K, Sawyer DC. Antinociceptive effects of oxymorphone-butorphanol-acepromazine combination in cats. Vet Surg. 1998; 27:466–472.
5. Scotto di Fazano C, Vergne P, et al. Preventive therapy for nausea and vomiting in patients on opioid therapy for non-malignant pain in rheumatology. Therapie. 2002; 57:446–449.
6. Stern LC, Palmisano MP. Frequency of vomiting during the postoperative period in hydromorphone-treated dogs undergoing orthopedic surgery. J Am Vet Med Assoc. 2012; 241(3):344–347.
7. Porreca F, Ossipov MH. Nausea and vomiting side effects with opioid analgesics during treatment of chronic pain: mechanisms, implications, and management options. Pain Med. 2009; 10(4):654–662.
8. Wilson DV, Evans AT, Miller R. Effects of preanesthetic administration of morphine on gastroesophageal reflux and regurgitation during anesthesia in dogs. Am J Vet Res. 2005; 66(3):386–390.
9. Wilson DV, Walshaw R. Postanesthetic esophageal dysfunction in 13 dogs. J Am Anim Hosp Assoc. 2004; 40(6):455–460.
10. Niedfeldt RL, Robertson SA. Post anesthetic hyperthermia in cats: A retrospective comparison between hydromorphone and buprenorphine. Vet Anaesth Analg. 2006; 3 (6):341–342.
11. Robertson SA. Pain management in the cat. In: Gaynor JS, Muir WM (Eds.). Handbook of veterinary pain management. St. Louis, 2009, Mosby.
12. Laviolette SR, Van Der Kooy D. GABA$_A$ receptors in the ventral tegmental area control bidirectional reward signalling between dopaminergic and non-dopaminergic neural motivational systems. Eur J Neurosci. 2001; 13(5):1009–1015.
13. Low Y, Clarke CF, Huh BK. Opioid-induced hyperalgesia: A review of epidemiology, mechanisms and management. Singapore Med J. 2012; 53(5):357.

14. Lee M, Silverman S, Hansen H, et al. A comprehensive review of opioid-induced hyperalgesia. Pain Physician. 2011; 14:145–161.

15. Taylor PM, Robertson SA. Morphine, pethidine and buprenorphine disposition in the cat, J Vet Pharmacol Therap. 2001; 24:391–398.

16. Robertson SA, Taylor PM, Lascelles BD, Dixon MJ. Changes in thermal threshold response in eight cats after administration of buprenorphine, butorphanol and morphine. Vet Rec. 2003; 153(15):462–465.

17. KuKanich B, Lascelles BD, Papich MG. Pharmacokinetics of morphine and plasma concentrations of morphine-6-glucuronide following morphine administration to dogs. J Vet Pharmacol Ther. 2005; 28(4):371–376.

18. KuKanich B, Lascelles BD, Papich MG. Use of a von Frey device for evaluation of pharmacokinetics and pharmacodynamics of morphine after intravenous administration as an infusion or multiple doses in dogs. Am J Vet Res. 2005; 66(11):1968–1974.

19. Lucas AN, Firth AM, Anderson GA, et al. Comparison of the effects of morphine administered by constant-rate intravenous infusion or intermittent intramuscular injection in dogs. J Am Vet Med Assoc. 2001; 218(6):884–891.

20. Guedes AG, Papich MG, Rude EP, Rider MA. Pharmacokinetics and physiological effects of intravenous hydromorphone in conscious dogs. J Vet Pharmacol Ther. 2008; 31 (4):334–343.

21. KuKanich B, Hogan BK, Krugner-Higby LA, Smith LJ. Pharmacokinetics of hydromorphone hydrochloride in healthy dogs. Vet Anaesth Analg. 2008; 35 (3):256–264.

22. Wegner K, Roberston SA, Kollias-Baker C, et al. Pharmacokinetic and pharmacodynamic evaluation of intravenous hydromorphone in cats. J Vet Pharmacol Therap 2004; 27:329–336.

23. Wegner K, Robertson JA. Dose-related thermal antinociceptive effects of intravenous hydromorphone in cats. Vet Anaesth Analg. 2007; 34(2):132–138.

24. Guedes AG, Papich MG, Rude EP, Rider MA. Comparison of plasma histamine levels after intravenous administration of hydromorphone and morphine in dogs. J Vet Pharmacol Ther. 2007; 30(6):516–522.

25. KuKanich B, Schmidt BK, Krugner-Higby LA, et al. Pharmacokinetics and behavioral effects of oxymorphone after intravenous and subcutaneous administration to healthy dogs. J Vet Pharmacol Ther. 2008; 31(6):580–583.

26. Siao KT, Pypendop BH, Stanley SD, Ilkiw JE. Pharmacokinetics of oxymorphone in cats. J Vet Pharmacol Ther. 2011; 34(6):594–598.

27. Robinson EP, Faggella AM, Henry DP, Russell WL. Comparison of histamine release induced by morphine and oxymorphone administration in dogs. Am J Vet Res. 1988; 49 (10):1699–1701.

28. Ingvast-Larsson C, Holgersson A, Bondesson U, et al. Clinical pharmacology of methadone in dogs. Vet Anaesth Analg. 2010; 37(1):48–56.

29. Ferreira TH, Rezende ML, Mama KR, et al. Plasma concentrations and behavioral, antinociceptive, and physiologic effects of methadone after intravenous and oral transmucosal administration in cats. Am J Vet Res. 2011; 72(6):764–771.

30. Erichsen HK, Hao JX, Xu XJ, Blackburn-Munro G. Comparative actions of the opioid analgesics morphine, methadone, and codeine in rat models of peripheral and central neuropathic pain. J Pain. 2005; 116(3):347–358.

31. KuKanich B, Borum SL. The disposition and behavioral effects of methadone in Greyhounds. Vet Anaesth Analg. 2008; 35(3):242–248.

32. Steagall PV, Carnicelli P, Taylor PM. Effects of subcutaneous methadone, morphine, buprenorphine or saline on thermal and pressure thresholds in cats. J Vet Pharmacol Ther. 2006; 29(6):531–537.

33. Ritschel WA, Neub M, Denson DD. Meperidine pharmacokinetics following intravenous, peroral, and buccal administration in beagle dogs. Methods Find Exp Clin Pharmacol. 1987; 12:811–815.

34. Slingsby LS, Taylor PM, Murrell JC. A study to evaluate buprenorphine at 40 µg kg(-1) compared to 20 µg kg(-1) as a post-operative analgesic in the dog. Vet Anaesth Analg. 2011; 38(6):584–593.

35. Steagall PV, Pelligand L, Giordano T, et al. Pharmacokinetic and pharmacodynamic modelling of intravenous, intramuscular and subcutaneous buprenorphine in conscious cats. Vet Anaesth Analg. 2013; 40(1):83–95.

36. Steagall PV, Mantovani FB, Taylor PM, et al. Dose-related antinociceptive effects of intravenous buprenorphine in cats. Vet J. 2009; 182(2):203–209.

37. Lascelles BD, Robertson SA, Taylor PM, et al. Proceedings of the 27th Annual Meeting of the American College of Veterinary Anesthesiologists. Orlando, Florida, October 2002.

38. Robertson SA, Taylor PM, Sear JW. Systemic uptake of buprenorphine by cats after oral mucosal administration. Vet Rec. 2003; 152(22):675–678.

39. Giordano T, Steagall PV, Ferriera TH, et al. Postoperative analgesic effects of intravenous, intramuscular, subcutaneous or oral transmucosal buprenorphine administered to cats undergoing ovariohysterectomy. Vet Anaesth Anal. 2010; 37 (4):357–366.

40. Abbo LA, Ko JC, Maxwell LK, et al. Pharmacokinetics of buprenorphine following intravenous and oral transmucosal administration in dogs. Vet Ther. 2008; 9(2):83–93.

41. Ko JC, Freeman LJ, Barletta M, et al. Efficacy of oral transmucosal and intravenous administration of buprenorphine before surgery for postoperative analgesia in dogs undergoing ovariohysterectomy. J Am Vet Med Assoc. 2011; 238(3):318–328.

42. Grimm KA, Tranquilli WJ, Thurmon JC, et al. Duration of nonresponse to noxious stimulation after intramuscular administration of butorphanol, medetomidine, or a butorphanol-medetomidine combination during isoflurane administration in dogs. Am J Vet Res. 2000; 61(1):42–47.

43. Sawyer DC, Rech RH, Durham RA, et al. Dose response to butorphanol administered subcutaneously to increase visceral nociceptive threshold in dogs. Am J Vet Res. 1991; 52 (11):1826–1830.

44. Wells SM, Glerum LE, Papich MG. Pharmacokinetics of butorphanol in cats after intramuscular and buccal transmucosal administration. Am J Vet Res. 2008; 69 (12):1548–1554.

45. Johnson JA, Robertson SA, Pypendop BH. Antinociceptive effects of butorphanol, buprenorphine, or both, administered intramuscularly in cats. Am J Vet Res. 2007; 68 (7):699–703.

46. Lascelles BDX, Robertson SA. Antinociceptive effects of hydromorphone, butorphanol, or the combination in cats. J Vet Intern Med. 2004; 18:190–195.

47. Howard JS. Nalbuphine in the successful long-term daily management of chronic severe pain: A first report. Am J Pain Manag. 2006; 16(1):29–33.

48. Copland VS, Haskins SC, Patz J. Naloxone reversal of oxymorphone effects in dogs. Am J Vet Res. 1989; 50(11):1854–1858.

49. Cepeda MS, Alvarez H, Morales O, et al. Addition of ultralow dose naloxone to postoperative morphine PCA: Unchanged analgesia and opioid requirements but decreased incidence of opioid side effects. Pain. 2004; 107:41–46.

50. LaVincenta SF, White JM, Somogyi AA, et al. Enhanced buprenorphine analgesia with the addition of ultra-low-dose naloxone in healthy subjects. Clin Pharm Ther. 2008; 83:144–152.

51. Gervitz C. Update on the management of opioid-induced constipation. Top Pain Manag. 2007; 23(3):1–5.

52. Veng-Pedersen P, Wilhelm JA, Zakszewski TB, et al. Duration of opioid antagonism by nalmefene and naloxone in the dog: An integrated pharmacokinetic/pharmacodynamic comparison. J Pharm Sci. 1995; 84:1101–1106.

53. Dyson DH, Doherty T, Anderson GI, et al. Reversal of oxymorphone sedation by naloxone, nalmefene, and butorphanol. Vet Surg. 1990; 19:398–403.

54. Li H, Zhao SF, Wang N, Ge ZH. [Pharmacokinetics of naltrexone hydrochloride and naltrexone glucuronide in the dog]. Yao Xue Xue Bao. 1996; 31(4):254–257. [Article in Chinese].

55. Day TK, Pepper WT, Tobias TA, et al. Comparison of intra-articular and epidural morphine for analgesia following stifle arthrotomy in dogs. Vet Surg. 1995; 24 (6):522–530.

56. Sammarco JL, Conzemius MG, Perkowski SZ, et al. Postoperative analgesia for stifle surgery: A comparison of intra-articular bupivacaine, morphine, or saline. Vet Surg. 1996; 25(1):59–69.

57. Stiles J, Honda CN, Krohne SG, Kazacos EA. Effect of topical administration of 1% morphine sulfate solution on signs of pain and corneal wound healing in dogs. Am J Vet Res. 2003; 64:813–818.

58. Thomson S, Oliver J, Gould D, et al. Preliminary investigations into the analgesic efficacy of topical ocular morphine in dogs and cats. Proceedings. British Small Animal Veterinary Congess: 2010.

59. Clark JS, Bentley E, Smith LJ. Evaluation of topical nalbuphine or oral tramadol as analgesics for corneal pain in dogs: A pilot study. Vet Ophthalmol. 2011; 14(6):358–364.

60. Bazin JE, Massoni C, Bruelle P, et al. The addition of opioids to local anesthetics in brachial plexus block: The comparative effects of morphine, buprenorphine, and sufentanil. Anaesthesia. 1997; 52(9):858–862.

61. Candido KD, Winnie AP, Ghaleb AH, et al. Buprenorphine added to the local anesthetic for axillary brachial plexus block prolongs postoperative analgesia. Reg Anesth Pain Med. 2002; 27(2):162–167.

62. Modi M, Rastogi S. Buprenorphine with bupivacaine for intraoral nerve blocks to provide postoperative analgesia in outpatients after minor oral surgery. J Oral Maxillofac Surg. 2009; 67:2571–2576.

63. Kyles AE, Hardie EM, Hansen BD, Papich MG. Comparison of transdermal fentanyl and intramuscular oxymorphone on post-operative behaviour after ovariohysterectomy in dogs. Res Vet Sci. 1998; 65(3):245–251.

64. Glerum LE, Egger CM, Allen SW, Haag M. Analgesic effect of the transdermal fentanyl patch during and after feline ovariohysterectomy. Vet Surg. 2001; 30(4):351–358.

65. Egger CM. Plasma fentanyl concentrations in awake cats and cats undergoing anesthesia and ovariohysterectomy using transdermal administration. Vet Anaesth Analg. 2003; 30:229–236.

66. Kyles AE, Papich M, Hardie EM. Disposition of transdermally administered fentanyl in dogs. Am J Vet Res. 1996; 57:715–719.

67. Lee DD, Papich MG, Hardie EM. Comparison of pharmacokinetics of fentanyl after intravenous and transdermal administration in cats. Am J Vet Res. 2000; 61(6):672–677.

68. Park I, Kim D, Song J, et al. Buprederm, a new transdermal delivery system of buprenorphine: Pharmacokinetic, efficacy and skin irritancy studies. Pharm Res. 2008; 25 (5):1052–1062.

69. Murrell JC, Robertson SA, Taylor PM, et al. Use of a transdermal matrix patch of buprenorphine in cats: Preliminary pharmacokinetic and pharmacodynamic data. Vet Rec. 2007; 160(17):578–583.

70. Andaluz A, Moll X, Ventrua R, et al. Plasma buprenorphine concentrations after the application of a 70-ug/h transdermal patch in dogs. Preliminary report. J Vet Pharmacol Ther. 2009; 32:503–505

71. Pieper K, Schuster T, Levionnois O, et al. Antinociceptive efficacy and plasma concentrations of transdermal buprenorphine in dogs. Vet J. 2011; 187(3):335–341.

72. Moll X, Fresno L, Garcia F, et al. Comparison of subcutaneous and transdermal administration of buprenorphine for preemptive analgesia in dogs undergoing elective ovariohysterectomy. Vet J. 2011; 187(1):124–128.

73. Linton DD, Wilson MG, Newbound GC, et al. The effectiveness of a long-acting transdermal fentanyl solution compared to buprenorphine for the control of postoperative pain in dogs in a randomized, multicentered clinical study. J Vet Pharmacol Ther. 2012; 35:53–64.

74. SR Veterinary Technologies. Buprenorphine. 2010. Retrieved from www.wildpharm. com/documents/Buprenorphine_info_sheet.pdf.

75. Veterinary Information Network Anesthesia & Analgesia Message Boards. International Veterinary Academy of Pain Management Listserve Forum.

76. SR Veterinary Technologies. Comparison of sustained-release buprenorphine and transmucosal buprenorphine in cats. Clin Res Bull. 2011.

77. SR Veterinary Technologies. Irritability and pharmacokinetics of two sustained release buprenorphine formulations (buprenorphine HCl SR TRI and buprenorphine HCl SR NMP) in cats. 2012.

78. Catbagan DL, Quimby JM, Mama KR, et al. Comparison of the efficacy and adverse effects of sustained-release buprenorphine hydrochloride following subcutaneous administration and buprenorphine hydrochloride following oral transmucosal administration in cats undergoing ovariohysterectomy. Am J Vet Res. 2011; 72(4):461–466.

79. Wildlife Pharmaceuticals: http://wildpharm.com/about-wildpharm.html.

80. SR Veterinary Technologies. Pharmacokinetic properties of novel sustained release buprenorphine and meloxicam formulations in rats. Clin Res Bull. 2011.

81. Foley PL, Liang H, Crichlow AR. Evaluation of a sustained-release formulation of buprenorphine for analgesia in rats. J Am Assoc Lab Anim Sci. 2011; 50(2):198–204.

82. Smith LJ, KuKanich B, Hogan BK, et al. Pharmacokinetics of a controlled-release liposome-encapsulated hydromorphone administered to healthy dogs. J Vet Pharmacol Ther. 2008; 31(5):415–422.

83. Krugner-Higby L, Smith L, Schmidt B, et al. Experimental pharmacodynamics and analgesic efficacy of liposome-encapsulated hydromorphone in dogs. J Am Anim Hosp Assoc. 2011; 47:185–195.

84. Krugner-Higby L, KuKanich B, Schmidt B, et al. Pharmacokinetics and behavioral effects of liposomal hydromorphone suitable for perioperative use in rhesus macaques. Psychopharmacology (Berl). 2011; 216(4):511–523.

85. Krugner-Higby L, KuKanich B, Schmidt B, et al. Pharmacokinetics and behavioral effects of an extended-release, liposome-encapsulated preparation of oxymorphone in rhesus macaques. J Pharmacol Exp Ther. 2009; 330(1):135–141.

86. Krugner-Higby L, Smith L, Clark M, et al. Liposome-encapsulated oxymorphone hydrochloride provides prolonged relief of postsurgical visceral pain in rats. Comp Med. 2003; 53(3):270–279.

87. Clark MD, Krugner-Higby L, Smith LJ, et al. Evaluation of liposome-encapsulated oxymorphone hydrochloride in mice after splenectomy. Comp Med. 2004; 54 (5):558–563.

88. Smith LJ, Krugner-Higby L, Clark M, et al. A single dose of liposome-encapsulated oxymorphone or morphine provides long-term analgesia in an animal model of neuropathic pain. Comp Med. 2003; 53(3):280–287.

89. Matsumoto AK. Oral extended-release oxymorphone: a new choice for chronic pain relief. Expert Opinion Pharmacother. 2007; 8(10):1515–1527.

90. Aragon CL, Read MR, Gaynor JS, et al. Pharmacokinetics of an immediate and extended release oral morphine formulation utilizing the spheroidal oral drug absorption system in dogs. J Vet Pharmacol Ther. 2009; 32(2):129–136.

91. Doohoo S, Tasker RA, Donald A. Pharmacokinetics of parenteral and oral sustained-release morphine sulphate in dogs. J Vet Pharmacol Ther. 1994; 17(6):426–433.

92. Doohoo SF, Tasker RA. Pharmacokinetics of oral morphine sulfate in dogs: A comparison of sustained release and conventional formulations. Can J Vet Res. 1997; 61(4):251–255.

93. KuKanich B. Pharmacokinetics of acetaminophen, codeine, and the codeine metabolites morphine and codeine-6-glucuronide in healthy greyhound dogs. J Vet Pharmacol Ther. 2010; 33(1):15–21.

94. KuKanich B, Paul J. Pharmacokinetics of hydrocodone and its metabolite hydromorphone after oral hydrocodone administration to dogs. ACVIM 2010

95. Barnhart MD, et al. Pharmacokinetics, pharmacodynamics, and analgesic effects of morphine after rectal, intramuscular, and intravenous administration in dogs. Am J Vet Res. 2000; 61:24–28.

96. Nakamura K, Nara E, Fuse T, Akiyama Y. Pharmacokinetic and pharmacodynamic evaluations of novel oral morphine sustained release granules. Biol Pharm Bull. 2007; 30 (8):1456–1460.

97. Vree TB, van Dongen RT, Koopman-Kimenai PM. Codeine analgesia is due to codeine-6-glucuronide, not morphine. Int J Clin Pract. 2000; 54(6):395–398.

98. Plumb DC. Plumb's veterinary drug handbook, ed. 7. Ames Iowa, 2011, Wiley Blackwell.

99. KuKanich B, Lascelles BD, Aman AM, et al. The effects of inhibiting cytochrome P450 3A, p-glycoprotein, and gastric acid secretion on the oral bioavailability of methadone in dogs. J Vet Pharmacol Ther. 2005; 28(5):461–466.

100. Gervitz C. Methadone's role in pain management: New dangers revealed. Top Pain Manag. 2007; 23(5):1–6.

101. McMillan CJ, Livingston A, Clark CR, et al. Pharmacokinetics of intravenous tramadol in dogs. Can J Vet Res. 2008; 72(4):325–331.

102. Giorgi M, Del Carlo S, Saccomanni G. Pharmacokinetics of tramadol and its major metabolites following rectal and intravenous administration in dogs. N Z Vet J. 2009; 57 (3):146–152.

103. KuKanich B, Papich MG. Pharmacokinetics and antinociceptive effects of oral tramadol hydrochloride administration in greyhounds. Am J Vet Res. 2011; 72(2):256–262.

104. Pypendop BH, Ilkiw JE. Pharmacokinetics of tramadol, and its metabolite O-desmethyl-tramadol, in cats. J Vet Pharmacol Ther. 2008; 31(1):52–59.

105. Brondani JI, Loureiro Luna SP, Beier SL, et al. Analgesic efficacy of perioperative use of vedaprofen, tramadol or their combination in cats undergoing ovariohysterectomy. J Feline Med Surg. 2009; 11(6):420–429.

106. Giorgi M, Meizler A, Mills PC. Pharmacokinetics of the novel atypical opioid tapentadol following oral and intravenous administration in dogs. Vet J. 2012; 194(3):309–313.

107. Australian Government Department of Health and Ageing, Therapeutic Goods Administration. Australian public assessment report for tapentadol. Retrieved from www.tga.gov.au/pdf/auspar/auspar-palexia.pdf, p. 9.

108. Pypendop BH, Ilkiw JE, Shilo-Benjamini Y. Bioavailability of morphine, methadone, hydromorphone, and oxymorphone following buccal administration in cats. J Vet Pharmacol Ther. 2013; doi: http://dx.doi.org/10.1111/jvp.12090. [Epub ahead of print.]

SUGGESTED READING

Hansen B. Pain. Semin Vet Med Surg (Small Anim)12 (2) (1997)55–142.

Mathews KA, ed. Update on management of pain. Vet Clin North Am Small Anim Pract. 2008; 38(6):xi-xiii.

Tranquilli WJ, Thurman JC, Grimm KA. Lumb and Jones' veterinary anesthesia and analgesia, ed 4. Hoboken, NJ, 2007, Wiley-Blackwell.

α_2-Agonists*

Bruno H. Pypendop

The α_2-agonists are a group of sedative-analgesic drugs (Box 10-1) that exert their clinical effects by interacting with α_2-adrenergic receptors in the central nervous system (CNS). They also decrease anesthetic requirements and produce muscle relaxation. Although not considered first-line analgesics like opioids or nonsteroidal anti-inflammatory drugs, α_2-agonists are increasingly used as analgesic adjuvants. In contrast to other classes of drugs used to manage pain, α_2-agonists are distinguished by their significant cardiovascular adverse effects.

HISTORICAL BACKGROUND

- 1962: Xylazine was synthesized in Germany for use as an antihypertensive agent in human beings; its sedative properties in animals were recognized soon afterward.
- Early 1970s: Xylazine and xylazine-ketamine combinations became popular for inducing sedation and general anesthesia in large animals; use in small animals soon followed.
- 1981: The sedative, analgesic, and muscle relaxant properties of xylazine were linked to stimulation of central α_2-adrenoceptors.[1]
- Late 1980s: New, more specific α_2-agonists (medetomidine, detomidine, and romifidine) were introduced; drug distribution and labeling varied widely from country to country.
- 1996: Medetomidine and the α_2-antagonist atipamezole became available in the United States (labeled for use in dogs only); veterinarians began using α_2-agonists in lower doses, often in combination with opioids, as anesthetic and analgesic adjuvants.
- 2006: Dexmedetomidine was approved in the United States for use in dogs and cats.
- Currently, dexmedetomidine is the most commonly used α_2-agonist for analgesia in small animal practice in the United States; medetomidine is not available, and romifidine and xylazine are rarely used as analgesic adjuvants.

*The author would like to acknowledge Leigh Lamont for her work on the previous edition.

BOX **10-1** α_2-Agonists

- Clonidine
- Detomidine
- Dexmedetomidine
- Medetomidine
- Romifidine
- Xylazine

MOLECULAR PHARMACOLOGY OF α_2-ADRENOCEPTORS

α_2-Adrenoceptor Structure

- All α_2-adrenoceptor proteins contain approximately 450 amino acids.[2]
- Each protein contains seven transmembrane domains with segments of lipophilic amino acids separated by segments of hydrophilic amino acids; these form an extracellular amino terminus and an intracellular carboxyl terminus with three small extracellular loops and three intracellular loops.

α_2-Adrenoceptor Subtypes

- Three distinct α_2-adrenoceptor subtypes have been recognized: α_{2A}, α_{2B}, and α_{2C}.[3]
- A fourth subtype (α_{2D}) has been identified and represents the rodent homologue of the human α_{2A}-adrenoceptor.[4]
- The genes for the three human subtypes have been cloned and are designated α_2-C10, α_2-C2, and α_2-C4 for the α_{2A}, α_{2B}, and α_{2C} subtypes, respectively.[3]
- Related subtypes have been cloned in other species including rat, mouse, pig, opossum, and fish; partial complementary DNA sequences from bovine and avian α_{2A}-receptors have also been identified.
- All three α_2 subtype genes share a common evolutionary origin; several key structural and functional domains are well conserved despite only 50% protein homology at the amino acid level.
- The α_2-agonists currently available do not exhibit selectivity for receptor subtypes.

α_2-Adrenoceptor Expression

- Expression is somewhat species specific, resulting in varied physiologic effects and pharmacologic activity profiles and making extrapolation of data among species difficult.[5]
- Distribution of α_2-adrenoceptor subtypes in several species is given in Table 10-1.

TABLE **10-1**	Expression and Distribution of α_2-Adrenoceptor Subtypes in Different Species	
	BRAINSTEM	**SPINAL CORD**
Rodents[6]	α_{2A}	α_{2A}, α_{2C}
Humans[6]	α_{2A}	α_{2A}, α_{2B}
Dogs[7,24,83]	α_{2A}	α_{2A}, α_{2C}

α_2-Adrenoceptor Subtype Functional Significance

- The sedative-hypnotic and anesthetic-sparing responses appear to be mediated by the α_{2A} subtype.[6–8]
- The analgesic responses are mediated by the α_{2A} and possibly the α_{2C} subtypes.
- Hypotensive and bradycardic actions are also mediated by the α_{2A} subtype.[9]
- Initial increase in systemic vascular resistance appears to be mediated by the α_{2B} subtype, with lesser contribution of the α_{2A} subtype in certain vascular compartments.[10]
- Hypothermic effects and modulation of dopaminergic activity are mediated by the α_{2C} subtype.[6]

Imidazoline Receptors

- All α_2-agonists commonly used in veterinary medicine, with the exception of xylazine, and atipamezole contain an imidazole moiety that binds to a second class of non-noradrenergic receptors called *imidazoline receptors*.[11]
- Imidazoline receptors are involved in central control of vasomotor tone and are located in the nucleus reticularis lateralis of the ventrolateral region of the medulla.[11]
- Central hypotensive effects observed after administration of imidazole α_2-agonists appear to result from activation of imidazoline receptors, α_{2A}-adrenoceptors, or both.[12–14]

Signal Transduction Mechanisms of α_2-Adrenoceptors

- The process by which any transmembrane receptor notifies the cell of receptor occupancy by a ligand is called *signal transduction*.
- α_2-Adrenoceptors are part of a larger receptor superfamily including dopaminergic, cholinergic, and serotonergic receptor systems that are coupled to guanine nucleotide binding proteins (G proteins) that function in signal transduction.
- G proteins link cell membrane receptors to intracellular effector mechanisms, amplify the signal, and transduce external chemical stimuli into cellular responses.

- Binding of a specific ligand (neurotransmitter, endogenous hormone, or exogenous drug) induces a conformational change in the α_2-adrenoceptor, which leads to activation of specific G proteins.[3]
- Activated G proteins then modulate the synthesis or availability of intracellular second messenger molecules or directly alter the activity of transmembrane ion channels.[3]
- Relevant α_2-adrenoceptor effector mechanisms include the following:
  1. Increased potassium conductance leading to hyperpolarization of membrane ion channels and a decreased firing rate of excitable cells in the CNS.[3]
  2. Inhibition of calcium influx through N-type voltage-gated calcium channels resulting in reduced fusion of synaptic vesicles with postsynaptic membranes and reduced neurotransmitter release.[15]
  3. Inhibition of the enzyme adenylate cyclase, resulting in decreased intracellular cyclic adenosine monophosphate accumulation and decreased phosphorylation of target regulatory proteins.[16]

MECHANISM OF ANALGESIC ACTION

- α_2-Adrenoceptors within the CNS are found on noradrenergic and non-noradrenergic neurons.
- Noradrenergic α_2-adrenoceptors are called *autoreceptors* and are located at supraspinal sites.
- Non-noradrenergic α_2-adrenoceptors are called *heteroreceptors* and are located in the dorsal horn of the spinal cord.[17,18]
- Both populations of receptors appear to be involved in α_2-agonist analgesia.

Analgesia Mediated at the Level of the Dorsal Horn

- α_2-Heteroreceptors are located presynaptically and postsynaptically on nociceptive neurons in the dorsal horn.
- Activation by norepinephrine or an exogenous α_2-agonist produces analgesia by one of two potential mechanisms:[19]
  1. Presynaptic α_2-heteroreceptors found on primary afferent C fibers bind the agonist. This causes a G protein–mediated decrease in calcium influx (see previous section), which results in decreased release of neurotransmitters and neuropeptides such as glutamate, vasoactive intestinal peptide, calcitonin gene–related peptide, substance P, and neurotensin.
  2. Postsynaptic α_2-heteroreceptors found on wide dynamic range projection neurons also bind the agonist. This produces neuronal hyperpolarization via G protein–coupled potassium channels (see previous section) and inhibits ascending nociceptive transmission.

Analgesia Mediated at the Level of the Brainstem

- Traditionally, it has been accepted that α_2-agonist–induced analgesia results from activation of dorsal horn α_2-heteroreceptors, whereas sedative-hypnotic effects are mediated by activation of supraspinal (brainstem) α_2-autoreceptors.
- It now appears that brainstem α_2-autoreceptors also contribute indirectly to analgesia.
- α_2-Autoreceptors are concentrated in three catecholaminergic nuclei in the pons: A5, A6 (also called the *locus ceruleus* [LC]), and A7.[20,21]
- The locus ceruleus (LC) is the most important of these, extending noradrenergic neurons to all segments of the spinal cord and modulating noradrenergic input from higher structures such as the periaqueductal gray matter (PAG) of the midbrain.
- Activation of α_2-autoreceptors in the LC by norepinephrine or an exogenous α_2-agonist results in neuronal inhibition and a decreased release of norepinephrine.
- Dampening of LC activity disinhibits activity in the adjacent cell bodies of A5 and A7 nuclei, resulting in increased release of norepinephrine from their terminals in the dorsal horn, which in turn activates spinal presynaptic and postsynaptic α_2-heteroreceptors to produce analgesia.[20]
- Higher supraspinal structures may also play a role. The PAG of the midbrain extends noradrenergic innervation to the LC and may lead to α_2-mediated decreases in LC norepinephrine release, which indirectly feeds back on spinal α_2-adrenoceptors to produce analgesia.[17]

CLINICAL PHARMACOLOGY OF α_2-AGONISTS

Xylazine

- Xylazine is the least selective α_2-agonist used clinically, with an α_2:α_1 binding ratio of only 160:1.[22]
- A variety of α_2-antagonists have been used to reverse the effects of xylazine, including yohimbine, tolazoline, idazoxan, and, more recently, atipamezole.
- Although still used extensively in large animal practice as a sedative-analgesic agent, xylazine is rarely used as an analgesic adjuvant in dogs and cats.

Clonidine

- An α_2-agonist approved in the United States in 1997 for use in humans as an antihypertensive agent.
- Possesses some α_1 effects, with an α_2:α_1 binding ratio of 220:1.[22]

- Has gained popularity as an analgesic adjuvant for certain types of pain syndromes in humans.
- Not currently used clinically in dogs and cats.

Dexmedetomidine

- Dexmedetomidine is the pure *S*-enantiomer of the racemic α_2-agonist medetomidine; it is considered to be twice as potent as medetomidine.[23]
- Dexmedetomidine was approved in the United States in 1999 for use in human beings as a continuous infusion to provide sedation in intensive care unit (ICU) settings; since that time its use has expanded into anesthesia and pain management practice.
- Dexmedetomidine was approved in the United States in 2006 for use in dogs and cats. Evidence suggests that equipotent doses of dexmedetomidine and medetomidine induce similar sedative, analgesic, and cardiovascular effects in these species.[23,24]

Medetomidine

- Medetomidine is an equal mixture of two optical enantiomers: dexmedetomidine (see previous discussion) and levomedetomidine.
- Dexmedetomidine is the active component, whereas levomedetomidine is considered pharmacologically inactive (although it may play a role in drug interactions).[23]
- Racemic medetomidine is lipophilic, facilitating rapid absorption after intramuscular administration; peak plasma concentrations are reached in approximately ½ hour.[25]
- Medetomidine and dexmedetomidine are the most specific α_2-agonists available clinically, with an α_2:α_1 binding ratio of 1620:1.[22]
- A specific α_2-antagonist, atipamezole, was marketed alongside medetomidine and rapidly reverses all sedative, analgesic, and cardiovascular effects associated with medetomidine, dexmedetomidine, and other α_2-agonists, if desired.
- Dexmedetomidine and medetomidine are presently the only α_2-agonists used routinely as analgesic adjuvants in dogs and cats, so further clinical discussions will focus on these agents.

Romifidine

- Romifidine is an imino-imidazolidine derivative of clonidine.
- Romifidine is a potent and reasonably selective α_2-agonist, producing sedative and analgesic effects comparable to those achieved with medetomidine.[26,27]
- Romifidine has a α_2:α_1 binding ratio of 340:1.
- Romifidine is not currently approved for use in dogs or cats in the United States and is not used commonly as an analgesic adjuvant at this time.

BOX 10-2 **Pharmacokinetic Properties of α_2-Agonists**

- Rapid absorption (intramuscular, subcutaneous, oral)
- Rapid hepatic metabolism and renal excretion
- Active metabolites possible

Detomidine

- A weakly basic, lipophilic imidazole derivative.
- Also possesses greater α_1 binding than medetomidine, with an α_2:α_1 binding ratio of 260:1.[22]
- Not commonly used as an analgesic adjuvant in dogs and cats (Box 10-2).

CONSIDERATIONS FOR VETERINARY PATIENT SELECTION

- α_2-Agonists may induce significant alterations in cardiopulmonary function (see the discussion of cardiovascular effects); these alterations, although somewhat dose dependent, are seen even after administration of a low dose.
- In most cases, use of α_2-agonists should be reserved for young to middle-aged animals without significant systemic disease.
- As a rule, α_2-agonists *should be avoided* in the following:
  1. Animals adversely affected by an increase in cardiac afterload or a decrease in cardiac output (e.g., mitral or tricuspid regurgitation or dilated cardiomyopathy)
  2. Animals with cardiac arrhythmias or conduction disturbances (e.g., premature ventricular contractions, atrioventricular block, or other bradyarrhythmias)
  3. Animals with preexisting hypertension
  4. Animals with an increased potential for arterial hemorrhage (e.g., traumatic arterial laceration)
  5. Animals for whom vomiting could have serious detrimental effects (e.g., upper gastrointestinal obstruction or corneal descemetocele)

CLINICAL USE AS ANALGESIC ADJUVANTS

See Box 10-3.

Sedation and Analgesia for Short, Noninvasive Procedures

- Medetomidine and dexmedetomidine are used extensively for short, noninvasive procedures in dogs and cats, whereas romifidine is used less frequently; dosage guidelines are presented in Table 10-2.

BOX **10-3** Clinical Use of α₂-Agonists

1. Sedative-analgesic agent for short, noninvasive procedures
2. Adjunct to general anesthesia
   a. Component of total injectable anesthesia protocols
   b. Preanesthetic sedative-analgesic agent
   c. Supplemental continuous infusion during inhalant anesthesia
3. Sedative-analgesic agent in postoperative or intensive care unit settings
4. Epidural or intrathecal administration
5. Intra-articular administration
6. Perineural administration

TABLE **10-2** Recommended Dosages of Selected α₂-Agonists for Routine Sedation and Analgesia

DRUG	DOSAGE
Dexmedetomidine*†	*Dog:* 0.005-0.01 mg/kg IM 0.0025-0.005 mg/kg IV *Cat:* 0.008-0.015 mg/kg IM 0.005-0.008 mg/kg IV
Medetomidine*†	*Dog:* 0.01-0.02 mg/kg IM 0.005-0.01 mg/kg IV *Cat:* 0.015-0.03 mg/kg IM 0.01-0.015 mg/kg IV
Romifidine*†	*Dog:* 0.02-0.04 mg/kg IM 0.01-0.02 mg/kg IV *Cat:* 0.03-0.06 mg/kg IM 0.015-0.03 mg/kg IV

*Often combined with an opioid to enhance sedation and analgesia.
†May be reversed with atipamezole at end of procedure.

- Medetomidine and dexmedetomidine can be used alone but are often combined with an opioid (e.g., hydromorphone, morphine, buprenorphine, or butorphanol) to enhance sedation and provide more intense analgesia.
- Examples of short, noninvasive procedures include radiographs, ultrasound examinations, minor laceration repair, wound debridement, bandage placement, ear canal examination and cleaning, skin biopsy, and oral examination.
- Despite the fact that many animals appear profoundly sedated with (dex)medetomidine-opioid combinations, it is crucial to recognize that they are not anesthetized and may be acutely aroused by any type of stimulation.
- If general anesthesia is required, an anesthetic agent must be titrated to effect (see next section).
- For intramuscular administration, medetomidine or dexmedetomidine is injected 20 minutes before initiation of the procedure.

- For intravenous administration, lower doses of medetomidine or dexmedetomidine are used; onset time is within minutes of injection.
- Duration of effect is relatively short, ranging from 30 to 180 minutes, depending in part on the dose administered. The addition of an opioid may prolong analgesia depending on the opioid chosen, the dose, and the route of administration.
- Some evidence suggests that high doses are required for the production of analgesia.
- Concurrent use of anticholinergics is not recommended when medetomidine or dexmedetomidine is administered.
- Basic hemodynamic parameters should be monitored closely when medetomidine or dexmedetomidine is used (see discussion of cardiovascular effects).
- Reversal of all α_2-mediated effects can be accomplished by intramuscular atipamezole administration if desired.

Adjunct to General Anesthesia

Component of Total Injectable Anesthesia Protocols

- Medetomidine and dexmedetomidine are often used in combination with injectable anesthetic agents such as ketamine, tiletamine-zolazepam, and propofol to produce short-term general anesthesia; opioids and benzodiazepines are also commonly included in such protocols.
- The addition of medetomidine or dexmedetomidine means that lower doses of anesthetic agents are required, analgesia is supplemented, and muscle relaxation is optimized.
- Numerous intramuscular and intravenous drug combinations involving medetomidine (or dexmedetomidine) have been used clinically in dogs and cats, and the reader is referred elsewhere for a review of these techniques.[28]

Preanesthetic Sedative-Analgesic Agent

- Medetomidine-opioid or dexmedetomidine-opioid combinations are commonly administered in the preanesthetic period before induction of anesthesia; dosage guidelines are given in Table 10-3.
- Addition of medetomidine or dexmedetomidine in the preanesthetic period greatly reduces the required dose of induction and maintenance agent (injectable or inhalant).[29-33]
- (Dex)medetomidine-opioid combinations can be administered intramuscularly (IM) or intravenously (IV).
- Concurrent administration of an anticholinergic is appropriate only in cases in which both severe bradycardia and hypotension are observed. It should be noted that in most cases, because of the vasoconstriction

TABLE **10-3**	**Recommended Dosages of Selected α_2-Agonists as Adjuncts to General Anesthesia**	
	PREANESTHETIC AGENT*	**SUPPLEMENTAL CRI DURING INHALANT ANESTHESIA**
Dexmedetomidine	*Dog:* 0.0025-0.005 mg/kg IM 0.0015-0.0025 mg/kg IV *Cat:* 0.005-0.01 mg/kg IM 0.0025-0.005 mg/kg IV	*Dog:* 0.0005 mg/kg/hr IV[25]
Medetomidine	*Dog:* 0.005-0.01 mg/kg IM 0.003-0.005 mg/kg IV *Cat:* 0.01-0.02 mg/kg IM 0.005-0.01 mg/kg IV	
Romifidine	*Dog:* 0.01-0.02 mg/kg IM 0.005-0.01 mg/kg IV *Cat:* 0.02-0.03 mg/kg IM 0.01-0.02 mg/kg IV	

Key: *CRI,* Constant rate infusion.
*Often combined with an opioid to enhance sedation and analgesia.

induced by α_2-agonists, blood pressure is normal or elevated. In addition, the accuracy of noninvasive blood pressure measurements may be compromised

- As with any general anesthesia protocol, hemodynamic monitoring (including heart rate, rhythm, and blood pressure) is essential (see discussion of cardiovascular effects).
- Reversal with atipamezole should be considered when excessive sedation and/or cardiovascular effects persist in the recovery period.

Supplemental Continuous Infusion During Inhalant Anesthesia

- The use of medetomidine or dexmedetomidine in continuous infusions as part of balanced anesthesia, typically in combination with inhalants, has been described.
- It has been proposed that the use of very low doses administered via continuous infusion concurrently with an inhalant anesthetic may attenuate the adverse cardiovascular effects seen when larger doses are administered as boluses.
- The cardiovascular effects of medetomidine in dogs anesthetized with sevoflurane have been evaluated. Medetomidine at 1, 2, and 3 µg/kg/hr produced significant cardiovascular depression. It was concluded that low-dose medetomidine constant rate infusion should be used with caution in dogs.[34]
- The effects of dexmedetomidine on inhalant requirements and on cardiorespiratory function have been evaluated in dogs and cats. In dogs, dexmedetomidine 0.5 and 3 µg/kg followed by 0.5 and 3 µg/kg/hr respectively

reduced the minimum alveolar concentration (MAC) of isoflurane by 18% and 59%.[35] The low dose resulted in a decrease in heart rate, whereas the higher dose produced more profound cardiovascular alterations.[35] In cats, dexmedetomidine decreased the MAC of isoflurane in a plasma concentration–dependent manner, by up to 86%.[33] However, it appeared that at plasma concentrations reducing MAC in a clinically relevant manner, the isoflurane-dexmedetomidine combination resulted in greater cardiovascular depression (decrease in cardiac output, increase in systemic vascular resistance) than an equipotent, higher concentration of isoflurane alone.[36]

- Additional studies are warranted to explore the potential use of medetomidine and dexmedetomidine as intravenous infusions in inhalant-anesthetized animals, alone or in combination with other adjunctive agents such as opioids, ketamine, and lidocaine.

Sedative-Analgesic Agent in Postoperative or Intensive Care Unit Settings

Based on experience with dexmedetomidine in human ICU patients, there is increasing interest in the use of low doses of medetomidine and dexmedetomidine administered as intravenous infusions in dogs and cats to provide extended periods of sedation and analgesia.

- Studies with dexmedetomidine infusions in humans show significant reductions in benzodiazepine and opioid requirements in intubated, mechanically ventilated patients without induction of serious impairment of cardiopulmonary function.[37,38]
- Also, a significantly improved cumulative nitrogen balance has been documented in patients receiving α_2-agonist infusions after surgery, probably as a result of stimulation of growth hormone release.[39]
- Evidence in cats suggests that low doses of dexmedetomidine administered intramuscularly may be ineffective at providing analgesia; it is, however, possible that low doses potentiate the analgesia induced by opioids.[40,41] Dexmedetomidine administered intravenously in cats, at doses ranging from 5 to 50 µg/kg produced antinociception. The duration of the effect appeared somewhat dose-dependent, and the effect was closely associated with the sedative effect.[42]
- Medetomidine (2 µg/kg followed by 1 µg/kg/hr or 4 µg/kg followed by 2 µg/kg/hr IV) caused typical cardiovascular alterations in dogs, with the higher dose producing more pronounced effects.[43] A study on dexmedetomidine in dogs suggested that analgesia was produced during administration of 3 and 5 µg/kg/hr IV; the cardiovascular effects were not characterized.[44]
- Additional studies are needed to characterize further the cardiovascular and sedative-analgesic effects of medetomidine and dexmedetomidine infusions before their routine use can be recommended for animals in the ICU.

Epidural and Intrathecal Administration

- The spinal site of action appears to be important in mediating α_2-agonist–induced analgesia.
- Stimulation of spinal cord cholinergic interneurons also may contribute to analgesia after neuraxial α_2-agonist administration.[45–47]
- Although intrathecal drug administration is not routinely used in veterinary medicine, epidural administration is common.
- Incorporation of a low dose of medetomidine combined with morphine for epidural administration prolonged the analgesia compared with use of morphine alone.[48] Other studies have found minimal or no benefits of adding (dex)medetomidine to epidural opioids or local anesthetics.[49–51]
- Medetomidine or dexmedetomidine may be combined with standard epidural doses of morphine, oxymorphone, buprenorphine, fentanyl, lidocaine, or bupivacaine and injected into the epidural space at the lumbosacral junction.
- The lipophilicity of medetomidine and dexmedetomidine means that it is rapidly cleared from the cerebrospinal fluid (CSF) in the vicinity of the spinal injection site; this anatomically restricts the action of the drug, and results in significant systemic absorption.
- The cardiovascular effects observed after epidural administration are comparable to those seen with systemic administration.[52]
- Clinical use of epidural medetomidine or dexmedetomidine in dogs and cats remains less common than that of morphine or local anesthetics. Additional studies are warranted to better characterize both benefits and adverse effects.

Intra-articular Administration

- α_2-Adrenoceptors are located in the peripheral nervous system on terminals of primary afferent nociceptive fibers; they appear to contribute to analgesia by inhibition of norepinephrine release at nerve terminals.[45]
- Studies in human beings have demonstrated a peripheral analgesic effect after intra-articular administration of α_2-agonists to patients undergoing arthroscopic knee surgery that is unrelated to vascular uptake of the drug and redistribution to central sites.[53]
- Addition of clonidine to bupivacaine or bupivacaine-morphine provided analgesic benefits after intra-articular administration in humans undergoing arthroscopic knee surgery.[54]
- Similarly, addition of dexmedetomidine to intra-articular ropivacaine improved quality and duration of analgesia in humans after arthroscopic knee surgery.[55]
- There is currently no study evaluating the intra-articular use of medetomidine or dexmedetomidine in dogs and cats.

Perineural Administration

- In human patients, clinical evidence suggests that α_2-agonists enhance peripheral nerve block intensity and duration when added to local anesthetics administered perineurally.
- Enhanced perineural blockade with α_2-agonists may be a result of the following:
  1. Hyperpolarization of C fibers through blockade of a specific type of potassium channel.[45]
  2. Local vasoconstriction that decreases vascular removal of local anesthetic surrounding neural structures and prolongs duration of action.
- A recent meta-analysis of the perineural use of dexmedetomidine in humans concluded that it may exhibit a facilitatory effect, but that insufficient safety data were available to support its use in the clinical setting.[56]
- One study reported that perineural administration of medetomidine prolonged the duration of mepivacaine-induced radial nerve block in dogs. Systemic administration of the same dose had a similar effect.[57] Similarly, dexmedetomidine prolonged the duration of vasodilation produced by sympathetic block with mepivacaine in dogs.[58]

CLINICAL ADVERSE EFFECTS OF α_2-AGONISTS

Comprehensive reviews of the physiologic adverse effects of α_2-agonists used in veterinary medicine are available elsewhere;[28,59] the following is a brief summary of relevant points.

Cardiovascular Effects

See Box 10-4.
- Immediately after administration, α_2-agonists bind vascular postsynaptic α_2-adrenoceptors, resulting in vasoconstriction.[60]

BOX 10-4 **Cardiovascular Effects of α_2-Agonists**

Immediate (Peripheral) Effects
↑ Systemic vascular resistance
↑ Arterial blood pressure
↓ Heart rate (baroreceptor reflex)
↓ Cardiac output

Delayed (Central) Effects
↓ Sympathetic activity
↓ Arterial blood pressure
↓ Cardiac output

- The increase in systemic vascular resistance produces a short-lived hypertensive phase accompanied by a compensatory baroreceptor-mediated reflex bradycardia.[60]
- The initial hypertension may be decreased or even absent after intramuscular administration, likely because of reduced peak plasma levels of the drug.
- Bradyarrhythmias as a result of increased vagal tone are not uncommon, with heart rates decreasing by as much as 70%.[60]
- Sinus arrhythmia, sinoatrial block, and first-degree and second-degree atrioventricular block are frequently seen; third-degree atrioventricular block and sinoatrial arrest occur rarely.
- Cardiac output decreases, typically in proportion to the decrease in heart rate.[60]
- Over time, heart rate and systemic vascular resistance return toward baseline; the duration of the effects is largely dose dependent.[60]

Respiratory Effects

See Box 10-5.

- Although respiratory rate, minute ventilation, and central respiratory drive decrease with administration of α_2-agonists, arterial pH, PaO_2, and $PaCO_2$ typically remain within a clinically acceptable range.[61,62]
- At high doses, especially in combination with other CNS depressants, decreases in mixed-venous PO_2 and oxygen content have been noted; venous desaturation is presumably related to increased tissue oxygen extraction associated with decreased cardiac output.

Gastrointestinal Effects

See Box 10-6.

- Up to 20% of dogs and up to 90% of cats vomit after medetomidine.[63] Dexmedetomidine likely has similar effects.

BOX 10-5   Respiratory Effects of α_2-Agonists

Low Doses (for Adjunctive Analgesia)
↓ Respiratory rate
↓ Normal minute ventilation
Normal $PaCO_2$, PO_2, and pH

High Doses (in Combination)
↓ Respiratory rate
↓ Tidal volume
↓ Minute ventilation
↑ CO_2, ↓ pH, ↓ $P\overline{v}O_2$,* possible ↓ PaO_2

*Partial oxygen pressure in mixed venous blood.

BOX 10-6 **Gastrointestinal Effects of α_2-Agonists**

↓ Salivation
↓ Gastric secretions
↓ Gastrointestinal motility
↑ Vomiting
↓ Swallowing reflex
Predisposition to gastric dilation (large-breed dogs)?

- Emesis is seen most often after subcutaneous and, less frequently, intramuscular administration.
- Medetomidine and dexmedetomidine also inhibit small intestinal and colonic motility in dogs.[64] They may decrease the lower esophageal sphincter tone and increase the likelihood of gastroesophageal reflux.

Renal Effects

See Box 10-7.
- Significant increases in urine output are seen transiently after administration of α_2-agonists to dogs and cats.[65,66]
- Increased urinary output may be the result of one or more of the following:
  1. Increased renal blood flow and glomerular filtration rate.[65,66] Such increases were observed following IV administration, while IM administration resulted in decreased renal blood flow and glomerular filtration rate.[65]
  2. Suppression of antidiuretic hormone (ADH) release centrally.[65]
  3. Antagonism of ADH at the level of the renal tubule.[67]

Endocrine Effects

- α_2-agonists cause hyperglycemia because of suppression of insulin secretion.[68]
- Cortisol and glucagon levels do not appear to change significantly,[68] but medetomidine has been shown to attenuate the stress response induced by other anesthetic agents (opioids and ketamine).[69] Dexmedetomidine likely produces similar effects.
- Medetomidine may blunt the perioperative stress response in dogs.[70,71]

BOX 10-7 **Renal and Endocrine Effects of α_2-Agonists**

Diuresis and natriuresis (↑ water and sodium excretion)
- Inhibition of ADH release
- Inhibition of rennin release
- Increase atrial natriuretic peptide
↓ Insulin release (hyperglycemia, glucosuria)

- Other hormonal changes include transient alterations in growth hormone, testosterone, prolactin, ADH, and follicle-stimulating hormone levels.

Miscellaneous Effects

- Increased myometrial tone and intrauterine pressure have been noted in several species after xylazine administration;[72-74] medetomidine, dexmedetomidine, and detomidine appear less likely to have this effect.
- Mydriasis has been reported after administration of xylazine and (dex) medetomidine because of central inhibition of parasympathetic innervation to the iris or direct sympathetic stimulation of α_2-receptors located in the iris and CNS.[75-78]
- Variable changes in intraocular pressure have been reported in some species after systemic administration of α_2-agonists.[79-83]

REFERENCES

1. Hsu WH: Xylazine-induced depression and its antagonism by alpha adrenergic blocking agents. J Pharmacol Exp Ther. 218:188–192, 1981.
2. MacDonald F, Kobilka BK, Scheinin M: Gene targeting—homing in on alpha 2-adrenoceptor-subtype function. Trends Pharmacol Sci. 18:211–219, 1997.
3. Aantaa R, Marjamaki A, Scheinin M: Molecular pharmacology of alpha 2-adrenoceptor subtypes. Ann Med. 27:439–449, 1995.
4. Blaxall HS, Heck DA, Bylund DB: Molecular determinants of the alpha-2D adrenergic receptor subtype. Life Sci. 53:PL255–259, 1993.
5. Ongioco RR, Richardson CD, Rudner XL, et al.: Alpha2-adrenergic receptors in human dorsal root ganglia: Predominance of alpha2b and alpha2c subtype mRNAs. Anesthesiology. 92:968–976, 2000.
6. Maze M, Fujinaga M: Alpha2 adrenoceptors in pain modulation: Which subtype should be targeted to produce analgesia? Anesthesiology. 92:934–936, 2000.
7. Schwartz DD, Jones WG, Hedden KP, et al.: Molecular and pharmacological characterization of the canine brainstem alpha-2A adrenergic receptor. J Vet Pharmacol Ther. 22:380–386, 1999.
8. Lakhlani PP, MacMillan LB, Guo TZ, et al.: Substitution of a mutant alpha2a-adrenergic receptor via "hit and run" gene targeting reveals the role of this subtype in sedative, analgesic, and anesthetic-sparing responses in vivo. Proc Natl Acad Sci U S A. 94:9950–9955, 1997.
9. MacMillan LB, Lakhlani PP, Hein L, et al.: In vivo mutation of the alpha 2A-adrenergic receptor by homologous recombination reveals the role of this receptor subtype in multiple physiological processes. Adv Pharmacol. 42:493–496, 1998.
10. MacMillan LB, Hein L, Smith MS, et al.: Central hypotensive effects of the alpha2a-adrenergic receptor subtype. Science. 273:801–803, 1996.
11. Bousquet P: Imidazoline receptors: From basic concepts to recent developments. J Cardiovasc Pharmacol. 26 Suppl 2:S1–S6, 1995.
12. Bousquet P, Bruban V, Schann S, et al.: Participation of imidazoline receptors and alpha(2-)-adrenoceptors in the central hypotensive effects of imidazoline-like drugs. Ann N Y Acad Sci. 881:272–278, 1999.
13. Head GA: Central imidazoline- and alpha 2-receptors involved in the cardiovascular actions of centrally acting antihypertensive agents. Ann N Y Acad Sci. 881:279–286, 1999.

14. Zhu QM, Lesnick JD, Jasper JR, et al.: alpha 2A-adrenoceptors, not I1-imidazoline receptors, mediate the hypotensive effects of rilmenidine and moxonidine in conscious mice. in vivo and in vitro studies. Ann N Y Acad Sci. 881(287–289), 1999.

15. Limbird LE: Receptors linked to inhibition of adenylate cyclase: Additional signaling mechanisms. FASEB J. 2:2686–2695, 1988.

16. Schwinn DA: Adrenoceptors as models for G protein-coupled receptors: Structure, function and regulation. Br J Anaesth. 71:77–85, 1993.

17. Budai D, Harasawa I, Fields HL: Midbrain periaqueductal gray (PAG) inhibits nociceptive inputs to sacral dorsal horn nociceptive neurons through alpha2-adrenergic receptors. J Neurophysiol. 80:2244–2254, 1998.

18. Millan MJ, Bervoets K, Rivet JM, et al.: Multiple alpha-2 adrenergic receptor subtypes. II. Evidence for a role of rat R alpha-2A adrenergic receptors in the control of nociception, motor behavior and hippocampal synthesis of noradrenaline. J Pharmacol Exp Ther. 270:958-972, 1994.

19. Buerkle H, Yaksh TL: Pharmacological evidence for different alpha 2-adrenergic receptor sites mediating analgesia and sedation in the rat. Br J Anaesth. 81:208–215, 1998.

20. Guo TZ, Jiang JY, Buttermann AE, et al.: Dexmedetomidine injection into the locus ceruleus produces antinociception. Anesthesiology. 84:873–881, 1996.

21. Peng YB, Lin Q, Willis WD: Involvement of alpha-2 adrenoceptors in the periaqueductal gray-induced inhibition of dorsal horn cell activity in rats. J Pharmacol Exp Ther. 278:125–135, 1996.

22. Virtanen R: Pharmacological profiles of medetomidine and its antagonist, atipamezole. Acta Vet Scand Suppl. 85:29–37, 1989.

23. Kuusela E, Raekallio M, Anttila M, et al.: Clinical effects and pharmacokinetics of medetomidine and its enantiomers in dogs. J Vet Pharmacol Ther. 23:15–20, 2000.

24. Savola JM, Virtanen R: Central alpha 2-adrenoceptors are highly stereoselective for dexmedetomidine, the dextro enantiomer of medetomidine. Eur J Pharmacol. 195:193–199, 1991.

25. Salonen JS: Pharmacokinetics of medetomidine. Acta Vet Scand Suppl. 85:49–54, 1989.

26. England GC, Flack TE, Hollingworth E, et al.: Sedative effects of romifidine in the dog. J Small Anim Pract. 37:19–25, 1996.

27. Lemke KA: Sedative effects of intramuscular administration of a low dose of romifidine in dogs. Am J Vet Res. 60:162–168, 1999.

28. Sinclair MD: A review of the physiological effects of alpha2-agonists related to the clinical use of medetomidine in small animal practice. Can Vet J. 44:885–897, 2003.

29. McSweeney PM, Martin DD, Ramsey DS, et al.: Clinical efficacy and safety of dexmedetomidine used as a preanesthetic prior to general anesthesia in cats. J Am Vet Med Assoc. 240:404–412, 2012.

30. Mendes GM, Selmi AL, Barbudo-Selmi GR, et al.: Clinical use of dexmedetomidine as premedicant in cats undergoing propofol-sevoflurane anaesthesia. J Feline Med Surg. 5:265–270, 2003.

31. Kojima K, Nishimura R, Mutoh T, et al.: Effects of medetomidine-midazolam, acepromazine-butorphanol, and midazolam-butorphanol on induction dose of thiopental and propofol and on cardiopulmonary changes in dogs. Am J Vet Res. 63:1671–1679, 2002.

32. Pascoe PJ, Raekallio M, Kuusela E, et al.: Changes in the minimum alveolar concentration of isoflurane and some cardiopulmonary measurements during three continuous infusion rates of dexmedetomidine in dogs. Vet Anaesth Analg. 33:97–103, 2006.

33. Escobar A, Pypendop BH, Siao KT, et al.: Effect of dexmedetomidine on the minimum alveolar concentration of isoflurane in cats. J Vet Pharmacol Ther. 35:163–168, 2012.

34. Carter JE, Campbell NB, Posner LP, et al.: The hemodynamic effects of medetomidine continuous rate infusions in the dog. Vet Anaesth Analg. 37:197–206, 2010.

35. Lin GY, Robben JH, Murrell JC, Aspegrén J, McKusick BC, Hellebrekers LJ. Dexmedetomidine constant rate infusion for 24 hours during and after propofol or isoflurane anaesthesia in dogs. Vet Anaesth Analg. 35(2):141–153, 2008.

36. Pypendop BH, Barter LS, Stanley SD, et al.: Hemodynamic effects of dexmedetomidine in isoflurane-anesthetized cats. Vet Anaesth Analg. 38:555–567, 2011.

37. Venn RM, Bradshaw CJ, Spencer R, et al.: Preliminary UK experience of dexmedetomidine, a novel agent for postoperative sedation in the intensive care unit. Anaesthesia. 54:1136–1142, 1999.

38. Hall JE, Uhrich TD, Barney JA, et al.: Sedative, amnestic, and analgesic properties of small-dose dexmedetomidine infusions. Anesth Analg. 90:699–705, 2000.

39. Mertes N, Goeters C, Kuhmann M, et al.: Postoperative alpha 2-adrenergic stimulation attenuates protein catabolism. Anesth Analg. 82:258–263, 1996.

40. Slingsby LS, Taylor PM: Thermal antinociception after dexmedetomidine administration in cats: A dose-finding study. J Vet Pharmacol Ther. 31:135–142, 2008.

41. Slingsby LS, Murrell JC, Taylor PM: Combination of dexmedetomidine with buprenorphine enhances the antinociceptive effect to a thermal stimulus in the cat compared with either agent alone. Vet Anaesth Analg. 37:162–170, 2010.

42. Pypendop BH, Ilkiw JE: Relationship between plasma dexmedetomidine concentration and sedation score and thermal threshold in cats. Am J Vet Res. In Press, 2014.

43. Lamont LA, Burton SA, Caines D, et al.: Effects of 2 different infusion rates of medetomidine on sedation score, cardiopulmonary parameters, and serum levels of medetomidine in healthy dogs. Can J Vet Res. 76:308–316, 2012.

44. van Oostrom H, Doornenbal A, Schot A, et al.: Neurophysiological assessment of the sedative and analgesic effects of a constant rate infusion of dexmedetomidine in the dog. Vet J. 190:338–344, 2011.

45. Eisenach JC, De Kock M, Klimscha W: alpha(2)-adrenergic agonists for regional anesthesia. A clinical review of clonidine (1984–1995). Anesthesiology. 85:655–674, 1996.

46. De Kock M, Eisenach J, Tong C, et al.: Analgesic doses of intrathecal but not intravenous clonidine increase acetylcholine in cerebrospinal fluid in humans. Anesth Analg. 84:800–803, 1997.

47. Eisenach JC, Hood DD, Curry R: Intrathecal, but not intravenous, clonidine reduces experimental thermal or capsaicin-induced pain and hyperalgesia in normal volunteers. Anesth Analg. 87:591–596, 1998.

48. Branson KR, Ko JC, Tranquilli WJ, et al.: Duration of analgesia induced by epidurally administered morphine and medetomidine in dogs. J Vet Pharmacol Ther. 16:369–372, 1993.

49. Pacharinsak C, Greene SA, Keegan RD, et al.: Postoperative analgesia in dogs receiving epidural morphine plus medetomidine. J Vet Pharmacol Ther. 26:71–77, 2003.

50. Steagall PV, Millette V, Mantovani FB, et al.: Antinociceptive effects of epidural buprenorphine or medetomidine, or the combination, in conscious cats. J Vet Pharmacol Ther. 32:477–484, 2009.

51. Smith LJ: A comparison of epidural analgesia provided by bupivacaine alone, bupivacaine + morphine, or bupivacaine + dexmedetomidine for pelvic orthopedic surgery in dogs. Vet Anaesth Analg. 40(5):527–536, 2013.

52. Duke T, Cox AM, Remedios AM, et al.: The cardiopulmonary effects of placing fentanyl or medetomidine in the lumbosacral epidural space of isoflurane-anesthetized cats. Vet Surg. 23:149–155, 1994.

53. Gentili M, Juhel A, Bonnet F: Peripheral analgesic effect of intra-articular clonidine. Pain. 64:593–596, 1996.

54. Joshi W, Reuben SS, Kilaru PR, et al.: Postoperative analgesia for outpatient arthroscopic knee surgery with intraarticular clonidine and/or morphine. Anesth Analg. 90:1102–1106, 2000.

55. Paul S, Bhattacharjee DP, Ghosh S, et al.: Efficacy of intra-articular dexmedetomidine for postoperative analgesia in arthroscopic knee surgery. Ceylon Med J. 55:111–115, 2010.

56. Abdallah FW, Brull R: Facilitatory effects of perineural dexmedetomidine on neuraxial and peripheral nerve block: A systematic review and meta-analysis. Br J Anaesth. 110:915–925, 2013.

57. Lamont LA, Lemke KA: The effects of medetomidine on radial nerve blockade with mepivacaine in dogs. Vet Anaesth Analg. 35:62–68, 2008.

58. Tezuka M, Kitajima T, Yamaguchi S, et al.: Addition of dexmedetomidine prolongs duration of vasodilation induced by sympathetic block with mepivacaine in dogs. Reg Anesth Pain Med. 29:323–327, 2004.

59. Murrell JC, Hellebrekers LJ: Medetomidine and dexmedetomidine: A review of cardiovascular effects and antinociceptive properties in the dog. Vet Anaesth Analg. 32:117–127, 2005.

60. Pypendop BH, Verstegen JP: Hemodynamic effects of medetomidine in the dog: A dose titration study. Vet Surg. 27:612–622, 1998.

61. Lerche P, Muir WW: Effect of medetomidine on breathing and inspiratory neuromuscular drive in conscious dogs. Am J Vet Res. 65:720–724, 2004.

62. Pypendop B, Verstegen J: Cardiorespiratory effects of a combination of medetomidine, midazolam, and butorphanol in dogs. Am J Vet Res. 60:1148–1154, 1999.

63. Vainio O: Introduction to the clinical pharmacology of medetomidine. Acta Vet Scand Suppl. 85:85–88, 1989.

64. Maugeri S, Ferre JP, Intorre L, et al.: Effects of medetomidine on intestinal and colonic motility in the dog. J Vet Pharmacol Ther. 17:148–154, 1994.

65. Saleh N, Aoki M, Shimada T, et al.: Renal effects of medetomidine in isoflurane-anesthetized dogs with special reference to its diuretic action. J Vet Med Sci. 67:461–465, 2005.

66. Grimm JB, Grimm KA, Kneller SK, et al.: The effect of a combination of medetomidine-butorphanol and medetomidine, butorphanol, atropine on glomerular filtration rate in dogs. Vet Radiol Ultrasound. 42:458–462, 2001.

67. Gellai M, Edwards RM: Mechanism of alpha 2-adrenoceptor agonist-induced diuresis. Am J Physiol. 255:F317–323, 1988.

68. Ambrisko TD, Hikasa Y: Neurohormonal and metabolic effects of medetomidine compared with xylazine in beagle dogs. Can J Vet Res. 66:42–49, 2002.

69. Ambrisko TD, Hikasa Y, Sato K: Influence of medetomidine on stress-related neurohormonal and metabolic effects caused by butorphanol, fentanyl, and ketamine administration in dogs. Am J Vet Res. 66:406–412, 2005.

70. Benson GJ, Grubb TL, Neff-Davis C, et al.: Perioperative stress response in the dog: Effect of pre-emptive administration of medetomidine. Vet Surg. 29:85–91, 2000.

71. Vaisanen M, Raekallio M, Kuusela E, et al.: Evaluation of the perioperative stress response in dogs administered medetomidine or acepromazine as part of the preanesthetic medication. Am J Vet Res. 63:969–975, 2002.

72. Wheaton LG, Benson GJ, Tranquilli WJ, et al.: The oxytocic effect of xylazine on the canine uterus. Theriogenology. 31:911–915, 1989.

73. Hodgson DS, Dunlop CI, Chapman PL, et al.: Cardiopulmonary effects of xylazine and acepromazine in pregnant cows in late gestation. Am J Vet Res. 63:1695–1699, 2002.

74. Schatzmann U, Jossfck H, Stauffer JL, et al.: Effects of alpha 2-agonists on intrauterine pressure and sedation in horses: Comparison between detomidine, romifidine and xylazine. Zentralbl Veterinarmed A. 41:523–529, 1994.

75. Hsu WH, Lee P, Betts DM: Xylazine-induced mydriasis in rats and its antagonism by alpha-adrenergic blocking agents. J Vet Pharmacol Ther. 4:97–101, 1981.

76. Hsu WH, Betts DM, Lee P: Xylazine-induced mydriasis: Possible involvement of a central postsynaptic regulation of parasympathetic tone. J Vet Pharmacol Ther. 4:209–214, 1981.

77. Jin Y, Wilson S, Elko EE, et al.: Ocular hypotensive effects of medetomidine and its analogs. J Ocul Pharmacol. 7:285–296, 1991.

78. Horvath G, Kovacs M, Szikszay M, et al.: Mydriatic and antinociceptive effects of intrathecal dexmedetomidine in conscious rats. Eur J Pharmacol. 253:61–66, 1994.

79. Rauser P, Pfeifr J, Proks P, et al.: Effect of medetomidine-butorphanol and dexmedetomidine-butorphanol combinations on intraocular pressure in healthy dogs. Vet Anaesth Analg. 39:301–305, 2012.

80. Artigas C, Redondo JI, Lopez-Murcia MM: Effects of intravenous administration of dexmedetomidine on intraocular pressure and pupil size in clinically normal dogs. Vet Ophthalmol. 15 Suppl 1:79–82, 2012.

81. Wallin-Hakanson N, Wallin-Hakanson B: The effects of topical tropicamide and systemic medetomidine, followed by atipamezole reversal, on pupil size and intraocular pressure in normal dogs. Vet Ophthalmol. 4:3–6, 2001.

82. Verbruggen AM, Akkerdaas LC, Hellebrekers LJ, et al.: The effect of intravenous medetomidine on pupil size and intraocular pressure in normotensive dogs. Vet Q. 22:179–180, 2000.

83. Potter DE, Ogidigben MJ: Medetomidine-induced alterations of intraocular pressure and contraction of the nictitating membrane. Invest Ophthalmol Vis Sci. 32:2799–2805, 1991.

CHAPTER 11

Local Anesthetics

Luis Campoy; Matt Read

PHYSIOLOGY OF NERVE CONDUCTION

The characteristics of nerve fiber size and the presence or absence of myelin have been shown to correlate with conduction velocity and function, with sympathetic fibers being the most sensitive to blockade, followed by sensory and motor fibers, respectively.

Membrane Potential and Action Potential

- A neuron's resting membrane potential is negative as a result of the disequilibrium of charged ions across its cell membrane.
- A membrane protein, the Na^+-K^+-ATPase pump, moves K^+ into the cell and Na^+ out of the cell in an active process that consumes energy.
- Because of the selective permeability of the membrane, K^+ "leaks" out of the cell along its concentration gradient, leaving a net negative charge inside the cell. As a result, the intracellular space is negative relative to the extracellular space, with the resting membrane potential being approximately -60 to -70 mV.
- In nociceptive neurons, mechanical, chemical, or electrical stimulation can cause the sodium channels to open.
- Sodium flows into the cell, reducing the voltage across the membrane.
- Once the potential difference reaches a threshold voltage (approximately 55 mV), it causes hundreds of contiguous sodium gates in that region of the membrane to open briefly. More sodium ions flow into the cell, completely depolarizing the membrane.
- This further opens more voltage-gated ion channels in the adjacent membrane, so a wave of depolarization courses along the cell (referred to as an *action potential*).
- Activation of voltage-gated Na^+ channels is very short-lived, and after only a few milliseconds these channels again become inactive and cannot be activated until they revert to their resting state (refractory period).
- After a slight delay, K^+ channels become activated, too, leading to an efflux of K^+ ions, which restores the resting membrane potential of the cell.
- During the process of repolarization, Na^+ and K^+ channels are reset to their resting state.

Mode of Action of Local Anesthetics

- Local anesthetics bind to sodium channels that are in their inactive state.
- This prevents subsequent channel activation and the influx of sodium that occurs with membrane depolarization.
- As a result, the action potential cannot be propagated because the threshold level is never attained.

PHARMACOLOGY

Local anesthetics consist of the following:

- A *lipophilic group*. The aromatic head, also known as a *benzene ring*, conveys liposolubility, which allows for diffusion through nerve sheaths and nerve cell membranes.
- A *hydrophilic group*. The amino tail conveys hydrosolubility. This characteristic permits molecular dissociation and binding of the drug molecules with the sodium channels.
- These two groups are separated by either an ester (e.g., procaine, tetracaine) or an amide linkage (e.g., lidocaine, mepivacaine, bupivacaine, ropivacaine). The intermediate chain (ester or amide) determines the synthesis and metabolism of the drug.

Clinical Tips

- Amide local anesthetics (e.g., lidocaine, mepivacaine, bupivacaine, ropivacaine) are most commonly used and are metabolized primarily by the liver.
- Most ester local anesthetics are metabolized by pseudocholinesterases in the blood.

COMMONLY USED LOCAL ANESTHETICS

Lidocaine

- One of the most frequently used local anesthetics.
- Amide-type anesthetic.
- Quick onset and short duration of action.
- Commonly used for local anesthesia of peripheral nerves, neuraxial anesthesia, local infiltration, and intravenous regional anesthesia (IVRA) and even for topical desensitization of mucosa or skin.
- For surgical anesthesia, concentrations of 1% to 2% are commonly used.
- Also used systemically as an intravenous agent for its analgesic, antiinflammatory, and antiarrhythmic effects.

Mepivacaine

- Amide-type anesthetic.
- Onset is similar to that of lidocaine; mepivacaine's duration of action is considered to be longer.

- Used in concentrations ranging from 1% to 2% for peripheral nerve blocks, epidural anesthesia, and local infiltration.

Bupivacaine

- Since its introduction into clinical practice in the early 1960s, bupivacaine has become one of the most commonly used local anesthetic agents.
- Slow onset of action.
- Significantly longer duration than lidocaine or mepivacaine.
- Bupivacaine is frequently used for nerve blocks and neuraxial anesthesia in a wide range of concentrations (0.125% to 0.75%), allowing for the development of differential blockade (sensory block without motor block).
- It is significantly more cardiotoxic than other local anesthetic agents should an overdose occur, and it should never be used for IVRA.

Levobupivacaine

- Amide-type anesthetic.
- Levobupivacaine is a formulation that includes one of the two enantiomers of bupivacaine, and therefore its actions are similar to the standard racemic mixture.
- The onset and duration of levobupivacaine do not significantly differ from those of bupivacaine.
- The main advantage is that levobupivacaine has a markedly reduced risk of cardiotoxicity when compared with bupivacaine.

Ropivacaine

- Amide-type anesthetic.
- At low concentrations (0.25% to 0.5%), ropivacaine has a relatively slow onset, similar to bupivacaine. At higher concentrations (0.75%), its onset may be as fast as that of mepivacaine.
- Long duration.
- At concentrations above 0.5%, ropivacaine produces sensory blockade similar to that obtained with bupivacaine, but there is less chance of inducing motor blockade.
- Ropivacaine has a lower potential for inducing cardiovascular and central nervous system (CNS) toxicity.
- As a result of these favorable characteristics, ropivacaine has gained wide acceptance and is being increasingly used for conduction and neuraxial anesthesia.

COMBINING LOCAL ANESTHETIC AGENTS BEFORE USE

- Local anesthetics are commonly combined before use, to maximize the desirable characteristics of individual drugs.

- For example, lidocaine (for its quick onset) and bupivacaine (for its longer duration) are commonly mixed in equal parts before injection.
- Few data are available regarding the safety, efficacy, or potentially altered pharmacokinetics of mixed local anesthetics.
  - The onset of action of a mixture of agents may be unpredictable because the resulting acid-base dissociation constant (pK_a) of the mixture is unknown.
  - In addition, a 50:50 mixture (e.g., lidocaine 2% and bupivacaine 0.5%) will result in half-strength concentrations of either drug (new concentrations of lidocaine 1% and bupivacaine 0.25%).
  - It is possible that the lower concentrations of the fast-acting drug and long-lasting drug will result in a slightly slower onset and a shorter duration than either individual agent by itself. In 2009, Cuvillon and colleagues[1] showed that when long-acting local anesthetics were mixed with lidocaine, although the onset of the block was faster, there was a decreased duration of action.
- Because of the lack of evidence to show a consistent advantage of mixing local anesthetics, a better approach is to simply select a single agent based on its desired, predictable, characteristics.

ADJUVANTS COMMONLY USED TO ENHANCE LOCOREGIONAL ANESTHESIA AND ANALGESIA

Adjunct agents are often combined with local anesthetics for techniques such as neuraxial anesthesia or peripheral nerve blockade. In the case of infiltration anesthesia, vasoconstrictors are frequently used.

Opioids

See Chapter 9 for more information on opioids.
- Morphine, hydromorphone, fentanyl, and buprenorphine are commonly added to local anesthetics to enhance epidural analgesia.
- The addition of opioids results in improved analgesia without affecting motor blockade.
- Morphine is the most widely used epidural opioid in veterinary medicine.
- Caution must be exercised because the administration of epidural morphine may result in urine retention. Other opioids such as tramadol and buprenorphine have been used with success through the epidural route in animals, but are less commonly used in clinical practice than morphine.
- Buprenorphine has been used as an adjunct to local anesthetics for epidural and peripheral nerve block and may enhance the quality of the nerve block through a local anesthetic–like mechanism of action involving Na^+ channel blockade, a property that other μ-agonists do not share.

Vasoconstrictors

The addition of epinephrine (1:100,000-1:200,000) to a local anesthetic solution may have several benefits:

- Longer duration of effect.
- Increased intensity of blockade.
- Reduced absorption of the anesthetic agent because of local vasoconstriction.
- Decreased surgical bleeding after infiltrative local anesthesia.
- In 2003, Neal[2] reviewed the existing literature and found that the potential for epinephrine to cause or potentiate nerve injury after peripheral block is exceedingly low in normal patients, whereas lower-than-normal peripheral nerve blood flow is apparently well tolerated.

It has been found that administration of epinephrine alone in the epidural space can cause segmental analgesia. The proposed mechanism is by interaction with α_2 receptors in the spinal cord. The increased intensity of blockade when epinephrine is added to a local anesthetic for epidural administration may therefore be the result of a combination of mechanisms:

- Local vasoconstriction causing reduced uptake of the primary local anesthetic agent into circulation
- Direct analgesic effect of the epinephrine

α_2-Adrenoceptor Agonists

- α_2-Agonist agents are commonly used to enhance the analgesia produced through both epidural anesthesia and peripheral nerve blocks.
- Clonidine and dexmedetomidine produce analgesia through supraspinal and spinal mechanisms (via adrenergic receptors) and have inhibitory effects on conduction of nerve impulses.
- Clinical benefits of the addition of dexmedetomidine to long-lasting amide-type local anesthetic agents have been shown. The addition of dexmedetomidine to ropivacaine administered to sciatic nerves in rats doubled the duration of the ropivacaine blockade.[3]

LOCAL ANESTHETIC TOXICITY

- High plasma levels of local anesthetics can occur after administration of an overdose or by unintentional intravascular administration.
- In addition, unanticipated high plasma levels of local anesthetics can be attained if biotransformation and/or elimination of the drug are slower than usual, as may occur in individuals with hepatic or renal insufficiencies.
- When the pharmacokinetic variables of lidocaine were calculated in dogs after partial hepatectomy and transplantation, the maximal plasma

BOX 11-1	Clinical Signs of Local Anesthetic Toxicity

- Nystagmus
- Muscular twitching
- Tonic-clonic convulsions
- Tremors or seizures (Increased levels of lactic acid and hypoxia may be observed after onset of seizures.)
- Generalized central nervous system depression (drowsiness, unconsciousness, coma)
- Hypotension (depressed systolic function, vasodilation, bradycardia, other arrhythmias)
- Electrocardiographic changes: widening of the QRS complex, inversion, bradycardia, ventricular premature complexes, ventricular tachycardia, ventricular fibrillation
- Death

concentration and area under the curve increased by almost 100% when compared with normal individuals.[4]

- Local anesthetic systemic toxicity typically manifests with CNS and cardiovascular system (CVS) complications (Box 11-1).
- Treatment of local anesthetic systemic toxicities consists of supportive therapy and pharmacologic treatment of the different clinical signs.
- More recently, specific agents have been developed that have the ability to chelate local anesthetics in plasma, reducing their circulating concentrations and minimizing their side effects.

Treatment

- Provide oxygen
- Intubate and ventilate with 100% O_2 if necessary
- Seizure control
  - Benzodiazepines (diazepam 0.25 to 0.5 mg/kg intravenously [IV])
  - Propofol (increments of 1 mg/kg IV)
  - Levetiracetam 20 mg/kg IV tid
- Intravenous fluids
- Vasopressors
  - Phenylephrine (bolus: 0.5 to 1 µg/kg IV; constant rate infusion [CRI]: 0.2 to 3 µg/kg/min IV)
  - Vasopressin (bolus: 0.003 IU/kg; CRI: 0.03 IU/kg/hr)
  - Epinephrine (increments of 1 µg/kg)
    - Epinephrine is not recommended for treatment of bupivacaine toxicity. The use of epinephrine may be limited because of the high incidence of serious ventricular dysrhythmias and lack of effectiveness on cardiac index and cardiac relaxation. Amrinone may be used instead.
- Inotropes
  - Dobutamine (CRI: 5 to 10 µg/kg/min)
  - Dopamine (CRI: 5 to 10 µg/kg/min)

- Anticholinergics
  - Atropine (0.02 to 0.05 mg/kg IV)
  - Glycopyrrolate (0.005 to 0.01 mg/kg IV)

If there is ventricular fibrillation or sustained ventricular tachycardia with severe hypotension (mean arterial pressure [MAP] <45 mm Hg)

- Cardiac massage
- Magnesium (0.3 to 0.6 mEq/kg IV over 5 minutes)
- Defibrillation (0.5 J/kg) may be considered
- "Lipid rescue" (Intralipid, Fresenius Kabi, Uppsala, Sweden) 1 mg/kg IV, can be repeated every 5 minutes or administered as a CRI at 0.25 mL/kg/min

Lipid Rescue

- Lipid emulsions have been the subject of multiple investigations and are now recommended for treatment of local anesthetic–induced cardiovascular collapse.[5]
- Administration of a 20% intravenous lipid emulsion (Intralipid, Fresenius Kabi, Uppsala, Sweden) has been shown to decrease mortality from 100% to 0% in rats after bupivacaine toxicity.[6]
- It is believed that a lipid emulsion creates a lipid plasma phase that extracts the lipid-soluble bupivacaine from the aqueous plasma phase, making it unavailable to tissues.[6]
- A 20% lipid emulsion is recommended to be administered as an initial bolus of 4 mL/kg followed by an infusion of 0.5 mL/kg/min for 10 minutes.

REFERENCES

1. Cuvillon P, Nouvellon E, Ripart J, et al. A comparison of the pharmacodynamics and pharmacokinetics of bupivacaine, ropivacaine (with epinephrine) and their equal volume mixtures with lidocaine used for femoral and sciatic nerve blocks: A double-blind randomized study. Anesth Analg. 2009; 108:641–649.
2. Neal JM. Effects of epinephrine in local anesthetics on the central and peripheral nervous systems: Neurotoxicity and neural blood flow. Reg Anesth Pain Med. 2003; 28:124–134.
3. Brummett CM, Hong EK, Janda AM, et al. Perineural dexmedetomidine added to ropivacaine for sciatic nerve block in rats prolongs the duration of analgesia by blocking the hyperpolarization-activated cation current. Anesthesiology. 2011; 115:836–843.
4. Perez-Guille BE, Villegas-Alvarez F, Toledo-Lopez A, et al. Pharmacokinetics of lidocaine and its metabolite as a hepatic function marker in dogs. Proc West Pharmacol Soc. 2011; 54:62–65.
5. RCA guidelines; www.spitalmures.ro/_files/protocoale_terapeutice/anestezie/anestezie__standarde_clinice.pdf.
6. Weinberg GL, VadeBoncouer T, Ramaraju GA, et al. (1998) Pretreatment or resuscitation with a lipid infusion shifts the dose-response to bupivacaine-induced asystole in rats. Anesthesiology 88, 1071–1075.

SUGGESTED READINGS

Almeida RM, Escobar A, Maguilnik S. Comparison of analgesia provided by lidocaine, lidocaine-morphine or lidocaine-tramadol delivered epidurally in dogs following orchiectomy. Vet Anaesth Analg. 2010; 37:542–549.

Eisenach JC, De Kock M, Klimscha W. Alpha(2)adrenergic agonists for regional anesthesia. A clinical review of clonidine: 1984-1995. Anesthesiology. 1996; 85:655–674.

Galindo A, Witcher T. Mixtures of local anesthetics: bupivacaine-chloroprocaine. Anesth Analg. 1980; 59:683–685.

Leffler A, Frank G, Kistner K, et al. Local anesthetic-like inhibition of voltage-gated Na+ channels by the partial mu-opioid receptor agonist buprenorphine. Anesthesiology. 2012; 116:1335–1346.

Pypendop BH, Siao KT, Pascoe PJ, et al. Effects of epidurally administered morphine or buprenorphine on the thermal threshold in cats. Am J Vet Res. 2008; 69:983–987.

Selander D, Brattsand R, Lundborg G, et al. Local anaesthetics: Importance of mode of application, concentration and adrenaline for the appearance of nerve lesions. An experimental study of axonal degeneration and barrier damage after intrafascicular injection or topical application of bupivacaine (Marcain). Acta Anaesth Scand. 1979; 23:127–133.

Weinberg G, Ripper R, Feinstein DL, et al. Lipid emulsion infusion rescues dogs from bupivacaine-induced cardiac toxicity. Reg Anesth Pain Med. 2003; 28:198–202.

Yoshitomi T, Kohjitani A, Maeda S, et al. Dexmedetomidine enhances the local anesthetic action of lidocaine via an alpha-2A adrenoceptor. Anesth Analg. 2008; 107:96–101.

CHAPTER 12

Local and Regional Anesthetic Techniques

Luis Campoy; Matt Read

GENERAL CONSIDERATIONS AND VETERINARY PATIENT PREPARATION

- For performance of the majority of nerve blocks in small animals, veterinary patients need to be either deeply sedated or anesthetized.
- Animals should be relaxed, easy to manipulate and position, and either minimally or completely unresponsive to needle advancement, electrolocation, and injection.
- Before any local or regional anesthetic technique is performed, the animal should be prepared properly.
  - Unless the block involves only subcutaneous injection of a local anesthetic solution (e.g., dental blocks, intratesticular blocks), the skin should be clipped free of hair and the skin surface should be scrubbed with a cleansing solution.
  - All other peripheral nerve blocks and epidural approaches should be treated as aseptic procedures, and sterile technique should be followed.

EQUIPMENT

There are many different needles, catheters, pumps, and specialized pieces of equipment that can be used to perform local or regional anesthetic techniques in small animal patients, and each has its own inherent advantages and disadvantages depending on the specific situation.

Needles

- Needles are generally selected based on their physical characteristics (e.g., tip design, length, gauge, absence or presence of insulation) and clinician preference.
- Needles that are used for local and regional anesthesia are typically designed for a single use.
- When possible, use of small-gauge needles is advisable to minimize the risk of nerve injury in the rare event that a nerve is inadvertently perforated during performance of a block.

- The design of the needle tip can affect the clinician's ability to appreciate the different tissue planes encountered as the needle is manipulated.
- As described for the majority of blocks in this chapter, if several different tissue planes will be crossed during performance of a particular regional anesthetic block, either short-bevel or Tuohy needles should be used.
  - These blunt needles convey more resistance to needle advancement, and the clinician is more likely to detect tactile "pops" as certain tissue planes are penetrated.
  - In addition, blunt (30- to 45-degree bevel, atraumatic) needle tips are less likely to penetrate the perineurium, especially if the needle approaches the nerve from a perpendicular orientation.
- Excessively long needles are more difficult to manipulate once they are in situ, especially if they are small gauge.
- Larger-gauge needles are less prone to bending, and their larger size allows for easier aspiration and injection, better appreciation of resistance to injection, and the potential to pass an indwelling catheter.
- Smaller-gauge needles tend to cause less pain in awake animals and carry less risk of causing nerve trauma.
- Based on these considerations, small-gauge needles (25 or 27 gauge) are typically used for infiltration anesthesia (e.g., incisional blocks) and superficial blocks (e.g., dental blocks), whereas large-gauge needles (19 to 22 gauge) are used for deeper blocks (e.g., brachial plexus, lumbar plexus, epidural).
- *Spinal needles* are characterized by sharpness. They have close-fitting, removable stylets that prevent tissue or fluid from entering the needle.
  - Designed for penetrating the dura mater during a spinal injection
- *Tuohy needles* are characterized by the presence of a curve at the distal tip of the needle that helps to "steer" the catheter in one particular direction along a peripheral nerve or into the epidural space.
  - Tuohy needles can be used to perform single-shot peripheral nerve or epidural injections or to facilitate placement of indwelling epidural or perineural catheters.
  - The tips of Tuohy needles are blunt, and as a result the clinician is able to better appreciate a tactile feeling as different tissue planes are penetrated.
- *Insulated nerve block needles* are coated with a thin layer of nonconducting material over the entire length of the needle except for a small area of metal that is exposed at the distal tip.
  - When the needle is connected to a peripheral nerve stimulator, the insulation on the needle prevents electric current from being released along the needle shaft into the surrounding tissues.
  - As a result, the current conducts down the length of the needle; thus a high-density current can be delivered at the exposed needle tip.

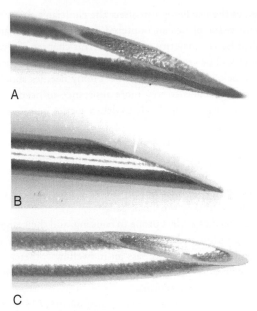

A

B

C

FIGURE 12-1   Close-up images of different types of needles. **A,** A 22-gauge hypodermic needle. **B,** A 22-gauge spinal needle. **C,** A 19-gauge Tuohy needle.

- When insulated needles are used for peripheral nerve blocks, low-intensity currents (0.2 to 0.5 mA) are used to stimulate motor fibers, helping in successful identification of the target nerves before injection of local anesthetic solutions (Figure 12-1).

PERIPHERAL NERVE STIMULATORS

- A peripheral nerve stimulator is a small piece of portable equipment that generates a square-wave electrical current.
- When a nerve stimulator is used with an insulated needle (see earlier discussion), the closer the needle is to the target nerve, the lower the electrical current required to elicit a muscle response.
- At sufficiently low currents (approximately 0.2 to 0.6 mA), if the stimulating needle is able to elicit contractions of the effector muscle or muscle group, it is assumed that the needle-to-nerve distance is small enough that if a local anesthetic solution is injected, sensory block will be achieved (Figure 12-2).

Use of Nerve Stimulation

1. Connect the negative electrode (*black*) to the insulated needle.
2. Connect the positive electrode (*red*) to the animal.

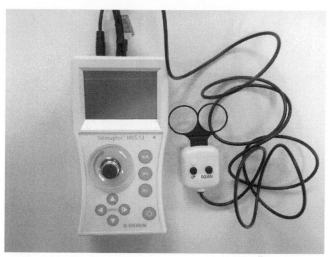

FIGURE 12-2   A peripheral nerve stimulator with a remote control for adjusting the delivered current.

3. Turn on the peripheral nerve stimulator and set the current at 1.0 to 1.5 mA.

4. Using anatomic landmarks, advance the insulated needle slowly toward the target nerve. When the nerve is exposed to enough current, depolarization of the nerve will occur, resulting in an observable or palpable muscle contraction (a twitch).

5. If motor responses are not encountered, carefully withdraw the needle to the level of the skin and redirect it.

6. Once a motor twitch is obtained, slowly decrease the current to zero, confirming that the twitches decrease in intensity.

7. Gradually increase the current from zero while making fine needle adjustments until a twitch is elicited at a final current of 0.5 mA or less (threshold current).

8. Aspirate the syringe. If blood is aspirated, reposition the needle.

9. Slowly inject the local anesthetic solution. As soon as the solution is injected, motor twitches will disappear as the local anesthetic (an electrolyte solution) expands the conductive area around the stimulating needle.

10. Ensure that there is no resistance to injection of the local anesthetic solution.

ULTRASOUND

• The combination of ultrasound technology and electrolocation is gaining popularity with veterinary clinicians.

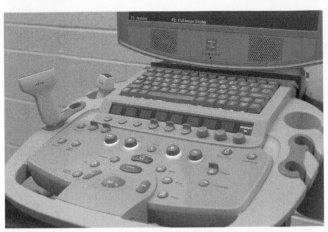

FIGURE 12-3   A sectorial\transducer ultrasound machine that can be used for performing regional anesthesia in small animal patients.

- Ultrasound allows for real-time visualization of the stimulating needle, as well as for identification of peripheral nerves and other important anatomic structures such as vessels, muscles, and fasciae.
- Although ultrasound guidance and electrolocation can be used separately for performing nerve blocks, they are very useful when used together.
- High-frequency linear array transducers (10 to 15 MHz) are most suitable for imaging superficial nerves that are less than 5 cm in depth (Figure 12-3).

Use of Ultrasound-Guided Peripheral Nerve Stimulation

1. Turn on the ultrasound machine and verify that the settings are optimized for nerve imaging.
2. Set the nerve stimulator to a frequency of 1 Hz (to minimally disturb the ultrasound image) and a current of 0.4 mA (threshold current).
3. Apply isopropyl alcohol (70%) to the area of the animal to be scanned to improve transducer-to-skin coupling and the quality of the resulting ultrasound image.
4. The non-dominant hand is used to place the transducer over the relevant area. Glide, rotate, or tilt the transducer until the target nerve (or nearby structures) can be identified in its short axis.
5. Insert the stimulating needle. Note that the long axis of the needle should be placed directly beneath the long axis of the ultrasound beam. This is known as the *in-plane technique* and allows the needle to be visualized while being advanced under the ultrasound beam.
6. Advance the needle toward the nerve, keeping the needle in the field of ultrasound view at all times.

7. Watch for the characteristic contractions of the appropriate muscle as the stimulating needle approaches the nerve.
8. Before administering the local anesthetic, aspirate the syringe. Positive aspiration of blood suggests that the needle has inadvertently penetrated a vessel and must be repositioned before drug administration.
9. If no blood is observed on aspiration, slowly begin to inject the local anesthetic. As you inject, use the ultrasound to monitor the fluid spreading around the nerve.
10. The anesthetic solution will appear as an anechoic (black) circumferential ring around the nerve. This is important to observe because it helps to rule out intravascular needle placement.
11. If at any point during the injection resistance is encountered, the presence of fluid accumulation around the nerve cannot be observed, or blood is aspirated, the needle position should be adjusted.

INFILTRATION AND WOUND CATHETERS

- Infiltration anesthesia is one of the oldest and most frequently used methods of providing local anesthesia and involves subcutaneous injection of local anesthetic solutions into different tissues.
- After injection, the injected drug diffuses into surrounding tissues and anesthetizes sensory nerves and nerve endings.
- Epinephrine (1:200,000) is often combined with local anesthetic solutions to reduce their absorption (thus reducing the risk of systemic toxicity) and to prolong their durations of action. This effect is more apparent when epinephrine is added to shorter-acting local anesthetics such as lidocaine.
- Bicarbonate can be added (approximately 0.3 mL bicarbonate to 9.7 mL local anesthetic) immediately before injection to minimize discomfort on injection in awake or lightly sedated animals.
- Local anesthetics have been investigated for their effects on wound healing in both in vitro and in vivo studies. Although results are equivocal, clinical experience suggests that the risk of complications is minimal when infiltration anesthesia is used in healthy animals and when aseptic techniques are followed.

INCISIONAL LINE BLOCK

- For its full benefits to be obtained, the incisional line block should be performed before surgery.
- Studies have shown that perioperative local infiltration along the planned incision line is associated with lower pain scores in the postoperative period and therefore reduced requirements for other analgesics.

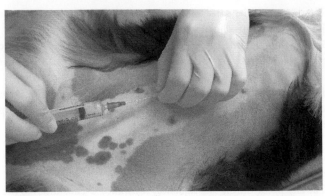

FIGURE 12-4 An incisional line block is being performed in a female dog before ovariohysterectomy.

- There is some evidence that unless muscle or linea alba is also blocked, infiltrating only the local subcutaneous tissue will not result in any perceived analgesic benefits.
- Although mild edema will be present in the injected tissues initially after administration, the tissues will return to normal by the time the abdominal incision is closed (Figure 12-4).

Step-by-Step Procedure

1. After preparation of the skin, insert a small-gauge needle (25- or 22-gauge hypodermic needle or spinal needle) subcutaneously along the linea alba.
2. Aspirate before injection of the anesthetic solution.
3. Inject the local anesthetic solution into the subcutaneous tissues and muscles until a noticeable bleb is created under the skin.
4. Remove the needle and reinsert it further along the anticipated incision line.
5. Aspirate and inject additional local anesthetic solution to extend the block.
6. Repeat this process until the length of the incision has been blocked.

Drugs and Dosage

Bupivacaine (0.5%) or lidocaine (2%), with or without epinephrine, are typically used at doses up to 2 mg/kg. If necessary, the local anesthetic solution can be diluted up to 50:50 with saline (0.9%) to increase the injectate volume.

INTRATESTICULAR BLOCKS

Studies have shown that intratesticular blocks lower inhalant anesthetic requirements during surgery and are associated with lower pain scores in the postoperative period (Figure 12-5).

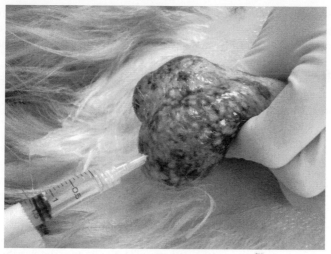

FIGURE 12-5   An intratesticular block is being performed in a male dog before castration.

Step-by-Step Procedure

1. After preparation of the skin, insert a small gauge needle (25- or 22-gauge hypodermic needle) into the body of the testis.
2. Aspirate before injection of the anesthetic solution.
3. Slowly inject the local anesthetic solution into the testis until the pressure within the testis is subjectively considered to increase (i.e., when the testis becomes palpably firm and swollen).

Drugs and Dosage

Bupivacaine (up to 1 mg/kg) or lidocaine (up to 2 mg/kg) without epinephrine is typically used, although the calculated volume is rarely necessary to reach the endpoint described previously.

WOUND CATHETERS

- Local infiltration techniques are limited by the duration of action of the particular local anesthetic that is used.
- The benefits of local anesthesia can be extended into the postoperative period by placement of a multi-fenestrated indwelling catheter into the operative field.
- Wound soaker (diffusion) catheters are technically easy to use, offer the potential for complete analgesia, and allow for repeated or continuous administration of local anesthetic solutions into painful wounds.

- Studies in animals and people have shown that use of wound soaker catheters is associated with lower pain scores, lowered requirements for other analgesics, and improved mobility and patient satisfaction (in humans).

Equipment

- Wound soaker catheter
- Suture
- PRN injection port
- Local anesthetic solution
- Infusion system (pump, syringes, and so on) can also be used

Step-by-Step Procedure

1. Place the catheter into the operative site at the end of the surgery, ideally near any visible nerves.
2. The fenestrations on the distal end of the catheter must all be placed into the wound; otherwise, local anesthetic will leak out onto the skin. Select a catheter with the appropriate length of fenestrations for the wound.
3. Close the surgical wound over the catheter (Figure 12-6).
4. Secure the catheter to the animal's skin using a suture wing or other method to prevent its dislodgment.
5. Connect the injection port or administration set to the catheter.
6. Administer the local anesthetic solution into the wound as required.
7. A sterile dressing can be used to cover the catheter insertion site to minimize infections.

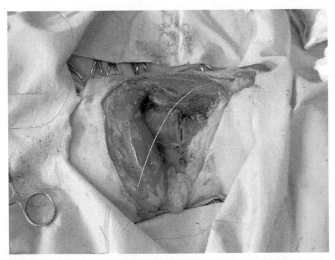

FIGURE 12-6   A wound soaker catheter is being placed into the surgical field after cancer surgery in a cat. The tissues will be closed over the catheter and it will be left in place as a means of providing local anesthesia for several days postoperatively.

HEAD

- Regional anesthesia is useful for providing anesthesia and analgesia to facilitate a variety of procedures on the head, or to treat preexisting painful conditions.
- The anatomic structures that are used to locate injection sites are easily identified in dogs and cats, making these blocks easy to perform in the majority of animals.

Infraorbital Nerve Block

- The infraorbital nerve is the rostral continuation of the maxillary nerve.
- When local anesthetic is injected only outside the infraorbital foramen, the block will anesthetize only the skin of the upper lip and nose but not the teeth.
- A 25-gauge, 2.5-cm (approximately 1 inch) hypodermic needle is adequate for most dogs and cats.

Step-by-Step Procedure

1. Palpate the infraorbital foramen on the lateral aspect of the maxilla, rostral to the medial canthus of the eye.
2. In larger animals, the infraorbital neurovascular bundle can be palpated under the skin as it leaves the infraorbital canal.
3. Insert the needle either percutaneously or intraorally after the upper lip is reflected dorsally.
4. Once the needle is located over the nerve, use a syringe to aspirate for blood.
5. Inject a small amount of local anesthetic (0.25 to 1 mL) over the infraorbital nerve.

Maxillary Foramen Block

- The maxillary nerve supplies the majority of sensory innervation to the upper jaw and its associated structures.
- When a local anesthetic solution is injected at the level of the maxillary foramen, this block will provide anesthesia and analgesia to all maxillary teeth and soft tissues, the hard and soft palate, and the lateral nasal mucosa.
- A 25-gauge, 2.5-cm (approximately 1-inch) hypodermic needle is adequate for most dogs and cats.

Step-by-Step Procedure

Three different approaches to the maxillary nerve have been described in dogs and cats.

Infraorbital Approach. See Figure 12-7.

1. Insert the needle as if performing an infraorbital nerve block (described earlier).

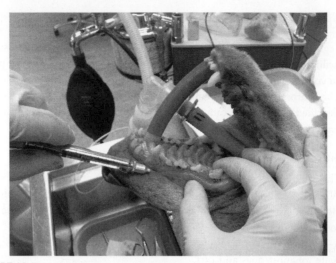

FIGURE 12-7 A maxillary block is being performed in a dog with use of a 27-gauge needle and an aspirating syringe. Note that a finger is used to press the skin overlying the infraorbital foramen to direct the injected local anesthetic into the infraorbital canal toward the maxillary nerve.

2. Inject a greater amount of local anesthetic (0.5 to 1 mL) into the infra-orbital canal and allow for proximal migration of the injectate toward the maxillary foramen while applying digital pressure over the foramen to prevent leakage out of the canal.

Subzygomatic Approach

1. Insert the needle transcutaneously ventral to the rostroventral border of the zygomatic arch, immediately caudal to the maxilla.
2. The needle is inserted perpendicular to the skin surface and is advanced toward the pterygopalatine fossa where the maxillary nerve courses before entering the maxillary foramen.
3. Use a syringe to aspirate for blood.
4. Inject a small amount of local anesthetic (0.25 to 1 mL).

Mental Nerve Block

- The mental nerve is the rostral continuation of the inferior alveolar nerve.
- When local anesthetic is injected at the level of the mental foramen, the block will anesthetize the rostral soft tissues of the lower lip but not the teeth.
- A 25-gauge, 2.5-cm (approximately 1-inch) hypodermic needle is adequate for most dogs and cats.
- In larger animals, the middle mental foramen can be palpated on the lateral aspect of the mandible, ventral to the mesial root of the second premolar tooth.

- The labial frenulum lies over the foramen and may also serve as a landmark if the foramen cannot be directly palpated.

Step-by-Step Procedure
1. Insert the needle under the skin or the mucosa of the labial frenulum over the mental foramen.
2. Use a syringe to aspirate for blood.
3. Inject a small amount of local anesthetic (0.25 to 1 mL) over the mental nerve.

Inferior Alveolar Nerve Block

- When local anesthetic is injected at the level of the mandibular foramen, the block will anesthetize the mandible and the mandibular teeth of the ipsilateral hemiarcade.
- The buccal nerve provides sensation to the soft tissue of the buccal aspect of the first, second, and third molars as well as the soft tissues of the chin and lower lip.
- Desensitization of the lingual gingiva, the floor of the mouth, and the rostral two thirds of the tongue may develop if the local anesthetic solution diffuses proximally to the lingual nerve.
- A 25-gauge, 2.5-cm (approximately 1-inch) hypodermic needle is adequate for most dogs and cats. Larger dogs may require a longer needle.
- The mandibular foramen can be palpated on the medial aspect of ramus, slightly dorsal to the vascular notch (concavity on the caudoventral aspect of the mandible).

Step-by-Step Procedure
The needle can be inserted either intraorally or transcutaneously, depending on the size of the animal and operator preference.

Intraoral Approach
1. Hold the mouth open using a mouth gag.
2. The mandibular foramen is localized with a finger of the free hand, and the needle is inserted through the mucosa medial to the mandible and lateral to the pterygomandibular raphe, at the level of the last mandibular molar tooth.
3. The needle is then directed ventrocaudally, toward the angular process, between the operator's fingers and the mandibular bone, to reach the mandibular foramen.
4. Once the needle is in the vicinity of the mandibular foramen, use a syringe to aspirate for blood.
5. Inject a small amount of local anesthetic (0.25 to 1 mL).

Extraoral Approach. See Figure 12-8.
1. This approach can be performed either by palpating the mandibular foramen (as described earlier) or blindly.

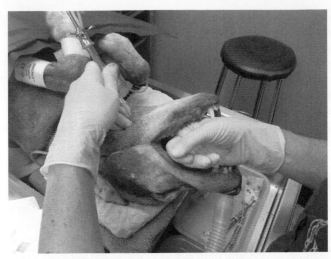

FIGURE 12-8 An inferior alveolar block is being performed in a dog with use of a 27-gauge needle and an aspirating syringe. Note that a mouth gag has been placed and a finger is being used to guide the needle into position beside the mandibular foramen on the medial aspect of the mandible.

2. In either case, place the needle perpendicular to the ventral margin of the mandible at the level of the vascular notch (immediately rostral to the angular process).
3. Place the needle by "walking off" the mandible medially and slowly advancing it to the level of the mandibular foramen (with or without it being palpated intraorally).
4. Once the needle is in the vicinity of the mandibular foramen, use a syringe to aspirate for blood.
5. Inject a small amount of local anesthetic (0.25 to 1 mL).

Retrobulbar Block

- The eye, adnexa, and orbit are richly innervated, suggesting that there is a high potential for pain associated with ophthalmic disease and surgery.
- Regional anesthesia is an effective means of minimizing the systemic side effects of other analgesic and anesthetic drugs during surgery, and for providing excellent postoperative pain control.

Positioning

- There are no specific requirements for positioning for administration of retrobulbar anesthesia to small animal patients.

- Positioning is based on operator preference and is often dependent on when the block is performed (preoperatively, intraoperatively, or postoperatively).
- Use the lateral canthus and the middle of the lower eyelid as landmarks.

Equipment
- 22-gauge, 1.5-inch spinal needle (bent in the middle of its shaft to create an approximately 20-degree angle)
- Local anesthetic solution

Step-by-Step Procedure
1. Position the needle midway between the lateral canthus and the middle of the lower eyelid (Figure 12-9).
2. Insert the needle along the inferior eyelid until it contacts the orbital rim.
3. Walk the needle off the orbital rim and direct it along the floor of the orbit, redirecting it dorsally to reach the apex of the orbit.
4. A slight popping sensation may be detected (occurs when the needle penetrates the orbital fascia).
5. Use a syringe to aspirate before injection.
6. Slowly inject the local anesthetic into the orbit. If resistance is encountered, withdraw and redirect the needle slightly.
7. If the block is successful, the pupil will dilate and the eye will rotate to a central orientation.

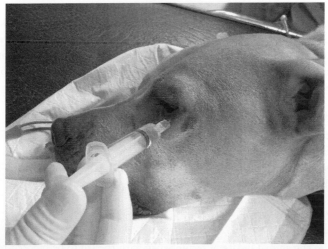

FIGURE 12-9   A retrobulbar block is being performed in a dog before enucleation surgery.

Drugs and Dosage

Use up to a maximum of 2 mL of local anesthetic solution (usually bupivacaine 0.5%).

THORACIC LIMB

Relevant Anatomy

- The ventral branches of the C6, C7, C8, and T1 spinal nerves provide sensory and motor innervation of the thoracic limb.
- The most relevant nerves, from cranial to caudal, are the suprascapular, subscapular, axillary, musculocutaneous, radial, median, and ulnar nerves.
- The axillary artery and vein are also located in the axillary space and are found immediately caudal to the median and ulnar nerves and cranial to the first rib.

Cervical Paravertebral Block

- Although it was originally described in 2000 and has been used clinically since then by some practitioners, the cervical paravertebral block is only now being critically investigated for use in small animals.
- Studies have shown that even when it is performed with ultrasound and/ or nerve stimulation, it is associated with important complications such as epidural spread of injectate and lack of efficacy. Until more detail is known about this block, it is not recommended for general use.

Brachial Plexus Block

- The brachial plexus block is considered to be an intermediate-level technique.
- Knowledge of relevant anatomy is required to increase the success rate and minimize the possible complications associated with this block.
- The brachial plexus block typically results in anesthesia of the distal humerus and structures distal to it (elbow, antebrachium, distal limb).
- Blind approaches to the brachial plexus are associated with low success rates and are therefore not recommended.

Use of Nerve Stimulation

Equipment

- Peripheral nerve stimulator
- Insulated needle (22-gauge, 50-mm needle for small or medium-sized animals; 21-gauge, 100-mm needle for larger animals)
- Local anesthetic solution

Positioning

Position the animal in lateral recumbency with the leg to be blocked placed uppermost and held in a natural position perpendicular to the longitudinal axis of the body.

Step-by-Step Procedure

1. Identify the acromion, point of the shoulder, first rib, and jugular vein.
2. The puncture site is located cranial to the acromion and medial to the subscapularis muscle.
3. Set the nerve stimulator to deliver a current of 1 mA at 1 to 2 Hz.
4. Insert the needle and carefully advance it in a caudal direction medial to the scapula (Figure 12-10).
5. When the tip of the needle approaches the musculocutaneous nerve, contractions of the biceps brachii muscle will result in flexion of the elbow. At this level, the musculocutaneous nerve is the most cranially located nerve of the brachial plexus (in a medium-sized dog, it is approximately 1 to 2 cm deep to the skin).
6. Extension of the elbow (from stimulation of the radial nerve) is also an acceptable end point. With this motor response, care must be taken because the axillary vessels lie just ventral to this position and any further needle advancement runs the risk of vascular puncture.
7. Pronation of the extremity (from stimulation of the median and ulnar nerves) should not be considered an acceptable end point because this response suggests that the needle has already been advanced past the major sensory nerves (radial, axillary). If this motor response is observed, the needle should be withdrawn until flexion or extension of the elbow is observed.
8. Once acceptable twitches are seen, incrementally decrease the nerve stimulator current to 0.4 mA, making sure that the same motor responses are elicited. Reposition the needle if necessary.

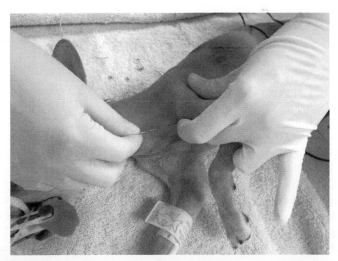

FIGURE 12-10 A brachial plexus block is being performed with a peripheral nerve stimulator before elbow surgery in a dog.

9. Before injection of the local anesthetic solution, it is important to verify that the needle is not positioned either intravascularly or intraneurally. Negative blood aspiration should be observed. It is imperative to ensure that no resistance during the injection is encountered.

Drugs and Dosage
- The recommended volume of local anesthetic to be injected is 0.25 to 0.3 mL/kg.
- Bupivacaine 0.5% is commonly combined with dexmedetomidine (0.5 μg/mL) to provide approximately 12 to 28 hours of blockade. Ropivacaine 0.75% combined with dexmedetomidine (0.5 μg/mL) can be used with similar results.

Use of Ultrasonography and Nerve Stimulation

Equipment
- Ultrasound machine with high-frequency linear array transducer (9 to 15 MHz)
- Peripheral nerve stimulator
- Insulated needle (22-gauge, 50-mm needle for small or medium-sized animals; 21-gauge, 100-mm needle for larger animals)
- Local anesthetic solution

Positioning
Position the animal in dorsal recumbency with the thoracic limbs flexed in a natural position.

Step-by-Step Procedure
See Figure 12-11.
1. The nondominant hand is used to place the ultrasound transducer over the axillary region in the depression that is created between the manubrium of the sternum and the supraglenoid tubercle of the scapula.
2. The transducer is oriented in a parasagittal plane and is glided, rotated, or tilted until the axillary vein and artery are observed in cross section (sometimes referred to as the "double-bubble" sign). These vessels will appear as anechoic (black) round structures and the artery will pulse.
3. Immediately dorsal to these vessels, identify the round hyperechoic (white or gray) root of C8 that is also observed in cross section.
4. Set the nerve stimulator to deliver a current of 1 mA at 1 Hz.
5. Once C8 has been identified, insert the stimulating needle dorsal to the cranial edge of the pectoralis muscle and lateral to the jugular vein. The needle should be advanced in-plane with the transducer to allow it to be observed approaching the target nerve root.
6. Advance the needle in a cranial-to-caudal direction, keeping the needle in the field of ultrasound view at all times. Aim the needle for the area

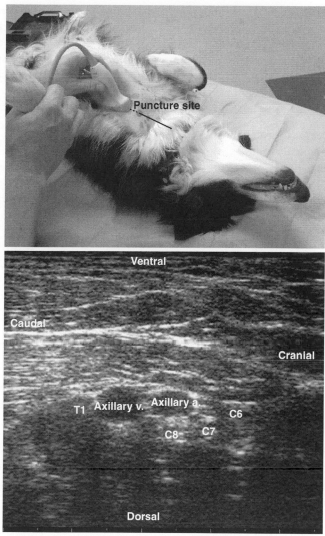

FIGURE 12-11   Ultrasound is being used to image the brachial plexus block of a sedated dog. Note the puncture site for a needle to be seen in-plane, and the important anatomic structures that must be identified before the block is performed.

directly dorsal to the axillary artery, in close proximity to the C8 root. Monitor for elbow extension resulting from triceps brachii muscle contraction as a result of C8 nerve root stimulation.

7. Once acceptable twitches are seen, incrementally decrease the nerve stimulator current to 0.4 mA, making sure that the same motor responses are elicited. Reposition the needle if necessary.

8. Before the local anesthetic solution is injected, verify that the needle is not positioned either intravascularly or intraneurally. Negative blood aspiration should be observed.

9. As the local anesthetic solution is injected, watch for fluid to spread around the target nerves (the anesthetic solution will appear anechoic). No resistance should be encountered during injection.

10. This approach should be repeated to block the other nerve roots that were observed close to the axillary artery.

Drugs and Dosage

The total volume of local anesthetic to be injected should be approximately 0.15 to 0.2 mL/kg; however, the final injection volume can be adjusted by monitoring the spread of the solution on the ultrasound image. The full volume does not need to be used if all of the target nerves appear to be surrounded by local anesthetic solution.

RUMM Block

Blockade of the radial, ulnar, median, and musculocutaneous nerves at the level of the mid-humerus will provide anesthesia of the distal limb, including the radius, ulna, carpus, and paw.

Relevant Anatomy

- The radial nerve is blocked on the lateral aspect of the distal humerus, between the lateral head of the triceps and the brachialis muscle.
- The ulnar, median, and musculocutaneous nerves are blocked on the medial aspect of the mid-humerus, cranial and caudal to the palpable pulse of the brachial artery.

Equipment

- Peripheral nerve stimulator
- Insulated needle (22-gauge, 50-mm needle)
- Local anesthetic solution

Positioning

- Position the animal in lateral recumbency with the leg to be blocked uppermost (for the radial nerve) or lowermost (for the other nerves).
- The elbow should be held in a flexed position.

Step-by-Step Procedure

1. Set the nerve stimulator to deliver a current of 1 mA at 1 to 2 Hz.
2. Insert the needle through the skin and carefully advance it toward the target nerve(s).
3. When the tip of the needle approaches the radial nerve, stimulation will result in extension of the carpus.

4. When the tip of the needle approaches the median nerve, stimulation will result in flexion and pronation of the antebrachium.

5. When the tip of the needle approaches the ulnar nerve, stimulation will result in flexion of the carpus and paw.

6. Once acceptable twitches are seen, incrementally decrease the nerve stimulator current to 0.4 mA, making sure that the same motor responses are elicited. Reposition the needle if necessary.

7. Before injection of the local anesthetic solution, it is important to verify that the needle is not positioned either intravascularly or intraneurally. Negative blood aspiration should be observed. It is imperative to ensure that no resistance during the injection is encountered.

Drugs and Dosage

• Bupivacaine (0.5%) is typically used for this block, with 0.1 mL/kg used for the radial nerve and 0.15 mL/kg used for the two injections to block the ulnar, median, and musculocutaneous nerves.

Blocks for the Manus in Cats

Local anesthesia can be provided to the distal limb to facilitate a variety of painful procedures including onychectomy surgery in cats, toe amputations, or any other surgery of the foot distal to the carpus.

Relevant Anatomy

Distal to the elbow:

• The radial nerve runs down the dorsomedial aspect of the limb.
• The ulnar nerve runs along the lateral aspect of the limb.
• The median nerve runs along the palmar aspect of the limb.

Equipment

• 25-gauge hypodermic needle
• Local anesthetic solution

Positioning

Position the animal in lateral recumbency or dorsal recumbency such that each of the thoracic limbs can be manipulated and all aspects of the distal limb may be accessed.

Step-by-Step Procedure

See Figure 12-12.

1. Injections are made at three specific locations on the distal limb. Alternatively, a ring block may be performed by injecting the calculated dose of local anesthetic around the entire limb at the level of the carpus. If both

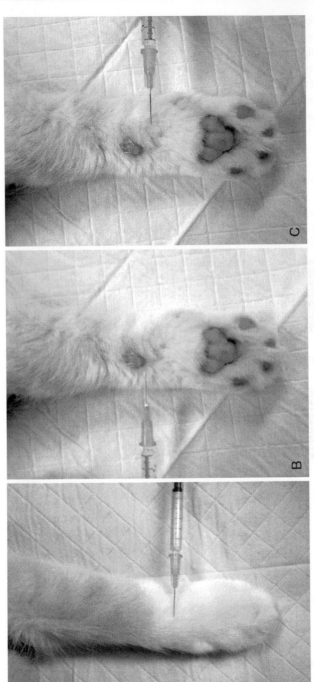

FIGURE 12-12 Locations for injections for distal limb analgesia in a cat. **A,** Radial nerve. **B,** Ulnar nerve. **C,** Median nerve.

legs are being blocked, the total dose of local anesthetic must be divided between the two limbs.

  a. *Radial nerve:* Insert the needle just distal to the carpus on the dorsomedial aspect of the metacarpus. Aspirate. Inject one third of the volume to be used for that limb.

  b. *Ulnar nerve:* Insert the needle on the lateral aspect of the limb at the level of the carpus. Aspirate. Inject one third of the volume to be used for that limb.

  c. *Median nerve:* Insert the needle just distal to the accessory carpal pad on the palmar aspect of the metacarpus. Aspirate. Inject one third of the volume to be used for that limb.

Drugs and Dosage

Bupivacaine (0.5%) is typically used for this block, up to a total dose of 2 mg/kg.

TRUNK

- Anesthesia and analgesia of the thoracic wall can be achieved by blocking the intercostal nerves.
- This can be accomplished by depositing local anesthetic solution adjacent to the nerves (intercostal block), near the point at which they leave the vertebral column (thoracic paravertebral block), or by injecting the solution into the pleural space so that it can diffuse across the parietal pleura to reach the intercostal nerves (interpleural block).
- Intercostal blocks and interpleural blocks are well described and are detailed here. Thoracic paravertebral blocks are commonly used in people, and are starting to be investigated for use in small animals.
- Anesthesia and analgesia of the abdomen are typically accomplished by use of epidural anesthesia or incisional line blocks. The transversus abdominis plane (TAP) block is a relatively new technique that has been recently investigated for use in small animals.

Intercostal Block

- The intercostal block is useful for providing analgesia before and after intercostal thoracotomy and chest tube placement and for desensitizing fractured ribs.
- It can be performed intraoperatively before closure of the thoracotomy incision, percutaneously before surgery, or in nonsurgical animal patients.
- This block is usually performed with use of anatomic landmarks and a regular needle, but it can also be performed with a nerve stimulator and an insulated needle (which is especially helpful in obese animals).

Equipment
- 25- or 22-gauge hypodermic or spinal needle
- Local anesthetic solution
- Peripheral nerve stimulator and insulated needle (22-gauge, 50-mm needle) can also be used

Positioning
Position the animal in lateral recumbency with the operative or affected side placed uppermost.

Step-by-Step Procedure
1. Blocks are performed two to three intercostal spaces cranial and caudal to the affected area (e.g., planned incision, fractured rib).
2. Each intercostal nerve is located on the caudal aspect of its associated rib, in close proximity to the intercostal vein and artery.
3. Insert the needle through the skin onto the rib, as far dorsally as the rib can be palpated.
4. Walk the needle off the caudal side of the rib until it enters the intercostal space. Do not advance the tip of the needle into the pleural space.
5. Use a syringe to aspirate for blood and air.
6. Slowly inject the desired volume of local anesthetic solution.

Drugs and Dosage
- The recommended volume of local anesthetic to be injected is 0.25 to 1.0 mL per nerve or site depending on animal size.
- Bupivacaine 0.5% is commonly used, up to a total dose of 2 mg/kg in small animals.
- For chronic administration, a wound soaker catheter may be tunneled subcutaneously along the intercostal space to facilitate continuous or repeated intermittent delivery of local anesthetics.

Interpleural Block
- The interpleural block is typically used to provide analgesia and anesthesia related to pain of thoracic origin.
- When used appropriately, it can also be used to treat pain related to the cranial abdomen, including pancreatitis.

Equipment
- Small gauge (22- or 20-gauge) butterfly catheter or through-the-needle catheter
- Local anesthetic solution
- If already placed, a preexisting chest tube can also be used to administer the local anesthetic solution

Positioning

Position the animal in lateral recumbency.

Step-by-Step Procedure

See Figure 12-13.

1. Connect the catheter to a syringe filled with 2 to 3 mL saline via a three-way stopcock.
2. Advance it onto the lateral aspect of the seventh or eighth rib at its midpoint (as measured from dorsal to ventral).
3. Walk the needle off the cranial border of the rib until it can be advanced through the intercostal space. Entering the thorax at the cranial border of

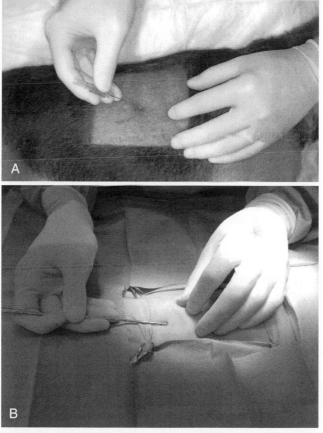

FIGURE 12-13 Interpleural analgesia can be administered by temporary placement of a catheter into the pleural space **(A)** or by placement of a chest tube **(B)**. A local anesthetic is injected into the interpleural space, and the animal is positioned such that the local anesthetic solution pools on the target intercostal nerves.

the rib helps minimize the risk of traumatizing the intercostal nerve and vascular bundle.

4. Once the parietal pleura is penetrated (often with a palpable pop or click), the column of saline in the syringe will slowly decrease in volume as the negative interpleural pressure aspirates it into the interpleural space.

5. If an over-the-needle catheter is used, advance the catheter off the needle stylet into the interpleural space.

6. A preloaded syringe with local anesthetic solution is then switched with the saline and the calculated volume of local anesthetic is slowly injected over 1 to 2 minutes through the catheter into the pleural space.

7. After injection of the local anesthetic, the catheter is withdrawn and the animal is maintained in a specific position for at least 10 minutes, allowing the local anesthetic to pool and block the underlying intercostal nerves.

   a. Blockade of the lateral thoracic wall is accomplished by placing the animal in lateral recumbency with the affected side down.

   b. Blockade of the sternum is accomplished by placing the animal in ventral recumbency.

8. If interpleural anesthesia does not appear to be effective, alter the animal's position to change the distribution of the local anesthetic.

9. Instead of use of a butterfly or over-the-needle catheter to perform a single-shot block, an indwelling catheter or chest tube can be placed into the pleural space to facilitate repeated injections.

Drugs and Dosage

Bupivacaine 0.5% is commonly used, up to a total dose of 2 mg/kg.

TAP Block

Based on research and clinical experiences in people, the TAP block is being investigated for use in small animals as a method for providing analgesia and anesthesia to the ventral abdominal wall.

Relevant Anatomy

- The abdominal wall consists of three muscle layers: the external abdominal oblique, the internal abdominal oblique, and the transversus abdominis, as well as their associated fascial sheaths.

- The ventral branches of the caudal thoracic and cranial lumbar nerves innervate the skin, muscles, and parietal peritoneum of the ventral abdominal wall.

- These nerves run ventrally through the fascial plane that exists between the internal abdominal oblique and transversus abdominis muscles.

- An ultrasound-guided technique allows for direct visualization of the different layers of the body wall, increasing the chances of block success while decreasing chances of peritoneal puncture (performing the TAP block blindly in small animals is unlikely to be successful and is therefore not recommended).

Equipment
- Ultrasound machine with high-frequency (9 to 15 MHz) linear array transducer
- Tuohy or spinal needles
- Local anesthetic solution
- Peripheral nerve stimulator and insulated needle (22-gauge, 50-mm needle) can also be used

Positioning
- Place the animal in lateral recumbency with the side to be blocked uppermost.
- The area of interest is found midway between the caudal aspect of the last rib and the iliac crest.

Step-by-Step Procedure
1. The nondominant hand is used to place the ultrasound transducer over the lateral body wall.
2. A clear image of the three muscle layers of the abdominal wall should be obtained before needle insertion.
3. Insert the needle in-plane through the skin and external and internal abdominal oblique muscles and into the fascial plane overlying the transversus abdominis muscle.
4. Inject a small (0.5 to 1 mL) test dose of local anesthetic solution into the potential space between the transversus abdominis and the internal abdominal oblique muscles.
5. Use the ultrasound image to visualize spread of the local anesthetic within the desired facial plane.
6. Once the needle is confirmed to be within the fascial plane, inject the remainder of the diluted local anesthetic solution for that side of the block.
7. After performance of the TAP block on one side, the animal is turned over into the other lateral recumbency and the procedure is repeated.

Drugs and Dosage
A dilute solution of bupivacaine is used, to a total volume of 1 mL/kg (ensuring that the animal does not receive more than 2 mg/kg of bupivacaine total, including what is used to block the contralateral side).

PELVIC LIMB

Relevant Anatomy

- The pelvic limbs of dogs and cats are innervated by the lumbar (femoral) and sacral (sciatic) nervous plexuses that arise from the L3, L4, and L5 and the L6, L7, and S1 spinal nerves, respectively.
- Both areas need to be blocked if surgical anesthesia and analgesia are to be provided to the entire pelvic limb.
- Femoral and sciatic nerve blocks are minimally invasive and are associated with few complications.

Femoral Nerve Block

- The femoral nerve block can be used to provide anesthesia for a wide range of surgical procedures and is commonly used in combination with a sciatic nerve block to achieve anesthesia of the pelvic limb.
- Use of a femoral nerve block will result in anesthesia of the femur (mid-diaphysis to distal femur), the femorotibial joint (medial aspect of the femorotibial joint capsule), and the skin of the dorsomedial tarsus and first digit.

Use of Nerve Stimulation

Equipment
- Peripheral nerve stimulator
- Insulated needle (22-gauge, 50-mm needle)
- Local anesthetic solution

Positioning
Position the animal in lateral recumbency with the limb to be blocked uppermost, abducted 90 degrees, and extended caudally.

Step-by-Step Procedure
See Figure 12-14.
1. Palpate the pectineus muscle, which is felt as a tight triangular muscular band on the medial aspect of the leg.
2. Palpate the femoral artery dorsal and cranial to the pectineus muscle.
3. Set the nerve stimulator to deliver a current of 1 mA at 1 to 2 Hz.
4. The puncture site is located within the femoral triangle, cranial to the femoral artery.
5. Insert the stimulating needle cranial to the femoral artery and advance it toward the iliopsoas muscle, maintaining a 20- to 30-degree angle to the skin.
6. Once the tip of the needle is close to the femoral nerve, contractions of the quadriceps muscle will result in stifle extension.

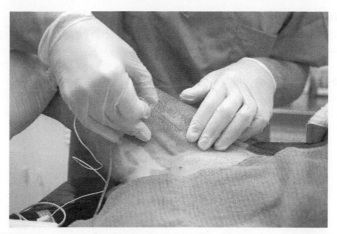

FIGURE 12-14   A femoral nerve block is being performed with a peripheral nerve stimulator before stifle surgery in a dog.

7. Once acceptable twitches are seen, incrementally decrease the nerve stimulator current to 0.4 mA, making sure that the same motor responses are elicited. Reposition the needle if necessary, ensuring that the fascia iliaca has been punctured (a pop or click will be felt).

8. Before injection of the local anesthetic solution, it is important to verify that the needle is not positioned either intravascularly or intraneurally. Negative blood aspiration should be observed. It is imperative to ensure that no resistance during the injection is encountered.

Drugs and Dosage

- The recommended volume of local anesthetic to be injected is 0.1 mL/kg
- Bupivacaine 0.5% is commonly combined with dexmedetomidine (0.5 μg/mL) to provide approximately 14 (6 to 24) hours (median [minimum to maximum]) of postoperative analgesia after cruciate surgery. Ropivacaine 0.75% combined with dexmedetomidine (0.5 μg/mL) can be used with similar results.

Use of Ultrasonography and Nerve Stimulation

Equipment

- Ultrasound machine with high-frequency linear array transducer (9 to 15 MHz)
- Peripheral nerve stimulator
- Insulated needle (22-gauge, 50-mm needle for small to medium-sized animals; 21-gauge, 100-mm needle for larger animals)
- Local anesthetic solution

Positioning

Position the animal in lateral recumbency with the limb to be blocked positioned uppermost, abducted 90 degrees, and extended caudally.

Step-by-Step Procedure

See Figure 12-15.

1. The nondominant hand is used to place the ultrasound transducer over the femoral triangle, perpendicular to the course of the femoral artery.

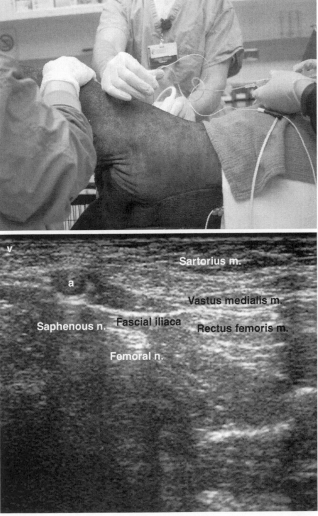

FIGURE 12-15   A femoral nerve block is being performed with use of ultrasound guidance and a peripheral nerve stimulator before stifle surgery in a dog.

2. Glide, rotate, or tilt the transducer until a short-axis view of the femoral vessels and the femoral and saphenous nerves is obtained. The vessels will appear as anechoic (black) round structures, and the artery will pulse.

3. Identify the round hyperechoic (white or gray, sometimes with a honeycomb-like structure) femoral and saphenous nerves in cross-section.

4. Set the peripheral nerve stimulator to deliver a current of 0.4 mA at 1 Hz.

5. Once the femoral nerve has been identified, insert the stimulating needle from a cranial-to-caudal direction through the sartorius and rectus femoris muscles. The needle should be advanced in-plane with the transducer to allow it to be observed approaching the femoral nerve.

6. Monitor for stifle extension that results from contraction of the quadriceps femoris muscles as the femoral nerve is stimulated.

7. Before the local anesthetic solution is injected, verify that the needle is not positioned either intravascularly or intraneurally. Negative blood aspiration should be observed.

8. As the local anesthetic solution is injected, watch for fluid to spread around the femoral nerve (the anesthetic solution will appear anechoic). No resistance should be encountered during injection.

Drugs and Dosage

- The total volume of local anesthetic to be injected is 0.1 mL/kg; however, the final injection volume can be adjusted by monitoring the spread of the solution on the ultrasound image. The full volume does not need to be used if the femoral and saphenous nerves appear to be surrounded by the local anesthetic solution.

- Bupivacaine 0.5% is commonly combined with dexmedetomidine (0.5 μg/mL) to provide approximately 14 (6 to 24) hours (median [minimum to maximum]) of postoperative analgesia after cruciate surgery. Ropivacaine 0.75% combined with dexmedetomidine (0.5 μg/mL) can be used with similar results.

Sciatic Nerve Block

A sciatic nerve block alone is sufficient for surgery of the foot and the hock. If the surgical procedure involves the tibia or the stifle, the femoral nerve should also be included in the block technique.

Use of Nerve Stimulation
Equipment

- Peripheral nerve stimulator
- Insulated needle (22-gauge, 50-mm needle)
- Local anesthetic solution

Positioning. Position the animal in lateral recumbency with the limb to be blocked uppermost and extended in a natural position.

Step-by-Step Procedure. See Figure 12-16.

1. Set the nerve stimulator to deliver a current of 1 mA at 1 to 2 Hz.
2. Identify the greater trochanter (GT) and ischial tuberosity (IT). The puncture site is located at a point one third of the distance from the GT to the IT.
3. Insert the stimulating needle perpendicular to the skin and advance it toward the sciatic nerve lying between the GT and IT.
4. Once the tip of the needle is close to the sciatic nerve, dorsiflexion or plantar extension of the foot will result.
5. Once acceptable twitches are seen, incrementally decrease the nerve stimulator current to 0.4 mA, making sure that the same motor responses are elicited. Reposition the needle if necessary.
6. Before injection of the local anesthetic solution, it is important to verify that the needle is not positioned either intravascularly or intraneurally. Negative blood aspiration should be observed. It is imperative to ensure that no resistance during the injection is encountered.

Drugs and Dosage

- The recommended volume of local anesthetic to be injected is 0.05 to 0.1 mL/kg
- Bupivacaine 0.5% is commonly combined with dexmedetomidine (0.5 µg/mL) to provide approximately 14 (6 to 24) hours (median [minimum to maximum]) of postoperative analgesia after cruciate surgery. Ropivacaine 0.75% combined with dexmedetomidine (0.5 µg/mL) can be used with similar results.

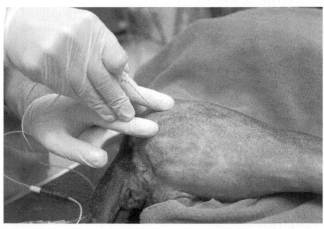

FIGURE 12-16 A sciatic nerve block is being performed with a peripheral nerve stimulator before stifle surgery in a dog.

Use of Ultrasonography and Nerve Stimulation

Equipment

- Ultrasound machine with high-frequency linear array transducer (9 to 15 MHz) with sterile sleeve when indicated
- Peripheral nerve stimulator
- Insulated needle (22-gauge, 50-mm needle for small to medium-sized animals; 21-gauge, 100-mm needle for larger animals)
- Local anesthetic solution

Positioning

Position the animal in lateral recumbency with the limb to be blocked uppermost and extended in a natural position.

Step-by-Step Procedure

See Figure 12-17.

1. The nondominant hand is used to place the ultrasound transducer in a craniocaudal position over the lateral aspect of the thigh immediately distal to the IT.
2. Glide, rotate, or tilt the transducer until a short-axis view of the sciatic nerve is obtained.
3. Set the peripheral nerve stimulator to deliver a current of 0.4 mA at 1 Hz.
4. Once the sciatic nerve has been identified, insert the stimulating needle in a caudal-to-cranial direction, guiding it through the semimembranosus muscle and medial to the fascia of the biceps femoris muscle. The needle should be advanced in-plane with the transducer to allow it to be observed approaching the sciatic nerve.
5. Monitor for plantar extension of the foot (corresponding to stimulation of the tibialis nerve component) or dorsiflexion of the foot (corresponding to stimulation of the peroneal nerve component).
6. Before the local anesthetic solution is injected, verify that the needle is not positioned either intravascularly or intraneurally. Negative blood aspiration should be observed.
7. As the local anesthetic solution is injected, watch for fluid to spread around the sciatic nerve (the anesthetic solution will appear anechoic). No resistance should be encountered during injection.

Drugs and Dosage

- The total volume of local anesthetic to be injected is 0.05 to 0.1 mL/kg; however, the final injection volume can be adjusted by monitoring the spread of the solution on the ultrasound image. The full volume does not need to be used if the sciatic nerve appears to be surrounded by the local anesthetic solution.

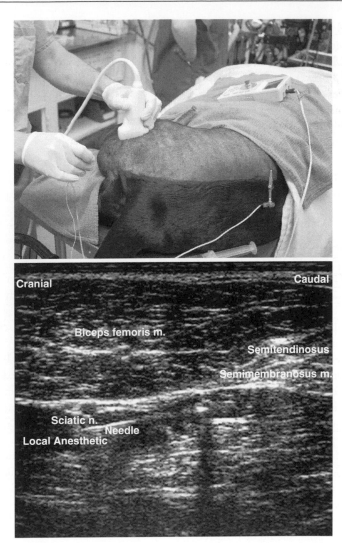

FIGURE 12-17 A sciatic nerve block is being performed with use of ultrasound guidance and a peripheral nerve stimulator before stifle surgery in a dog.

- Bupivacaine 0.5% is commonly combined with dexmedetomidine (0.5 µg/mL) to provide approximately 14 (6 to 24) hours (median [minimum to maximum]) of postoperative analgesia after cruciate surgery. Ropivacaine 0.75% combined with dexmedetomidine (0.5 µg/mL) can be used with similar results.

Epidural Anesthesia and Analgesia

Relevant Anatomy

- The administration of agents with analgesic properties via the epidural route has been used for many years to provide highly effective, localized anesthesia and analgesia.
- The *epidural space* is located between the dura mater and the wall of the vertebral canal. It contains adipose and connective tissue, as well as the internal vertebral venous plexus.
- Epidural anesthesia is typically performed in dogs and cats at the lumbosacral intervertebral space, because the epidural space is typically largest at this location (the dural sac tapers off in this area).
- After being administered by the epidural route, local anesthetics bathe the spinal nerve roots and block their conduction. When opioids, α_2-adrenoceptor agonists, and other agents are administered, their primary actions are through interaction with receptors in the spinal cord itself.
- As a result of blocking spinal nerve roots, use of epidural local anesthetics will result in sensory, motor, and sympathetic blockade. When opioids are used, only sensory pathways are blocked, while motor and sympathetic functions are preserved.
- Local anesthetics and opioids may be used in combination and result in excellent analgesia.

Equipment

- Tuohy needle
- Local anesthetic solution

Positioning

- Epidural lumbosacral anesthesia in dogs and cats is performed with the animal positioned in either sternal or lateral recumbency. The spine is often easier to palpate when the animal is positioned in sternal recumbency, especially in obese animals.
- When the animal is positioned in sternal recumbency, the pelvic limbs should be pulled forward, as opposed to being frog-legged or directed caudally.

Identification of the Epidural Space

- *Hanging drop:* The animal must be positioned in sternal recumbency. If a drop of saline or local anesthetic solution is placed in the hub of the Tuohy needle, the solution will usually be aspirated when the tip of the needle enters the epidural space. Use of the hanging-drop technique is useful in medium- to large-breed dogs but is less reliable in smaller dogs and cats.

- *Loss of resistance:* Until the tip of the needle is correctly located in the epidural space, there will be some degree of resistance if pressure is applied to the plunger of a syringe while the needle is being advanced through the intervertebral ligaments. If pressure is applied to the plunger of the syringe, a pop and a sudden loss of resistance to injection is usually appreciated as the needle punctures the ligamentum flavum and enters the epidural space.

- *Nerve stimulation:* Similar to the use of nerve stimulation to identify peripheral nerves, an insulated needle can be used to correctly identify when the tip of the needle penetrates the ligaments and enters the epidural space. Once the tip of the needle reaches the epidural space, twitches in the pelvic limbs and tail will be observed, providing immediate, objective feedback about needle position before any drugs are administered.

- It is possible to obtain a *false-negative* response if foreign material (e.g., blood clot, fat, periostium, skin) fills the needle shaft and causes obstruction. With use of the loss-of-resistance technique, a *false positive* may result if the needle is located within the intervertebral fat and the drug solution can be injected without any appreciable resistance.

Step-by-Step Procedure

See Figures 12-18 and 12-19.

1. The puncture site is located between the spinous processes of L7 and S1 on the dorsal midline of the animal.
2. After the area has been clipped and the skin prepared for injection, the needle is advanced through the skin and into the subcutaneous tissue.

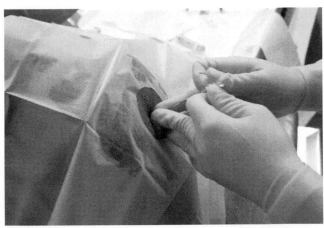

FIGURE 12-18   A Tuohy needle is being placed into the epidural space in a dog.

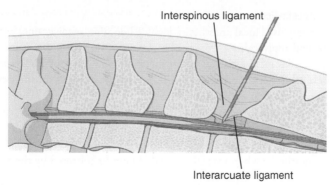

Interspinous ligament

Interarcuate ligament

FIGURE 12-19   Representation of the relevant anatomy for performance of epidural anesthesia in a dog.

Usually there is no palpable resistance to needle advancement in these tissues.

3. The needle is then advanced through the interspinous ligament until it is thought to be embedded in the ligament. Resistance to needle advancement will be appreciated as the needle penetrates this ligament.

4. Depending on personal preference and available equipment, use of the hanging-drop, loss-of-resistance, or nerve stimulator techniques can be used to identify when the needle penetrates the ligamentum flavum and enters the epidural space.

5. If during any of these manipulations the needle comes into contact with bone, it should be withdrawn and redirected caudally or cranially as applicable. Walking the needle off of the adjacent bones will help to identify the lumbosacral intervertebral space. Movements should be gentle and controlled to minimize the risks of causing tissue trauma.

6. The dural sac extends further caudally in cats and small dogs. When performing the technique in these animals, to minimize the chances of performing a spinal block (with the needle tip in the cerebrospinal fluid), the anesthetist should focus on stopping needle advancement as soon as the epidural space is entered.

7. After the epidural space is correctly identified, the needle hub should be inspected for the presence of cerebrospinal fluid or blood. If either fluid is observed, the needle should be removed from the animal and the procedure should be repeated with use of a new needle.

8. Check the label on the syringe to make sure the correct solution will be injected. Inject the drug solution slowly over 1 minute.

Drugs and Dosage

Two main classes of drugs are used for epidural anesthesia and analgesia in dogs and cats: local anesthetics and opioids.

Local Anesthetics

- Commonly used local anesthetics include lidocaine, mepivacaine, bupivacaine, and ropivacaine.
- Because all local anesthetics result in comparable levels of analgesia and muscle relaxation, the choice of local anesthetic depends on the desired onset and the desired duration of action.
- When local anesthetics are used epidurally, they will block sensory, motor, and sympathetic innervation to the blocked dermatomes. The clinician should anticipate arterial hypotension and avoid use of epidural local anesthetics when vasodilation would not be tolerated by the animal (e.g., uncorrected hypovolemia).
- The total volume of injected local anesthetic solution determines how far cranial the block will be obtained.
- For caudal procedures (of the tail, anus, perianal areas), approximately 0.1 mL/kg of solution is adequate. This volume can also be administered by the sacrococcygeal intervertebral space to facilitate passage of urinary catheters in cats with lower urinary obstructions (Figure 12-20).
- For procedures of the pelvic limbs, approximately 0.2 mL/kg is required for the local anesthetic solution to reliably block spinal nerve roots up to and including the level of L3 (where the femoral nerve originates).
- For abdominal procedures, even larger volumes are required, up to approximately 0.4 mL/kg to block up to the level of T9. Side effects such as arterial hypotension are more profound in these cases.
- Effects last only up to the expected duration of the local anesthetic (e.g., 6 to 8 hours for the longest-acting drugs).

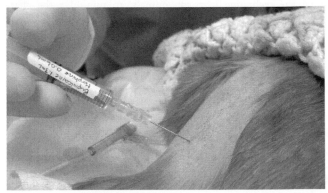

FIGURE 12-20 Epidural anesthesia being performed at the sacrococcygeal intervertebral space in a cat.

Opioids

- Commonly used opioids include morphine (0.1 mg/kg) and hydromorphone (0.05 mg/kg). Lately the use of fentanyl (1 to 5 µg/kg) is gaining popularity.

- Opioids are typically diluted in either saline or in local anesthetic solutions to encourage distribution along a broader area of the spinal canal.

- Opioids only modulate sensory transmission, and spare motor and sympathetic functions. As a result, they may still be used safely in animals that should not receive a local anesthetic (e.g., those with cardiovascular instability).

- Opioids must diffuse across the meninges and into the dorsal horn of the spinal cord to have an effect. As a result, they have slower onset times than local anesthetics (e.g., morphine takes up to 1 to 2 hours for its effects to be seen).

- Beneficial effects last much longer than with local anesthetics, with the analgesic effects of hydromorphone lasting up to 10 to 12 hours, and the effects of morphine lasting up to 18 to 24 hours.

- Urinary retention may occur when opioids are administered epidurally and should be monitored for and treated appropriately.

INTRAVENOUS REGIONAL ANESTHESIA

- Intravenous regional anesthesia (IVRA) is relatively straightforward to perform. A tourniquet is applied to a limb proximal to the planned surgical site, and a local anesthetic is injected intravenously distal to the tourniquet.

- After intravenous injection, the local anesthetic spreads from the vessels into the nearby tissues to reach the nerve trunks.

- IVRA can be used to provide analgesia and anesthesia for surgical procedures lasting no longer than 90 minutes that involve the distal extremities (distal to the elbow and the hock).

- Prolonged application of a tourniquet must be avoided because of the potential for tissue ischemia underneath and distal to the tourniquet and possible ischemic pain associated with the compression of these tissues.

Step-by-Step Procedure

See Figure 12-21.

1. Catheterize a vein in the distal limb with use of a small-gauge catheter (e.g., 24 or 22 gauge), and secure it in place.
2. Identify a peripheral arterial pulse in the distal limb, and mark with a pen the area where the pulse is readily palpable.
    a. Following exsanguination of the limb and application of the tourniquet, the absence of a pulse at this location should be verified to confirm appropriate application of the tourniquet.

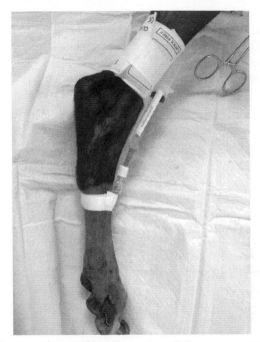

FIGURE 12-21 Intravenous regional anesthesia being performed in a dog before toe amputation surgery. Note that the limb has been exsanguinated, the tourniquet has been inflated, and a lidocaine neat solution is being administered into a preplaced catheter that is directed distally.

3. If a pneumatic tourniquet is to be employed, it is useful to determine the lower occlusion pressure for the cuff.
   a. This measurement corresponds to the lowest pressure in the cuff that will prevent arterial flow distal to the tourniquet.
   b. The cuff pressure will need to be maintained above (i.e., 100 mm Hg higher) the lower occlusion pressure during the procedure.
4. Exsanguinate the limb by elevating the leg for 3 to 5 minutes to allow for passive venous drainage.
5. Next, apply an elastic bandage concentrically around the limb from distal to proximal, being careful not to dislodge the intravenous catheter that was previously placed.
6. Apply the tourniquet to the limb above the level of exsanguination.
   a. If a pneumatic tourniquet is used, the cuff should be inflated to a pressure 50 to 100 mm Hg above the previously measured lower occlusion pressure.
   b. In the case of a non-pneumatic rubber tourniquet, the band should be placed above the elastic wrap that was used for exsanguination and secured tightly to prevent inadvertent release.

7. Document the time that the tourniquet is applied on the animal's anesthetic chart.
   a. The remaining procedures should be limited to 90 minutes from the time that the tourniquet was applied, to avoid complications from prolonged ischemia and compression of tissues under the tourniquet.
8. Once the tourniquet is in place, carefully remove the elastic bandage that was used to exsanguinate the limb.
9. Confirm that the previously identified peripheral pulse is now absent. Never proceed with the block if an arterial pulse is detected.
10. Inject the local anesthetic solution slowly over 2 to 3 minutes.
    a. Avoid high injection pressure that might increase venous pressure and cause leakage of the local anesthetic under the tourniquet into systemic circulation.
11. Document the time of local anesthetic administration on the animal's anesthetic chart, and observe the animal for several minutes for potential signs of systemic toxicity.
    a. After injection of the lidocaine, the catheter can be removed.
12. At the end of the procedure the tourniquet can be removed slowly. Because there should have been no arterial blood flow during the surgical procedure, the surgical site should be evaluated for hemorrhage.

Drugs and Dosage

- Lidocaine is the only local anesthetic that is recommended for IVRA.
- It is used at doses of 2.5 to 5 mg/kg with concentrations of 0.25% to 2%.
  - In dogs and cats, a 0.5% lidocaine solution up to a total injected volume of 0.6 mL/kg works well for most situations.
- Even though a tourniquet is used to keep the local anesthetic in the distal limb, there is always a possibility of leakage under the cuff whereby inadvertent systemic distribution of the injected local anesthetic solution can occur.
  - For this reason, formulations that contain epinephrine or preservatives should be avoided.
- Bupivacaine has a very narrow therapeutic index between the dose that is required for its local anesthetic effects and the dose that results in systemic toxicity.
  - When bupivacaine has been used for IVRA in people it has been associated with severe complications including death.
  - For this reason, *bupivacaine should never be used for IVRA*.

SUGGESTED READINGS

Abelson AL, McCobb EC, Shaw S, et al. Use of wound soaker catheters for the administration of local anesthetic for post-operative analgesia: 56 cases. Vet Anaesth Analg. 2009; 36:597–602.

Accola PJ, Bentley E, Smith LJ, et al. Development of a retrobulbar injection technique for ocular surgery and analgesia in dogs. J Am Vet Med Assoc. 2006; 229:220–225.

Almeida TF, Fantoni DT, Mastrocinque S, et al. Epidural anesthesia with bupivacaine, bupivacaine and fentanyl, or bupivacaine and sufentanil during intravenous administration of propofol for ovariohysterectomy in dogs. J Am Vet Med Assoc. 2007; 230:45–51.

Beckman BW, Legendre L. Regional nerve blocks for oral surgery in companion animals. Compend Contin Educ Small Anim Pract. 2002; 24:439–442.

Brower MC, Johnson ME. Adverse effects of local anesthetic infiltration on wound healing. Reg Anesth Pain Med. 2003; 28:233–240.

Campoy L, Bezuidenhout AJ, Gleed RD, et al. Ultrasound-guided approach for axillary brachial plexus, femoral nerve, and sciatic nerve blocks in dogs. Vet Anaesth Analg. 2010; 37:144–153.

Campoy L, Martin-Flores M, Looney AL, et al. Distribution of a lidocaine-methylene blue solution staining in brachial plexus, lumbar plexus and sciatic nerve blocks in the dog. Vet Anaesth Analg. 2008; 35:348–354.

Campoy L, Martin-Flores M, Ludders JW, et al. Comparison of bupivacaine femoral and sciatic nerve block versus bupivacaine and morphine epidural for stifle surgery in dogs. Vet Anaesth Analg. 2012; 39:91–98.

Campoy L, Read M, (Eds.) Small animal regional anesthesia and analgesia. Ames, Iowa, 2013, Wiley-Blackwell.

Duggan J, Bowler GM, McClure JH, et al. Extradural block with bupivacaine: Influence of dose, volume, concentration and patient characteristics. Br J Anaesth. 1988; 61:324–331.

Echeverry DF, Gil F, Laredo F, et al. Ultrasound-guided block of the sciatic and femoral nerves in dogs: a descriptive study. Vet J. 2010; 186:210–215.

Freire CD, Torres ML, Fantoni DT, et al. Bupivacaine 0.25% and methylene blue spread with epidural anesthesia in dog. Vet Anaesth Analg. 2010; 37:63–69.

Ford DJ, Pither C, Raj PP. Comparison of insulated and uninsulated needles for locating peripheral nerves with a peripheral nerve stimulator. Anesth Analg. 1984; 63:925–928.

Futema F, Fantoni DT, Auler JOC, et al. A new brachial plexus technique in dogs. Vet Anaesth Analg. 2002; 29:133–139.

Lee I, Yamagishi N, Oboshi K, et al. Distribution of new methylene blue injected into the lumbosacral epidural space in cats. Vet Aneaeth Analg. 2004; 31:190–194.

Lemke KA, Creighton CM. Paravertebral blockade of the brachial plexus in dogs. Vet Clin North Am Small Anim Pract. 2008; 38:1231–1241.

Liu SS, Richman JM, Thirlby RC, et al. Efficacy of continuous wound catheters delivering local anesthetic for postoperative analgesia: A quantitative and qualitative systematic review of randomized controlled trials. J Am Coll Surg. 2006; 203:914–932.

Mahler SP, Adogwa AO. Anatomical and experimental studies of brachial plexus, sciatic, and femoral nerve-location using peripheral nerve stimulation in the dog. Vet Anaesth Analg. 2008; 35:80–89.

Naganobu K, Hagio M. The effect of body position on the 'hanging drop' method for identifying the extradural space in anaesthetized dogs. Vet Anaesth Analg. 2007; 34:59–62.

Perlas A, Niazi A, McCartney C, et al. The sensitivity of motor response to nerve stimulation and paresthesia for nerve localization as evaluated by ultrasound. Reg Anesth Pain Med. 2006; 31:445–450.

Portela DA, Otero PE, Tarragona L, et al. Combined paravertebral plexus block and parasacral sciatic block in healthy dogs. Vet Anaesth Analg. 2010; 37:531–541.

Rioja E, Sinclair M, Chalmers H, et al. Comparison of three techniques for paravertebral brachial plexus blockade in dogs. Vet Anaesth Analg. 2012; 39:190–200.

Rochette J. Regional anesthesia and analgesia for oral and dental procedures. Vet Clin North Am Small Anim Pract. 2005; 35:1041–1058.

Schroeder CA, Snyder LBC, Tearney CC, et al. Ultrasound-guided transversus abdominis plane block in the dog: an anatomical evaluation. Vet Anaesth Analg. 2011; 38:267–271.

Shilo Y, Pascoe PJ, Cissell D, et al. Ultrasound-guided nerve blocks of the pelvic limb in dogs. Vet Anaesth Analg. 2010; 37:460–470.

Steinfeldt T, Nimphius W, Werner T, et al. Nerve injury by needle nerve perforation in regional anaesthesia: does size matter? Br J Anaesth. 2010; 104:245–253.

Tsai TP, Vuckovic I, Dilberovic F, et al. Intensity of the stimulating current may not be a reliable indicator of intraneural needle placement. Reg Anesth Pain Med. 2008; 33:207–210.

Tsui BCH, Hadzic A. Peripheral nerve stimulators and electrophysiology of nerve stimulation. In: Hadzic A (Ed.). Textbook of regional anesthesia and acute pain management. New York, 2007, McGraw Hill Medical.

Tsui BCH, Wagner A, Finucane B. Electrophysiologic effect of injectates on peripheral nerve stimulation. Reg Anesth Pain Med. 2004; 29:189–193.

Valverde A. Epidural analgesia and anesthesia in dogs and cats. Vet Clin North Am Small Anim Pract. 2008; 38:1205–1230.

CHAPTER 13

Glucocorticoids

Mark G. Papich

Glucocorticoids have an important role in many of the treatments we provide as veterinarians. The list of conditions and diseases that are treated with glucocorticoids is long and includes immune-mediated disease, inflammation of various tissues, hormonal replacement (glucocorticoid deficiency), neurologic disease, and cancer. The role of these agents in treating pain is less understood. Glucocorticoids do not have a direct effect on nociception and are not primary analgesics. However, because many painful conditions are mediated by inflammatory conditions, glucocorticoids can be beneficial as an adjunct in overall management. Glucocorticoids produce many important pharmacologic effects, but these must be weighed against the long list of side effects and adverse reactions they produce.

PHARMACOLOGY OF GLUCOCORTICOIDS

Corticosteroids are the steroid molecules released from the adrenal gland in response to various stimuli. The mineralocorticoids (e.g., aldosterone) control the salt-retaining properties and will not be discussed in this chapter (although many of the synthetic corticosteroids used in therapy have some degree of mineralocorticoid activity). Glucocorticoids have their primary effect on metabolism, glucose, and inflammatory properties. This chapter will focus on those drugs. The other major corticosteroids are those that affect reproduction and have androgenic or estrogenic activity. These will not be discussed in this chapter.

Cortisol is the major naturally occurring glucocorticoid in animals (also called *hydrocortisone*). Its natural functions in the body are many, including intermediary metabolism. Cortisol is synthesized from cholesterol, and via a series of steps and intermediary steroids, it is eventually converted from cholesterol. Cortisol is secreted in the blood and is largely bound (>90%) to plasma proteins, primarily corticosteroid-binding globulin. A smaller amount is bound to albumin, but with less affinity. Only the unbound portion is active for physiologic and pharmacologic actions, but the fraction bound to albumin is more readily available because of the low binding affinity.

By contrast, synthetic glucocorticoids (e.g., dexamethasone) are bound to albumin rather than the corticosteroid-binding globulin.

Secretion of cortisol in people is estimated to be 10 to 20 mg/day (equivalent to 0.15 to 0.30 mg/kg/day) with peaks and troughs throughout the day that follow a circadian rhythm. These levels can rise 10-fold in the face of severe stress. Despite older reports that suggested diurnal rhythms in dogs and cats (and perhaps a reverse pattern in cats), no such pattern has been identified.[1] In animals, the daily cortisol production in a nonstressed animal is approximately 1 mg/kg according to Ferguson and colleagues.[1] These daily rates of production are important to note because this is the amount that must be replaced when states of adrenal insufficiency are treated.

Cortisol secretion in healthy animals is under tight regulatory control. Figure 13-1 shows the normal feedback and regulation. Secretion of cortisol exerts a negative feedback, ultimately reducing the secretion of cortisol. It is important to note that exogenous glucocorticosteroids (prednisolone, dexamethasone) also produce the same feedback, sometimes for several hours. Long-term treatment with glucocorticoids can therefore produce adrenal atrophy.

Cellular Action

Glucocorticoids are the most consistently effective drugs available for the treatment of various forms of inflammation in animals. However, their potent anti-inflammatory effects and immunosuppressive actions must be

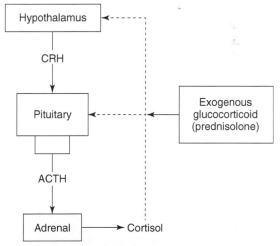

FIGURE 13-1   Hypothalamic-pituitary-adrenal axis. Control of cortisol secretion. Cortisol is secreted naturally from the adrenal in response to adrenocorticotropic hormone *(ACTH)*. ACTH in turn is under regulatory control from corticotropin-releasing hormone *(CRH)* from the hypothalamus, and negative influences from endogenous and exogenous steroids *(dashed line)*.

balanced by their multiple side effects and adverse effects. In the past, clinicians referred to the action of glucocorticoids simply by saying that they "stabilize cell membranes." Such a simplistic (and inaccurate) description of their cellular action no longer is appropriate. Glucocorticoids exert their action via binding to intracellular receptors, translocating to the nucleus, and binding to receptor sites on responsive genes, where they modulate the transcription of glucocorticoid-responsive genes[2-7] (Figure 13-2). Through regulation of glucocorticoid-responsive genes, protein synthesis is altered, which affects cell function. These effects may be mediated by the interaction of glucocorticoids with activator protein 1 (AP-1) and nuclear factor κB (NF-κB) (see Figure 13-2). For control of inflammation, the major effect of corticosteroids is to inhibit synthesis of inflammatory mediators. This action of glucocorticoids is not immediate and may not become apparent for several hours. This is an important consideration if pharmacologic glucocorticoids are used in an acute or critical care situation in a veterinary hospital.

The action of glucocorticoids is complex and involves interactions with intracellular receptors and subsequent modulation of gene expression. Figure 13-3 shows the concept of *transrepression* and *transactivation*.

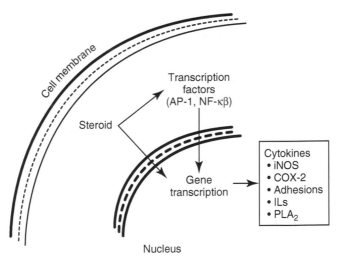

FIGURE 13-2 Action of corticosteroids. Glucocorticoids translocate to the cell where they bind to glucocorticoid receptors. After binding to these receptors, they may enter the nucleus, where they bind to glucocorticoid-responsive elements on genes that subsequently affect the transcription of inflammatory products (*iNOS*, inducible nitric oxide synthase; *COX-2*, cyclooxygenase-2; cellular adhesions; *ILs*, interleukins; and *PLA$_2$*, phospholipase A$_2$). Glucocorticoids also may act through intermediary mechanisms to influence the function of other transcription factors such as activator protein–1 *(AP-1)* and nuclear factor–κB *(NF-κB)*, which act on non–glucocorticoid responsive elements to regulate the transcription of genes that control inflammatory products. (See text for more details.)

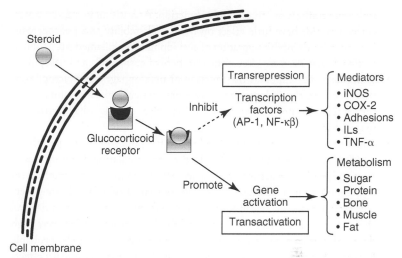

FIGURE 13-3   Action of glucocorticoids. The action of glucocorticoids is a balance between transrepression and transactivation. After binding to the glucocorticoid receptor and translocating, these drugs either inhibit or promote synthesis of proteins that are responsible for activity. Transrepression is responsible for the anti-inflammatory actions, suppressing mediators (iNOS, COX-2, ILs, and TNF-α). Transactivation, on the other hand, is responsible for many of the metabolic effects, including changes that can be adverse when these drugs are used for a long time. (See text for more details.) (Key: *AP-1,* Activator protein–1; *iNOS,* inducible nitric oxide synthase; *COX-2,* cyclooxygenase-2; *ILs,* interleukins; *NF-κB,* nuclear factor–κB; *TNF-α,* tumor necrosis factor-α.)

Transrepression suppresses ("turns off") expression of inflammatory products, such as cytokines, and cyclooxygenase-2 (COX-2), the enzyme that produces inflammatory prostaglandins. But glucocorticoids also cause transactivation, which produces metabolic changes that are responsible for many of the adverse effects of these agents. Although there have been many attempts over the years, no one has successfully produced a synthetic glucocorticoid that produces the beneficial changes (transrepression) while at the same time eliminating the negative effects (transactivation).

CLINICAL EFFECTS OF GLUCOCORTICOIDS

Anti-inflammatory Effects

- Leukocytes: Corticosteroids increase the circulating numbers of mature neutrophils. There is a release of cells from the marginal pool of neutrophils and decreased migration and egress into inflammatory tissue. This effect is attributed to decreased expression of adhesion molecules, reduced adherence to the vessel endothelium, and reduced diapedesis from the vessels. Subsequently, there is decreased movement of inflammatory cells into tissues in response to chemotactic stimuli. Glucocorticoids affect leukocyte traffic more than cellular function. At anti-inflammatory doses, glucocorticoids have little effect on lysosomal stability and phagocytosis.

- Glucocorticoids inhibit migration of eosinophils into inflamed sites. Glucocorticoids also decrease circulating numbers of eosinophils and basophils.
- Glucocorticoids suppress the function of macrophages. In macrophages, they decrease the inflammatory response, generation of cytokines, and the ability to process antigens. They also inhibit phagocytosis of macrophages.
- Glucocorticoids decrease the numbers of lymphocytes in the peripheral circulation—caused by a redistribution of circulating lymphocytes—depress lymphocyte activation, and decrease participation of lymphocytes in inflammation. T cells are affected more than B cells. B cells are generally resistant to the immunosuppressive effects of glucocorticoids, and there is minimal effect on immunoglobulin synthesis. However, high doses of corticosteroids may decrease immunoglobulin levels, probably because of increased catabolism, as well as through the secondary effects to suppress accessory cells and cytokine synthesis. At anti-inflammatory doses, glucocorticoids do not decrease an animal's ability to mount a normal immune response (e.g., from vaccinations).[8]
- Effects on cytokines: Glucocorticoids inhibit release of inflammatory cytokines from leukocytes (e.g., interleukin [IL]–1, tumor necrosis factor–α [TNF-α], prostaglandins). Glucocorticoids decrease expression of cytokines from lymphocytes (e.g., IL-2).
- Effects on vessels: Corticosteroids improve microvascular integrity, decrease vessel permeability, and improve microvascular circulation. Some of the stabilizing effect on vessels may be attributable to an antagonism of vasoactive substances (e.g., histamine, 5-HT), decreasing release of histamine from basophils and mast cells, or decreased synthesis of inflammatory mediators (e.g., prostaglandins, TNF-α).
- Effects on arachidonic acid metabolism: Corticosteroids inhibit the synthesis of the isoform of cyclooxygenase (PG synthase-2, also called COX-2) responsible for prostaglandin synthesis during inflammation. Corticosteroids also may produce a dual blockade of the arachidonic acid cascade by an inhibition of phospholipase A_2, resulting in lower concentrations of prostaglandins, prostacyclin, thromboxane, and leukotrienes. Despite this evidence, it is not fully understood if the glucocorticoid effect on arachidonic acid metabolism, prostaglandin synthesis inhibition, or leukotriene metabolism is clinically relevant.[9]

Clinical Use: Planning Corticosteroid Therapy

- Short-term therapy (less than 2 weeks): Glucocorticoids can be administered daily at anti-inflammatory doses without serious long-term side effects.

- Long-term therapy: If long-term therapy is not needed, the medication can be discontinued abruptly with little chance of a rebound effect from adrenal suppression. For long-term, chronic therapy, glucocorticoid doses should be titrated to the lowest effective dose and, if possible, administered every other day (EOD).

Choice of a Corticosteroid

- The comparison of glucocorticoids is shown in Table 13-1. Glucocorticoids are ranked according to their potency, duration of action, and mineralocorticoid (sodium-retaining) activity.
- Prednisolone, prednisone, and methylprednisolone are the most common choices because they are intermediate-acting steroids and can be used on an EOD schedule. Initial (induction) dosages (prednisone or prednisolone) for anti-inflammatory activity are approximately 1 mg/kg/day for 5 to 10 days, then the dosage is gradually lowered (tapered) to approximately 1 mg/kg EOD for another 5 to 10 days and eventually to 0.5 mg/kg EOD. These are typical anti-inflammatory maintenance dosages, although in some animals it may be possible to lower the dosage further. There can be wide variation of response among individuals, and dosages should be titrated to the response for each animal.
- Prednisone and prednisolone can be used interchangeably in dogs. Horses and cats should receive prednisolone. There is either a deficiency in converting prednisone to its active metabolite prednisolone or a problem with oral absorption of prednisone (see later discussion).

TABLE 13-1   Comparison of Various Glucocorticoid Bases

DRUG	DURATION OF ACTION (HR)*	COMPARATIVE POTENCY†	MINERALOCORTICOID EFFECTS
Hydrocortisone (cortisol)	8-12	1	2
Prednisolone	12-36	4	1
Prednisone	12-36	4	1
Methylprednisolone	12-36	5	2
Triamcinolone‡	12-36	5	0
Flumethasone	32-48	15	0
Dexamethasone	32-48	25	0
Betamethasone	32-48	25	0
Deoxycorticosterone (DOCA)	0	0	200
Fludrocortisone (Florinef)	Not applicable	10	250

*Based on duration of hypothalamic-pituitary-adrenal (HPA)–axis suppression.
†Potency is listed by arbitrarily assigning cortisol a potency of 1.0; as the value increases, so does the potency.
‡Some authors of veterinary glucocorticoid reviews and those reporting their clinical experience suggest that in animals, anti-inflammatory potency of triamcinolone may be equal to that of dexamethasone. Clinical studies have also supported this higher potency level for triamcinolone—approximately seven times more potent than prednisolone.

- Methylprednisolone is sometimes used by clinicians as an alternative to prednisolone or prednisone for long-term oral use. There is some belief, although completely anecdotal, that it is better tolerated in some animals.
- Dexamethasone is often used for short-term treatment in the hospital because it is readily available as a concentrated water-soluble solution (dexamethasone sodium phosphate) that can be injected intravenously (IV) or intramuscularly (IM) or added to IV fluids. Other water-soluble formulations are also available (see later discussion). Because dexamethasone is considerably more potent than prednisolone (see Table 13-1), the dosage should be adjusted accordingly.

Corticosteroid Formulations

- Phosphate and succinate esters: These esters are highly soluble and associated with a rapid onset of action. These esters may be given IV to achieve rapid, high serum concentrations. Examples include prednisolone sodium succinate (Solu-Delta-Cortef), methylprednisolone sodium succinate (MPSS; Solu-Medrol), and dexamethasone sodium phosphate (Azium SP and other brands).
- Acetate and acetonide esters: These esters are poorly soluble and are given IM, subcutaneously (SC), or intra-articularly for a prolonged effect. Absorption occurs slowly, in days to weeks. Examples include methylprednisolone acetate (Depo-Medrol) and triamcinolone acetonide (Vetalog).
- Aqueous suspensions: These are not soluble in water and exist as injectable suspensions. They can be rapidly absorbed after IM or SC injection.
- Solutions: These forms are solutions in propylene glycol or alcohol. An example is dexamethasone solution. Solutions are not recommended for rapid IV bolus administration and are not soluble if added to fluid solutions.

Differences Among Species

- Cats often require higher dosages than dogs, sometimes twice as much as dogs, possibly because of differences in receptors.[10] Prednisolone is preferred over prednisone in cats. In cats, some evidence indicates that either oral absorption of prednisone is poor, or once it is absorbed there is a deficiency in the ability to convert to prednisolone. This has been primarily an anecdotal observation and reported only in an abstract from conference proceedings.[11]
- Horses are also deficient in their ability to convert prednisone to prednisolone.[12]
- Methylprednisolone (1 to 2 mg/kg/day, tapered to 0.5 mg/kg q48h) and triamcinolone (0.2 mg/kg/day tapered to 0.1 mg/kg q48h) also have been used in cats and have been shown to be effective for treatment of allergic pruritus. Cats are also more resistant to the adverse effects than are dogs, but that does not alleviate all concerns about the long-term

metabolic effects (increased risk of diabetes, liver changes, catabolic effects, increased risk of heart disease).

Rationale for Every-Other-Day Therapy

- When an intermediate-acting glucocorticoid is used (duration of action of 12 to 36 hours), the hypothalamic-pituitary-adrenal (HPA) axis has an opportunity to recover before the next dose.
- Select a glucocorticoid that does not have a long duration of action for EOD therapy (e.g., dexamethasone is unacceptable because its duration is at least 36 to 48 hours). After receiving prednisolone 1 mg/kg every 48 hours, the level of adrenocorticotropic hormone (ACTH) was suppressed in dogs for 18 to 24 hours and returned to normal until the next scheduled dose.[13]
- EOD therapy will minimize but *will not prevent* adrenal atrophy and other adverse effects such as those on the immune system and the effects on metabolism.

Adrenal Recovery Following Glucocorticoid Therapy

- After short-term glucocorticoid therapy, HPA axis recovery occurs quickly, and the medication can be discontinued abruptly. After long-term therapy it may take longer for adrenal gland recovery from suppression, and a withdrawal syndrome may be observed in animals after glucocorticoids are discontinued.
- After chronic treatment, adrenocortical recovery occurs within a few weeks. In healthy dogs, complete recovery of the HPA axis was evident 2 weeks after cessation of daily prednisone administration.[14] In another study, recovery occurred 1 week after discontinuation of EOD prednisolone administration.[13]
- Because recovery of adrenal function after glucocorticosteroid therapy can vary among animals, veterinarians should advise animal owners of the possibility of adrenal suppression after discontinuation of corticosteroid therapy. Animals should be monitored for signs of adrenocortical insufficiency (e.g., lethargy and weakness), and animals should be supplemented with physiologic doses of a short- to medium-acting corticosteroid as needed, especially at times of stress.[15] Because the usual physiologic secretion of cortisol is 1 mg/kg/day, this translates to a daily dosage for glucocorticoid supplementation of 0.2 to 0.25 mg/kg of prednisolone.

ADVERSE EFFECTS OF GLUCOCORTICOIDS

The benefits of corticosteroids must be weighed against the potential adverse effects. Glucocorticosteroid receptors are found in practically every cell of the body. Therefore, effects in various tissues and organ systems are sometimes unavoidable. Some of the adverse effects are as follows.

Central Nervous System

- Polyphagia
- Euphoria
- Behavior changes (e.g., increased restlessness or excitability)

Metabolic Effects

- Lipolysis
- Hyperlipidemia
- Protein catabolism
- Fatty infiltration of liver
- Steroid hepatopathy

Musculoskeletal System

- Osteoporosis
- Decreased growth
- Muscle weakness and/or loss of muscle mass
- Skeletal muscle wasting (steroid myopathy)
- Fibroblast inhibition
- Decreased intestinal calcium absorption

Endocrine System

- Decreased thyroid hormone synthesis
- Anti-insulin effects
- HPA axis suppression
- Increased parathyroid hormone synthesis

Gastrointestinal System

- Gastrointestinal (GI) ulceration
- Pancreatitis
- Colonic perforation

Host Defenses (Immune System)

- Decreased bacterial killing
- Increased risk of septicemia
- Increased risk of infection
- Recurrent septic cystitis (urinary tract infection)
- Recurrent bacterial pyoderma

Fluid Balance

- Sodium and fluid retention
- Polyuria and polydipsia

Cardiovascular Effects

- Fluid overload (water retention)
- Increased risk of cardiac failure in cats

SPECIFIC CLINICAL APPLICATIONS

Anti-inflammatory Use

The most common use of glucocorticoids is for systemic or local inflammatory conditions involving the musculoskeletal system (e.g., arthritis), skin (e.g., atopic dermatitis), respiratory system (e.g., bronchitis and asthma), intestine (e.g., inflammatory bowel disease), central nervous system (CNS), and allergic conditions. The treatment approach is rather similar in each situation (see the earlier discussion of choice of a glucocorticoid). Prednisolone, prednisone, and methylprednisolone are the most common choices because they are intermediate-acting steroids and can be used on an EOD schedule. Initial (induction) dosages (prednisone or prednisolone) for anti-inflammatory activity are approximately 1 mg/kg/day for 5 to 10 days, then the dosage is gradually lowered (tapered) to approximately 1 mg/kg EOD for another 5 to 10 days, and eventually to 0.5 mg/kg EOD. These are typical anti-inflammatory maintenance dosages, although in some animals it may be possible to lower the dosage further. There can be wide variation of response among individuals, and dosages should be titrated to the response for each animal.

For some diseases (e.g., ocular diseases or skin inflammation), topical forms of these agents may be used. Topical preparations exist in creams, ointments, and solutions, often in combination with other agents (e.g., antibacterial and antifungal medications).

Immunosuppression

Corticosteroids (glucocorticoids) are usually the primary drugs used to treat or manage immune-mediated disorders involving various organ systems and tissues. As reviewed by Cohn,[16] corticosteroids suppress the ability of macrophages to engulf cells and process antigens that are necessary to stimulate an immune response. Corticosteroids also profoundly affect lymphocytes. A complex series of interactions among antigens, macrophages, T cells, and cytokines is important for immunologic expression. Glucocorticoids suppress the activity of macrophages and the synthesis of IL-2. Glucocorticosteroids appear to have the most effect on T lymphocytes. Therefore, effects can be seen from suppression of helper cells to cell-mediated immunity. Direct effects on antibody synthesis do not occur. In clinical veterinary medicine the action of glucocorticoids is dose dependent.

There is no evidence from a well-controlled study in animals to show that one glucocorticoid is superior to another with regard to efficacy. Nor is there any documentation to show that injectable therapy is more effective than oral treatment. The choice of corticosteroid becomes a practical one: dexamethasone sodium phosphate is the most common injectable formulation in veterinary hospitals, and prednisolone (or prednisone) tablets are the most common oral forms. For long-term therapy, intermediate-acting steroids (e.g., prednisolone) should be used to reduce adverse effects. During short-term treatment, dexamethasone can be used.

Initial (induction) dosage regimens employed are in the range of daily doses of 2.2 to 4.4 mg/kg (prednisolone). A commonly used immunosuppressive dosage of prednisolone for dogs is 2 mg/kg orally q12h. During the initial induction period the daily dose can be divided into a twice-daily regimen to lessen (but not eliminate) some of the acute effects, such as GI problems or behavioral changes. After the induction treatment phase the dosage interval can be extended to once daily for another period of time until it is determined that the animal's condition is stable. If this is possible, the long-term maintenance dosage should be 0.5 to 1 mg/kg EOD. The optimal dosage that balances adverse effects and clinical response should be determined by titration. Immune-mediated diseases can vary greatly with respect to the level of glucocorticoids necessary to control clinical signs. A maintenance dosage of 0.5 to 1 mg/kg q48h is possible in some animals, but a higher dosage or the addition of other drugs may be necessary in animals with disease that is more refractory. Cats often require a higher dosage, sometimes twice as much as dogs.

Spinal Trauma

Corticosteroids, specifically MPSS, have been administered to prevent further injury to the spinal cord caused by ischemia and inflammation from trauma. The review by Olby[17] provided an excellent summary of the studies in experimental animals and the human clinical trials that have evaluated the potential benefit of corticosteroids for this indication.

The action of corticosteroids was reviewed by Hall and others.[18-20] The action of corticosteroids that appears to be most important for protection of spinal cord tissue from injury after trauma is that of inhibition of lipid peroxidation of membranes caused by oxygen-derived free radicals.[18-20] This action is unrelated to the hormone effects of these drugs. A high dosage of MPSS (30 mg/kg) is required. Platt and Olby[21] provide full details of recommended dosing protocols for MPSS in spinal cord injury. These dosages far exceed the amount necessary to produce a typical corticosteroid effect from binding to glucocorticosteroid cellular receptors.

Lower dosages are not effective for treating spinal cord trauma, even though at those dosages all the corticosteroid receptors are probably occupied. A secondary beneficial effect may occur through the ability of corticosteroids to inhibit synthesis of inflammatory cytokines and suppress generation of arachidonic acid products (vasoactive prostaglandins), which may cause ischemia of the neural tissue. MPSS is not as effective if treatment is delayed for more than 8 hours, and may actually be harmful. Administration of high doses of MPSS has been associated with side effects that can be serious, such as GI perforation and infection. Therefore its use is not recommended unless the animal has complete loss of voluntary motor function, because paretic animals have a good prognosis.

Current recommendations support the use of MPSS as the superior corticosteroid for spinal cord trauma rather than prednisolone or dexamethasone. MPSS is a hemisuccinate ester that is converted to a sodium salt to make it more water soluble. Hydrocortisone is much less active, or is in fact ineffective, even at dosages of 120 mg/kg.[18-20] The 1,2 double bond of prednisolone (which is lacking in hydrocortisone) appears to be a requirement for the anti–lipid peroxidation effect. There is also evidence that dexamethasone is not as effective as methylprednisolone for preventing lipid peroxidation.[22] It is not recommended to simply increase the amount of dexamethasone to achieve the desired effect because this would likely increase the risk of adverse effects. Intestinal perforation has been reported from administration of high doses of dexamethasone for treating spinal cord trauma. Despite the research studies and extrapolations from human medicine, the efficacy of glucocorticoids is questionable, and there is no current evidence that it is beneficial in the treatment of canine spinal cord injury.[21] Glucocorticosteroids are not recommended for treatment of head trauma.[21]

Cancer

Glucocorticoids are commonly used in cancer chemotherapy and are a component of some of the combination protocols. Prednisone or prednisolone has been used as the sole drug for some tumors (e.g., mast cell tumors [MCTs]), but most often it is used in combination with other drugs. Usually prednisolone or prednisone is the drug of choice in anticancer protocols. A usual starting dosage is 40 mg/m^2 orally every day. When tumor remission occurs, the dosage is frequently decreased to 20 mg/m^2 EOD. The effects of glucocorticoids are related to the following:

- Cytolysis of lymphoid cells. Glucocorticoids appear to be cytolytic for malignant lymphoid cells. The mechanism may be related to the synthesis of an endonuclease that disrupts DNA. Glucocorticoids have been used for therapy of lymphoma as a single drug, but tumor resistance develops rapidly.
- Decrease in the inflammation associated with tumors and chemotherapy.
- Decrease in the adverse effects associated with chemotherapy. For example, the polyuria-polydipsia induced by prednisone and prednisolone in dogs may be beneficial for reducing the risk of cyclophosphamide-induced cystitis.

- Improvement in the animal's appetite and production of an antiemetic effect. Dexamethasone is used in some chemotherapy protocols for its antiemetic action.
- Decrease in the effects of TNF.
- Reduction in the edema and inflammation associated with some CNS tumors. Glucocorticoids are capable of crossing the blood-brain barrier.

REFERENCES

1. Ferguson DC, Dirikolu L, Hoenig M. Glucocorticoids, mineralocorticoids, and adrenolytic drugs. In: JE Riviere JE, MG Papich (Eds.). Veterinary pharmacology and therapeutics, ed. 9, Ames, Iowa, 2009, Wiley-Blackwell Publishing.
2. Boumpas DT, Chrousos GP, Wilder RL, et al. (1993) Glucocorticoid therapy for immune-mediated diseases: Basic and clinical correlates. Ann Intern Med. 1993; 119:1198-1208.
3. Barnes PJ. Adcock I (1993) Anti-inflammatory actions of steroids: Molecular mechanisms. Trends Pharmacol Sci. 1993; 14:436–441.
4. Barnes PJ. Corticosteroids: The drugs to beat. Eur J Pharmacol. 2006; 533:2–14.
5. Barnes PJ. Molecular mechanisms of corticosteroids in allergic diseases. Allergy. 2001; 56:928–936.
6. Hayashi R, Wada H, Ito K, Adcock IM. Effects of glucocorticoids on gene transcription. Eur J Pharmacol. 2004; 500:51–62.
7. Rhen T, Cidlowski JA. Antiinflammatory action of glucocorticoids—new mechanisms for old drugs. New Engl J Med. 2005; 353:1711–1723.
8. Nara PL, Krakowka S, Powers TE: Effects of prednisolone on the development of immune response to canine distemper virus in Beagle pups. Am J Vet Res. 1979; 40:1742–1747.
9. Peters-Golden M, Henderson WR Jr. Leukotrienes. N Engl J Med. 2007; 357 (18):1841–1854.
10. Van den Broek AHM, Stafford WL: Epidermal and hepatic glucocorticoid receptors in cats and dogs. Res Vet Sci. 1992; 52:312–315.
11. Graham-Mize CA, Rosser EJ. Bioavailability and activity of prednisone and prednisolone in the feline patient. Vet Dermatol. 2004; 15(s1):7–10.
12. Peroni DL, Stanley S, Kollias-Baker C, Robinson NE. Prednisone per os is likely to have limited efficacy in horses. Equine Vet J. 2002; 34(3):283–287.
13. Brockus CW, Dillon AR, Kemppainen RJ: Effect of alternate-day prednisolone administration on hypophyseal-adrenocortical activity in dogs. Am J Vet Res. 1999; 60:698–702.
14. Moore GE, Hoenig M: Duration of pituitary and adrenocortical suppression after long-term administration of anti-inflammatory doses of prednisone in dogs. Am J Vet Res. 1992; 53:716–720.
15. Romatowksi J: Iatrogenic adrenocortical insufficiency in dogs. J Am Vet Med Assoc. 1990; 196:1144–1146.
16. Cohn L. The influence of corticosteroids on host defence mechanisms. J Vet Intern Med. 1991; 5:95–104.
17. Olby N. Current concepts in the management of acute spinal cord injury. J Vet Intern Med. 1999; 13:399–407.
18. Brown SA, Hall ED. Role of oxygen-derived free radicals in the pathogenesis of shock and trauma, with focus on central nervous system injuries. J Am Vet Med Assoc. 1992; 200:1849–1858.
19. Hall ED. Neuroprotective actions of glucocorticoid and nonglucocorticoid steroids in acute neuronal injury. Cellular Molecular Neurobiology. 1993; 13:415–432.

20. Hall ED. The neuroprotective pharmacology of methylprednisolone. J Neurol. 1992; 76:13–22.

21. Plat S, Olby N. Neurological emergencies. In: S Platt S, N Olby (Eds.). BSAVA manual of canine and feline neurology, ed. 4, Gloucester UK, 2013, British Small Animal Veterinary Association.

22. Hoerlein BF, Redding RW, Hoff EJ, McGuire JA. Evaluation of naloxone, crocetin, thyrotropin releasing hormone, methylprednisolone, partial myelotomy, and hemilaminectomy in the treatment of acute spinal cord trauma. J Am Anim Hospl Assoc. 1985; 21:67–77.

CHAPTER 14

Alternative Drugs and Novel Therapies Used to Treat Pain

James S. Gaynor; William W. Muir III

Many drugs are capable of modifying an animal's response to pain but are not routinely administered in veterinary practice. Most drugs used for this purpose can be considered adjuvant therapy and reduce hypersensitivity (see Chapter 16). Evidence substantiating their efficacy is often speculative and not based on blinded randomized controlled trials in animals with naturally occurring pain.

INJECTABLE DRUGS

Ketamine

 Microdoses of ketamine can be used to provide analgesia for severe pain, particularly if central sensitization is suspected.

Mechanism of Action

Ketamine has traditionally been considered a dissociative anesthetic. Ketamine is a nonspecific N-methyl-D-aspartate (NMDA) receptor antagonist that reduces central sensitization (antihyperalgesic effect) and activates descending inhibitory nerve activity (antinociceptive effect). Ketamine is also known to produce a short-term (1- to 20-minute) local anesthetic effect.

Efficacy/Use

NMDA receptor stimulation is associated with central neuronal sensitization and the wind-up phenomenon. Blockade of NMDA receptors results in antihyperalgesia, less dysphoria, and lower opioid requirements. Ketamine is effective therapy for both acute pain— and chronic pain—producing conditions.

- Microdoses of ketamine, much lower than those used to produce anesthesia, can be administered as an adjunct to analgesia protocols and general anesthesia.
- Ketamine dosages ranging from 0.2 to 0.5 mg/kg intravenously (IV) or subcutaneously (SC) can be administered before surgical stimulation.

- Infusion doses at rates ranging from 10 to 50 µg/kg/min can be administered perioperatively or for the treatment of severe pain conditions.
- Lower infusion rates, 1 to 10 µg/kg/min, are used in conjunction with opioids or α_2-agonists to improve multimodal analgesic protocols.
  - In the absence of an infusion pump, 0.6 mL (60 mg) of ketamine can be added to a 1-liter bag of crystalloid solution to be administered at 10 mL/kg/hr to achieve the intraoperative administration rate of 10 µg/kg/min.
  - Ketamine, 2 µg/kg/min, can be administered without a syringe pump by adding 0.6 mL (60 mg) of ketamine to a 1-liter bag of crystalloid solution to be administered at 2 mL/kg/hr.

Pharmacology
The pharmacology and analgesic effects of microdose ketamine have not been established in conscious dogs. Low doses (microdoses) of ketamine are likely to produce minimal cardiovascular stimulatory effects.

Side Effects and Toxicity
Microdose ketamine has not been reported to produce side effects. Anecdotal accounts indicate that some animals develop tachycardia.

Special Issues
Microdose ketamine administered alone has not been demonstrated to produce analgesia. Ketamine is best used in conjunction with other analgesics as part of a multimodal analgesic protocol. Microdose tiletamine (in amounts similar to those of ketamine) can be administered as an alternative to ketamine but is likely to produce mild sedative effects.

Magnesium

Mechanism of Action
Central sensitization, or wind-up, is mediated by a cascade of events, including neuronal depolarization and NMDA receptor phosphorylation, resulting in an increase in nerve cell excitability. Activation of the NMDA receptor involves removal of magnesium blockade. Magnesium administration may decrease wind-up and act independently to block and suppress calcium currents and neuronal excitability. Intrathecal magnesium administration may also potentiate the effect of morphine and delay the onset of opioid tolerance.

Efficacy/Administration
- The efficacy of IV magnesium administration for the treatment of pain in animals is unsubstantiated. Magnesium has been administered intravenously to humans for treatment of headache and postoperative and neuropathic pain and subarachnoidally for allodynia and as an adjunct to intrathecal morphine administration.

- Dosages ranging from 5 to 15 mg/kg IV have been extrapolated from the dosage used in humans. This dosage is used with no apparent side effects to treat refractory cardiac dysrhythmias in dogs.
- Humans have been given up to 50 mg/kg IV bolus followed by 8 mg/kg/hr as an adjuvant to perioperative fentanyl analgesia.

Pharmacology
Physiologic concentrations of magnesium modulate cell membrane calcium flux. Magnesium deficiency may amplify pain.

Side Effects and Toxicity
Side effects include depression, vasodilation that may predispose to hypotension, and tachycardia.

Special Issues
Measurement of plasma magnesium may be misleading because it may not reflect intracellular magnesium concentration.

Clonidine

Mechanism of Action
Clonidine is relatively nonspecific α_2-agonist. Clonidine hyperpolarizes nerve cell membranes, blocks the conduction of nerve fibers, and may induce enkephalin-like substance release at peripheral sites.

Efficacy/Administration
- Clonidine has been administered intrathecally to dogs, cats, and humans.
- Studies conducted in humans have shown that clonidine provides effective analgesia.
- Clonidine may be used as part of a multimodal approach to treat chronic pain in animals that have developed a tolerance to nonsteroidal anti-inflammatory drugs (NSAIDs) or opioids or those with pain that is unresponsive to opioid treatment.
- Epidural clonidine (200 to 300 μg/kg/hr) in dogs produced good analgesia and mild cardiorespiratory effects typical of α_2-agonists.

Pharmacology
Clonidine produces effects typical of α_2-agonists, including central nervous system (CNS) depression, respiratory depression, bradycardia, and transient hypertension followed by normotension or mild hypotension. These effects are less pronounced than with dexmedetomidine.

Side Effects and Toxicity
Sedation bradycardia and hypotension may develop after clonidine administration. People have reported experiencing dry mouth after clonidine administration.

Special Issues

Clonidine is not antagonized by naloxone. Dosages for treating pain in dogs and cats have not been developed.

Ziconotide

Mechanism of Action

Ziconotide is a potent, selective, reversible blocker of neuronal N-type voltage-sensitive calcium channels.

Efficacy/Administration

- Ziconotide is an intrathecal analgesic indicated for the treatment of severe chronic pain.
- Intrathecal administration of 1 µg/kg to dogs inhibits thermal skin sensation but induces modest trembling.

Pharmacology

- Ziconotide maintains its analgesic efficacy over months and does not cause tolerance, dependence, or respiratory depression in humans.
- The median half-life is 4.5 hours in dogs.

Side Effects and Toxicity

Side effects include trembling, ataxia bradycardia, dizziness, nausea, and confusion. These side effects are mild to moderate in severity, resolve over time, and reverse after drug discontinuation.

Special Issues

Clinically relevant dosages of ziconotide have not been determined in dogs and cats.

ORAL DRUGS

Tramadol

Mechanism of Action

Tramadol is an atypical opioid that produces analgesia by activation of mu (µ) opioid receptors (MORs) and inhibition of reuptake of serotonin (5-hydroxytryptamine [5-HT]; selective serotonin reuptake inhibitor [SSRI]) and norepinephrine (NE; norepinephrine reuptake inhibitor [NERI]). Tramadol is a racemate with active enantiomers; each has a different profile of activity. Noradrenergic (NA) and 5-HT reuptake inhibition are predominantly the actions of the (−) and (+) enantiomers of the parent compound, respectively. The opioid effect of tramadol is believed to be, at least in part, related to its major metabolite, O-desmethyltramadol (M1) which is considerably more potent than the parent compound.

Efficacy/Administration

- Tramadol is effective for the treatment of mild to moderate pain and ineffective for the treatment of severe pain and is best used as part of a multimodal analgesic protocol.
- Tramadol has been used to alleviate pain associated with osteoarthritis, fibromyalgia, diabetic neuropathy, and neuropathic pain in humans.

Tramadol can provide mild to moderate pain control and works especially well in conjunction with a nonsteroidal anti-inflammatory drug.

- Tramadol may useful for the treatment of allodynia.
- Clinical doses range from 2 to 4 mg/kg bid to qid for dogs and 2 to 4 mg/kg bid for cats.
- Tramadol can be combined with NSAIDs for the treatment of chronic pain.

Pharmacology

- Oral administration of tramadol in dogs results in rapid absorption with approximately 75% bioavailability. Administration with or without food seems to make no difference.
- O-desmethyltramadol (M1) has 300-fold greater affinity for μ opioid receptors than the parent compound.
- Modulation of NE and serotonin in the CNS may be responsible for central pain modulation.
- The median half-life is 1 to 2 hours in dogs and approximately 2.5 hours in cats. The M1 metabolite (more active component) has a half-life of approximately 5 hours in cats.

Side Effects and Toxicity

- Side effects are somnolence, trembling, ataxia, bradycardia, nausea, and loss of appetite. Seizures are a rare event. These side effects are mild to moderate in severity, resolve over time, and reverse after drug discontinuation.
- Short-term administration of tramadol may cause some nausea and vomiting, although this is unlikely at recommended doses.
- Long-term administration may cause constipation or diarrhea. This occurs infrequently in dogs. The likelihood is unknown in cats.

Special Issues

- Drug interactions may occur between tramadol monoamine oxidase inhibitors (MAOIs) and NERIs and SSRIs (serotonin syndrome) (see Chapter 7).
- Tramadol is less likely to induce tolerance in animals and humans compared with morphine because of its nonopioid mechanism of action.

Tapentadol

Mechanism of Action

Tapentadol is a μ opioid receptor agonist and a noradrenaline (norepinephrine) reuptake inhibitor. These opioidergic and noradrenergic activities are believed to account for the analgesic effects of the drug. Tapentadol is also a weak serotonin reuptake inhibitor; however, this weak serotonergic activity is not thought to be relevant with regard to the drug's analgesic activity.

Efficacy/Administration

- Tapentadol is similar to tramadol and is best used as part of a multimodal analgesic protocol.
- Clinical dosage ranges from 5 to 10 mg/kg bid to qid.
- Tapentadol can be combined with NSAIDs for the treatment of chronic pain.

Pharmacology

- Pharmacology is similar to that of tramadol. Modulation of NE and serotonin in the CNS may be responsible for central pain modulation.
- The median half-life of tapentadol is 0.5 to 1.0 hour in dogs

Side Effects and Toxicity

- Side effects are similar to those of tramadol and include somnolence, trembling, ataxia, bradycardia, nausea, and loss of appetite. Seizures are a rare event. These side effects are mild to moderate in severity, resolve over time, and reverse after drug discontinuation.

Special Issues

- Drug interactions may occur between tramadol monoamine oxidase inhibitors (MAOIs) and NERIs and SSRIs (serotonin syndrome) (see Chapter 7).

Amantadine

Amantadine was developed as an antiviral drug for use in humans. Amantadine and memantine have been shown to have efficacy for treatment of drug-induced extrapyramidal effects and for Parkinson disease.

 Amantadine may help to reduce allodynia and opioid tolerance in animals with chronic pain.

Mechanism of Action

Amantadine and memantine block NMDA receptors.

Efficacy/Administration
- Amantadine and memantine are administered for the treatment of neuropathic pain.
- Amantadine and memantine can be administered to animals suffering from wind-up, allodynia, and opioid tolerance and may permit a lower dose of opioid administration. Dogs with problem osteoarthritis and decreased responsiveness to NSAID therapy generally benefit from the coadministration of amantadine for 21 days as needed.
- Amantadine appears to be helpful in maintaining comfort in dogs with musculoskeletal pain or osteosarcoma.
- In humans, amantadine significantly reduced fentanyl use during surgery, and also reduced postoperative pain and morphine consumption.
- The dosage of both drugs for dogs and cats is approximately 3 to 5 mg/kg orally (PO) once daily.

Pharmacology
The pharmacology of amantadine and memantine in dogs and cats has not been well established, although the pharmacology of rimantadine, a similar drug, is known for dogs. In humans, amantadine is well absorbed, is not metabolized, and is excreted in the urine.

Side Effects and Toxicity
- The feline toxic dose is 30 mg/kg.
- Dogs may develop high anxiety, restlessness, and dry mouth as the daily dose approaches 6 mg/kg or if there is impaired renal excretion.
- Behavioral effects in dogs and cats begin at 15 mg/kg PO.

Special Issues
The duration of action of amantadine and memantine may be prolonged in animals with renal insufficiency.

Gabapentin

Gabapentin is a structural analogue of γ-aminobutyric acid (GABA). Gabapentin was originally introduced as an antiepileptic drug.

Mechanism of Action
- Although gabapentin is related to GABA, it does not appear to have any analgesic effect at GABA receptors.
- Gabapentin produces antinociceptive effects by activating hyperpolarizing-activated cation channels and the $\alpha_2\delta$ subunit of spinal N-type Ca^{2+} channels, thereby modulating calcium influx in nerve terminals and reducing the release of prostimulatory neurotransmitters including glutamate and substance P.

Efficacy/Administration

Gabapentin is useful for helping control pain related to neuropathic conditions, osteoarthritis, and cancer.

- Gabapentin is effective therapy for neuropathic pain, hyperalgesia, and allodynia.
- Gabapentin appears to be best suited for treatment of hypersensitivity.
- Gabapentin dose-dependently inhibits dorsal horn responses to inflammation-induced pain.
- Gabapentin decreases allodynia related to mechanical pressure and cold but does not affect nociceptive thresholds.
- Gabapentin reduces hyperalgesia when given systemically or intrathecally.
- Gabapentin, given prophylactically, can inhibit hyperalgesia related to incisional, peripheral nerve, and thermal injury.
- Initial doses range from 2.5 to 10 mg/kg PO bid.
  - Dosage may be able to be increased up to 50 mg/kg PO bid or tid.

Pharmacology
Gabapentin is highly bioavailable in dogs. Gabapentin is metabolized by the liver and almost exclusively excreted by the kidneys. The pharmacokinetics of gabapentin are not changed by multiple doses. The half-life is about 3 to 4 hours.

Side Effects
- Sleepiness
- Muscle weakness and fatigue
- Weight gain with chronic administration

Special Issues
- Gabapentin may be useful as part of a multimodal approach for controlling surgical pain and as an adjunct to NSAIDs for the control of problem osteoarthritis pain. Gabapentin can also be administered as part of a multimodal approach for control of cancer pain.
- Gabapentin is synergistic with opioids, enhancing both analgesic and sedative effects.

Pregabalin

Mechanism of Action
Like gabapentin, pregabalin produces antinociceptive effects by activating hyperpolarizing-activated cation channels and the $\alpha_2\delta$ subunit of spinal N-type Ca^{2+} channels, thereby modulating calcium influx in nerve terminals and reducing the release of prostimulatory neurotransmitters including glutamate and substance P.

Efficacy/Administration

- The efficacy of pregabalin is similar to that of gabapentin, and pregabalin is best used as part of a multimodal analgesic protocol.
- Initial clinical dosage ranges from 1 to 3 mg/kg bid to qid.
- Pregabalin can be combined with NSAIDs or tramadol for the treatment of chronic pain.

Pharmacology

- Pregabalin is a neuroactive drug that can be used to treat partial-onset (focal) seizure disorders, neuropathic pain, and anxiety. Like gabapentin, pregabalin seems to work as a close structural relative to GABA.
- The median half-life of pregabalin is approximately 3 to 4 hours in dogs.

Side Effects and Toxicity

Side effects are similar to those of gabapentin and include somnolence, trembling, muscle weakness, and listlessness.

Special Issues

Both pregabalin and gabapentin are synergistic with opioids, enhancing both analgesic and sedative effects.

Mexiletine

Mechanism of Action

Mexiletine inhibits nerve conduction by blocking sodium channels.

Efficacy/Administration

In humans, mexiletine is administered to treat cardiac arrhythmias and neuropathic pain.

Pharmacology

- Mexiletine reduces the rate of rise of the action potential by inhibiting the inward sodium current.
- Mexiletine is relatively well absorbed from the gut and has a low first-pass effect.
- Mexiletine can be administered to dogs at 5 to 8 mg/kg PO bid or tid. Mexiletine is contraindicated in cats.

Side Effects and Toxicity

Side effects are similar to those produced by lidocaine. Nausea and vomiting are the most likely effect in dogs and cats. CNS effects (tremors, dizziness), shortness of breath, premature ventricular contractions, and chest pain have been reported in humans. Seizures, agranulocytosis, and thrombocytopenia are rare but may occur.

Special Issues

Mexiletine should be administered cautiously to animals with liver or heart disease.

Alendronate

Mechanism of Action

Alendronate is a bisphosphonate that inhibits osteoclast-mediated bone reabsorption.

Efficacy/Administration

- Alendronate is administered to reduce inflammation from pathologic fractures caused by osteosarcoma.
- The efficacy of bisphosphonates for reducing pain is speculative and likely dependent on their secondary ability to reduce inflammation.
- The effective dosage for pain reduction in dogs is speculative: 0.5 to 1.0 mg/kg PO once daily. No dosage has been determined for cats.

Pharmacology

- Renal excretion is the only route of elimination, and the half-life is measured in weeks.
- Alendronate should not be given with food. Feeding should be delayed for a minimum of 30 minutes after administration.
- Alendronate should not be administered with other medications that may contain calcium.

Side Effects and Toxicity

Gastrointestinal effects are common in humans. Osteonecrosis of the jaw has also been reported.

Special Issues

Alendronate should not be administered to animals with kidney disease.

Nimodipine

Mechanism of Action

Nimodipine enhances the antinociceptive properties of morphine by blocking calcium channels.

Efficacy/Administration

In humans, nimodipine is administered perioperatively to decrease postoperative morphine requirements.

Pharmacology

Nimodipine is an L-type dihydropyridine calcium channel blocker with relatively high penetration of the blood-brain barrier.

Side Effects and Toxicity
Hypotension has been reported in humans.

Special Issues
Research is lacking on the use of nimodipine to treat pain in dogs and cats.

Nifedipine

Mechanism of Action
Nifedipine is a calcium channel blocker.

Efficacy/Administration
In humans, nifedipine has been administered sublingually in conjunction with epidural morphine to decrease morphine requirements and improve analgesia.

Pharmacology
In humans, nifedipine is used to treat hypertension. Calcium channel blocking activity may help ameliorate smooth muscle spasmodic contractures and reduce visceral pain.

Side Effects and Toxicity
Hypotension has been reported in humans.

Special Issues
Research is lacking regarding the administration of nifedipine to treat pain in dogs and cats; therefore therapeutically relevant dosages to treat pain are not available.

Cannabis

Cannabis sativa has been used for centuries for its psychoactive and potentially medicinal effects. There is little to no evidence in the refereed literature that cannabis has a beneficial use in dogs and cats. The extrapolation of data from the human medical field, however, is promising, especially from a pain management perspective.

Mechanism of Action
- There are more than 60 cannabinoids that can be derived from the *C. sativa* plant.
  - THC (Δ9-tetrahydrocannabinol) is the major psychoactive compound.
  - Cannabinol and cannabidiol are also active components, with less than ten times the potency of THC.
- Cannabinoid receptors CB_1 (CNS) and CB_2 (peripheral tissues) have been identified in dogs.

- CB_1 receptors are distributed throughout the brain, especially in the basal ganglia, substantia nigra, globus pallidus hippocampus, cerebellum, and frontal regions of the cerebral cortex.
  - Typically presynaptic.
  - Stimulation inhibits adenyl cyclase and stimulates potassium channel conductance.
  - May inhibit acetylcholine, L-glutamate, GABA, NE, dopamine, and serotonin.
  - Responsible for centrally mediated analgesia.
- CB_2 receptors are found in splenic macrophages, peripheral nerve terminals, vas deferens, tonsils, and thymus.
  - Stimulation inhibits adenyl cyclase and stimulates potassium channel conductance.
  - Possibly involved in immune regulation and induction of an anti-inflammatory effect.
- There appear to be endogenous cannabinoid receptor ligands as well as agonists and antagonists.
- All active cannabinoid compounds bind to both types of receptor.

Efficacy/Administration

- In humans, medical marijuana is prescribed for chronic conditions, as an adjunct therapy, or if other treatments have been inadequate.
- Provides symptomatic relief of pain and anxiety (especially neuropathic pain).
- Used as an analgesic in painful disease states such as diabetic neuropathy and arthritis because of its anti-inflammatory properties.
- Relieves spasticity in spinal cord injuries.
- Antiemetic (antivomiting) therapy for patients receiving cancer chemotherapy.
- Stimulates appetite.
- Used to treat behavioral disorders such as separation anxiety, neurosis, and dementia.
- Medical marijuana is available in several forms—smokable, edible, and tinctures—with one product currently designed specifically for dogs and cats.
- Three products have been produced by pharmaceutical companies for use in humans.
  - Nabilone (Cesamet) is a Schedule II synthetic cannabinoid.
  - Dronabinol (Marinol) is a Schedule III synthetic THC.
  - Sativex is made of multiple extracts of THC and cannabidiol, but is not available in the United States.
- Extrapolation of data from humans implies a THC dosage of approximately 0.05 mg/kg.

- To help prevent vomiting, THC should not be administered on an empty stomach.
- Therapy should always begin with a low dosage and increase to achieve desired efficacy.

Pharmacology
- Onset after ingestion is approximately 60 minutes and is likely dose related.
- Fifteen percent of THC is excreted in the urine, and the rest in the feces.
- THC accumulates in adipose tissue, inducing a half-life of about 30 hours. In dogs, about 80% of THC is cleared over 5 days.

Side Effects and Toxicity
- Minimum lethal dose is 3 g/kg, implying a very high safety margin.
- Side effects include ataxia, hypersalivation, sedation, disorientation, mydriasis, bradycardia, vomiting, and tremors.
- Caution should be used under the following circumstances.
  - Pregnancy.
  - Respiratory or cardiovascular diseases.
  - Liver failure, although sublingual administration may be a good option.
- Potential adverse drug interactions, although definitive evidence is lacking.
  - Chlorpromazine: cannabis may necessitate administration of larger therapeutic doses of chlorpromazine.
  - Cyclosporine: cannabidiol may increase cyclosporine levels.
  - Cisplatin: one documented case report of a fatal stroke in a young man who had received cisplatin and smoked cannabis.
  - Caution should be used when administering with any other sedatives and CNS depressants.
  - Fluoxetine: mania may occur when fluoxetine is administered in combination with cannabis.
  - Nicotine (secondhand smoke, smoking household): possible increase in the stimulant effect of cannabis, particularly increasing the heart rate.
  - Opioids: low doses of cannabis enhance the effects of morphine and other opioids. Animal studies have shown that cannabinoids may enhance the potency of opioids. This is perhaps the most clearly documented interaction.
  - Phenytoin: one in vitro study suggests that Δ9-tetrahydrocannabinol, a major constituent of cannabis, might induce phenytoin metabolism.
  - Theophylline: cannabis increases clearance of theophylline and may necessitate administration of larger therapeutic doses of theophylline.
  - Tricyclic antidepressants: tachycardia has been described in patients taking tricyclic antidepressants who smoked cannabis.

Special Issues
- Medical use of marijuana is still illegal from a federal perspective in the United States.
- There are no jurisdictions with statutes making medical use of marijuana legal for animals. However, some jurisdictions permit legal possession.
- Practitioners should check local laws before prescribing any cannabinoids to animals.

Nutraceuticals

Many nutraceuticals available over the counter are used in animals. These include glucosamine sulfate, glucosamine hydrochloride, chondroitin sulfate, *Perna canaliculus*, methylsulfonylmethane, microlactin, and buffered vitamin C. Some dosages and potential side effects have been determined (Table 14-1).

Nutraceutical formulations are not controlled by the U.S. Food and Drug Administration (FDA). Therefore there is no oversight of quality or quantity of ingredients in the various products available.

- Glucosamine-chondroitin
  - Many glucosamine-chondroitin supplements are available for humans and animals. There seem to be few formulations for which there are data for efficacy in pets.
    - The combination of glucosamine hydrochloride, low-molecular-weight chondroitin, and manganese can induce biosynthetic activity in canine cartilage.
    - This combination also has a protective effect when administered before an acute joint injury. Individuals who received this combination before joint injury healed more quickly than those administered the combination after injury.
- Data support supplementation with *P. canaliculus* based on the effects in a rat model and in humans with arthritis.
- No clinical data support the use of methylsulfonamethane or buffered vitamin C in animals for the relief of pain. These products may be beneficial, but well-controlled studies have not been performed to document this.
- Emerging data indicate that the combination of glucosamine hydrochloride, *P. canaliculus*, methylsulfonylmethane, and manganese may be effective at ameliorating the clinical signs of osteoarthritis in dogs.
- Microlactin is thought to be a potent inhibitor of neutrophil adherence, migration, and participation in the immune response to musculoskeletal conditions including arthritis. Unpublished data show efficacy for pain relief in dogs with osteoarthritis.
- Buffered vitamin C is believed to have chondroprotective, antiinflammatory, and immunoresponsive effects that may provide pain control for animals with osteoarthritis. No documented evidence exists for its efficacy in veterinary patients.

TABLE 14-1 Commonly Administered Nutraceuticals: Concerns and Dosages

NUTRACEUTICAL	CONCERNS	DOSAGE	
		DOGS	CATS
Glucosamine sulfate Glucosamine hydrochloride	Minor gastrointestinal (GI) disturbance	*Large dogs*: Up to 750 mg PO bid	250 mg PO bid
Glucosamine + chondroitin sulfate	Minor GI disturbance	13-15 mg/kg chondroitin PO sid	15-20 mg/kg chondroitin PO sid
Perna canaliculus	Allergic reactions, fluid retention, skin rash, and upset stomach. In addition, Perna mussel supplements should not be given to people or animals with allergies to fish or shellfish.	*1-20 kg*: Loading dose (10 days): two tablets per day; maintenance dose: one tablet per day *21-40 kg*: Loading dose: three tablets per day; maintenance dose: two tablets per day *40 kg and over*: Loading dose: four tablets per day; maintenance dose: three tablets per day (one tablet = 600 mg)	
Methylsulfonylmethane	Sulfur toxicity at extreme doses	*Large dogs*: Up to 2 g PO bid	100-250 mg PO bid
Microlactin	Vomiting, diarrhea	*Less than 40 lb*: 500 mg PO bid *40-80 lb*: 1000 mg PO bid *81-120 lb*: 1500 mg PO bid	*Up to 12 lb*: 200 mg PO bid *Over 12 lb*: 300 mg PO bid
Buffered vitamin C	Minor GI disturbance at high doses; should not be administered with anesthetics	Gradually increase dose to 250-1000 mg PO bid	Gradually increase dose to 250 mg PO bid
Elk velvet antler	Minor GI disturbance at high doses	250 mg/30 lb PO daily	125 mg / cat PO daily
Hyaluronic acid (HA)	None	*Under 30 lb*: 1 mg PO daily *31-45 lb*: 2 mg PO daily *45-60 lb*: 3 mg PO daily *>45 lb*: 4-5 mg PO daily (based on near-identical HA)	1 mg PO daily (based on near-identical HA)

- Elk velvet antler
  - Components:
    - Glucosamine
    - Chondroitin
    - Hyaluronic acid (HA)
    - Omega-3 and omega-6 fatty acids
    - Calcium
    - Phosphorus
    - Growth factors
    - Magnesium
    - Copper
    - Zinc
    - Selenium
    - Collagen
  - Elk velvet antler is the fastest growing living tissue of any animal.
  - The FDA allows the claim, substantiated by scientific evidence, that velvet antler provides nutritional support for joint structure.
  - Increases function in dogs with osteoarthritis
    - Daily life activity
    - Gait
    - Force plate data
    - Increased muscle building
    - Possible anti-inflammatory effects
- Hyaluronic acid (HA)
  - Injectable HA is a drug, but in oral form it is considered a supplement.
  - HA is the most abundant lubricant in the body, present in joints, muscles, tendons, skin, eyes, and myocardium.
  - HA is composed of high molecular weight, long chain molecules. The only way to produce near-bioidentical HA is by bacterial fermentation.
  - Most products are derived from powdered rooster comb or chicken cartilage, resulting in low to medium molecular weight and short to medium chain molecules.
  - HA molecules of all sizes are absorbed easily.
  - Absorption of HA molecules that are not nearly bioidentical may produce two effects:
    - Lack of efficacy
    - Decreased lubrication as a result of induction of hyaluronidase activity leading to destruction of endogenous HA
- Homeopathy
  - Complex homeopathic preparation (Zeel) has documented efficacy in dogs.
  - Comparable effectiveness to carprofen in dogs with osteoarthritis.

- Symptomatic effectiveness
- Lameness
- Stiffness
- Pain on palpation
- No detected side effects, which is in accordance with the concept of homeopathy.

Stem Cell Therapy

Stem cell therapy (SCT) has been investigated for clinical use since the 1950s. Pharmacologic interventions in pain management are mainly palliative, and although they temporarily relieve the pain, they do not address the core underlying mechanisms of the pain. Neurotropic factors are critical in the development and survival of neurons and they participate in the regeneration and repair of nerves. Mesenchymal stem cells have been shown to produce a wide array of cytokines and growth factors (more than 84), including many neurotropic factors, and have therefore been the subject of considerable research to determine the detailed mechanism by which stem cells support the functioning of nervous system and to formulate clinical protocols for their use in pain management. SCT provides a new tool for practitioners in dealing with refractory pain cases. SCT is broadly being deployed as a mechanism to reduce tissue damage from many injuries and diseases and therefore the stimulation of pain sensation. More recently, the findings that SCT can produce direct effects on normal and injured neurons via neurotropic cytokines bring a new paradigm in the treatment of pain. Lastly, recent studies have shown that stem cells can produce drugs that have direct effects on receptors such as opioid receptors, adding yet another tool in the therapeutic arsenal of the pain practitioner. The modern practitioner is well advised to consider this modality in handling complex cases requiring pain management and regeneration of neural function.

Mechanism of Action
- Homing to inflammation or ischemia
- Anti-inflammation
- Antiapoptosis
- Neurotropic factor production
- Stimulation of mitosis of neuroprogenitors
- Antifibrosis
- Angiogenesis
- SCT delivers a population of cells able to communicate with other cells in their local environment. Until recently, differentiation was thought to be the primary function of stem cells.

- The functions of regenerative cells are now known to be much more diverse, including immune modulation and secretion of cell signaling factors and cytokines that influence both local and remote cell populations. These cellular functions are implicated in a highly integrated and complex network.
- Cellular therapy should be viewed as a complex, yet balanced, approach to a therapeutic goal where the cells take their signals from the microenvironment of the injured tissue.
- Unlike traditional medicine, in which one drug targets one or a few receptors, a single SCT can be applied in a wide variety of injuries and diseases.

Efficacy/Administration

In a clinical sense, the functions of stem cells can be categorized as having an indirect or direct effect on the nervous system.

Indirect Effects
- Anti-inflammatory: reduce overall tissue inflammation
- Antiapoptotic: reduce tissue damage and cell death
- Antifibrotic: reduce fibrosis in damaged tissue
- Angiogenic: increased blood flow to damaged tissues

Direct Functions
- Neurotropic growth factor secretion
- Antiapoptosis: prevents cell death
- Stimulation of mitosis of neuroprogenitors
- Differentiation into neural phenotype cells
- Opioid receptor agonist
- Angiogenesis: increased blood flow to neurons
- Recent studies have shown a profound effect of SCT on mechanical allodynia and thermal hyperalgesia. The mechanisms are proposed to be a reduction in proinflammatory interleukin (IL)–1β and IL-17 and an increase in anti-inflammatory cytokine IL-10 as well as a reduction in the overactivity of β-galactosidase. These effects have been seen with local as well as systemic administration of stem cells.
- Beyond peripheral neuropathic pain, a recent case report has shown promising results in human spinal cord crush injury and in two controlled studies in beagles with severe spinal cord damage.
- In diabetic neuropathy, animal model studies have shown a reduction in progression of disease, improvement in motor nerve conduction velocity, and improvement in blood flow to nerves.

Sources of Clinical Grade Adult Stem Cells
- For use of SCT, a source of stem cells must be chosen. In veterinary medicine, there are two primary sources.

- Bone marrow
- Adipose tissue: the only tissue with adequate concentrations of adult mesenchymal stem cells for direct (uncultured) use
- All other sources need to be expanded ex vivo to obtain a therapeutic dose to treat a veterinary patient.
- Use of in-clinic systems for veterinary stem cell processing has not been ruled on by the FDA and presents challenges to the practitioner with regard to sterility, dose determination (cell counting), and storage.
- Central laboratory service businesses provide solutions to the sterility, cell count, and cryostorage needs without capital investment and can ensure that quality control measures are in place before administration.

Administration

- Stem cells can be delivered to the animal by nearly every typical route.
  - Intravenous
  - Intra-articular
  - Intrathecal
  - Intraperitoneal
  - Regional perfusion
  - Locally administered
- Cells have a peripheral and central effect in modulating neuropathic pain.
- Systemic administration has a profound effect in reducing inflammation.
- Equine practitioners have adopted regional perfusion to deliver SCT to soft-tissue and bone injuries in peripheral locations.
- Intrathecal and intracord administration has been reported effective in multiple diseases.
  - Spinal cord trauma
  - Immune-mediated neural diseases such as multiple sclerosis
  - Modulation of pain and inflammation from rheumatoid arthritis
    - Canine osteoarthritis pain and inflammation have been treated effectively with intra-articular administration of adipose-derived stem cells as demonstrated in clinical efficacy studies.

Side Effects and Toxicity
Special Issues: Food and Drug Administration Regulation of Stem Cell Therapy in Veterinary Medicine

- In the United States, the FDA Center for Veterinary Medicine regulates all veterinary drugs. Stem cell products are considered to be drugs and are regulated as such by the FDA.
- Service businesses that separate and isolate stem cells from autologous tissues are being allowed to operate by the FDA under regulatory discretion, but any products such as allogeneic cells must be approved under the New Animal Drug Application (NADA) approval process.

Autologous Platelet Therapy

Intra-articular injection of autologous platelets may be a potential treatment for osteoarthritis in dogs. Growth factors present in platelets enhance regenerative processes in osteoarthritic joints. Elaboration of growth factors, including platelet-derived growth factors from the α-granules of platelets, can directly promote healing and recruit stem cells to the site, facilitating tissue repair. Intra-articular administration of autologous platelet concentrates derived from whole blood is efficacious in human patients with osteoarthritis. A single intra-articular injection of autologous platelets in 20 client-owned dogs with osteoarthritis involving a single joint produced significant improvements at 12 weeks.

Gene Therapy

Neuropathic pain is associated with nerve injury, chronic pain, and surgery, particularly if tissue damage is extensive. IL-10 is an anti-inflammatory molecule that has achieved interest as a therapeutic agent for neuropathic pain. Non-neuronal glial cells within the spinal cord parenchyma become activated in response to inflammation or trauma and play a major role in the development and maintenance of neuropathic pain by producing proinflammatory cytokines that sensitize pain pathways and enhance pain processing. The anti-inflammatory cytokine IL-10 is a candidate to suppress proinflammatory cytokines released by activated glia. Intrathecal administration of an unencapsulated nonviral plasmid DNA (pDNA) IL-10 protein has been shown to provide relief from pain in rats and dogs, enabling long-term reversal of neuropathic pain.

Monoclonal Antibodies

Nerve growth factor (NGF) is essential for the survival of sensory neurons and is expressed locally at sites of injury and inflammation, thereby promoting pain and hyperalgesia. It is also produced by a variety of inflammatory and immune cells, including joint chondrocytes. NGF causes immediate and long-term excitability by activating the transient receptor potential vanilloid receptor (TRPV1) and neurotransmitters such as substance P and brain-derived neurotrophic factor (BDNF). NGF also causes nerve endings to sprout into the site of inflammation. Neutralizing antibodies to NGF provide highly effective analgesia for pain caused by inflammation, arthritis, cancer, and bone fracture in animal models and humans. Monoclonal antibodies are a major class of biologic therapies currently in development (www.nexvet.com/science) for the treatment of pain in dogs and cats. Anti–nerve growth factor (anti-NGF) monoclonal antibodies (mAbs) hold promise for reducing acute and chronic pain in dogs and cats.

ACKNOWLEDGMENTS

The authors would like to acknowledge Dr. Bob Harman, CEO Vet-Stem, Poway, California, for his assistance in preparing the stem cell therapy portion of this manuscript.

SUGGESTED READINGS

Allen MR, Kubek DJ, Burr DB. Cancer treatment dosing regimens of zoledronic acid result in near-complete suppression of mandible intracortical bone remodeling in beagle dogs. J Bone Miner Res. 2010; 25:98–105.

Black L, Gaynor J, Harman R, et al.: Effect of adipose-derived mesenchymal stem and regenerative cells on lameness in dogs with chronic osteoarthritis of the coxofemoral joints: a randomized, double-blinded, multicenter controlled trial. Vet Ther. 2007; 8(4):272–284.

Black L, Gaynor J, Harman R, et al.: Effect of intraarticular injections of autologous adipose-derived mesenchymal stem and regenerative cells on clinical signs of chronic osteoarthritis of the elbow joint in dogs. Vet Ther. 2008; 9:3.

Bujak-Giżycka B, Kącka K, Suski M, et al.: Beneficial effect of amantadine on postoperative pain reduction and consumption of morphine in patients subjected to elective spine surgery. Pain Medicine. 2012; 13:459–465.

Canapp SO, McLaughlin RM, Hoskinson JJ, et al.: Scintigraphic evaluation of glucosamine hydrochloride and chondroitin sulfate as a treatment for acute synovitis in dogs. Am J Vet Res. 1999; 60:1552–1557.

Caplan A: Mesenchymal stem cells as trophic mediators. J Cell Biochem. 2006; 98:1076–1084.

Crosby V, Wilcock A, Corcoran R: The safety and efficacy of a single dose (500 mg or 1 g) of intravenous magnesium sulfate in neuropathic pain poorly responsive to strong opioid analgesics in patients with cancer. J Pain Symptom Manag. 2000; 19:35–39.

De Kock M, Crochet B, Morimont C, Scholtes JL: Intravenous or epidural clonidine for intra and postoperative analgesia. Anesthesiology. 1993; 79:525–531.

Fahie MA, Ortolano GA, Guercio V, et al.: A randomized controlled trial of the efficacy of autologous platelet therapy for the treatment of osteoarthritic in dogs. J Am Vet Med Assoc. 2013; 243:1291–1297.

Felsby S, Nielsen J, Arendt-Nielsen L, et al.: NMDA receptor blockade in chronic neuropathic pain: A comparison of ketamine and magnesium chloride. Pain. 1996; 64:283–291.

Fortino RF, Pelaez D, Cheung HS: Concise review: Stem cell therapies for neuropathic pain. Stem Cells Trans Med. 2013; 2:394–399.

Gene therapy treatment showing promise for dogs with chronic pain. Retrieved from www.aahanet.org/blog/NewStat/post/2012/12/19/845594/Gene-therapy-treatment-showing-promise-for-dogs-with-chronic-pain.aspx.

Gourion-Arsiquaud S, Allen MR, Burr DB, et al.: Bisphosphonate treatment modifies canine bone mineral and matrix properties and their heterogeneity. Bone. 2010; 46:666–672.

Guercio A, Marco P, Casella S, et al.: Production of canine mesenchymal stem cells from adipose tissue and application in dogs with chronic osteoarthritis of the humeroradial joints. Cell Bio Internat. 2012; 36(2):189–194.

Ichim T, Solano F, Lara F, et al.: Feasibility of combination allogeneic stem cell therapy for spinal cord injury: A case report. Int Arch Med. 2010; 3:30.

Kroin JS, McCarthy RJ, Von Roenn N, et al.: Magnesium sulfate potentiates morphine antinociception at the spinal level. Anesth Analg. 2000; 90:913–917.

Koinig H, Wallner T, Marhofer P, et al.: Magnesium sulfate reduces intra- and postoperative analgesic requirements. Anesth Analg. 1998; 87:206–210.

KuKanich B, Cohen RL: Pharmacokinetics of oral gabapentin in Greyhound dogs Vet J. 2011; 187:133–135.

Lawson BR, Belkowski SM, Whitesides JF, et al.: Immunomodulation of murine collagen-induced arthritis by N, N-dimethylglycine and a preparation of Perna canaliculus. BMC Complement Altern Med. 2007; 7:20.

Lascelles BD, Gaynor JS, Smith ES, et al.: Amantadine in a multimodal analgesic regimen for alleviation of refractory osteoarthritis pain in dogs. J Vet Intern Med. 2008; 22:53–59.

Lehmann KA: Tramadol for the management of acute pain. Drugs. 1994; 47(suppl 1):19–32.

Lin JH, Russell G, Gertz B: Pharmacokinetics of alendronate: An overview. Int J Clin Pract. Suppl. 1999; 101:18–26.

Mahani SE, Motamedi F, Ahmadiani A: Involvement of hypothalamic adrenal axis on the nifedipine-induced antinociception and tolerance in rats. Pharmacol Biochem Behav. 2006; 85:422–427.

Mama KR, Golden AE, Monnet E, et al: Plasma and cerebrospinal fluid concentrations and NMDA receptor binding activity associated with intraoperative administration of low-dose ketamine. In Proceedings 7th World Congress of Veterinary Anaesthesia, Berne, 2000; p 78, (abstract).

Martinez SA, McCormick DJ, Powers MY, et al.: The effect of Glyco-Flex III on a stable stifle osteoarthritis model in dogs: A pilot study. Presented at the Veterinary Orthopedic Society Annual Scientific Meeting, Sun Valley, Idaho, 2007.

Minto CF, Power I: New opioid analgesics: An update. Int Anesthesiol Clin. 1997; 35:49–65.

Miranda HF, Pinardi G: Antinociception, tolerance, and physical dependence comparison between morphine and tramadol. Pharmacol Biochem Behav. 1998; 61:357–360.

Mao J, Chen LL: Gabapentin in pain management. Anesth Analg. 2000; 9:680–687.

Moreau M, Dupuis J, Bonneau N, et al.: Clinical evaluation of a powder of quality elk velvet antler for the treatment of osteoarthrosis in dogs. Can Vet J. 2004; 45:133–139.

Ortiz L, DeTreil M, Fattman C, et al.: Interleukin 1 receptor antagonist mediates the anti-inflammatory and antifibrotic effect of mesenchymal stem cells during lung injury. Proc Natl Acad Sci. 2007; 104:11002–11007.

Pud D, Eisenberg E, Spitzer A, et al.: The NMDA receptor antagonist amantidine reduces surgical neuropathic pain in cancer patients: A double blind, randomized, placebo controlled trial. Pain. 1998; 75:349–354.

Pypendop BH, Ilkiw JE: Pharmacokinetics of tramadol, and its metabolite O-desmethyltramadol, in cats. J Vet Pharmacol Ther. 2008; 31:52–59.

Pypendop BH, Siao KT, Ilkiw JE: Effects of tramadol hydrochloride on the thermal threshold in cats. Am J Vet Res. 2009; 70:1465–1470.

Radulovic LL, Turck D, von Hodenberg A, et al.: Disposition of gabapentin (neurontin) in mice, rats, dogs, and monkeys. Drug Metab Dispos. 1995; 23:441–448.

Rodriguez J, Murphy M, Madrigal M, et al.: Autologous stromal vascular fraction therapy for rheumatoid arthritis: Rationale and clinical safety. Int Arch Med. 2012; 5:5.

Salazar V, Dewey CW, Schwark W, et al.: Pharmacokinetics of single-dose oral pregabalin administration in normal dogs. Vet Anaesth Analg. 2009; 36:574–580.

Sindrup SH, Anderson G, Madsen C, et al.: Tramadol relieves pain and allodynia in polyneuropathy: A randomised, double-blind, controlled trial. Pain. 1999; 83:85–90.

Soderquist RG, Sloane EM, Loram LC, et al.: Release of plasmid DNA-encoding IL-10 from PLGA microparticles facilitates long-term reversal of neuropathic pain following a single intrathecal administration. Pharm Res. 2010; 27:841–854.

Thomopoulos S, Matsuzaki H, Zaegel M, et al.: Alendronate prevents bone loss and improves tendon-to-bone repair strength in a canine model. J Orthop Res. 2007; 25:473–479.

CHAPTER 15

Factors Influencing Analgesic Drug Selection, Dose, and Routes of Drug Administration

William W. Muir III

CHOICE OF ANALGESIC THERAPY

The choice of analgesic therapy, whether pharmacologic or nonpharmacologic, should be tailored to each animal's needs with the following goals:
- Improving the animal's quality of life (QOL) (see Chapter 6)
- Eliminating or suppressing pain
- Eliminating or suppressing pain behavior and promoting normal behavior
- Making the animal more comfortable
- Returning the animal to maximum function despite residual pain
- Removing stress or distress

The pain experience is always multidimensional and incorporates physiologic (nociception, autonomic responses, endocrine effects), sensory (location, intensity, quality), postural (stance, gait), and behavioral (activity, mood, appetite) responses. Pharmacologic approaches to the treatment of pain should be carefully considered, given the diverse effects and potential side effects of the various methods that are used to treat pain. Determining the cause, location, severity, and duration of pain in relation to current pain therapies and the animal's medical status are the most important factors in the design of a therapeutic plan. For example, the choice and administration of analgesic drugs for the treatment of pain produced by an elective surgical procedure is likely to be considerably different from that prescribed for the treatment of osteoarthritis from hip dysplasia. Similarly, the treatment of pain caused by acute inflammatory conditions (abscesses) or abrasions is likely to be different from therapy designed to reduce or eliminate pain caused by multiple trauma. Analgesic therapies, particularly drug and dosage recommendations, must be individualized according to the cause and severity of the animal's pain. "Therapeutic" plasma concentrations do not guarantee analgesic efficacy. The animal's physical status, medical history, and behavior pattern, in addition to the pet owner's compliance and understanding of therapeutic consequences, must be considered in prescribing pain therapy. Ultimately, the treatment of pain is only as good as one's understanding of its mechanisms and the use of therapeutic approaches that target the causes. (Procedure-based pain management is discussed in Chapter 16.)

Anamnesis

The dog's or cat's age, weight, sex, breed, physical status, concurrent diseases, and associated therapies are important determinants of drug selection and dose (Box 15-1).

Age

Young (younger than 12 weeks) and older animals generally require reduced dosages of drugs. Drug metabolism and elimination pathways may not be fully developed in the very young or may be impaired by aging or concurrent disease (reduced renal or hepatic function) in older animals. Most nonsteroidal anti-inflammatory drugs (NSAIDs), for example, are not recommended for administration to animals younger than 8 to 10 weeks of age and preferably not younger than 4 months of age and should be administered cautiously to aged dogs and cats. Young and older animals frequently demonstrate more pronounced calming or sedative effects when administered opioids or α_2-agonists.

Weight

The animal's weight should be used as a guide for determining dose, particularly if the drug has a narrow therapeutic range. Calculation of drug dose based on body surface area (BSA) is much more accurate. Body surface area (BSA) in square meters $= K$ (body weight [kg]$^{0.67}$): $K = 10.1$ for dogs and 10.4 for cats. Animals that are obviously overweight or underweight generally require lower dosages than are recommended. Overweight cats are particularly susceptible to drug overdose because of difficulty estimating their true lean body weight (bw). Regardless, all animals, particularly small ones (<5 kg), should be weighed as accurately as possible before initiation of drug therapy.

BOX 15-1   **Factors to Consider Before Prescribing Analgesic Drugs**

- Animal: Age, weight, sex, breed, physical status, medical behavior, drug history, and environment
- Mechanism of pain (inflammatory, neuropathic, cancer, other)
- Location and severity of pain
- Duration of pain
- Consequences of pain (physical, behavioral)
- Type (pharmacologic, physical, complementary) and benefits of therapy
- Route of administration (drug delivery)
- Efficacy and safety of therapy
- Potential side effects or toxicity
- Potential for therapeutic (drug) interactions
- Clinical experience

Sex

Some drugs display sex-related differences in drug dose-response characteristics. Clinically, however, no studies to date support clinically relevant sex-related differences in the response of animals to standard analgesic therapies.

Breed

Breed differences can have a significant impact on drug selection and dose. Veterinary textbooks should be consulted, and the package insert for veterinary-approved drugs carefully reviewed before prescription of any drug. Doberman Pinschers, for example, are predisposed to the extrapyramidal side effects produced by most opioid drugs. Some Boxer dogs have demonstrated pronounced side effects and may have died after administration of acepromazine. Himalayan cats frequently demonstrate increased locomotor activity and hyperexcitability when administered standard doses of opioids for pain control. Collies and other herding breeds demonstrate a deletion mutation of the *mdr* gene, predisposing them to drug side effects. The deletion mutation generates a premature stop codon in the *mdr* gene, resulting in a severely truncated, nonfunctional P-glycoprotein (P-gp). P-gp does not have intrinsic metabolic functions but is an important component of intestinal drug metabolism, drug excretion in renal tubular cells and bile canalicular cells, and the integrity of the blood-brain barrier (i.e., in pumping drugs out of the central nervous system [CNS]).

Physical Status

The animal's physical status and the physical examination findings are major determinants of drug dose and the technique selected to produce analgesia. Dogs and cats in pain generally derive more benefit and demonstrate fewer side effects from analgesic therapies (preventative, constant rate infusion [CRI]) and nonconventional routes (epidural [ED], transcutaneous) of drug administration. Vigilant monitoring must be provided when animals are unconscious or demonstrate signs of cardiorespiratory compromise.

History

The animal's medical, pharmacologic, and pain history are key factors for determining analgesic therapies and the development of short- and long-term pain therapy protocols (see Chapter 5). Although typically not emphasized, nonpharmacologic approaches should always be considered as an alternative or in addition to the administration of drugs for the treatment of acute and chronic pain (see Chapters 22 and 23).

Medical History

The medical history may alter drug selection and dosage. The development of adverse effects after the administration of adjunctive or adjuvant drugs (see Chapter 14) in herding dogs with multidrug resistance gene 1 (MDR-1) mutation may become problematic. The mutation results in nonfunctional P-gp and is associated with multiple drug sensitivity. Dogs or cats with a history of significant CNS or behavioral disorders (seizures, aggression, separation anxiety) may demonstrate pronounced CNS or behavioral changes when administered drugs that are known to produce depression or somnolence in addition to analgesia. For example, the administration of relatively low doses of opioids to older dogs that have become less social may produce depression, periods of disorientation, or episodes of aggression. The administration of tramadol in conjunction with gabapentin is likely to produce disorientation, drowsiness, and decreased sociability in dogs and cats. Similarly, dogs or cats with diseases that affect drug metabolism (liver) and elimination (liver, renal) may demonstrate drug-related side effects after administration of standard doses of drugs.

Pharmacologic History

The animal's response to previous drug therapy, particularly the response to analgesic and sedative drugs, should be determined. Drug dosages are published as guidelines and should be used only as a starting point. Many animals experience a "first-dose effect" that may include one or more side effects (e.g., vomiting, nervousness, disorientation) when drugs are first administered. Dogs or cats that are being administered NSAIDs or behavior-modifying drugs (tricyclic antidepressants [TCAs]), for example, are more likely to demonstrate exaggerated drug-related side effects and toxicity than animals that are not receiving these medications. Tramadol should be avoided or used with caution in dogs or cats that are being administered monoamine oxidase inhibitors (MAOIs), selective serotonin reuptake inhibitors (SSRIs), S-adenosylmethionine (SAMe), or TCAs. Elevated serotonin levels can lead to "serotonin syndrome," indicated by restlessness, altered mentation, muscle twitching, hyperthermia, shivering, diarrhea, sedation, loss of consciousness, and death (see Chapter 7). Ultimately, analgesic therapy must be tailored to meet the animal's needs, and knowledge of the animal's response to previous analgesic therapies can be helpful in this regard.

Pain History and Behavior

The choice of analgesic therapy and the development of an analgesic plan depend on the duration (acute, chronic), severity, and cause of pain. The animal's pain history is always important in the initial design of an analgesic plan. Some dogs and cats, for example, seem to overreact to mild noxious events, demonstrating exaggerated signs or responses (hyperresponsivness) to what would otherwise be considered minimally painful events. Other dogs and cats demonstrate little or no response to painful stimuli. For example, small-breed dogs that have lived the majority of their lives indoors generally demonstrate exaggerated responses to minor traumatic events, including physical manipulation, when compared with larger, more sedentary outside dogs. Although a generalization, the last statement emphasizes the importance of knowing the animal's history and response to pain (e.g., aggressive when hurt). Hyperexcitable, hypersensitive animals often benefit from drugs that produce analgesia and mild sedation.

Environment
The animal's environment may provide insight into the factors responsible for producing pain and pain-associated behaviors. Older osteoarthritic dogs required to climb up or down stairs may refuse to move and become agitated when coerced. Similarly, younger animals (dogs or cats) that are in pain may become aggressive if disturbed or forced to play.

Owner Expectations
The owners' opinions and expectations regarding the animal's sociability, pain intensity, pain behavior, and pain therapies should be determined. Their ability to administer medications or perform nonpharmacologic therapeutic techniques must be determined. The advantages, disadvantages, and cost of the pain therapy should be explained. Owners who are unfamiliar with or unsure of the drugs and techniques used for the treatment of pain are much less likely to comply with therapeutic recommendations.

Cause, Severity, and Duration of Pain

General guidelines regarding the cause (inflammatory, neuropathic, dysfunctional), severity (mild, moderate, severe), and duration (transient, acute, chronic) of pain should be developed and should guide the development of a therapeutic plan (see Chapters 21, 22, and 23).

Cause
Knowing or determining the cause of pain provides insight into potential therapeutic approaches. For example, gastric distention (visceral pain) with or without displacement (bloat) requires gastric decompression, the administration of potent opioids, surgical intervention, and vigilant postoperative monitoring. Similarly, severe visceral pain with respiratory distress caused by thoracic trauma and pneumothorax may not respond to anti-inflammatory medications and chest tubes, particularly if there are fractured or displaced ribs. Dogs with cervical disk disease (neuropathic pain) may temporarily benefit from anti-inflammatory drugs (glucocorticosteroids) and analgesic agents (opioids) but eventually require surgery for long-term relief of pain. Determining the cause of pain therefore helps determine the importance of the mechanical (use dependent), inflammatory, and neuropathic components and suggests appropriate remedies (surgery, anti-inflammatory medications, analgesics).

Severity

Animals demonstrating signs of severe pain attract attention. Regardless of individual animal variability, the more pronounced the signs, the more pronounced the pain. With this in mind, severe pain requires the administration of pain-relieving techniques that provide immediate, efficacious, and sustained analgesic effects. In other words, the severity of the pain determines what analgesic drugs and techniques are used. To this end, many pain scoring systems and variations of these systems have been developed to quantitate, categorize, and evaluate pain and the severity of pain in animals (see Chapters 5 and 6). Pain scoring systems are an integral part of animal evaluation and serve as the basis for drug selection, dose determination, and choice of route of administration. For example, a dog or cat with severe pain resulting from tissue trauma caused by an automobile accident generally requires the administration of potent intravenous (IV) opioids (e.g., hydromorphone) for the immediate onset of analgesia. Oral (PO) anti-inflammatory drugs (firocoxib, carprofen, deracoxib, robenacoxib), when appropriate, or combination (multimodal) therapies are administered for longer-term analgesia. In contrast, a dog or cat subjected to intense transient pain associated with the placement of a large-gauge IV needle (jugular catheter) or the placement of a chest tube may benefit more from the administration of a local anesthetic (lidocaine). Less severe forms of pain generally respond to less aggressive methods for producing analgesia (e.g., cold compresses), thereby decreasing the potential for drug-related side effects and toxicity.

Duration

The duration for which pain has been present helps to determine the most appropriate analgesic therapy. The injection of a local anesthetic may provide adequate analgesic therapy for an otherwise normal, healthy dog or cat subjected to acute transient pain. Animals that have experienced moderate to severe pain for extended periods, however, generally require extensive physical and targeted analgesic therapy and frequent reevaluation because of the upregulation or adaptation of the sensory nervous system. Both severe and chronic pain can be responsible for the production of "wind-up," central sensitization, and allodynia (see Chapter 2). Animals with chronic pain frequently derive more benefit from a multimodal approach—drugs that act by different pharmacologic mechanisms—than from larger doses of a single drug. Some drug combinations offer the advantage of drug synergism and a reduction in drug-related side effects and toxicity (see Chapter 16). The choice of drug, drug dosage, and therapeutic plan (pharmacologic and/or nonpharmacologic) should be periodically reassessed for maintenance of adequate analgesia and limitation of the possibility for drug toxicity or the development of drug tolerance.

FACTORS THAT DETERMINE DRUG DOSE

Knowledge of the general principles that define drug doses, dosage regimens, and routes of administration is required for optimization of drug therapy. This knowledge includes an understanding of pharmacokinetics (PK) and pharmacodynamics (PD) and the factors that determine them: drug absorption, distribution, metabolism, and elimination (ADME), and the relationship between drug concentration and drug effect. PK-PD data help to determine the selection of drug dosage regimens, the route of drug administration, and the magnitude and duration of drug effect.

Pharmacokinetics

Pharmacokinetic analysis of drug behavior provides a quantitative approach to the determination of drug and drug metabolite disposition in the body. The time course of drug elimination is determined from blood or plasma, although other fluids such as cerebrospinal fluid (CSF), tears, and saliva have been used to determine whether therapeutically relevant drug concentrations have been achieved. Once administered, drugs distribute into theoretic compartments (i.e., central, peripheral) that do not necessarily correspond to any physiologically relevant space (Figure 15-1, *A*). Once in the body, all drugs are subjected to a multitude of metabolic and excretory processes that result in their inactivation and elimination. Drug plasma concentration (Cp) versus time data provide a graphic representation of the disposition of a drug in the body (Figure 15-1, *B* and *C*).

- The rates of drug ADME are used to mathematically determine key pharmacokinetic variables (volume of distribution [V_d], total clearance [CL_T], half-life [$t_{1/2}$]) that are used to describe the disposition of a drug in the plasma and to determine standard drug doses and dosage regimens.
- Plasma is the most commonly assayed fluid for the detection of a drug (parent compound) and its major metabolite(s). The rate of drug elimination from the plasma for most (not all) drugs is dependent on the concentration of drug in the plasma, so-called "first-order elimination" (one exponential term) (see Figure 15-1). In other words, the rate of drug elimination from the plasma decreases as the concentration of drug in the plasma decreases. A plot of the log concentration of the drug versus time produces a straight line. More complex multiple-compartment models are used when the plot of the drug log concentration versus time curve is not linear (Figure 15-2). Nonlinear drug log concentration-time profiles suggest complex drug metabolism or elimination processes.
- Physiologically based pharmacokinetic modeling is a quantitative attempt to model drug disposition in the body in terms of physiologically identifiable compartments to predict tissue concentrations (effect-site) within specific organs (liver, kidney), tissues (skin, muscle), and fluids (blood, CSF, urine).

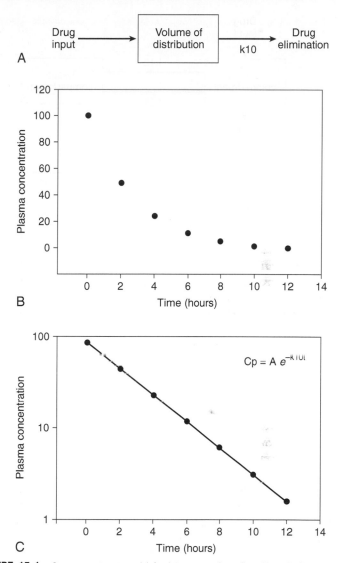

FIGURE 15-1   One-compartment model for intravenous drug disposition. **A,** Pharmacokinetic models are used to describe drug disposition (drug concentration vs. time profiles). **B,** The disposition of many drugs can be described by a first-order or one-compartment mode (e.g., ketoprofen), in which the rate of drug elimination depends on the drug plasma concentration *(Cp)*. **C,** A plot of the log concentration of *Cp* is a straight line.

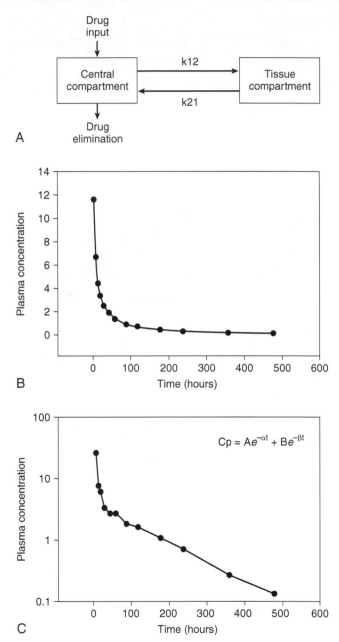

FIGURE 15-2 Two-compartment model of intravenous drug disposition. **A,** Multiple-compartment models are used when **B,** a plot of the plasma concentration *(Cp)* versus time, and **C,** log of *Cp* versus time, curves show curvature. Two-compartment models are common for many drugs (opioids, α_2-agonists).

Factors Affecting Drug Uptake (Absorption) and Distribution

Drugs administered by routes other than the IV route (e.g., transcutaneous, sub-cutaneous [SC], intramuscular [IM], or PO) must be absorbed into the body so that they can be distributed to the effect site. Drugs that are administered intra-venously depend on the injection technique used (bolus, intermittent injection, infusion) and factors that promote (increased tissue blood flow) or limit (high protein binding) drug access to the effect site. The distribution of a drug to the effect site is governed by four factors: *drug binding, ionization, perfusion,* and *diffusion.* Once a drug enters the blood, it is distributed throughout all the tissues of the body based on their total blood flow. The tissues can be cate-gorized based on the percentage of cardiac output they receive into vessel-rich group (e.g., heart, lung, brain, liver, and kidney), muscle group, fat group, and vessel-poor group (e.g., tendons, ligaments, and joint spaces). Skin can be a vessel-rich or vessel-poor group tissue, depending on temperature and prevailing autonomic (sympathetic) tone. Vessel-rich group tissues receive the majority (greatest percentage) of the cardiac output and are expected to receive the greatest amount of drug in the shortest time. A decrease in cardiac output pro-longs the time necessary for drug distribution and, as a result of compensatory homeostatic responses, alters drug distribution. Animals in shock, for example, have a greater percentage of their cardiac output (and therefore any IV admin-istered drug) delivered to vessel-rich group tissues (heart, lungs, and brain).

Absorption

A drug must pass through several different membranes to reach the effect site. The nature of the membrane and total surface area exposed to the drug, drug concentration (concentration gradient,) and temperature *(Fick's law of diffusion)* are key factors that determine the rate of passage of the drug through them and, consequently, the rate at which the drug response occurs. The rate of passage of a drug through a membrane can range from zero (i.e., no movement of drug across the membrane) to the rate of blood flow to the membrane (i.e., the drug moves across the membrane as fast as it is deliv-ered). Biologic membranes are composed of a bimolecular layer of lipid mol-ecules coated on both sides by a protein layer. Hydrophilic drugs have a difficult time crossing lipid (hydrophobic) membranes. Many biologic mem-branes appear to contain pores that permit passage of small molecules. Some biologic membranes have mechanisms that transport specific molecules across the membrane. Examples of various transport mechanisms include dif-fusion, ultrafiltration, and carrier-mediated transport.

Diffusion

Diffusion across biologic membranes is determined as follows.
* Membrane characteristics (anatomic and structural characteristics) and the permeability of different membranes vary considerably. For example,

most capillary membranes are highly permeable, but capillary membranes of the brain are much less permeable to the diffusion of less lipophilic molecules. The blood-brain barrier is not a barrier to the diffusion of lipophilic molecules. *Drugs that have a low molecular weight, are not electrically charged, or are highly lipophilic readily diffuse into the various tissue compartments (e.g., extracellular space, intracellular space, and CSF).*

- Concentration gradient: The drug concentration difference across a biologic membrane determines the direction (high concentration to low concentration) and rate (i.e., the rate of diffusion is directly proportional to the concentration difference) of diffusion.

- The rate of diffusion of a drug across a membrane depends on the membrane permeability characteristics if the membrane is a barrier to drug passage; this is known as *membrane-limited diffusion.*

- Drugs are delivered rapidly to highly perfused (vessel-rich group) tissues and slowly to poorly perfused (fat group) tissues. The rate of diffusion of a drug across a membrane also depends on its rate of drug delivery to the tissue if the drug rapidly passes through the membrane; this is known as *blood-flow rate-limited diffusion.*

- Lipid solubility: *Lipophilicity* is a term used to describe the solubility of the drug in fatty or oily solutions and is measured by determining the oil-water partition coefficient ($P = lipophilicity$). The lipophilicity is determined by the number and type of chemical constituents that are attached to the primary chemical molecule (Table 15-1). The oil-water partition coefficient of a drug is a major determinant of the rate of drug diffusion across biologic (lipid-hydrophobic) membranes.

  - The ED or intrathecal (IT) administration of analgesic drugs provides a good example of the practical importance of lipophilicity. Highly lipid-soluble drugs (e.g., fentanyl and hydromorphone) rapidly diffuse

TABLE 15-1	Relative Lipophilicity of Drugs	
DRUG	**KEY CHEMICAL SUBSTITUENTS**	**RELATIVE P**
Most NSAIDs	COO—, COOH	Poor
Procaine, xylazine	NH_2	
Morphine	OH	Intermediate
Lidocaine, bupivacaine	$NHCH_2 H_5$	
Oxymorphone	$=O$	Good
Butorphanol	CH_2-cyclobutyl	
Fentanyl	CH_3, $N(CH_3)_2$	
Naloxone	$CH_2CH=CH_2$	Excellent

Key: *NSAIDs,* Nonsteroidal anti-inflammatory drugs; *P,* lipophilicity.

out of the ED space or CSF into surrounding tissues, producing a relatively short duration of analgesic effect. Morphine is less lipid soluble than fentanyl or hydromorphone and therefore produces a longer duration of analgesia when administered by the ED or IT route.

- Small molecules (e.g., electrolytes, water, and ethanol) can diffuse through membranes via aqueous pores. Very large molecules do not readily diffuse through membranes.
- Protein binding: Many drugs bind reversibly to macromolecules such as plasma proteins (e.g., albumen, α_1-acid glycoprotein) and tissue proteins (Drug + Protein = Drug-protein complex). A bound drug is not free to diffuse or interact with receptors; some active transport processes remove bound drugs from binding sites. Hypoproteinemia can markedly enhance the effect of drugs that are otherwise highly protein bound (e.g., fentanyl, methadone).
  - Drug protein binding in the blood reduces the concentration of *free drug* available for diffusion across membranes; therefore the rate of diffusion across the membrane is decreased when a drug is extensively protein bound.
  - At equilibrium, the concentration of free drug is the same on both sides of the membrane; however, the concentration of the total drug (bound and unbound) may be different on the two sides of the membrane, depending on how much of it is bound to proteins.
- Differential ionization: Ionized substances do not *diffuse* across biologic membranes. Differences in pH exist across many biologic membranes (e.g., the pH of gastric contents ranges from about 2 to 3, and that of plasma is approximately 7.4). These differences lead to accumulation of drug (i.e., ionized plus nonionized) on that side of the membrane where the drug is more ionized.
  - The partitioning (tissue-to-plasma ratio [$R_{T/P}$] of a drug between two regions of differing pH) is described by the Henderson-Hasselbalch equation:

  $$R_{T/P} = \frac{(1 + \text{antilog } [pK_a - pH_T])}{(1 + \text{antilog } [pK_a - pH_P])}$$

  where pH_T and pH_P are the pH values of a tissue and plasma, respectively, and pK_a is the dissociation constant of the drug. Although the pH of the plasma is maintained within narrow limits, the pH of injured or infected tissues varies considerably, generally becoming more acidic. Basic drugs (opioids) in an acidic environment will ionize, reducing their ability to diffuse.
- Ultrafiltration: Water and relatively small molecules (molecular weight <500 Da) easily pass through membranes (e.g., glomerular filtration) by the hydrostatic pressure of the blood. Drug molecules bound to plasma proteins are not filtered because most proteins (e.g., albumin: 60 kDa) are generally too large to pass through the membrane.

- Carrier-mediated transport: Most membranes possess specialized transport mechanisms that regulate the movement of drugs and other molecules. These transport mechanisms generally use a carrier molecule that may or may not require energy. Carrier-mediated transport is particularly important for the transfer of drugs across the renal tubules, biliary tract, gastrointestinal tract, and blood-brain barrier.
  - Carrier-mediated transport may or may not limit diffusion but often has a maximum value (becomes saturated). Competitive inhibition of transport may occur if a second molecule binds to the carrier, thereby interfering with the transport of the first molecule.
- Active transport is usually coupled to an energy source such as adenosine triphosphate and can transport molecules against an electrochemical gradient (e.g., transport of essential nutrients from the gastrointestinal tract against a concentration gradient). Active transport is usually specific and competitive.
- Specificity: The transport mechanism is usually specific for a single substance or a group of closely related substances (e.g., transport of anions from the blood into the renal tubule in the nephron).
- Competitive: The transport process is competitively inhibited by other molecules also transported by the system.
- Facilitated transport promotes the equilibration of the transported substance—for example, the transport of a molecule in the same direction as its electrochemical gradient (Na^+ flux into renal tubules).

Drug Elimination

Metabolism and excretion determine drug elimination from the body. The liver and kidneys are the two major organs of elimination for most drugs, although the plasma (Hoffman elimination) and lungs are potential sites for the metabolism and elimination of some gases (nitrous oxide [N_2O]) and vapors (inhalant anesthetics). The metabolism of drugs and other foreign substances is a protective mechanism that encompasses bodily responses that decrease drug lipophilicity and increase drug protein binding or ionization. P-gp is a large protein that functions as a transmembrane efflux pump and is deficient in genetically predisposed animals (see the discussion of medical history). It transports chemicals from inside the cell to outside the cell, facilitating excretion. P-gp is normally expressed in the apical border of intestinal epithelial cells, brain capillary endothelial cells, biliary canalicular cells, renal proximal tubular epithelial cells, placenta, and testes. Occasionally, drug metabolism results in the production of drugs that are more potent than the parent (prodrug) compound (e.g., O-desmethyltramadol) or more toxic (metabolites of lidocaine).

Metabolism in the Liver

Liver metabolism depends highly on the cytochrome P-450 enzyme system, a heterogeneous group of highly active and efficient enzymes. Synthesis of some of these enzymes is induced by exposure to drugs such as phenobarbital and rifampin, and some are inhibited by exposure to drugs (chloramphenicol). The capacity of the cytochrome P-450 enzyme to metabolize drugs is very high; therefore most drugs administered at therapeutic concentrations rarely saturate the system. Consequently, the rate of drug metabolism is generally proportional to drug concentration (first order); however, in cases of poisoning, the enzyme system may saturate and the rate of metabolism is slowed.

- Drugs absorbed from the gastrointestinal tract pass through the liver before reaching the systemic circulation. If the drug is rapidly and extensively metabolized by the liver it is considered to undergo *first-pass metabolism* (Figure 15-3) with only a small fraction of the parent drug reaching the systemic circulation (e.g., morphine and lidocaine). First-pass metabolism (elimination) is the reason many drugs, particularly opioids, are relatively ineffective when administered orally to dogs and cats.
- Major metabolic pathways in mammals include the following:
  - Phase 1 pathways: Oxidation, reduction, hydrolysis (Esterases are also found in plasma). Cytochrome P-450 3A (CYP3A) is the major phase 1 drug-metabolizing enzyme family in mammals. Genetic studies have

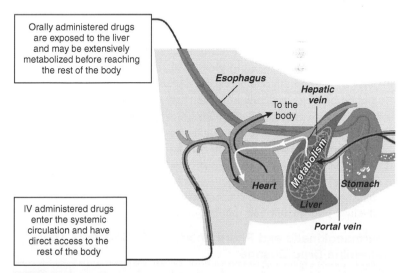

Orally administered drugs are exposed to the liver and may be extensively metabolized before reaching the rest of the body

Esophagus

Hepatic vein

To the body

Metabolism

Heart

Stomach

Liver

Portal vein

IV administered drugs enter the systemic circulation and have direct access to the rest of the body

FIGURE 15-3　First-pass elimination. The effects of many drugs are greatly reduced (e.g., oral opioids) by metabolism in the liver or by biliary excretion.

documented *mdr* gene deletion and decreased expression of P-gp in 10 breeds of dogs including Collies, Australian sheepdogs, Shetland sheepdogs and Old English sheepdogs. Cytochrome P-450 3A and P-gp are expressed at high levels in the villus tip of enterocytes in the gastrointestinal tract. P-gp is also found in renal tubular cells, bile canalicular cells, and brain capillary endothelial cells (blood-brain barrier), where it limits absorption or facilitates the excretion of many drugs including antihistamines (H_1 and H_2 antagonists), phenothiazines, corticosteroids, and some opioids (e.g., butorphanol, morphine).

- Phase 2 pathways: Conjugation (e.g., reaction of a drug or phase 1 metabolite with glucuronic acid). Differences in drug metabolism between species are frequently a result of the absence of a particular enzyme system in one species versus another; for example, in cats the ability to conjugate most substances with glucuronic acid is deficient.
- Spontaneous decomposition occurs in the plasma at physiologic pH and near-normal temperature by means of a base-catalyzed reaction (Hoffman elimination). In this reaction, protons (H^+) are cleaved from the α-carbon atom of the molecule, resulting in subsequent metabolism and inactive by-products (e.g., etomidate and atracurium).

Excretion of Drugs and Drug Metabolites

Excretion of drugs and drug metabolites involves the kidneys (urine), biliary mechanisms (bile), and other routes (tears, sweat, saliva, feces).

Renal Excretion. Renal excretion is important for the *elimination* of drugs and their metabolites (e.g., ketamine, fentanyl). It involves three mechanisms: glomerular filtration, tubular secretion, and passive reabsorption.

- *Glomerular filtration* of unbound drug: Highly bound drugs such as the NSAIDs are not excreted by glomerular filtration.
- *Tubular secretion* of anions (e.g., NSAIDs, glucuronic acid conjugates) and cations (e.g., cimetidine) occurs with many drugs.
- *Passive reabsorption* of lipophilic drugs: The pH of urine can have profound effects on the extent of tubular reabsorption.

Biliary Excretion. Biliary excretion is an active process usually restricted to drugs or metabolites above a species-specific molecular size; drug conjugates are frequently secreted in the bile.

Enterohepatic cycling involves the intestinal reabsorption of a drug excreted by the liver into the bile and the intestine.

Pharmacokinetic and Pharmacodynamic Concepts That Determine Drug Dosage

Pharmacodynamic analysis describes the relationship between drug *Cp* and drug effect. Pharmacologic effects require that drug molecules be bound to constituents of cells or tissues to produce an effect. Most drugs exert their effects by combining with regulatory proteins, including enzymes (NSAIDs), carrier molecules, ion channels (local anesthetics), and receptors (opioids, α_2-agonists). The term *receptor* is commonly used to describe any macromolecule (generally a protein) that the drug combines with to produce its effects. The drug concentration at the receptor site is assumed to be related to the concentration of drug in blood or plasma. The drug concentration at the receptor site, however, is generally not identical to its concentration in blood because of a number of factors, including drug binding to plasma and tissue proteins, ion trapping of the drug, and slow passage of the drug through membranes. Equilibration of drug between the plasma and the receptor site generally produces a predictable relationship between Cp and effect (dose-effect relationship). The clinical goal is to develop and administer a therapeutic regimen that establishes and maintains an effective drug Cp and effect for as long as required.

Pharmacokinetic variables help determine drug disposition and the duration of drug action in the body. The basic variables include V_d, clearance (usually considered as total clearance: CL_T), and half-life ($t_{1/2}$). These data are used to determine loading dose, maintenance dose, and dosage interval. Additional variables such as mean resonance time (MRT) and bioavailability are used to adjust and refine initial calculations.

Receptor Pharmacology

In the body there are many different types of drug receptors that when occupied by drugs are capable of producing cellular effects, including analgesia (Table 15-2). The pharmacologic response that follows drug (ligand) occupation of receptors is proportional to the number or fraction of receptors occupied.

TABLE 15-2	Transmitters and Receptors
TRANSMITTERS	**RECEPTOR SUBTYPES**
Analgesic Transmitters	
Opioid	μ, κ, δ
α_2	α_{2A}, α_{2B}, α_{2D}
Cannabinoid	CB_1, CB_2
Algesic Transmitters	
Prostaglandin	EP_1 to EP_4
Histamine	H_1
Calcium	N and L type
Substance P	NK_1
NMDA	NR_1
AMPA	$iGluR_1$ to $iGluR_3$
Kainate	KA_1, KA_2, $GluR_5$ to $GluR_7$

Key: *AMPA*, α-Amino-3-hydroxy-5-methyl-4-isoxazolepropionic acid; *NMDA*, N-methyl-D-aspartate.

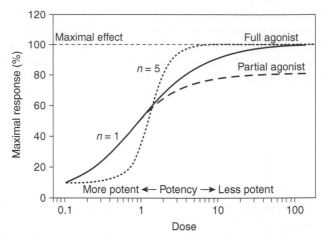

FIGURE 15-4 The dose-response curve relates plasma concentration *(Cp)* to the effect produced. Drugs that act at receptor sites (e.g., opioids, α_2-agonists) and produce the maximum effect possible are called *full agonists* (e.g., morphine, hydromorphone, and fentanyl). *Partial agonists* produce less than the maximal effect (e.g., buprenorphine). Drugs that produce a maximal effect at lower *Cp* or doses are more potent than drugs that require higher *Cp*. The shape (slope) of the *Cp*-effect curve *(n)* is important for estimating the therapeutic range of the drug.

Agonist. An agonist is a drug that binds to and activates a receptor and produces a biologic effect (Figure 15-4). Drugs that produce the maximal response possible (dose-response curve) are called *full agonists* (i.e., the intrinsic activity is 1).

Agonist-Antagonist. An agonist-antagonist is a drug that exhibits some properties of an agonist (a substance that fully activates the receptor) and some properties of an antagonist (a substance displaces [competitive antagonism] an agonist at that receptor), thereby reversing the effect of the agonist. Antagonistic effects are usually dose dependent.

Antagonist. An antagonist is a drug that binds to a receptor and produces no biologic effect. Drug antagonists block, interfere with, or reverse the effects of agonists. A pure antagonist is assumed to produce no agonistic effects and has an intrinsic activity of zero.

- Competitive receptor antagonists compete for the receptor site. Their effects are said to be *surmountable* or *reversible* because they can be overcome by a higher dose of the agonist. Competitive antagonists shift the dose-effect curve to the right (e.g., most opioid antagonists and α_2-antagonists [opioid: naloxone, naltrexone; α_2-antagonists: tolazoline, yohimbine, atipamezole]).
- Noncompetitive receptor antagonists produce an effect that cannot be overcome by increasing concentrations of the agonist (e.g., buprenorphine

acts as a noncompetitive antagonist to other opioids). Effects of noncompetitive receptor antagonists are irreversible until the drug is completely eliminated.

Partial Agonist. A partial agonist is a drug that interacts with a receptor but produces less than the maximal effect (see Figure 15-4). A partial agonist produces less than full agonist effects (i.e., intrinsic activity is between 0.0 and 1.0) and is by definition less efficacious than a full agonist. Partial agonists may also act as antagonists (e.g., buprenorphine).

Intrinsic Activity (Efficacy). The term *intrinsic activity* refers to the maximal possible effect that can be produced by a drug. Intrinsic activity is determined by the drug-receptor relationship for a drug that acts on receptors. Receptor pharmacology assumes that the effect of a drug is proportional to the number of receptors occupied, implying that a greater effect is produced by occupation of more receptors and that a maximal effect can be produced without occupation of all the receptors of the drug. Low-efficacy opioids (e.g., butorphanol) or partial agonists (e.g., buprenorphine) must by definition occupy more receptors to produce a given effect than higher-efficacy opioids (e.g., fentanyl) because of their lower intrinsic activity. Intrinsic efficacy for opioids is as follows: fentanyl > hydromorphone > morphine > buprenorphine > butorphanol > nalbuphine.

Potency. Potency is the intensity of effect produced for a given drug dose. Two drugs can be equally efficacious (i.e., produce the same maximal response) but vary in potency (dose required to produce the response). The drug that requires the larger dose to produce the desired effect is said to be less potent.

Racemic Mixtures. Some drug molecules have two or more three-dimensional structures. Drugs that have the same chemical formula but two different structures are termed *isomers* of each other. Isomers that have different structures as a result of the interchange of any two groups around a central carbon atom are termed *enantiomorphs*. A drug that has an asymmetric carbon atom (asymmetric center is termed a *center of chirality*) and exists as an equimolar mixture of optical (mirror image) isomers is called a *racemic mixture*. The two components of racemic mixtures may have similar or different receptor effects. Medetomidine is a racemic mixture of dexmedetomidine and levomedetomidine. Levomedetomidine is believed to be pharmacologically inactive but may alter the PK (elimination) of dexmedetomidine.

Pharmacodynamic Models

The most commonly used and simplest model for describing the dose-effect relationship over a range of drug concentrations is derived from the Hill equation, which relates the drug effect to the maximum drug effect (E_{max}), Cp, and the drug concentration required to produce 50% of the maximum effect (EC_{50}):

$$E = \frac{E_{max} \times Cp}{EC_{50} + Cp}$$

This equation usually produces a hyperbolic or sigmoid drug Cp-effect curve, which permits the estimation of drug effects at differing drug doses and provides insight into the PD of the drug (Figure 15-5).

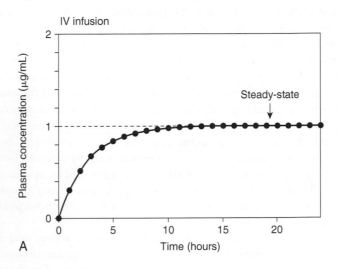

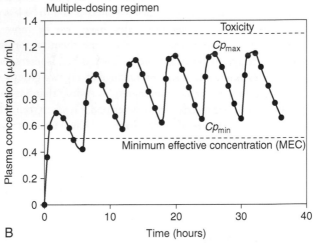

FIGURE 15-5 **A,** Drugs administered intravenously by constant rate infusion (CRI) reach a steady-state value that can be predicted by their half-lives (i.e., 90% of steady state in 3.3 half-lives). **B,** The plasma concentration (Cp) varies between a Cp_{max} and Cp_{min} when drugs are administered at regular intervals (hours). Fluctuations between Cp_{max} and Cp_{min} at steady state increase as the dosage interval increases and can be predicted by the half-life of the drug. The Cp_{max} is equal to two times the Cp_{min} when the dosage interval is equal to the half-life of the drug.

Key Pharmacokinetic Variables

Volume of Distribution. The V_d is the apparent volume within which the drug is distributed. The word *apparent* is used because some drugs are bound to tissues, resulting in V_d much larger than the total volume of body water in which they are distributed. For example, if a 10-mg dose of a drug is injected into the body and the plasma concentration (Cp) is 0.002 mg/mL, then the V_d would be 5000 mL (5 L: 10 mg/0.002 mg/mL). The V_d of morphine is 6.1 L/kg in the dog and 1.35 L/kg in the cat. The V_d of lidocaine is 4.9 L/kg in the dog and 3.6 L/kg in the cat. These examples emphasize species differences and the much smaller V_d of morphine in the cat compared with that in the dog. The V_d calculated during the elimination phase is described by the relationship between the amount of drug injected into the body and the plasma concentration (Cp) of the drug before elimination begins or at time 0 (Cp_0):

$$V_d = \frac{\text{Amount injected into body}}{Cp_0}$$

The V_d calculated at steady-state equilibrium (V_{dss}) defines the extent of drug dilution at the peak of drug distribution and is a more accurate assessment of drug dilution in the body. The V_{dss} is calculated as follows:

$$V_{dss} = \frac{\text{Dose}}{AUC}$$

where AUC is area under the curve.

- Units of V_d are volume (e.g., milliliter or liter) or volume per unit of bw (e.g., milliliter per kilogram of bw).
- A large V_d implies extensive distribution of the drug to tissues, whereas a small V_d implies more limited distribution.
- The *mean resonance time* is a term used to describe the average time that the drug stays in the body or the time it takes for 63.2% of a drug injected into the body to be eliminated. The MRT can be used to calculate V_{dss}:

$$V_{dss} = \frac{\text{Dose}}{AUC \times MRT}$$

Clearance. The total clearance (CL_T) of drug from plasma is the volume of biologic fluid (blood, plasma) that is completely freed (cleared) of drug by all routes of elimination. Units for clearance are flow (e.g., milliliters per minute) or flow per unit of bw (e.g., milliliters per minute per kilogram bw). These units (milliliters per minute per kilogram) emphasize that clearance is not the amount of drug being removed from the body but the amount of biologic fluid "cleared" of drug. Clearance can be calculated as the rate of elimination of the drug by all routes divided by the Cp of the drug:

$$CL_T = \frac{\text{Rate of elimination}}{C_p}$$

- The lower limit for clearance by an organ of elimination is zero. The upper limit is the plasma flow to the organ. Individual organ clearances can be added together for the total body clearance:

$$CL_T = CL_H + CL_R + CL_{Other}$$

where CL_T is the total clearance, CL_H is the hepatic clearance, CL_R is the renal clearance, and CL_{Other} represents the sum of all other clearance processes.

- Total clearance (CL_T) is an indicator of organ function and can be used to predict the average concentration or steady-state concentration of drug in the blood or plasma. For example, if the CL_T is 0.1 mL/min/kg and the rate of drug administration is 0.1 μg/kg/min, then the average drug concentration of the plasma is 1.0 μg/mL (0.1 μg/min/kg ÷ 0.1 mL/min/kg).

- The total clearance of a drug by all the elimination processes in the body is calculated by dividing the dose administered by the total area under the Cp time curve (AUC) from the time of administration until the drug concentration in the plasma can no longer be measured ($CL_T =$ Dose/AUC). In other words, if the target steady-state Cp and clearance for a drug are known, then the dose rate can be calculated: Dose rate $= Cp \times CL_T$. For example, if the target Cp is 80 μg/mL and the clearance is 0.125 mL/min/kg, then the dose rate will be 10 μg/min/kg (80 μg/mL × 0.125 mL/min/kg) or 3.6 mg/kg every 6 hours (10 μg/min/kg × 60 min = 0.6 mg/kg × 6 hr = 3.6 mg/kg every 6 hours [q 6 hr]).

Half-Life. The elimination half-life ($t_{1/2}$) is the time required for the Cp of the drug to decrease to 50% of an earlier value (Box 15-2). Half-life is expressed in units of time (minutes, hours).

- The half-life of a drug can also be used to determine the time required for an infused drug to reach steady state (Box 15-3; see Figure 15-5, *A*).

BOX 15-2 **Estimated Time for Drug Removal**

1 Half-life: 50% eliminated
2 Half-lives: 75% eliminated
3 Half-lives: 87.5% eliminated
3.3 Half-lives: 90% eliminated
4 Half-lives: 93.75% eliminated
5 Half-lives: 97% eliminated

BOX 15-3 **Estimated Time Required to Reach Steady State**

1 Half-life: 50% of steady state
2 Half-lives: 75% of steady state
3 Half-lives: 87.5% of steady state
3.3 Half-lives: 90% of steady state

- The $t_{1/2}$, total clearance, and V_d are related to one another by the following equation:

$$t_{1/2} = \frac{0.693 \times V_d}{CL_T}$$

- Changes in total clearance or V_d alter the $t_{1/2}$. For example, reduced renal clearance resulting from renal or liver disease will decrease total clearance and increase $t_{1/2}$.

Bioavailability

The term *bioavailability (F)* indicates the amount of drug that reaches the systemic circulation after administration by a non-IV route. For example, the bioavailability of many opioids is relatively low in dogs after PO administration because of metabolism by the liver (first-pass effect) before the drug reaches the systemic circulation. Most opioids and α_2-agonists are buccally absorbed, but their individual bioavailabilities vary considerably. Buprenorphine is almost 100% absorbed across the buccal membranes of cats but is only 50% absorbed in dogs.

Bioequivalence

Bioequivalence is a term that is used when two drugs are compared. Two drugs are considered to be bioequivalent when the C*p* versus time profiles and pharmacologic, therapeutic, and toxic effects are the same after administration of equal doses by the same route. Although the peak and trough C*p*s of two drugs may not necessarily be exactly the same, they are considered to be bioequivalent when the maximum and minimum C*p*s and the time required to produce a predetermined response are the same.

Calculation of Dosage Regimens

The ability to estimate and calculate drug dosage regimens is critical to producing a desired therapeutic effect and preventing adverse drug effects.

Maintenance Dose

The maintenance dose is the dose administered to maintain therapeutic drug concentrations (see Figure 15-5, *B*). The maintenance dose (MD) is equal to the desired C*p* times the total body clearance.

$$MD = Cp \times CL_T$$

- For example, calculate the maintenance dose for a drug with a V_d of 2000 mL/kg and clearance of 20 mL/min/kg to be administered to a 10-kg dog to achieve a steady-state plasma drug concentration of 2 μg/mL.

$$\text{MD} = 2\,\mu g/mL \times 20\,mL/min/kg$$
$$\text{MD} = 40\,\mu g/min/kg$$
$$\text{MD} = 40\,\mu g/min \times 10\,kg = 400\,\mu g/min$$
$$\text{or } (60\,min \times 6\,hr \times 40\,\mu g/min/kg)\ 14.4\,mg\ q\ 6\ hr$$

- The time required to reach a steady-state drug concentration is determined by the $t_{1/2}$ of the drug (50% of final steady-state drug concentration is achieved in one half-life, 75% in two half-lives, 87.5% in three half-lives, 90% in 3.3 half-lives) (see Box 15-2). Delay in achieving desired plasma drug concentrations may be critical for certain drugs (e.g., transcutaneous fentanyl patch, buprenorphine).

Loading Dose

The loading dose (LD) is administered at the start of a dosage regimen to achieve effective Cp rapidly. The LD is equal to the desired or target Cp multiplied by the V_d:

$$\text{LD} = Cp \times V_d$$

For example, calculate the LD required to achieve a Cp of 2 µg/mL for a drug with a V_d of 2000 mL/kg bw and clearance of 20 mL/min/kg bw to be administered to a 10-kg dog:

$$\text{LD} = 2\,\mu g/mL \times 2000\,mL/kg$$
$$\text{LD} = 4000\,\mu g/kg\ bw \times 10\,kg$$
$$\text{LD} = 40,000\,\mu g/1000\,\mu g = 40\,mg$$

NOTE: The value of the clearance term was provided but was not needed for this calculation.

Dosing Interval

The dosing interval is the period between doses. An infinitely small dosing interval is a constant rate infusion (CRI). The time taken to achieve 90% of the final steady-state Cp during CRI is 3.3 half-lives. A drug with a 2.5-hour half-life would take approximately 8.25 hours to reach 90% of its final steady-state Cp if administered by CRI (see Figure 15-5, B). Fluctuations between the maximum plasma concentration (Cp_{max}) and minimum plasma concentration (Cp_{min}) at steady state increase as the dosage interval increases. $Cp_{max} = 2 \times Cp_{min}$ when the dosage interval equals the half-life.

For example, calculate the maximum dosage interval for a drug with a V_d of 2000 mL/kg and a clearance of 20 mL/min/kg to achieve a Cp_{max} no more than twice Cp_{min}:

$$\text{Dosing interval} = t_{1/2} = 0.693 \times V_d / CL_T$$
$$\text{Dosing interval} = 0.693 \times (2000\,mL/kg\ bw) / (20\,mL/min/kg)$$
$$\text{Dosing interval} = 69.3\,min$$

Pharmacokinetic-Pharmacodynamic Models

Pharmacokinetic-pharmacodynamic models are valuable for defining the therapeutic index and lethal dose of a drug (Figure 15-6).

Median Effective Dose

The median effective dose (ED_{50}) is the dose of drug required to produce a predetermined specified effect in 50% of treated animals.

Median Lethal Dose

The median lethal dose (LD_{50}) is the dose of drug required to cause death in 50% of treated animals.

Therapeutic Index

The therapeutic index (TI) is a measure of the margin of safety of a drug and is determined by dividing the LD_{50} by the ED_{50}:

$$TI = \frac{LD_{50}}{ED_{50}}$$

The TI may vary depending on the predetermined pharmacologic end-point desired (e.g., analgesia versus sedation). In many instances, the ED_{50} increases while the LD_{50} stays the same, resulting in a decrease in the TI.

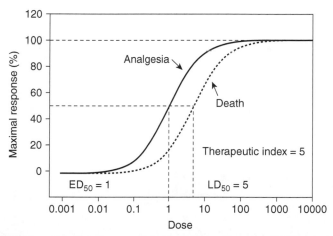

FIGURE 15-6   The therapeutic index is determined by dividing the median lethal dose (LD_{50}) by the median effective dose (ED_{50}) and provides a measure of the margin of safety for that drug.

ROUTES OF DRUG ADMINISTRATION

Choosing the appropriate route for drug administration can be the deciding factor in producing adequate analgesia, obtaining owner compliance, and avoiding drug-related side effects or toxicities (Figure 15-7). Dogs or cats that are sick or that demonstrate signs of CNS depression, cardiovascular or respiratory compromise, or chronic renal disease may not adequately absorb, distribute, or eliminate many medications. The route of drug administration determines peak plasma drug concentration and may be more important than the drug administered (Box 15-4 and Figure 15-8).

Oral

Oral (PO) administration of drugs is preferred for the treatment of most types of chronic and many types of acute pain. Occasionally nasogastric (NG), gastrostomy, and jejunostomy routes of drug administration are considered in animals that cannot take PO drugs. These last routes are subject to the same considerations as drugs administered orally. Analgesic drugs (NSAIDs) can be administered orally for preemptive or preventative analgesia or administered in conjunction with injectable analgesics to produce additive or synergistic effects. PO administration of drugs can be accomplished in the hospital or at home with minimal to no supervision. Drug effects may require several hours to become apparent and are relatively

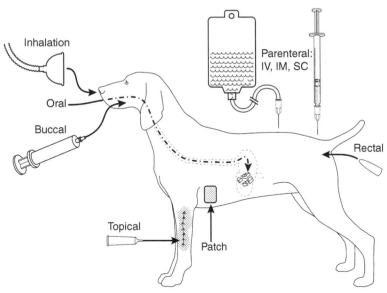

FIGURE 15-7 Routes of drug administration. Inhalation, buccal (sublingual), oral (PO), intravenous *(IV)*, intramuscular *(IM)*, subcutaneous *(SC)*, topical (cream, patch), and rectal.

BOX 15-4	Routes of Analgesic Drug Administration
ROUTE	**ONSET OF ACTION**
Epidural or subarachnoid	5-10 min
Intra-articular	3-5 min
Intramuscular	10-20 min
Intranasal or inhalational	1-3 min
Intraperitoneal	3-5 min
Intravenous or intraosseous	30-60 sec
Oral	30-90 min
Rectal	5-30 min
Subcutaneous	15-30 min
Sublingual, buccal, or transmucosal	3-5 min (can be variable)
Topical	Variable (minutes to hours)
Transcutaneous or topical	Variable (minutes to hours)
Transdermal	Variable (minutes to hours)

prolonged after PO administration. Drug side effects, other than nausea and vomiting, especially after the first dose, are comparatively uncommon. Orally administered drugs are subject to first-pass metabolism in the liver, which limits their bioavailability and clinical efficacy (see Figure 15-4). Diet, eating behavior, drug formulation, and concurrent diseases can produce prolonged absorption from the gastrointestinal tract and erratic absorption patterns, leading to an inadequate analgesic response. Finally, the owner must comply with administration schedules for therapy to be effective.

Intravenous

Intravenous (IV) drug administration provides the most rapid, immediate, and predictable effects. Drugs can be administered intravenously as a bolus, slow injection, or CRI. After IV administration, the animal must be closely monitored for immediate or delayed adverse drug effects. Drug plasma concentrations are the highest immediately after IV drug administration, increasing the potential for drug-related side effects and toxicity. Sites of venous access in dogs or cats receiving CRI should be evaluated for signs of extravasation, thrombophlebitis, and generalized inflammation.

Intramuscular and Subcutaneous

Drug administration via the intramuscular (IM) and subcutaneous (SC) routes is easily performed and provides relatively rapid (5 to 20 minutes) onset of effect and a longer duration of effects (see Figure 18-8, A). SC drug administration is relatively painless if small needles are used. Analgesic drugs can be administered less frequently than required for IV injections, and plasma concentrations are not as high, reducing the potential for side effects

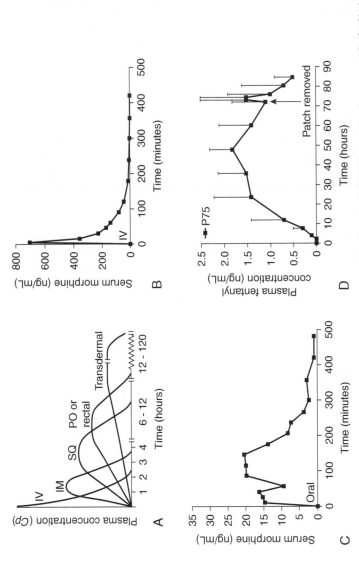

FIGURE 15-8 **A,** The plasma concentration (*Cp*) time curve for a drug is dependent on the route of administration. **B,** The *Cp* for morphine decreases rapidly after IV administration in dogs. **C,** Morphine *Cp* increases more gradually and is sustained for a longer period after oral administration. **D,** The *Cp* of fentanyl (fentanyl patch; 75 μg/hr) in dogs increases slowly before reaching a steady-state concentration (up to 24 hours). (From Dohoo SE, Tasker RAR: Pharmacokinetics of oral morphine sulfate in dogs: A comparison of sustained release and conventional formulations. Can J Vet Res, 1997; 61:251-255; Egger CM, Duke T, Archer J, Cribb PH: Comparison of plasma fentanyl concentrations by using three transdermal fentanyl patch sizes in dogs. Vet Surg, 1998; 27:159-166.)

and drug-related toxicity. The IM administration of drugs can be painful, particularly when larger volumes are administered or if the drug pH and other formulation excipients are irritating. Drug absorption is occasionally erratic after IM or SC drug administration, producing more variable drug effects than after IV administration. Erratic drug absorption is more likely to occur in dogs and cats with poor peripheral circulation (dehydration, hypovolemia, hypothermia).

Epidural and Intrathecal

Various drug combinations (e.g., opioids and local anesthetics) are administered epidurally (ED) or intrathecally (IT) in dogs and cats. Although the ED route was originally used only for administration of local anesthetics (lidocaine) and opioids (morphine), recent clinical trials have investigated the analgesic effects of ED administration of NSAIDs (e.g., ketoprofen), dissociative anesthetics (e.g., ketamine), and α_2-agonists (e.g., xylazine, medetomidine, dexmedetomidine). ED drug administration produces good to excellent analgesia for extended periods (>10 hours) with relatively small drug doses, thereby limiting the potential for side effects and toxicity. The ED administration of opioids, α_2-agonists, and NSAIDs also avoids the loss of motor control associated with larger doses of local anesthetic drugs. Epidurally administered drugs should be sterile and preservative free and ideally should have relatively poor lipid solubility to limit absorption and prolong effects. The ED or IT administration of drugs must be performed by appropriately trained and skilled personnel and requires sterile technique.

Topical

Analgesic drugs are available for both topical (TOP) and transdermal (TD) administration. Drugs administered by these routes are generally if not always formulated with penetration enhancers to improve drug bioavailability (Table 15-3). Alternative methods for improving drug skin penetration include liposomes, ultrasound, and electric current. TOP and TD drug absorption and kinetics are dependent on multiple factors (Box 15-5). The word *topical* is defined as pertaining to a specific area. The therapeutic effect of TOP drugs extends only to the local area (e.g., cornea, superficial skin lesion) and should produce no or minimal systemic effects. A eutectic mixture of local anesthetics (lidocaine-prilocaine [EMLA] cream), multiple concentrations of lidocaine cream (4% or 5% lidocaine), and a 5% lidocaine patch (Lidoderm) are available.

Transdermal

Transdermally (TD) delivered drugs are applied to the skin, but the effects are produced systemically, not just at the site of drug administration. The drug is absorbed into the blood, bypassing liver metabolism (first-pass

TABLE 15-3	Penetration Enhancers for Topical or Transdermal Drug Delivery

Chemical

- Solvents: water, alcohols, alkyl methyl sulfoxides (dimethyl sulfoxide), dimethyl acetamide, dimethyl formamide, and others
- Azones
- Terpenes, terpenoids and essential oils
- Fatty acids and esters
- Surfactants
- Bile salts
- Miscellaneous chemicals
- Prodrug approach

Physical

- Abrasion
- Electroporation
- Iontophoresis
- Laser radiation
- Sonophoresis, phonophoresis
- Microneedle devices
- Needleless injection
- Magnetophoresis

BOX 15-5	Factors Affecting Drug Penetration of Skin

- Site of application
- Thickness and integrity of the stratum corneum epidermidis
- Size of the molecule
- Permeability of the membrane of the transdermal drug delivery system
- State of skin hydration
- pH of the drug
- Drug metabolism by skin flora
- Lipid solubility
- Depot of drug in skin
- Alteration of blood flow in the skin by additives and body temperature

elimination), and effects persist for as long as the patch contains drug and remains in contact with the skin. TD drug delivery is an excellent method for providing preemptive, preventative or "background" analgesia before major surgery and as primary or adjunct analgesic after a major traumatic event. Fentanyl has been formulated for nasal, intranasal (ITN), transmucosal (TM), buccal (BUC), sublingual (SL), PO, inhaled, and TD drug delivery, although the IV and TD routes are the most frequently employed in veterinary medicine. The high potency, lipophilicity, low molecular weight, and excellent skin flux properties (1000 times that of morphine) of fentanyl

(Duragesic, Recuvyra) make it ideal for TD administration. TOP fentanyl (Recuvyra) is a TD solution approved for use in dogs that is rapidly absorbed through the skin. The recommended dose is 2.6 mg fentanyl per kilogram bw (i.e., 0.052 mL/kg, 50 mg/mL), applied topically to the dorsal scapular area 2 to 4 hours before surgery. The manufacturers state that "it is imperative that Recuvyra is only applied to the dorsal scapular area, as absorption has been shown to vary between different locations on the skin." TD absorption is enhanced by addition of the penetration enhancer octyl salicylate. Buprenorphine patches (Butrans) are also available for TD drug delivery, but clinical experience in dogs and cats suggests that they are less efficacious than fentanyl patches. The potential for drug-related side effects and toxicity is low because of slow drug absorption and comparatively lower drug plasma concentrations compared with the IV and IM routes of administration. Slow drug absorption also prolongs the time to produce analgesia, making it difficult to predict drug effects and titrate drug dosage (see Figure 15-8, A). Skin irritation may develop in some dogs and cats.

Sublingual, Buccal, and Transmucosal

Like TD drug delivery, the sublingual (SL), buccal (BUC), and transmucosal (TM) routes of drug delivery depend on drug absorption from the body surface, in this case the mucous membranes. Mucous membrane absorption also includes drug absorption from the conjunctiva, nasal mucosa, and vagina and rectal walls, although these routes are generally discussed individually. The absorbed drug is not subjected to first-pass liver metabolism. Although potentially having the same advantages as TD drug delivery, the SL and BUC routes of drug administration require animal cooperation. The influence of saliva on drug absorption and the unfamiliar taste produced by many drugs can be problematic. Regardless, the PO administration of various opioid-containing syrups (e.g., codeine, morphine, and buprenorphine) and dextromethorphan results in absorption of drug through the mucous membranes, producing analgesic effects that can last for several hours. The BUC absorption of opioids depends on pH and may be limited by an acidic environment. Buprenorphine, a weak base ($pK_a = 8.24$), demonstrates close to 100% bioavailability in cats and up to 50% bioavailability in dogs. Experimental and clinical studies examining analgesic efficacy in cats suggest comparable or superior analgesic efficacy to other opioids in cats but variable effects in dogs. Meloxicam is available as a TM PO spray (Oro-CAM) for the control of pain and inflammation associated with osteoarthritis in dogs. Ethanol is added as a penetration enhancer.

Intranasal or Inhalational

Intranasal (ITN) and inhalational (INH) drug delivery are similar to SL and BUC administration and require minimal cooperation. Drug absorption is rapid, producing almost immediate drug effects. Few analgesic drugs other than butorphanol and buprenorphine have been investigated for ITN administration. This route of drug administration should be considered for administering opioids when venous access in limited. Inhalation of analgesic drugs has not been adequately evaluated in dogs or cats, although drugs have been administered through an endotracheal tube, when appropriate, during emergencies or if no established IV route is available.

Intra-articular

Intra-articular (IA) administration of a drug has the potential for producing immediate local and systemic effects. The increased vascularity and surface area of a properly placed injection facilitate drug effects. The administration of local anesthetics, corticosteroids, and opioids has been particularly successful in this regard.

Intrathoracic, Intraperitoneal, Intravesical

The intrathoracic (ITr), intraperitoneal (IP), and intravesical (IVC, bladder) routes provide an alternative to more conventional methods for drug administration. The onset of drug effects is relatively rapid because of the large surface area for drug absorption but ultimately dependent on the drug's physical and chemical properties (e.g., lipid solubility, pH). These routes are popular in laboratory animals but not commonly employed in dogs and cats. They can be useful when venous access is compromised or of limited availability or when an analgesic drug, generally a local anesthetic, is administered to limit or prevent pain initiated by thoracic, abdominal, or bladder surgery and/or inflammation.

Rectal

The rectal (PR) route of administration of drugs to dogs and cats is occasionally considered but rarely used. Although rectal (intravesicular) administration of drugs can be performed, the bioavailability and drug absorption are highly variable. Furthermore, drugs administered rectally are generally absorbed slowly, and drug absorption can be disrupted by fecal material, defecation, or straining to defecate.

SUGGESTED READING

Andaluz A, Moll X, Ventura R, et al.: Plasma buprenorphine concentrations after the application of a 70 µg/hr transdermal patch in dogs. Preliminary report. J Vet Pharmacol Ther, 2009; 32:503–505.

Baheti SR, Wadher KJ, Umekar MJ: A recent approach towards transdermal drug delivery by physical and chemical techniques. Internationale Pharmaceutica Sciencia, 2011; 1:42–53.

Batrakova EV, Gendelman HE, Kabanov AV: Cell-mediated drugs delivery. Expert Opin Drug Deliv, 2011; 8:414–433.

Beckman BW: Pathophysiology and management of surgical and chronic oral pain in dogs and cats. J Vet Dent, 2006; 23:50–60.

Becker DE: Adverse drug interactions. Anesth Prog, 2011; 58:31–41.

Benson HAE: Transdermal drug delivery: Penetration enhancement techniques. Curr Drug Deliv, 2005; 2:23–33.

Bushnell TG, Justins DM: Choosing the right analgesic. Drugs, 1993; 46:394–408.

Cascorbi I: Drug interactions: Principles, examples and clinical consequences. Dtsch Arztebi Int, 2012; 109:546–556.

Challa R, Ahuja A, Ali J, et al.: Cyclodextrins in drug delivery: An updated review. AAPS Pharm Sci Tech, 2005; 6:E329–E357. Retrieved from www.aapspharmscitech.org.

Clark TP: The clinical pharmacology of cyclooxygenase-2-selective and dual inhibitors. Vet Clin North Am Small Anim Pract, 2006; 36:1061–1085.

Coelho JF, Ferreira-Patricia Alves PC: Drug delivery systems: Advanced technologies potentially applicable in personalized treatments. EPMA J, 2010; 1:164–209.

Committee on Drugs: Alternative routes of drug administration: Advantages and disadvantages. Pediatrics, 1997; 100:143–152.

Dowling P: Pharmacogenetics: It's not just about ivermectin in collies. Can Vet J, 2006; 47:1165–1168.

Giuliano EA: Nonsteroidal anti-inflammatory drugs in veterinary ophthalmology. Vet Clin North Am Small Anim Pract, 2004; 34:707–723.

Hare JE, Niemuller CA, Petrick DM: Target animal safety study of meloxicam administered via transdermal oral spray (Promist technology) for 6 months in dogs. J Vet Pharmacol Ther, 2012; Sept 25:1–5.

Henrotin Y, Sanchez C, Balligand M: Pharmaceutical and nutraceutical management of canine osteoarthritis: Present and future perspectives. Vet J, 2005; 170:113–123.

Hopfensperger MJ, Messenger KM, Papich MG, Sherman BL: The use of oral transmucosal detomidine hydrochloride gel to facilitate handling in dogs. J Vet Behav, 2013; 8:114–123.

Jorge LL, Feres CC, Teles VEP: Topical preparations for pain relief: Efficacy and patient adherence. J Pain Res, 2011; 4:11–24.

Ko JCH, Mawell LK, Abbo LA, et al.: Pharmacokinetics of lidocaine following the application of 5% lidocaine patches to cats. J Vet Pharmacol Ther, 2008; 31:359–367.

KuKanich B, Clark TP: The history and pharmacology of fentanyl: Relevance to a novel, long-acting transdermal fentanyl solution newly approved for use in dogs. J Vet Pharmacol Ther, 2012; 35(Suppl 2):3–19.

Lascelles BD, McFarland JM, Swann H: Guidelines for safe and effective use of NSAIDs in dogs. Vet Ther, 2005; 6:237–251.

Mathews KA, Dyson DH: Analgesia and chemical restraint for the emergent patient. Vet Clin North Am Small Anim Pract, 2005; 35:481–515.

Mealey KL: Adverse drug reactions in herding-breed dogs: The role of P-gp. Compendium of Continuing Education, 2006; 28:23–33.

Mealey KL: Therapeutic implications of the MDR-1 gene. J Vet Pharmacol Ther, 2004; 27:257–264.

Muir WW III, Woolf CJ: Mechanisms of pain and their therapeutic implications. J Am Vet Med Assoc, 2001; 219:1346–1356.

Practice guidelines for acute pain management in the perioperative setting. A report by the American Society of Anesthesiologists Task Force on Pain Management, Acute Pain Section. Anesthesia, 1995; 85:1071–1081.

Robertson SA: Managing pain in feline patients. Vet Clin North Am Small Anim Pract, 2005; 35:129–146.

Robertson SA, Taylor PM: Pain management in cats: Past, present and future. 2. Treatment of pain: Clinical pharmacology. J Feline Med Surg, 2004; 6:321–333.

Shojaei AH: Buccal mucosa as a route for systemic drug delivery: A review. J Pharm Pharmaceut Sci, 1998; 1:15–30.

Taylor PM, Robertson SA: Pain management in cats: Past, present and future. 1. The cat is unique. J Feline Med Surg, 2004; 6:313–320.

Toutain PJ, Rerran A, Bousquet-Melou A: Species differences in pharmacokinetics and pharmacodynamics. In: F Cunningham, J Elliott, P Lees (Eds.): Comparative and veterinary pharmacology, New York, 2010, Springer.

Toutain PL: Pharmacokinetics/pharmacodynamics integration in dosage regimen optimization for veterinary medicine. In: JE Riviere, M Papich (Eds.): Veterinary pharmacology and therapeutics, ed 9, Ames, Iowa, 2009, Wiley-Blackwell.

Verma P, Thakur AS, Deshmukh K, et al. Routes of drug administration. Int J Pharm Sci Res, 2010; 1:54–59.

CHAPTER 16

Drug Interactions, Analgesic Protocols and Their Consequences, and Analgesic Drug Antagonism

William W. Muir III

P ain is a multidimensional sensory experience that normally functions to protect the organism, prevent tissue injury, and promote healing. Most acute injuries (trauma, surgery) produce this type of so-called "adaptive" pain. Pain that occurs in the absence of tissue injury or that persists well beyond the healing process is considered pathologic and "maladaptive," serving no protective or beneficial physiologic function. This type of pain can be caused by nerve damage, alterations, or disease in the nervous system (see Chapter 2). The mechanisms responsible for the production of adaptive and maladaptive pain continue to be elucidated and provide potential targets for therapeutic approaches. Many of these approaches take advantage of the drug's mechanism of action and beneficial drug interactions (i.e., additivity, synergism) with other drugs, which serve as the basis for *multimodal analgesic* drug combinations. The terms *multimodal preemptive* and *preventative* are routinely employed in the clinical pain literature and designate current thinking regarding therapeutic approaches for the treatment of most painful conditions. Each term has a specific meaning, although the terms preemptive and preventative are often confused.

DRUG INTERACTIONS

The ability of one drug to alter the effects of another, thereby producing a different drug effect, is frequently encountered and often expected during drug therapy. Drug interactions can be pharmacokinetic or pharmacodynamic in origin and may produce beneficial, untoward, or toxic effects. Pharmacokinetic drug interactions occur when one drug alters the plasma concentration (Cp) and therefore the maximum duration of effect of another drug. Infusions of lidocaine, for example, are known to slow the metabolism and elimination of drugs that depend on liver metabolism (opioids, α_2-agonists), thereby intensifying and prolonging their effects. Pharmacodynamic drug interactions occur when one drug alters the effects of a second drug without changing the Cp or elimination (pharmacokinetics) of the second drug.

Pharmacokinetic Drug Interactions

Pharmacokinetic drug interactions occur when one drug alters the concentration and therefore the effects of another. Most pharmacokinetic drug interactions occur when one drug changes the absorption, distribution, metabolism, elimination, or protein binding of another drug. (Protein-bound drugs are inactive.)

Pharmacodynamic Drug Interactions

Pharmacodynamic drug interactions occur when one drug alters the effects of another drug without altering its Cp. The most common causes of pharmacodynamic drug interactions include the various types of drug antagonism (competitive, noncompetitive) or agonism (*potentiation, additivity,* and *synergism [supra-additivity]*). Elaborate mathematical and statistical methods have been developed to determine whether various drug mixtures produce additive or supra-additive (synergistic) effects. The *isobologram* is derived by comparing the effects of two drugs alone and in combination at several fixed dosages or ratios and, in its simplest form, illustrates when a drug combination is additive, antagonistic, or synergistic (Figure 16-1).

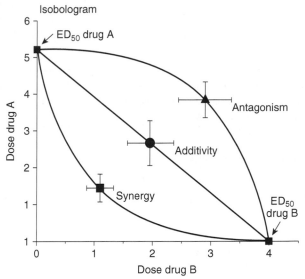

FIGURE 16-1   Isobolograms are one method used to determine whether or not drug combinations are additive, synergistic, or antagonistic. The median effective doses (ED_{50}) for two drugs are plotted on the x- and y-axes. The line that connects them is the line of additivity: A dose of drug A that produces a 25% effect and a dose of drug B that produces a 25% effect should produce a 50% effect. If lower doses than anticipated produce a 50% effect, the drug combination is said to be supra-additive or synergistic (concave curve); if higher doses are required to produce a 50% effect, then the drugs are antagonistic (convex curve).

Potentiation

The ability of one drug to potentiate the effects of another is common in anesthetic practice and the administration of analgesic drugs. The administration of drugs not known for their analgesic activity (e.g., acepromazine, diazepam) will potentiate the analgesic effects of opioids.

Additivity

Additivity or summation of drug effects occurs when the effects of one drug are simply additive to those of another drug. For example, if two drugs that produce analgesia are mixed together and administered, the analgesia produced is the sum of the individual analgesic activity of each drug. This is generally the case when two full opioid agonists (e.g., morphine and fentanyl) are mixed together and administered. The drug doses need not be the same because of differences in drug potency. It is interesting to note that full opioid agonists (e.g., hydromorphone) and lower doses of butorphanol are also additive.

Drug Additivity. Evidence for drug additivity occurs when a proportional increase in the concentration of one drug exactly compensates for a proportional reduction in the concentration of a second drug.

Supra-additivity. Supra-additivity or synergism occurs when a mixture of two or more drugs produces a greater response than expected (i.e., greater than the sum of their individual effects; see Figure 16-1). Drug synergism can be expected when drugs that act by different mechanisms of action are mixed together. Various drug combinations (e.g., nonsteroidal anti-inflammatory drugs [NSAIDs] and opioids; opioids and α_2-agonists; opioids and local anesthetics; opioids and dissociative anesthetics) frequently demonstrate synergistic effects. Synergistic drug combinations are the basis for many multimodal drug combinations but must be administered carefully because unwanted and potentially toxic effects may also be potentiated (e.g., respiratory depression and bradyarrhythmias).

Drug Synergism. Drug synergy (supra-additivity) occurs if the combined concentrations of two drugs required to produce the desired effect are significantly less than predicted by additivity.

Drug Infra-additivity. Drug infra-additivity results if the combined concentrations of both drugs required to produce the desired effect is significantly greater than predicted by additivity.

TECHNIQUES FOR ANALGESIC DRUG ADMINISTRATION

The medical practices adopted for drug administration can be as important as the drug selected in determining the therapeutic efficacy of analgesic drug therapy (Box 16-1). The efficacy of buprenorphine patches, for example, remains controversial. Similarly, the analgesic effects of more potent opioids

BOX 16-1 **Drug Administration Techniques**

- Local or regional anesthesia
- Preemptive analgesia
- Constant rate infusion
- Multimodal
- Drug rotation schedules

(e.g., morphine and fentanyl) are generally enhanced by the concurrent administration of NSAIDs and α_2-agonists, frequently reducing the total amount of opioid required to produce effective analgesia.

Local and Regional Anesthetic Nerve Blocks

Local and regional anesthetic nerve blocks (e.g., infiltration, epidural, and intercostal) are valuable adjuncts to the administration of parenteral analgesic medications. Most regional anesthetic techniques can be markedly enhanced by ultrasound-guided nerve blocks, which, when performed properly, provide excellent analgesia that lasts for several hours with a low potential for serious side effects (see Chapters 11 and 12).

Preemptive versus Preventative Analgesia

The term *preemptive analgesia* (or *preemptive antihyperalgesia*) was coined by Patrick Wall to describe the potential benefits of the preoperative administration of analgesic drugs for preventing the development of acute and chronic postoperative pain caused by the central sensitization induced by surgical incision. The concept is a rational extension of the belief that prior administration of analgesic drugs will prevent or attenuate peripheral or central sensitization and their consequences. The production of adequate analgesia during a surgical (or any painful) procedure is considered important because most anesthetic drugs are known to suppress motor activity to an equal or greater degree as sensory activity. The presumption that the administration of an analgesic drug or drugs (multimodal analgesia) before surgery can limit intraoperative nociception, stress, and subsequent analgesic (opioid) consumption, however, has not always been realized and has prompted alternative terms (*preventive analgesia, balanced analgesia, broad versus narrow preemptive analgesia, protective analgesia*) and reconsideration of the design of clinically conducted analgesic trials. Data collected from randomized clinical trials in humans on the timing of analgesic drug administration (i.e., initiation of analgesia before versus during or after the noxious stimulus) have produced confusing results. Preprocedural (preemptive) analgesic drug administration is clearly better than giving no analgesic, but few well-controlled studies have compared preprocedural versus procedural or postprocedural (preventative) analgesic strategies. Adding to this dilemma are studies conducted in humans that have demonstrated that preoperative administration of an NSAID is no better than administration of the drug after surgery.

Preemptive Analgesia

Preemptive analgesia is a pharmacologic intervention performed before a noxious event (e.g., surgery) that is intended to minimize the impact of the stimulus by preventing peripheral and/or central sensitization.

Preventative Analgesia

The term *preventive analgesia* has been proposed as a more comprehensive approach to pain therapy than *preemptive analgesia*. Data generated in humans suggests that blocking the peripheral nociceptive barrage that occurs in the hours after a painful event or procedure decreases pain at later time periods, whereas blocking the nociceptive barrage during the procedure does not, thereby implicating the role of postoperative factors in the development of outcome and chronic pain production. These studies highlight the shortcoming of the classic view of preemptive analgesia: analgesic treatment that is initiated before a procedure to reduce the consequences of nociceptive transmission initiated by the procedure. The goal of preventative analgesia is to minimize sensitization induced by noxious perioperative stimuli including those arising before, during, and after the procedure. A preventive analgesic effect is produced if or when postprocedural pain and/or analgesic consumption are decreased relative to a placebo treatment or compared with no treatment and the analgesic effect extends for a period of time that outlasts the pharmacologic effects (>5.5 half-lives) for the drug in question. Preventive analgesia does not focus on the relative timing of analgesic interventions (e.g., preemptive analgesia), but on prevention of noxious periprocedural stimuli from producing peripheral and/or central sensitization. Evidence from human surgical candidates suggests that the provision of effective analgesia in the early postoperative period may lead to clinically important benefits with respect to long-term recovery (e.g., less chronic pain). For example, studies in humans have demonstrated that perioperative administration of pregabalin, a drug that modulates voltage-dependent calcium channels via binding to their $\alpha_2\delta$ subunit, reduces pain for weeks to months after lumbar diskectomy and total knee arthroplasty. Pregabalin modulates neurotransmitter release by changing the intrinsic activation-inactivation properties in nociceptive pathways. Perioperative pregabalin administration was associated with less pain intensity and improved functional outcomes 3 months after surgery versus epidural blockade. Blockade of the peripheral nociceptive barrage in the hours after surgery decreases pain at later time periods, whereas blocking the intraoperative nociceptive barrage does not, suggesting that postoperative factors contribute to a greater extent to the outcomes than intraoperative factors. Such studies highlight the shortcoming of the classic definition of preemptive analgesia.

Constant Rate Infusion

A constant rate infusion (CRI) can be used to provide continuous adjustable anesthesia or analgesia for extended periods (Figure 16-2). The use of a CRI to produce a steady-state plasma concentration of drug avoids the peaks (potential toxicity) and troughs (potential loss of drug effect) associated with repeated injectable or oral drug administration. Opioids, local anesthetics, and some anesthetic drugs (e.g., ketamine and tiletamine-zolazepam [Telazol]) can be administered by CRI to provide excellent analgesia for hours or days. One or two intravenous (IV) bolus drug doses (loading dose) are usually administered in conjunction with the initiation of CRI to help establish and sustain therapeutic plasma drug concentrations until steady-state drug concentrations are reached.

Frequent Low Dosing

The frequent (every 3 to 4 hours) administration of low doses of analgesic drugs by IV or intramuscular (IM) injection is similar to CRI because a lower dose of drug is administered more frequently, thus minimizing peak and trough drug concentrations and the potential for toxicity and ineffective drug plasma concentrations, respectively. This technique can be used when CRI cannot be used or is technically difficult to perform, and it is well suited for high-risk animals in which higher-dose bolus administration is more likely to produce unwanted side effects. This technique, however, is labor intensive and more disturbing to the animal than CRI.

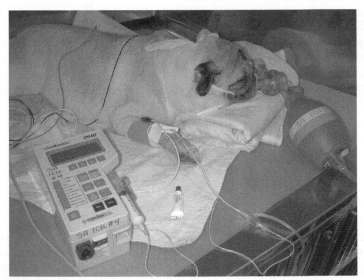

FIGURE 16-2 The quantitative and accurate infusion of drugs (analgesics, anesthetics) can be facilitated by programmable syringe infusion pumps.

Multiple Routes

The same or different analgesic drugs can be administered by multiple routes to produce immediate and sustained drug effects. The IV administration of a drug in conjunction with its IM or subcutaneous (SC) administration produces immediate drug effects, which are sustained for a longer duration, depending on the rate of absorption and pharmacokinetics of the drug administered. This technique is particularly useful for drugs that have intermediate (1 to 2 hours) to short (<30 minutes) half-lives. Repeated IM administration of hydromorphone in conjunction with the placement of a fentanyl patch (transcutaneous drug delivery), for example, can be used to initiate opioid analgesia (morphine) until effective plasma concentrations of fentanyl are reached, which may take 6 to 12 hours (see Chapter 9).

Multiple Drug Administration

The administration of two or more analgesic drugs (multimodal therapy; see the discussion of multimodal analgesia), sequentially or together, is an effective method of improving and enhancing analgesic drug effects. Generally speaking, drugs that act by different mechanisms of action are additive and frequently supra-additive (synergistic) when administered at the same time. Synergism has the potential to reduce the doses of each drug to be administered, decreasing the potential for the development of drug related side effects or toxicity.

Drug Rotation Schedules

The rotation of drugs that act by the same general mechanism or different mechanisms (e.g., opioids and NSAIDs) may help prevent the development of drug tolerance and drug-related toxicities. Intermittent dosage schedules (e.g., 3 days on, 2 days off) and alternate administration of carprofen with deracoxib or codeine, for example, may help to sustain analgesic drug effects and avoid toxicities unique to single-drug therapy.

Multimodal Analgesia

The identification of multiple pain-initiating mechanisms prompted the practice of administering multiple drugs that produce effects by different mechanisms (multimodal analgesia). Multimodal analgesia—also referred to as *opioid-sparing, balanced, preemptive* (before procedure), or *preventative* analgesia—relies on the theory that different classes of drugs acting by different mechanisms produce superior analgesia because of additive or synergistic drug effects. Theoretically this approach should improve the efficacy and safety of pain therapy and potentially reduce the dose of the individual drugs used in a multimodal cocktail compared with the need for a higher dose if a single medication is administered. Several issues, however, have confounded the multimodal approach to pain management, including inadequate knowledge regarding which mechanisms are responsible for the production of pain, inadequate knowledge regarding which drugs and drug doses are most likely to produce clinically relevant additive or synergistic drug effects, great interanimal variability, and the potential for multidrug additive or synergistic side effects. Although opioid-related side effects (e.g., nausea, vomiting, urinary retention, ileus, constipation, sedation, ventilatory depression, hyperthermia, agitation-aggression, hyperalgesia) have been described, nonopioid analgesics (ketamine, gabapentinoids) and cyclooxygenase-selective NSAIDs also produce drug-related side effects (e.g., hepatotoxicity and renal toxicity, coagulopathy, confusion, sedation, and disorientation), which can be exacerbated when these drugs are administered as a part of a multimodal regimen. Recent evidence suggests that the efficacy of analgesic therapy and the benefit-risk ratio for the various drug combinations advocated is more likely to be dependent on the type of procedure being performed (e.g., orthopedic, abdominal, thoracic, endoscopic) than the analgesic efficacy of the drug combinations selected. This evidence suggests that procedure- or disease-specific, evidenced-based pain management protocols are more successful for treating and controlling pain in humans than administering the same multimodal analgesic protocol (whether additive or synergistic) to every animal (Table 16-1). As an example, continuous epidural analgesia after a major abdominal procedure in humans provides more benefit for reducing dynamic pain, ileus, and postoperative nausea and vomiting than the combination of an NSAID and an opioid. This approach is inherently simple, targets pain at the site of origin before centrally mediated (neuroplastic) changes can occur, and is less likely to produce side effects (see Chapters 11 and 12).

Most clinicians inherently expect that better pain prevention or relief will lead to improved clinical outcomes including reduced organ dysfunction, decreased morbidity, and a shorter hospital stay. There are few if any controlled studies in veterinary medicine to confirm this expectation, and a review of the published literature from humans does not support a major benefit with respect to these outcome measures. Future studies, particularly in animals

TABLE 16-1	Treatments That Reduce Hypersensitivity or Decrease Basal Pain Sensitivity	
REDUCE HYPERSENSITIVITY	**DECREASE BASAL PAIN SENSITIVITY**
Anticonvulsants	Local anesthetics
Antidepressants	Opioids
NSAIDs	Neurectomy
Capsaicin	

Key: *NSAID,* Nonsteroidal anti-inflammatory drug.

with naturally occurring pain, should focus on more meaningful end points (e.g., resumption of dietary intake, recovery of bowel and bladder function, resumption of normal physical activities, and reduced hypervigilance). Furthermore, updated evidence-based principles need to be employed.

DEVELOPING A TREATMENT PLAN

The development and periodic reassessment of a therapeutic treatment plan for pain are essential for producing adequate and effective short- or long-term analgesia in dogs and cats (Box 16-2). A rational approach to the treatment of pain is most logically based on a clinical diagnosis and an understanding of the various mechanisms responsible for producing pain. Some drugs are more effective for reducing pain hypersensitivity, whereas others decrease basal sensitivity to noxious stimuli (see Table 16-1). Notably, the treatment of severe pain with drugs that are capable of producing only mild analgesic effects not only is likely to be ineffective, but may make pain harder to treat, increasing the likelihood of drug-related side effects.

Therapeutic protocols should be designed for the treatment of mild, moderate, and severe pain. In addition to drug-related issues, the cost of therapy should be integrated into these plans (Box 16-3). Nonpharmacologic therapies should be considered and incorporated into the therapeutic plan whenever appropriate. Educational materials describing the consequences of pain,

---

BOX 16-2   Key Components of Analgesic Drug Therapy

- Drug or method for alleviating pain
- Pain-prevention program
- Analgesic technique
- Outcome goals
- Methods for assessing pain and analgesia
- Documentation of success or failure
- Pain diary
- Education of staff and pet owner

BOX 16-3   Key Drug Issues

- Mechanism of action
- Analgesic potency
- Duration of effect
- Central nervous system depression
- Anti-inflammatory effects
- Side effects and toxicity
- Drug interactions
- Cost

the advantages of pain therapy, and the advantages and disadvantages of different therapeutic approaches should be made available to help educate pet owners.

Drugs

Drug selection and therapeutic technique should be based on the cause, severity, and duration of pain (see Chapters 5 and 7). Drugs should be thought of and categorized based on their mechanism of action, analgesic potency, and potential to produce unwanted side effects. A pain scoring system should be used in conjunction with a quality-of-life rating system to assess the severity of pain and the success or failure of therapy (see Chapter 5). Clinical experience and familiarity with a select group of drugs is important in achieving a beneficial drug effect.

Clinical Efficacy

Clinical efficacy refers to the ability of a drug to produce the desired clinical effect, regardless of the intrinsic activity (maximal effect) and the dose required to produce the effect (potency), while avoiding (minimizing) side effects or toxicity. Fentanyl, for example, may be totally ineffective in the treatment of severe pain produced by a herniated disk. This example has important clinical implications for the administration of analgesic drugs because it implies that the severity of the disease, or in this case the intensity of pain, determines the clinical efficacy of the drug. When the intensity of pain increases, the effectiveness of any drug decreases, and in the case of opioids, more receptors need to be occupied to produce a therapeutic effect. Eventually a point is reached at which no matter how many receptors are occupied, analgesia may be difficult to produce. In other words, the intensity of the pain dictates which analgesic drugs should be used first. Low-efficacy opioids (e.g., codeine, butorphanol, tramadol) may be adequate for the treatment of most causes of mild to moderate pain and can be used in combination with higher-efficacy opioids (e.g., morphine and oxymorphone) to enhance analgesic effects. The treatment of severe pain usually requires a multimodal technique that employs full opioid agonists, α_2-agonists, local anesthetics, and nonanesthetic doses of dissociative anesthetics (e.g., ketamine).

Tolerance

Tolerance occurs when increasing drug doses are required over time to maintain a desired effect. Drug tolerance can develop acutely (within hours) or chronically (over days, weeks, months) and may be attributed to pharmacokinetic changes (e.g., liver enzyme induction and increased clearance) or pharmacodynamic changes (altered cellular responses reducing the effects of the drug). One potential mechanism for opioid tolerance is *receptor desensitization* caused by a decrease in functional opioid receptors after chronic

opioid administration. Regardless of cause, the development of drug tolerance presents a significant problem in the treatment of pain, generally requiring that drug therapy be discontinued and that alternative analgesic therapy
be implemented.

Drugs that require occupancy of a smaller number of receptors to produce
an effect (e.g., fentanyl) are less likely to produce tolerance than less potent
drugs (e.g., codeine, butorphanol, meperidine).

Physical Dependence

Physical dependence is characterized by the development of untoward effects
when a drug is acutely withheld or withdrawn.

WHAT TO DO WHEN THE THERAPEUTIC PLAN DOES NOT WORK

Anyone who has treated dogs, cats, or any animal in pain is familiar with
therapeutic failure. Many causes for pain exist, and many factors influence
the animal response to painful sensations and the effects of analgesic therapies (Box 16-4). Physical therapy (see Chapter 19), complementary techniques (see Chapter 18), and behavior-modifying drugs (see Chapter 14)
or techniques in conjunction with changes in the animal's environment
may be required to treat pain effectively in some animals. Lack of owner compliance with prescribed recommendations should be considered as one possible cause of therapeutic failure.

CONCERNS REGARDING PROFOUNDLY EFFECTIVE ANALGESIC THERAPIES

The concern that the production of analgesia, particularly for extended
periods of time, may accelerate tissue damage including osteoarthritic
changes is not supported by evidence. Alternatively, drugs that produce
somnolence (e.g., anticonvulsants, antidepressants) can lead to muscle

---

BOX 16-4	Therapeutic Failure

- Reevaluate the animal.
- Reevaluate treatment plan: Drug(s), dose(s), technique(s).
- Reevaluate pet owner's compliance.
- Reevaluate animal's environment.
- Reevaluate nonpharmacologic treatments.
- Consider alternative or adjunctive therapies.
- Consider drug tolerance and interactions.
- Consider behavioral modification.

weakness, listlessness, and depression. Therefore, medications capable of providing profound analgesia (profoundly effective analgesic therapy [PEAT]) should be considered in relationship to their potential to mask clinical signs or predispose the animal to serious adverse consequences including the consideration for euthanasia (Box 16-5). Analgesic therapy performs at its best when it returns pain sensitivity to its normal set point (Figure 16-3). For example, NSAIDs reduce inflammation and pain but do not reliably alter sensitivity to otherwise painful stimuli. Antidepressants and anticonvulsants share this same property, though they work by different mechanisms. Alternatively, opioids and α_2-agonists can be administered at doses that reduce pain sensitivity and allodynia but are also used to provide near-complete anesthesia.

BOX **16-5** **Potential Adverse Consequences of Profoundly Effective Analgesic Therapy (PEAT)**

- Muscle weakness, listlessness, and depression
- Injuries: Orthopedic (fractures, degenerative disease of the joints); integument, soft tissue, and dentition (lacerations, bruises, corneal abrasion)
- Infection: Sepsis, unrecognized intra-abdominal pathology, septic joints, osteomyelitis
- Quality of life: May be reduced because of listlessness and depression

---

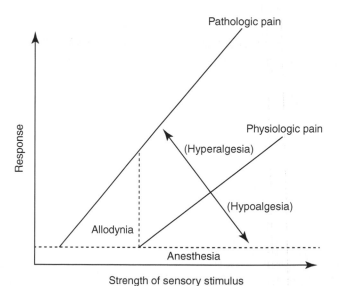

FIGURE 16-3 The normal stimulus-response relationship for pain. Shifts to the left produce hyperalgesia and allodynia; shifts to the right produce hypoalgesia or complete analgesia.

PREVENTING DRUG-RELATED EFFECTS AND TOXICITY

Drug-related side effects and toxicity are common consequences of drug administration, even when recommended drug doses and administration schedules are followed. Some side effects are easily eliminated (e.g., opioid-induced bradycardia and central nervous system [CNS] depression), whereas others may be irreversible and fatal (e.g., NSAID-induced acute renal failure). Many of the drugs used to produce analgesia (e.g., opioids, α_2-agonists, and local anesthetics) have the potential to produce a wide variety of side effects and toxicity. Opioids are notorious for their ability to induce vomiting, bradycardia, and augmentation of the respiratory depressant effects of anesthetics. α_2-Agonists can produce bradycardia, respiratory depression, and excessive CNS depression in otherwise normal healthy dogs or cats, even when relatively low doses are administered. The IV bolus administration of benzodiazepines (e.g., diazepam and midazolam), drugs usually considered to be relatively free of side effects or toxicity, can induce acute collapse, bradycardia, and unconsciousness. The initial response to a drug-related side effect, once identified, should focus on its clinical significance and the most appropriate means for its elimination. Fortunately, a variety of drugs and pharmacologic techniques can be used to antagonize or eliminate unwanted drug side effects (Box 16-6).

DISCONTINUING DRUG ADMINISTRATION

Stopping the administration of a drug, slowing the rate of drug administration, and decreasing the frequency of intermittent drug administration are simple and effective methods for minimizing unwanted drug-related side effects. Animals that are receiving drugs chronically (NSAIDs) should be monitored periodically for signs of substantiated toxicities (e.g., gastric ulcers; renal and liver failure).

Drug Administration

The dose, rate of drug administration, and frequency and route of drug administration can be changed to help decrease the possibility of drug-related side effects. Decreasing the drug dosage or rate of administration or incrementally administering the dose decreases peak plasma drug concentrations,

---

BOX **16-6**   **Drug Antagonism**

- Change in method of drug administration (stop or reduce dose)
- Pharmacokinetic antagonism (prevent absorption; hasten metabolism and elimination)
- Competitive antagonism (bind or inactivate receptors)
- Physiologic antagonism (counteract adverse effect)

thereby decreasing the potential for the development of drug-related side effects.

Route of Administration

Administering drugs by routes that delay drug absorption (e.g., oral or transdermal) prolongs the time from the onset to peak drug effect but decreases peak plasma drug concentrations, thereby decreasing the potential for the development of drug-related side effects.

PHARMACOKINETIC ANTAGONISM

Pharmacokinetic antagonism is the use of therapies and techniques that decrease the plasma concentration of the drug. Therapies that decrease or inhibit drug absorption or increase drug elimination should be considered.

Decreasing Drug Absorption

The absorption of orally administered drugs can be decreased or inhibited by the administration of substances that interfere with drug absorption from the gastrointestinal tract (kaolin, pectin, activated charcoal). Alternatively, drugs that induce vomiting (apomorphine) can be administered to limit the amount of drug that is absorbed from the gastrointestinal tract.

Increasing Drug Elimination

Drug elimination can be enhanced by improving or ensuring adequate blood supply to the major organs of elimination (liver, kidneys, lungs) for the drug in question. This may require subcutaneous or IV administration of fluids and cardiovascular stimulants (dopamine, dobutamine, alkalinizing solutions). The renal excretion of drugs can be increased by administering fluids, optimizing pH (e.g., alkaline urine pH), and promoting diuresis (furosemide).

RECEPTOR BLOCKADE (DRUG ANTAGONISTS)

Opioids, α_2-agonists, and benzodiazepines produce their effects by combining with and activating receptors. Drugs that combine with receptors and produce less than the expected maximal response are referred to as *partial agonists* (e.g., buprenorphine). Furthermore, two drugs with the same ability to combine (affinity) with a receptor could produce different degrees of analgesia (activity). The drug that produces the maximal effect is termed *a full agonist*, whereas the drug that produces less than the maximal effect is termed *a partial agonist*. Pure drug *antagonists* combine with receptors without causing their activation, thereby preventing the effects of agonists. The affinity of the antagonist for the receptor determines how much drug is necessary to produce an antagonistic effect (high affinity = low amounts of drug).

Some drugs combine with, activate, and inhibit the receptor occupation of other drugs. These drugs are called *agonists-antagonists*. Some drug antagonists and agonist-antagonists compete for receptors with the agonist or partial agonist, implying that the receptor binds to one drug at a time and that the effects of the antagonist or agonist-antagonist are surmountable if enough agonist or partial agonist is administered (see Chapter 7). Butorphanol, for example, is an opioid agonist-antagonist that is additive with full opioid agonists when administered at low doses. Larger doses (>0.2 mg/kg) of butorphanol can be used to antagonize the effects of the pure opioid agonists morphine and hydromorphone. Low doses ("microdoses") of the opioid antagonists naloxone, naltrexone have been administered in conjunction with hydromorphone to humans to minimize opioid-related side effects (delirium, depression, vomiting, constipation, urine retention) without interfering with opioid agonist–induced analgesia. Most drug antagonists are generally administered in doses far in excess of what is required to overcome agonist effects. This is an important point, considering the administration of a drug antagonist reverses toxic and analgesic effects of another drug. Special consideration should be given to the antagonist selected, its dosage, and route of administration. Drug antagonists should be administered incrementally (titrated) to achieve the desired effect whenever possible unless used in a life-or-death situation. Finally, caution is advised whenever a drug antagonist is administered to reverse CNS depression because the return to consciousness may produce CNS and cardiovascular consequences (excitement, agitation, aggression, hypertension, cardiac arrhythmias).

Opioid Antagonists

Naloxone and naltrexone are pure opioid antagonists (i.e., produce no opioid effects) that have high affinity for μ, κ, and σ opioid receptors. Relatively small doses of either drug can be used to rapidly reverse unwanted or lingering CNS, respiratory, and cardiac (bradycardia) effects produced by opioid agonists or partial agonists. Naloxone is rapidly metabolized and eliminated in dogs and cats, producing relatively short-lived (10 to 20 minutes) effects and predisposing to renarcotization and respiratory depression. Naltrexone produces effects similar to those of naloxone but has a much longer duration of action (several hours). Both drugs produce few direct, drug-related effects when administered IV at currently recommended doses. Conventional doses of naloxone and naltrexone will reverse the analgesic effects of systemic and parenteral opioid administration and inhibit acupuncture analgesia. The IV administration of large doses of naloxone or naltrexone may produce a state of hyperalgesia because of interference with the protective effect of endogenous opioids (e.g., endorphin and enkephalin). IV bolus administration of naloxone generally produces rapid reversal of opioid-related side effects but may cause some animals to become excited, delirious, or aggressive. Unless an emergency

TABLE 16-2	Opioid and Benzodiazepine Antagonists	
DRUG	**RECOMMENDED USE**	**EMERGENCY USE**
Naloxone	5-15 µg/kg IV	50-100 µg/kg IV
Naltrexone	50-100 µg/kg SC	—
Nalorphine	0.05-0.1 mg/kg IV	—
Flumazenil*	0.2 mg total dose IV	—
Butorphanol[†]	0.05-1.0 mg/kg IV	—
Pentazocine[†]	0.1-0.5 mg/kg IV	—
Buprenorphine[†,‡]	5-10 µg/kg IV	—

*Benzodiazepine antagonist.
[†]Opioid with opioid antagonistic effects (see Chapter 9).
[‡]Monitor for respiratory depression; drug is a partial agonist.

situation exists, small doses of either drug should be incrementally administered to produce the desired effect (e.g., consciousness; Table 16-2).

Opioid Partial or Mixed Agonists-Antagonists

Nalorphine, nalbuphine, pentazocine, and butorphanol are opioids classified as agonists-antagonists. Buprenorphine, a partial agonist, produces less than the maximal response ("ceiling effect") and produces opioid antagonist effects because of high affinity for the µ opioid receptor (see Chapter 9). These drugs are occasionally administered to reverse the unwanted effects (e.g., prolonged sedation) of pure opioid agonists (e.g., morphine and hydromorphone). Butorphanol, for example, can be administered during recovery from anesthesia to antagonize the effects produced by the preanesthetic administration of hydromorphone. Butorphanol administration may restore consciousness and prevent respiratory depression after surgery. Evidence also exists that the administration of small doses of opioid agonist-antagonists (e.g., nalorphine, pentazocine, or butorphanol) in conjunction with or after the administration of a pure opioid agonist (e.g., morphine or hydromorphone) may produce additive analgesia. This suggests that analgesia is improved postoperatively when the sedative effects of morphine are partially antagonized. Care must be taken in the selection of partial agonists or agonist-antagonists to antagonize the effects of a pure opioid agonist (morphine, hydromorphone) because some partial agonists (buprenorphine) may antagonize analgesic effects and have been demonstrated to exaggerate the respiratory depressant effects of pure opioid agonists (meperidine). This effect could become problematic in animals that do not regain consciousness after the administration of buprenorphine.

α₂-Agonists

Yohimbine, tolazoline, and atipamezole are α_2-receptor antagonists that are administered to antagonize the central and peripheral effects of α_2-agonists

TABLE **16-3**	α_2-Antagonists
DRUG	**DOSAGE**
Yohimbine	0.1-0.3 mg/kg IV
	0.3-0.5 mg/kg IM
Tolazoline	0.5-1.0 mg/kg IV
	2-5 mg/kg IM
Atipamezole	0.05-0.2 mg/kg IV
	2-5 times medetomidine dose

(Table 16-3). Yohimbine ($\alpha_2/\alpha_1 = 40/1$) and tolazoline ($\alpha_2/\alpha_1 = 4/1$) are relatively nonspecific α_2-antagonists compared with atipamezole ($\alpha_2/\alpha_1 = 8500/1$) and occasionally produce hypotension (α_1 blockade) and reflex tachycardia. Tolazoline is also noted for producing histamine release, which may contribute to hypotension. All three drugs are recommended for the reversal of α_2-agonist–induced (xylazine, medetomidine, dexmedetomidine, detomidine, romifidine) side effects, including sedation, respiratory depression, and bradycardia. The intramuscular administration of atipamezole produces rapid and complete reversal of α_2-agonist effects, including the elimination of analgesia. The IV bolus administration of manufacturer-recommended doses of α_2-agonists should be reserved for emergency or life-threatening situations. α_2-Agonist administration can initiate involuntary muscle twitching (jactitations), myoclonus, excitement, delirium, and aggression associated with vomiting, urination, and defecation. Clinically, the IM or subcutaneous administration of atipamezole produces rapid uneventful recovery from α_2-agonist sedation and respiratory depression without significant untoward effects.

Benzodiazepine Antagonists

Diazepam and midazolam are centrally acting muscle relaxants that are frequently combined with opioids to produce calming and muscle relaxation before surgery. Diazepam and midazolam can induce dose dependent disorientation, delirium, and on rare occasions profound CNS and associated respiratory depression. On rare occasions, the IV bolus administration of diazepam can also produce bradycardia and hypotension. Flumazenil is a rapidly acting and specific competitive antagonist of diazepam- and midazolam-induced CNS and respiratory depression. Clinical dosages range from 0.1 mg/kg IV to 0.3 mg/kg IM. IV administration is rarely associated with emergence delirium or signs of excitement.

PHYSIOLOGIC ANTAGONISM

Physiologic antagonism refers to the administration of drugs that do not act as specific receptor antagonists but are administered to produce effects that

TABLE 16-4	Therapy for Analgesic Drug-Related Side Effects	
PROBLEM	THERAPY	DOSAGE
Sedation, depression	Analeptics	
	Doxapram	0.2-0.5 mg/kg IV
	Aminophylline	2-10 mg/kg IV
Excitement, seizures	Tranquilizers, muscle relaxants	
	Acepromazine	0.01-0.05 mg/kg IV, IM
	Droperidol	0.1-0.03 mg/kg IV, IM
	Dexmedetomidine	0.005-0.02 mg/kg IV, IM
	Diazepam	0.1-0.5 mg/kg IV, CRI
	Phenobarbital	1-3 mg/kg IV
	Propofol	1-3 mg/kg IV; 0.1-0.2 mg/kg/min
Vomiting	Antiemetics	
	Ondansetron	0.5 mg/kg IV
	Metoclopramide	0.1-0.3 mg/kg IV
Bradycardia	Anticholinergics	
	Atropine	0.01-0.02 mg/kg IV, IM
	Glycopyrrolate	0.005-0.01 mg/kg IV, IM
Respiratory depression	Respiratory stimulants	
	Doxapram	0.2-0.5 mg/kg IV
	Ventilation	
Hypotension	Catecholamines	
	Dopamine	0.001-0.005 mg/kg/min IV
	Dobutamine	0.001-0.010 mg/kg/min IV
	Ephedrine	0.1-0.5 mg/kg IM

oppose or cancel the effects of the problem drug (Table 16-4). For example, anticholinergics (atropine, glycopyrrolate), fluids, or dopamine are administered to oppose the bradycardic and hypotensive effects of opioids or inhalant anesthesia. The administration of atropine or glycopyrrolate to treat opioid or α_2-agonist bradycardia should be carefully considered because coadministration may result in the production of sinus tachycardia or cardiac arrhythmias.

Analeptics

Sedation and behavioral changes are common side effects of many analgesic drugs. Excessive sedation or depression can produce an unresponsive, listless pet, a reduction in appetite, and the potential for significant respiratory depression. This type of response to centrally acting analgesic drugs is best treated by reducing the analgesic drug dose or selecting an analgesic that produces minimal CNS effects. Animals recovering from anesthesia may demonstrate good analgesia but have significant cardiorespiratory depression. Doxapram is a respiratory stimulant that increases CNS activity in dogs and cats. Although not a specific antagonist, doxapram can counteract the CNS depressant effects of low to moderate doses of α_2-agonists, opioids, and injectable or inhalant anesthetics. Once conscious, most animals remain conscious, but because doxapram has a relatively short half-life, animals should be closely monitored to avoid a relapse to CNS and respiratory depression. Aminophylline, although noted for its bronchodilatory effects, also stimulates the CNS. The IV or IM administration of aminophylline to dogs and cats can shorten recovery from anesthesia, increase alertness, and counteract mild to moderate sedation without antagonizing the effects of analgesic drugs. Aminophylline has a much longer duration of action than doxapram.

Tranquilizers and Muscle Relaxants

Nervousness, apprehension, agitation, seizures, and involuntary muscle twitching are potential side effects associated with the use of traditional centrally acting analgesic medications. These side effects are more frequent when large doses are administered or when analgesic drugs are given to animals with preexisting CNS disorders. Acepromazine is an excellent tranquilizer that produces adjunctive analgesic and antiemetic effects when combined with opioids. Relatively low doses (<0.01 mg/kg) given IV or IM can be used to calm nervous or agitated dogs and cats. Droperidol and haloperidol are butyrophenone tranquilizers noted for their mild calming and antiemetic effects and can be used as alternatives to acepromazine. Droperidol and haloperidol are frequently used as behavior modifiers, and either drug can be used to reduce or eliminate apprehension and agitation in dogs and cats. Drug doses should be titrated to the desired effect, and initial doses of droperidol should not exceed 0.1 mg/kg IV or IM. Diazepam and midazolam are excellent centrally acting neuromuscular blocking drugs that can be used to control involuntary muscle twitching or spasms and seizures. Repeated IV administration (0.1 mg/kg) or infusion (0.1 to 0.5 mg/kg/hr) may be required to control involuntary muscle spasms or seizures in some animals. Dogs and cats with seizures that do not respond to diazepam or midazolam therapy should be administered phenobarbital (1 to 3 mg/kg IV) or anesthetized with propofol (1 to 3 mg/kg IV; 0.1 to 0.2 mg/kg/min).

Antiemetics

Nausea and vomiting are common but self-limiting side effects associated with the use of opioid and α_2-agonist drugs. Occasionally, vomiting may persist and result in dyspnea, bradycardia, and potentially aspiration. Vomiting is particularly problematic when it occurs in association with the induction, maintenance, or recovery from anesthesia. As noted previously, acepromazine or droperidol can be used before or in combination with opioids or α_2-agonists to reduce vomiting. Ondansetron (0.5 mg/kg IV), metoclopramide (0.2 to 0.5 mg/kg IM) or maropitant (0.1 to 0.3 mg/kg) can be administered to prevent or eliminate acute vomiting without producing sedation. Persistent vomiting in dogs has been treated by infusing metoclopramide (0.01 to 0.02 mg/kg/hr).

Anticholinergics

Sinus bradycardia, first- and second-degree atrioventricular block with ventricular escape beats, and, rarely, third-degree atrioventricular block may occur after the administration of opioids and particularly α_2-agonists. Opioid-induced bradyarrhythmias are generally caused by increases in parasympathetic tone and are readily responsive to treatment with atropine (0.01 to 0.02 mg/kg IV) or glycopyrrolate (0.005 to 0.01 mg/kg IV). α_2-Agonist–induced bradyarrhythmias may also be caused by increases in parasympathetic tone but can be augmented by decreases in sympathetic tone. Cardiac rhythm disturbances (ventricular arrhythmias) can occur or may be exaggerated by the coadministration of an α_2-agonist and an anticholinergic, and this should be avoided. The administration of anticholinergics 20 to 30 minutes after the administration of an α_2-agonist is generally inconsequential.

Respiratory Stimulants

Respiratory depression is an underappreciated and significant side effect associated with IV or long-term analgesic drug administration; it is most common when opioids and α_2-agonists are administered in conjunction with injectable or inhalant anesthetics. Signs of respiratory depression are often subtle, unless significant decreases in respiratory rate or apnea are observed. Respiratory rate and depth should be closely monitored after the IV administration of opioids, α_2-agonists, and benzodiazepines. Doxapram is an excellent but short-acting CNS and respiratory stimulant but is not a specific drug antagonist. Significant respiratory depression may follow a period of transient respiratory stimulation if consciousness does not improve, because carbon dioxide concentrations (the principal drive to breathing) may have been significantly reduced. Respiratory depression therefore is best treated by careful monitoring, oxygen supplementation, periodic stimulation, and techniques that hasten drug elimination. If necessary, assisted or mechanical ventilation should be used to maintain breathing and normal pH and blood gas values.

Catecholamines

Arterial blood pressure should be monitored in any animal in which hypotension is suspected. Hypotension and poor tissue perfusion may occur as a consequence of loss of consciousness, bradyarrhythmias, vasodilation, and low cardiac output. Clinically, hypotension may result in lethargy, depression, muscle weakness, and considerable delays in recovery from anesthesia. Acute hypotension should be treated with appropriate fluids (10 to 20 mL/kg IV lactated Ringer's solution; 5 to 10 mL/kg IV hydroxyethyl starch) or the administration of dopamine (1 to 4 µg/kg/min), dobutamine (1 to 10 µg/kg/min), or ephedrine (0.1 to 0.5 mg/kg IV to effect).

SUGGESTED READINGS

Andaluz A, Moll X, Ventura R, et al.: Plasma buprenorphine concentrations after the application of a 70 microg/h transdermal patch in dogs. Preliminary report. J Vet Pharmacol Ther, 2009; 32:503–505.

Argoff C: Mechanisms of pain transmission and pharmacologic management. Curr Med Res Opin, 2011; 27:2019–2031.

Buvanendran A, Kroin JS: Multimodal analgesia for controlling acute postoperative pain. Curr Opin Anaesthesiol, 2009; 22:588–593.

Clark JD: The pitfalls of profoundly effective analgesic therapies. Clin J Pain, 2008; 24:825–831.

Dahl JB, Moiniche S: Pre-emptive analgesia. Brit Med Bulletin, 2004; 71:13–27.

Elvir-Lazo OL, White PF: The role of multimodal analgesia in pain management after ambulatory surgery. Curr Opin Anaesthesiol, 2010; 23:697–703.

Hendricks JFA, Eger EI, Sonner JM, et al.: Is synergy the rule? A review of anesthetic interactions producing hypnosis and immobility. Anesth Analg, 2008; 107:494–506.

Katz J, Clarke H, Seltzer Z: Preventive analgesia: Quo vadimus? Anesth Analg, 2011; 113:1242–1253.

Leavitt SB. Opioid antagonists, naloxone & naltrexone: Aids for pain management. Pain Treatment Topics, 2009. Retrieved from http://stew202.home.comcast.net/~stew202/media/OpioidAntagonistsForPain.pdf.

Moll X, Fresno L, García F, et al.: Comparison of subcutaneous and transdermal administration of buprenorphine for pre-emptive analgesia in dogs undergoing elective ovariohysterectomy. Vet J, 2011; 187:124–128.

Practice guidelines for acute pain management in the perioperative setting: An updated report by the American Society of Anesthesiologists Task Force on Acute Pain Management. Anesthesiology, 2012; 116:248–273.

Shafer SL, Hendricks JFA, Flood P, et al.: Additivity versus synergy: A theoretical analysis of implications for anesthetic mechanisms. Anesth Analg, 2008; 107:507–524.

Vadivelu N, Mitra S, Narayan D: Recent advances in postoperative pain management. Yale J Biol Med, 2010; 83:11–25.

White PF, Kehlet H, Meal JM, et al.: The role of the anesthesiologist in fast-track surgery: From multimodal analgesia to perioperative medical care. Anesth Analg, 2007; 104:1380–1398.

Woolf CJ. Pain: moving from symptom control towards mechanism-specific pharmacologic management. Ann Intern Med. 2004; 140:441–451.

Young A, Buvanendran A: Recent advances in multimodal analgesia. Anesthesiology Clin, 2012; 30:91–100.

CHAPTER 17

Energy Modalities

Therapeutic Laser and Pulsed Electromagnetic Field Therapy

James S. Gaynor

THERAPEUTIC LASER

Laser therapy is the application of nonablative laser radiation to injured or dysfunctional physiologic systems to modulate cell signaling and metabolism and to stimulate healing within the tissues.

Laser Therapy Basics

- The term *laser* is an acronym for "light amplification by stimulated emission of radiation."
- The light energy is absorbed by the cells within the tissue, resulting in physiologic and metabolic changes involved in the healing process and pain relief.
- Laser therapy is based on photochemical but not thermal effects. The following is a list of proposed mechanisms for the treatment modality:
  - The laser energy is absorbed by cytochrome c oxidase in the mitochondria. This energy transfer stimulates the respiratory chain, leading to increased adenosine triphosphate (ATP) production and modulation of cell signaling.
  - Low concentrations of reactive oxygen species (ROSs) are generated during the absorption of laser energy, leading to modulated cell metabolism and signaling.
  - Liberation of nitric oxide (NO) via photo-dissociation leads to increased circulation and changes in inflammatory signaling.
- Laser parameters
  - *Wavelength* is the color of the light emitted expressed in nanometers (nm). This quality of the light emitted by the device determines the ability of the therapeutic energy to penetrate the tissue. Most laser therapy devices operate in a "therapeutic window" between 650 nm and 1000 nm.
  - *Power* is the rate at which energy is emitted from the device expressed in watts (W). The average power output of a device determines the amount of time necessary to deliver the desired dose. Class IIIb devices

have a maximum average power output of up to 0.5 W, and class IV devices have a maximum average power output of more than 0.5 W.

- *Pulsing frequency*, expressed in hertz (Hz), describes the ability to turn the laser emission on and off at desired intervals. Theory suggests that synchronizing aspects of pulsing with the frequency of biologic reactions could optimize laser therapy treatments. However, there is currently no agreement in the literature regarding optimal pulsing parameters for specific conditions, and continuous wave treatment remains the gold standard for laser therapy efficacy.
- Lasers produce the following effects:
  - Improved cell respiration
  - Increased tissue perfusion and neovascularization
  - Collagen and protein synthesis
  - Leukocyte phagocytosis
  - Stimulation of the immune system
  - Reduced inflammation
  - Increased cell migration and proliferation
  - Analgesia

Common Laser Therapy Applications for General Practice

- Pain management
- Wound healing
- Rehabilitation
- Dermatology—lick granulomas
- Musculoskeletal injuries

Laser Therapy Dosage Considerations

1. The dose is established as the energy density applied to the tissue. This is typically expressed in units of joules (J) per centimeter squared.
2. Superficial conditions (e.g., wounds) should be treated with 2 to 6 J/cm^2.
3. Deep conditions (e.g., arthritis, tendon injury) should be treated with 6 to 10 J/cm^2.

Laser Therapy Treatment Techniques

- Point treatment
  - Advantage: Can apply recommended dose quickly with most available devices.
  - Disadvantage: Requires precise location of treatment points for optimal results.
- Treatment of large areas
  - Advantage: Application of effective dose to a large area can provide more consistent results across multiple clinicians.

- Disadvantage: Application can be done only in a reasonable amount of time with a higher-power device.
- On-contact treatment
  - Standard convex optic: This treatment is typically held in one location for the duration of the treatment.
  - Laser-massage optic: This treatment is typically applied over an area in conjunction with tissue manipulation or massage.
  - Advantage: Contact treatment enhances laser penetration by limiting reflection at the surface of the tissue and by displacing interstitial fluid to effectively decrease the treatment depth.
  - Disadvantage: Contact treatment is not desirable over open wounds, contusions, or bony prominence.
- Off-contact treatment
  - This treatment is generally applied using diverging optics over a large area.
  - Advantage: This treatment allows the user to vary the energy density of the treatment.
  - Disadvantages: This treatment technique is more variable, and some laser energy is lost because of reflection at the tissue interface.

Equipment

- Two types of laser units are commonly used in veterinary medicine:
  - Helium-neon gas tube (a red light emitter): It produces a wavelength of 632 to 650 nm, which can penetrate tissues to a depth of 0.8 to 15 mm.
  - Gallium arsenite diode (an infrared light emitter): It produces a wavelength of 904 nm, which can penetrate to a depth of 10 mm to 5 cm.
- The exact protocols in already programmed or programmable lasers aid in the following:
  1. Optimal energy density
  2. Maximum power
  3. Exact frequency information
  4. Precise application optics (resonance phenomenon)
- Variable equipment is on the market and is advocated for management of the following:
  1. Open wounds
  2. Burns
  3. Ulcers
  4. Pressure sores
  5. Preventing proud flesh formation
  6. Resolving swelling from inflammation
  7. Treatment of musculoskeletal conditions

- - Back pain and injury
  - Tendinitis
  - Suspensory injuries
  - Ligament injuries
  - Sprains
  - Arthritis
- Failed treatment responses are most likely attributable to delivery of inadequate doses of energy.
- Advantages
  1. Laser therapy is a noninvasive, safe, and painless form of therapy.
  2. It requires short treatment periods.
  3. Minimal animal restraint during the treatment is necessary.
  4. Laser therapy is a versatile modality that is effective for many conditions encountered in veterinary medicine.
- Disadvantages
  1. The cost for the unit is from $2000 to tens of thousands of dollars if an option to lease is not available.
  2. Lasers have a reduced ability to stimulate and balance acupuncture points in comparison to needles.
  3. Few studies have compared the efficacy of one type of laser with another.

PULSED ELECTROMAGNETIC FIELD THERAPY

- Pulsed magnetic field therapy (PMFT) is a method of applying a magnetic field with an extremely low range of frequencies to the cell to change the electrical potentials of nerves and other cells and normalize the flow of ions and nutrients in the cell to promote the healing of damaged tissues.
- The concept of using magnets for healing the body goes back thousands of years to ancient Greece, Egypt, and China.
- Recent studies on repair of bone fractures and delayed union fractures have suggested that acupuncture analgesia and healing properties may be mediated by changing electromagnetic fields in the body.
- Pulsating magnetic fields have been used since the 1970s on dogs, small animals, and performance horses, such as show horses and thoroughbred racehorses.
- Indications for using PMFT were primarily to alleviate pain originating from various tissues:
  1. Acute and chronic sore backs
  2. Arthritic joints
  3. Inflamed tendons
  4. Inflamed tendon sheaths

- The size and composition of the magnet determine the strength of the magnetic field, which subsequently determines the depth of tissue penetration.
- During magnetic therapy, the hydrogen and oxygen molecules in the water of blood and iron become magnetically polarized and align with other components in the blood. The charged molecules and aggregates then travel throughout the body more efficiently, thus allowing the blood's nourishing energy to more effectively support healing and recovery.
- Magnetic field therapy for pain management and healing is effective at very low power.
- Magnetic field therapy systems use multiform pulses of alternating (oscillating positive and negative) electromagnetic induction fields (EMIFs).
- The EMIFs mimic the body's waveforms
- Frequencies ranging from 0.5 to 5 Hz are beneficial for:
  - Reducing blood loss
  - Infections
  - Inflammation
  - Degenerative joint diseases
  - Generalized pain
- Frequencies of 5 to 18 Hz aid in:
  - Muscle toning
  - Improving circulation
- Various equipment to deliver pulsating magnetic therapy has been manufactured. Accessories include:
  1. Applicator pads
  2. Generator
  3. Magnetic field tester
  4. Jackets for dogs and small animals
  5. Beds for dogs and small animals
  6. Blankets, neck wraps, hocks, and leggings for horses

Targeted Pulsed Electromagnetic Field Therapy

- Targeted pulsed electromagnetic field therapy (tPEMF) can produce significant effects with the following attributes:
  - Proprietary signals (tPEMF)
  - *A priori* targeting of electrochemical activity
  - Decreased power, increased efficacy compared with PEMF
  - Treats through dressings, clothing, casts, and so on
  - Specific effects of tPEMF include (Figure 17-1):
    - Targeting of calcium-calmodulin binding (Ca/CaM)
    - Anti-inflammatory cascade

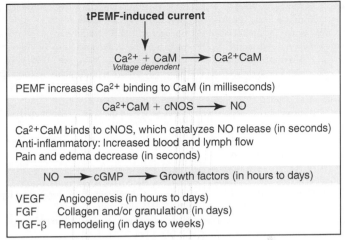

FIGURE 17-1 Mechanism of action of targeted pulsed electromagnetic (tPEMF) field therapy. Key: Ca^{2+}, calcium ion; *CaM*, calmodulin; *cNOS*, constitutive nitric oxide synthase; *NO*, nitric oxide; *VEGF*, vascular endothelial growth factor; *FGF*, fibroblast growth factor; *TGF-β*, transforming growth factor β.

- Signal configuration that couples to Ca^{2+} binding
- In general, tPEMF targets inflammation and accelerates anti-inflammatory activity.
- There are significant amounts of published data regarding tPEMF in humans and laboratory animals—much more than for PEMF alone.
  - Arthritis pain control
  - Pain management
  - Edema resolution
  - Wound healing

ACKNOWLEDGMENTS

I would like to acknowledge Jason T. Smith, PhD, Director of Clinical Affairs, LiteCure LLC, Newark, Delaware, for his help in compiling information on therapeutic laser and pulsed electromagnetic field therapy.

SUGGESTED READINGS

Becker RO, Selden G: The ticklish gene. In The body electric. Electromagnetism and the foundation of life, New York, 1985, William Morrow.

Basford JR: Low-energy laser therapy: Controversies and new research findings. Lasers Surg Med, 1989; 9(1):1–5.

Boopalan PRJVC, Chittaranjan SB, Balamurugan R, et al.: Pulsed electromagnetic field (PEMF) treatment for fracture healing, Curr Orthop Pract, 2009; 20(4):423–428.

Brosseau L, Robinson V, Wells G, et al.: Low level laser therapy (classes I, II and III) for treating rheumatoid arthritis. Cochrane Database Syst Rev, 2005; (4):CD002049.

Brosseau L, Robinson V, Wells G, et al. Low level laser therapy (class III) for treating osteoarthritis. Cochrane Database Syst Rev, 2007; (1):CD002046.

Hellyer PW, et al.: The use of pulsed electromagnetic field (PEMF) therapy to provide postoperative analgesia in the dog. Proceedings of the annual meeting of the American College of Veterinary Anesthesia and Analgesia (abstract), Dallas, Tex., 1999, p 41.

Hug K, Röösli M: Therapeutic effects of whole-body devices applying pulsed electromagnetic fields (PEMF): A systematic literature review. Bioelectromagnetics, 2011; 33(2):95–105. [Epub ahead of print].

Markov MS: Expanding use of pulsed electromagnetic field therapies. Electromagn Biol Med, 2007; 26(3):257–274.

Marks R, de Palma F: Clinical efficacy of low power laser therapy in osteoarthritis. Physiother Res Int, 1999; 4(2):141–157.

Posten W, Wrone DA, Dover JS, et al.: Low-level laser therapy for wound healing: Mechanism and efficacy. Dermatol Surg, 2005; 31(3):334–340.

Puett DW, Griffin MR: Published trials of nonmedicinal and noninvasive therapies for hip and knee osteoarthritis. Ann Intern Med, 1994; 121(2):133–140.

Schneider WL, Hailey D: Low level laser therapy for wound healing. Alberta Heritage Foundation for Medical Research (AHFMR), 1999; 1–23.

Yousefi-Nooraie R, Schonstein E, Heidari K, et al.: Low level laser therapy for nonspecific low-back pain. Cochrane Database Syst Rev, 2008; (2):CD005107.

PART THREE

Application of Concepts and Therapy

CHAPTER 18

Acupuncture

Leilani Alvarez

Acupuncture is a safe and effective means for complementary pain relief. It is a sophisticated and complex form of medicine that employs a whole-body approach and incites the body's endogenous healing mechanisms. It has been practiced for thousands of years and has very few, if any, significant side effects. Acupuncture can be used to treat a variety of medical conditions (Figure 18-1), and there is a growing number of evidence-based studies to support its use. This chapter will focus on the use of acupuncture for pain relief.

HISTORY

Acupuncture has been practiced for over 4000 years in China and other Asian countries. Western cultures rejected acupuncture for many centuries because of discordance with medical knowledge at the time that seemed to contradict philosophical and metaphoric theories of acupuncture. It is only with our more current understanding of neurophysiology that acupuncture has gained acceptance in the Western world. Acupuncture was introduced to the United States in the 1950s but gained popular interest in the 1970s when diplomatic relations with the People's Republic of China improved.[1] The International Veterinary Acupuncture Society was formed in 1974 and has been training veterinarians in acupuncture ever since, along with other organizations.

Traditional Chinese veterinary medicine (TCVM), which encompasses acupuncture, herbal medicine, and other disciplines, states that disease is caused by an imbalance of energy. When the body is balanced (understood as homeostasis in conventional medicine) health is achieved. There are two principle approaches in TCVM acupuncture: the Eight Principles approach, which is a derivation of *yin-yang*, and the Five Elements approach.[2] Unimpeded flow of *qi* (loosely translated as life force or energy) through channels or pathways, called *meridians*, is essential for health. Acupuncture points along these meridians have specific physiologic functions. Point prescriptions

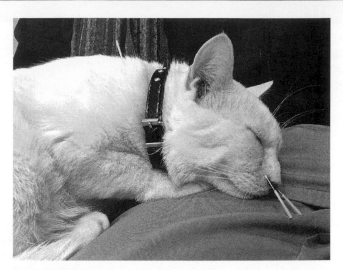

FIGURE 18-1   Demonstration of acupuncture treatment in a cat.

TABLE 18-1	Acupuncture Point Selection for Specific Painful Conditions*
PAINFUL CONDITION	**ACUPUNCTURE POINT**
Mouth or tooth pain	LI 4, ST 4, ST 6, SI 19, TH 10, TH 17, GB 20, ST 44
Neck pain or cervical intervertebral disk disease (IVDD)	GV 14, GV 16, GB 20, BL 10, BL 11, SI 15, TH 10, SI 3, LI 4, TH 5, BL 23, LI 15
Shoulder pain	LI 15, TH 14, BL 11, LI 11, SI 9, SI 3
Elbow pain	LU 5, LI 10, LI 11, TH 10
Carpal pain	LI 4, TH 5, LU 7
Metacarpal phalangeal (MCP) pain	LI 4, TH 3, *Baxie*
Back pain or thoracolumbar IVDD	Local points on the bladder meridian, BL 62, SI 3
Lumbar pain or lumbosacral disease	*Bai-hui, shen-shu, shen-peng, shen-jiao,* BL 23
Coxofemoral pain	GB 29, GB 30, BL 54, *jian-jiao*
Stifle pain	ST 36, ST 35, GB 34, BL 21, *xi-yan*
Tibiotarsal pain	BL 60, KID 3, LIV 3
Metatarsal phalangeal (MTP) pain	LIV 3, ST 44, *Bafeng,* GB 41

*See Appendix 1 for description of point locations.

can be used to address particular painful regions (Table 18-1). There are more than 360 documented acupuncture points in the body, with more than 150 points identified in companion animal medicine. Each point has a specific anatomic location and characteristic effects (see Appendix 1). Acupuncture was studied classically in humans and horses. Acupuncture points in dogs, cats, and other species are transpositional points, in which comparative anatomy was used to identify their location.

EVIDENCE-BASED MEDICINE

Critically reviewed, well-designed studies are largely lacking in the field of veterinary complementary and alternative medicine. As the popularity of acupuncture has grown in human medicine, so has the interest in judicious scientific research to support its efficacy. Several recent randomized controlled trials (RCTs) in humans have demonstrated the effectiveness of acupuncture for specific painful conditions.[3-5]

There is a growing body of evidence for the use of acupuncture as a complementary treatment modality in companion animals. Often the challenges in reporting valid data with regard to acupuncture involve studies with too few subjects, subjective parameters, absence of appropriate blinding, and difficult-to-replicate treatment protocols.[6] There is also the challenge of an appropriate control group, as sham acupuncture has multiple physiologic effects and does not accurately represent a control group.[7]

Human Evidence

Several Cochrane reviews have demonstrated the effectiveness of acupuncture for a wide variety of painful conditions.[4] A systematic review of 29 human RCTs involving acupuncture for the relief of chronic pain conditions including chronic headaches and back, neck, shoulder, and osteoarthritic pain found that acupuncture was superior to sham and no acupuncture control groups.[3] A systematic review of knee osteoarthritis also found that acupuncture was superior to sham acupuncture and standard treatment.[8] Similarly, a Cochrane systematic review of 16 RCTs involving nearly 3500 patients with peripheral joint osteoarthritis showed that patients receiving acupuncture had statistically significant benefits over sham control groups; however, the authors concluded that the benefits were small and likely a result of a placebo effect.[9] A systematic review in 2010, however, concluded that acupuncture is more effective than placebo for chronically occurring painful conditions.[5]

Veterinary Evidence

In a recent randomized controlled clinical trial, dogs that received electroacupuncture (EA) were less likely to require rescue analgesia than dogs receiving sham acupuncture or morphine alone.[10]

In another small study, dogs receiving EA had significantly elevated β-endorphin levels 1 and 3 hours after elective ovariohysterectomy, and effects of analgesia persisted at least 24 hours.[11] In a study comparing 80 paraplegic dogs with thoracolumbar disk herniation that did not undergo surgery, dogs receiving EA and steroids had a faster and higher return to ambulation, reduced back pain, and reduced relapse incidence compared with dogs receiving prednisone alone.[12]

In a controlled clinical trial, dogs undergoing hemilaminectomy for acute disk herniation that received EA in addition to conventional analgesics required significantly lower doses of fentanyl in the first 12 hours postoperatively compared with control groups receiving conventional analgesics alone.[13]

Earlier studies also demonstrated the effectiveness of EA in conjunction with standard care over surgery and conventional treatments alone in dogs with intervertebral disk disease.[14,15] Rigorous evidence-based medicine continues to be insufficient and often inadequate in the veterinary field of complementary and alternative medicine; however, evidence is mounting, especially in the area of acupuncture, and should continue to expand.[16]

MECHANISM OF ACTION

The effects of acupuncture on body systems are vast and complex, and involve multiple pathways that influence the neurologic, musculoskeletal, endocrine, cardiovascular, and immune systems. The focus in this section will be on the pain-relieving and analgesic effects of acupuncture.[17–20]

Anatomy of Acupoints

Acupuncture points are distinct loci in the body that are known to cause specific physiologic effects. They are shallow depressions in the body, typically overlying borders between muscles, tendons, or bones. There has been no definitive evidence demonstrating that acupuncture points (or acupoints) are specific anatomic entities. Many points, however, correlate with known anatomic structures, such as motor end points, and may be classified according to their association with neural structures.[21] Histologically, many acupoints are associated with larger accumulations of mast cells, nerve bundles and plexuses, capillaries, venules, and lymphatics as compared with surrounding tissues.[17] For example, several acupoints along the bladder meridian correspond to branches of the median cutaneous nerve as it enters the dermis along the thoracolumbar spine (Figure 18-2). Acupoints are also known to have lower electrical impedance than surrounding tissues. For this reason, hand-held electric point finders are used for locating and stimulating acupoints. Finally, many acupoints correlate with known trigger point locations.[22]

Local Effects

- Tissue trauma leading to local inflammatory effects including stimulation of the coagulation cascade and release of inflammatory mediators including prostaglandins, leukotrienes, bradykinin, and platelet activating factor (Figure 18-3)
- Release of histamine, heparin, and kinin protease from mast cells, leading to vasodilation
- Stimulation of nociceptive afferent sensory nerve fibers Aδ (group III) and C (group IV)
- Release of trigger points

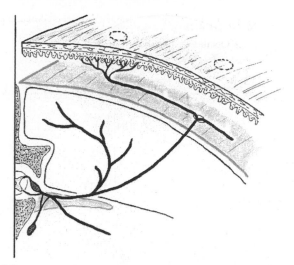

FIGURE 18-2   Cutaneous nerve entering the dermis at an acupuncture point along the bladder meridian. (From Schoen AM: Veterinary acupuncture: ancient art to modern medicine, ed 2, St Louis, 2001, Mosby.)

Neural Mechanisms

Peripheral Nervous System

Nociceptors respond to the noxious mechanical stimulation of needle insertion by transmitting sharp pain (pinprick) sensations via thinly myelinated small diameter Aδ afferent nerve fibers and aching or burning pain via unmyelinated slower-conducting C polymodal fibers (see Figure 18-3). These set off inhibitory pathways along with Aβ afferent stimulation from percutaneous stimulation that block further pain transmission to the brain, as explained by the gate-control theory (see Chapter 3).

Central Nervous System

Stimulation of specific acupuncture points has been shown via magnetic resonance imaging (MRI) to incite changes in focal neuronal activity in the hippocampus, hypothalamus, and other areas of the brain.[23]

The following is a simplistic outline of the central nervous system (CNS) effects of acupuncture (see Figure 18-3):

- Nociceptive Aδ (fast-conducting) and C (slow-conducting) nerve fibers send a signal to the dorsal horn of the spinal cord.
- The message travels up the spinothalamic tract (STT) and spinoreticular tract (SRT) to the brainstem and thalamic nucleus.
- Stimulation of the periaqueductal gray (PAG) and thalamus causes release of multiple endogenous opiate neurotransmitters (endorphins, enkephalins, and dynorphin).

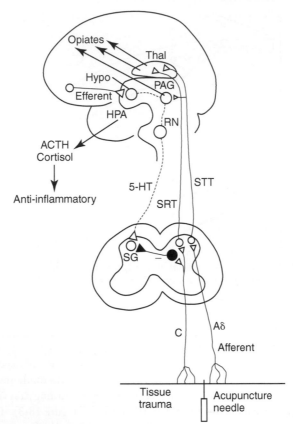

FIGURE 18-3 Acupuncture mechanism of action. When an acupuncture needle pierces the skin, it causes micro tissue trauma, setting off the coagulation cascade and releasing multiple anti-inflammatory mediators. Nociceptive afferent nerves, Aδ (fast conducting) and C polymodal (slow conducting), send signals to the dorsal horn of the spinal cord, synapsing and traveling via the spinothalamic tract *(STT)* and the spinoreticular tract *(SRT)*, respectively, to the thalamus *(Thal)*. The periaqueductal gray *(PAG)* and Thal release opiate peptides in response to ascending nociceptive pathways. Efferent nerves from the prefrontal cortex synapse at the hypothalamus *(Hypo)* and project down the PAG and nucleus raphe *(RN)*, releasing inhibitory mediators serotonin *(5-HT)* and monoamines. These stimulate the substantia gelatinosa *(SG)* region of the dorsal horn of the spinal cord to release enkephalin or dynorphin and inhibit transmission of nociceptive fibers. (Key: *ACTH*, Adrenocorticotropic hormone; *HPA*, hypothalamic-pituitary-adrenal axis.)

- Activation of the hypothalamic-pituitary-adrenal (HPA) axis releases adrenocorticotropic hormone (ACTH), cortisol, and anti-inflammatory mediators with multiple humoral effects.
- Efferent nerves synapse at the hypothalamus and project down the PAG and nucleus raphe (NR), releasing monoamines, serotonin (5-hydroxytryptamine [5-HT]), and norepinephrine.

- Descending pathways activate inhibitory interneurons in the substantia gelatinosa (lamina II) of the dorsal horn of the spinal cord, releasing enkephalin or dynorphin binding to opioid receptors of incoming peripheral nociceptors.
- Activation of opioid receptors inhibits release of substance P and further blocks pain.

Autonomic Nervous System

Stimulation of certain acupuncture points is thought to stimulate internal organs via the sympathetic and parasympathetic nervous systems. Afferent impulses from somatic nerve endings conduct signals to the spinal cord ascending to the hypothalamus and activating a somato-autonomic reflex, which leads to multiple autonomic responses including vasodilation and changes in cardiac output. The acupoint, GV 26, can be used as a resuscitation point because of its sympathetic effects on increasing cardiac output. Auricular acupuncture and ST 36 (overlying the peroneal nerve motor point) have strong parasympathetic effects and positively influence gastrointestinal (GI) transit time. These effects are inhibited with the administration of atropine.[24]

ACUPUNCTURE ANALGESIA

EA may be used effectively to induce analgesia during surgical procedures and postoperatively to reduce the dosage and frequency of pharmaceutical drug administration (Figure 18-4). Effects are thought to result primarily from descending inhibitory pathways. Low-frequency high-intensity EA (2 to 20 Hz) is opioid peptide mediated and has a cumulative effect. High frequency EA (80 to 200 Hz) induces the sympathoadrenal medullary axis, leading to release of serotonin, epinephrine, and norepinephrine, and is noncumulative.[22,25] In addition, EA can effectively control neuropathic pain by disinhibiting central sensitization and wind-up pain.[26,27]

Acupuncture analgesia may be inhibited via the following[19,22]:
- Administration of naloxone for low-frequency EA
- Administration of drugs that block serotonergic receptors
- Local anesthetics injected at the site of acupuncture needle insertion
- Needle insertion in areas of segmental nerve damage

ACUPUNCTURE FOR SPECIFIC CONDITIONS

The practice of acupuncture involves detailed study and advanced clinical training. Point prescriptions afford ease of treatment, especially for the inexperienced acupuncturist; however, the most successful treatments will also take into account TCVM theories and incorporate knowledge of concurrent

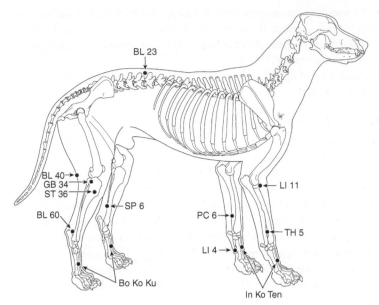

FIGURE 18-4   Locations of various acupuncture points to induce analgesia in dogs.

diseases and a whole-body approach. The information in Table 18-1 is only a guideline for possible treatment strategies for specific painful conditions; other approaches may be successful for particular animals. For all conditions involving musculoskeletal pain, local trigger points should be treated.

FORMS OF ACUPUNCTURE

Dry Needle

A sterile acupuncture needle is inserted into a known acupuncture location. Needles may be stainless steel or silicone coated and may come in individual packages or in bundles of 5 or 10 needle packs (Figure 18-5). A wide variety of needles is available and range in size from 28 to 36 gauge (which is less than a millimeter) and ½ inch to 2 inches long for small animals, and 20 to 32 gauge, ½ inch to 3½ inches long for large animals (Figure 18-6).

Aquapuncture

In aquapuncture, sterile solution is injected into acupuncture points via large-gauge hypodermic needles (typically 25 gauge) to provide prolonged stimulation to the point. The point is distended with the solution and swells the point, providing a more subtle but longer-lasting type of stimulation to the acupoint. Effects are likely to last as long as it takes the body to resorb the solution, in many cases up to 24 hours (Figure 18-7).

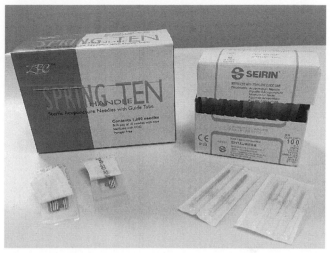

FIGURE 18-5 Examples of acupuncture needles. Acupuncture needles may be stainless steel *(left)* or silicone coated *(right)* and may come in bulk packages *(left)* or individually packaged *(right)*.

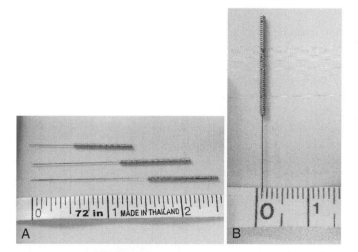

FIGURE 18-6 Acupuncture needle sizes.

Any sterile solution may be employed. Examples include the following:
- Vitamin B_{12}
- Adequan
- Lidocaine or other analgesics
- Saline
- Homeopathic solutions
- Autologous blood products

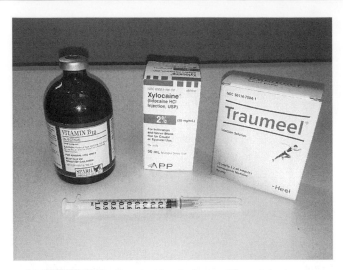

FIGURE 18-7 Examples of medications used for aquapuncture.

Electroacupuncture

Electrical leads are attached to stainless steel acupuncture needles that are already in place, and an electric current is applied to provide increased stimulation to the acupuncture points. The current (direct or alternating), frequency (Hz), mode (continuous, intermittent, dispense or disperse), and amplitude are set according to the specific condition being treated. Electroacupuncture (EA) affords a longer-lasting treatment than dry-needle treatment alone and can provide profound analgesic effects (Figure 18-8).

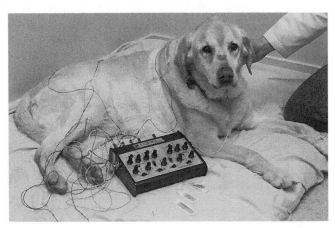

FIGURE 18-8 Demonstration of a dog receiving electroacupuncture treatment.

Trigger Point Acupuncture

Myofascial trigger points (MTrPs) are hyper-reactive taut bands or nodules found in skeletal muscles that elicit a characteristic twitch response on palpation and cause referred pain.[6,28] MTrPs may be caused by multiple factors including direct trauma, chronic or repetitive overuse of the muscle, or psychological stress. The noxious stimuli relayed by trigger points are known to be one of the most common causes of musculoskeletal pain, yet they are largely underdiagnosed and undertreated.[22] Inactivation of MTrPs can be achieved via insertion of an acupuncture needle directly at the site of the trigger point. Dry needling of MTrPs can offer immediate and long-lasting relief of chronic soft-tissue pain. Needling of sensitive areas in the body such as MTrPs may correlate with the acupuncture technique of needling "*Ashi*" points, which are defined as tender or sensitive points. As demonstrated by studies by Melzack and colleagues in 1981 and Dosher in 2006, there is significant overlap between MTrPs and acupuncture points.[28] Although MTrPs can vary in location, there are well documented areas in the body where trigger points commonly occur. Many acupuncture points have been found to correlate with common trigger point locations (Table 18-2). In addition, it is likely that most Ashi points are actually trigger points. Sterile solutions may be injected into MTrPs to deactivate them in the same manner as aquapuncture.

Laser Acustimulation

Low-level laser therapy (LLLT) devices may be used to stimulate individual acupuncture points in patients and animals that do not tolerate needling. Typically, 1 to 2 Joules/cm^2 are administered per point, using wavelengths in the range of 660 to 904 nm. Treatments times are fast, and treatment is effective and well tolerated. LLLT may also be used to treat trigger points.

Moxibustion

The process of moxibustion involves burning the herb *Artemisia vulgaris* or "mugwort," a species of chrysanthemum. A tightly wound roll, called a *moxa stick,* or other forms may be used to provide heat stimulation directly to the

TABLE 18-2	Acupuncture Points in the Dog Correlating With Trigger Points[1]
ACUPOINT	**LOCATION OF TRIGGER POINT CORRELATE**
GB 34	Peroneus longus trigger point
GB 29	Gluteus medius trigger point
ST 36	Cranial tibialis trigger point
SI 9	Triceps trigger point
Local bladder points	Longissimus thoracis and lumborum trigger points
LIV 10 and LIV 11	Adductor-pectineus trigger point

acupoint or applied to the needle for secondary warming. Care must be used to avoid overheating or burning the skin surface.

Acupressure

Digital pressure is applied to the acupoint to stimulate the area. Pressure should be applied for several minutes to each point. Effects are generally shorter lasting than with other methods.

Implantation

Gold beads or other sterile products may be implanted at the site of acupoints for permanent stimulation. Prospective, double-blind clinical trials in veterinary medicine have failed to demonstrate the benefit of gold wire or gold bead implantation for the treatment of canine hip dysplasia.[29,30]

SIDE EFFECTS AND PRECAUTIONS

Acupuncture when practiced by certified and qualified veterinarians is one of the safest medical modalities for pain relief. Adverse events are rare.

The most common side effects include the following:

- Early return to function and possible overuse of injured or traumatized limb
- Sedation
- Masking of symptoms
- Local pain, soreness, numbing, or a tingling sensation, commonly called the *"de-qi" effect*, which is short lasting and usually resolves immediately after treatment
- Erythema and local skin reaction; less commonly, minor bleeding at the site of needle insertion

  Contraindications and precautions include the following[6,27]:

- Bleeding tendencies (coagulopathy, thrombocytopathy)
- Needling infected or highly inflamed skin
- Electroacupuncture in those with pacemakers, arrhythmias, or seizure tendency
- Needling directly through or around a known malignant tumor (NOTE: Distant needling for palliative pain relief or relief of side effects of chemotherapy and radiation is effective and indicated for those with cancer.)
- Caution should be used in fractious or resistant animals to prevent inappropriate needle placement that could lead to tissue trauma, organ puncture, or nerve or blood vessel laceration

ACUPUNCTURE TRAINING

Acupuncture on animals should be practiced by qualified veterinarians who have successfully completed training and acquired certification. Veterinary

TABLE **18-3**	Programs for Veterinary Acupuncture Certification		
NAME	**LOCATION**	**COURSE LEADER**	**CONTACT**
International Veterinary Acupuncture Society (IVAS)	Varies every year nationwide Also offered internationally	Multiple	1730 South College Ave, Suite 301 Fort Collins, CO 80525 (970) 266-0666 Fax: (970) 266-0777 office@ivas.org www.ivas.org
Chi Institute	Reddick, Florida	Huisheng Xie	9700 West Hwy 318 Reddick, FL 32686 (800) 891-1986 Fax: (866) 700-8772 register@tcvm.com www.tcvm.com
Medical Acupuncture for Veterinarians	Colorado State University College of Veterinary Medicine	Narda Robinson	Colorado Veterinary Medical Association 191 Yuma St Denver, CO 80223 (303) 318-0447 Fax: (303) 318-0450 Narda.Robinson@colostate.edu www.colovma.org

acupuncture is practiced exclusively by licensed veterinarians, unlike human acupuncture, in which licensed acupuncturists are generally not medical doctors. The training involves approximately 6 months of study and additional clinical practice and may be completed at one of three institutions (Table 18-3).

CONCLUSION

In a world of rapidly developing pharmaceutical drugs for pain management, an animal may be subjected to medications that have been used for less than a decade. The medication may lack formal study in the species receiving the medication, and often the drug interactions and side effects are significant or poorly understood. In contrast, acupuncture embodies thousands of years of safe and effective use, and a growing number of evidence-based studies support its use. Acupuncture should be part of a multimodal pain management program standard for all veterinary patients.

REFERENCES

1. Schoen AM. Veterinary acupuncture: Ancient art to modern medicine, ed 2, St. Louis, 2001, Mosby.
2. Maciocia G. The foundations of Chinese medicine: A comprehensive text for acupuncturists and herbalists, ed 2, London, 2005, Churchill Livingstone.

3. Vickers AJ, Cronin AM, Maschino AC, et al. Acupuncture for chronic pain: Individual patient data meta-analysis. Arch Intern Med. 172:1444–1453, 2012.

4. Lee MS, Ernst E. Acupuncture for pain: An overview of Cochrane reviews. Chin J Integr Med. 17:187–189, 2011.

5. Hopton A, MacPherson H. Acupuncture for chronic pain: Is acupuncture more than an effective placebo? A systematic review of pooled data from meta-analyses. Pain Pract. 10:94–102, 2010.

6. Filshie J, White A. Medical Acupuncture: A Western scientific approach, London, 1998, Churchill Livingstone.

7. Maciocia G. The practice of Chinese medicine: The treatment of diseases with acupuncture and Chinese herbs, ed 2, 2008, Churchill Livingstone.

8. Cao L, Zhang XL, Gao YS, Jiang Y. Needle acupuncture for osteoarthritis of the knee. A systematic review and updated meta-analysis. Saudi Med J. 33:526–532, 2012.

9. Manheimer E, Cheng K, Linde K, et al. Acupuncture for peripheral joint osteoarthritis. Cochrane Database Syst Rev: Art. No. CD001977.

10. Gakiya HH, Silva DA, Gomes J, et al. Electroacupuncture versus morphine for the postoperative control pain in dogs. Acta Cir Bras. 26:346–351, 2011.

11. Groppetti D, Pecile AM, Sacerdote P, et al. Effectiveness of electroacupuncture analgesia compared with opioid administration in a dog model: A pilot study. Br J Anaesth 107:612–618, 2011.

12. Han HJ, Yoon HY, Kim JY, et al. Clinical effect of additional electroacupuncture on thoracolumbar intervertebral disc herniation in 80 paraplegic dogs. Am J Chin Med. 38:1015–1025, 2010.

13. Laim A, Jaggy A, Forterre F, et al. Effects of adjunct electroacupuncture on severity of postoperative pain in dogs undergoing hemilaminectomy because of acute thoracolumbar intervertebral disk disease. J Am Vet Med Assoc. 234:1141–1146, 2009.

14. Joaquim JG, Luna SP, Brondani JT, et al. Comparison of decompressive surgery, electroacupuncture, and decompressive surgery followed by electroacupuncture for the treatment of dogs with intervertebral disk disease with long-standing severe deficits. J Am Vet Med Assoc. 236:1225–1229, 2010.

15. Hayashi AM, Matera JM, Fonseca Pinto AC. Evaluation of electroacupuncture treatment for thoracolumbar intervertebral disk disease in dogs. J Am Vet Med Assoc. 231:913–918, 2007.

16. Arlt S, Heuwieser W. Evidence-based complementary and alternative veterinary medicine—a contradiction in terms? Berl Munch Tierarztl Wochenschr. 123:377–384, 2010.

17. Steiss JE. The neurophysiologic basis of acupuncture. In: Schoen AM, editor: Veterinary acupuncture: Ancient art to modern medicine, ed 2, St. Louis, 2001, Mosby.

18. Kendall DE. Parts I and II. A scientific model of acupuncture. Am J Acupunct. 17:251–268, 343–360, 1989.

19. Bowsher D. Mechanisms of acupuncture. In Filshie J and White A, editor: Medical acupuncture: A Western scientific approach, New York, 2006, Churchill Livingstone.

20. Ma YT, Ma M, Cho ZH. Biomedical acupuncture for pain management: An integrative approach, Philadelphia, 2005, Elsevier.

21. Gunn CC. Acupuncture loci: A proposal for their classification according to their relationship to known neural structures. Am J Clin Med. 4:183–195, 1976.

22. Baldry PE. Acupuncture, trigger points and musculoskeletal pain. Brookline, 2000, Churchill Livingstone.

23. Chiu JH, Cheng HC, Tai CH, et al. Electroacupuncture-induced neural activation detected by use of manganese-enhanced functional magnetic resonance imaging in rabbits. Am J Vet Res. 62:178–182, 2001.

24. Li H, Wang YP. Effect of auricular acupuncture on gastrointestinal motility and its relationship with vagal activity. Acupunct Med. 31:57–64, 2013.

25. Gaynor JS, Klide AM. Acupuncture for surgical analgesia and postoperative analgesia. In Schoen AM, editor: Veterinary acupuncture: Ancient art to modern medicine, ed 2, St. Louis, 2001, Mosby.

26. Tian S, Wang XY, Ding GH. Repeated electro-acupuncture attenuates chronic visceral hypersensitivity and spinal cord NMDA receptor phosphorylation in a rat irritable bowel syndrome model. Life Sci. 83:356–363, 2008.

27. Cantwell SL. Traditional Chinese veterinary medicine: The mechanism and management of acupuncture for chronic pain. Top Companion Animal Med. 25:53–58, 2010.

28. Dommerholt J, Huijbregts PA: Myofascial trigger points, pathophysiology and evidence-informed diagnosis and management, Sudbury, Mass., 2011, Jones and Bartlett Publishers.

29. Hielm-Bjorkman A, Raekallio M, Kuusela E, et al: Double-blind evaluation of implants of gold wire at acupuncture points in the dog as a treatment for osteoarthritis induced by hip dysplasia. Vet Rec. 149:452–456, 2001.

30. Bolliger C, DeCamp CE, Stajich M, et al: Gait analysis of dogs with hip dysplasia treated with gold bead implantation acupuncture. Vet Comp Orthop Traumatol. 15:116–122, 2002.

31. Xie H, Preast V: Traditional Chinese veterinary medicine: Fundamental principles, 2005, Jing Tang.

APPENDIX 1	Select Small Animal Acupuncture Point Locations and Indications[1,31]	
POINT	**LOCATION**	**INDICATION**
Lung (LU) 5	On the transverse cubital crease, on the lateral side of the biceps brachii tendon (elbow flexed)	Local point for elbow pain, weakness or paralysis of the front leg, fever, respiratory problems
Lung (LU) 7	Medial carpus, proximal to the styloid process of the radius and medial to the tendon of the extensor carpi radialis	Master point of the head and neck Respiratory disorders, neck pain and stiffness, local point for carpal problems
Large intestine (LI) 4	Between the second and third metacarpal (MC) bones, approximately at the middle of the third MC bone on the radial side (Dr. Xie location)	Master point of the face and mouth Strong analgesic and anti-inflammatory point Local point for MC and carpal problems
Large intestine (LI) 10	One sixth the distance from the elbow joint to the carpus, between the extensor carpi radialis and the common digital extensor muscles	Shoulder, elbow, and leg pain
Large intestine (LI) 11	Lateral depression cranial to the flexed elbow, in the transverse cubital crease	Immune stimulation Local point for elbow and shoulder pain
Large intestine (LI) 15	At the shoulder, cranial and distal to the acromion, on the cranial margin of the acromial head of the deltoid muscle	Local point for shoulder pain, atrophy, and paralysis of the forelimb, cervical stiffness
Stomach (ST) 4	On the face, at the lateral corner of the mouth	Toothache, trigeminal neuralgia, facial paralysis
Stomach (ST) 6	On the face, in the depression at the middle of the masseter muscle belly	Toothache, facial paralysis, masseter myositis
Stomach (ST) 35	In the depression below the patella and lateral to the patellar ligament	Local point for stifle pain, cruciate injuries, patellar luxation, rear limb weakness
Stomach (ST) 36	1 cun* from the cranial crest of the tibia, in the belly of the cranial tibialis muscle	Master point of the abdomen All gastrointestinal (GI) disorders, strong analgesic point, local point for stifle problems, rear limb weakness and paralysis
Stomach (ST) 44	In the foot, proximal to the web margin between the second and third toes, in the depression distal and lateral to the second metatarsophalangeal (MTP) joint	Trigeminal neuralgia, local point for MTP joints and rear paws
Small intestine (SI) 3	Proximal to the metacarpal phalangeal (MCP) joint on the lateral side, fifth MC	Cervical, neck, and forelimb pain Combine with BL 62 to treat entire back
Small intestine (SI) 9	In the large depression caudal to the proximal humerus, along the caudal border of deltoid muscle, between the long and lateral heads of the triceps muscle	Shoulder pain, forelimb lameness or paralysis, correlates with common trigger point location

APPENDIX 1	**Select Small Animal Acupuncture Point Locations and Indications—cont'd**	
POINT	**LOCATION**	**INDICATION**
Small intestine (SI) 19	In the face, rostral to the tragus (center) below TH 21 at the caudal border of the mandible	Temporomandibular joint (TMJ) problems, deafness
Bladder (BL) 10	On dorsal aspect of the neck, in the depression at the atlantoaxial junction, medial to the wing of the atlas	Local point for cervical, shoulder, and back pain
Bladder (BL) 11	Midpoint between the spinous process (SP) of the first thoracic vertebra and the medial border of the scapula, 1.5 cun lateral to the SP	Influential point for bone. Arthritis anywhere in the body; neck, shoulder, and back pain
Bladder (BL) 23	1.5 cun lateral to the SP of the second lumbar vertebra	Kidney association point Low back pain, any arthritis, rear limb weakness, IVDD, kidney disease
Bladder (BL) 54	Dorsal to the greater trochanter of the femur	Coxofemoral pain, sciatica, hindlimb weakness and paralysis
Bladder (BL) 60	Large depression between the lateral malleolus of the fibula and the common calcaneal tendon level	Pain or paralysis of the rear limb, low back pain, local point for tarsal pain
Bladder (BL) 62	In the depression directly distal to the lateral malleolus of the fibula	Pain or paralysis of the rear limb, combine with SI 3 to treat entire back
Kidney (KID) 3	In the depression between the medial malleolus of the fibula and the common calcanean tendon (opposite and slightly ventral to BL 60)	Similar to BL 62; kidney problems, deafness, ear problems
Triple heater (TH) 3	On the dorsum of the paw between MC 4 and 5 bones, in the depression proximal to the MCP joint	Local point for carpal and MCP joint pain, deafness, ear problems
Triple heater (TH) 5	2 cun proximal to the carpus, at the distal end of the interosseous space between the radius and ulna	Pain and paralysis of the forelimb, neck and TMJ pain, carpal arthritis, fever
Triple heater (TH) 10	Along the caudal border of the antebrachium, in a depression proximal to the olecranon process	Head, neck, and forelimb disorders, local point for elbow problems, fever, forelimb paralysis
Triple heater (TH) 14	Caudal and distal to the acromion, on the caudal margin of the acromial head of the deltoid muscle	Local point for shoulder problems, radial nerve paralysis
Triple heater (TH) 17	On the face, ventral to the ear in the depression between the mandible and the mastoid process	Pain in TMJ and upper cervical regions, facial paralysis, deafness, ear problems
Gall bladder (GB) 20	At the dorsocranial neck, caudal to the occipital bone, in the depression between the sternomastoideus and sterno-occipitalis muscles	Neck pain and stiffness, cervical IVDD, seizures, and brain disorders

Continued

APPENDIX 1	Select Small Animal Acupuncture Point Locations and Indications—cont'd	
POINT	**LOCATION**	**INDICATION**
Gall bladder (GB) 29	At the hip, one third the distance between the greater trochanter and the cranial dorsal iliac spine	Local point for all hip problems, hindlimb atrophy and paralysis; correlates with gluteus medius trigger point
Gall bladder (GB) 30	At the hip, midway between the greater trochanter and the tuber ischii	Hip problems, sciatic nerve pain or paralysis, biceps femoris muscle problems
Gall bladder (GB) 34	In the depression anterior and distal to the head of the fibula on the lateral side of the hind leg	Influential point for tendons Muscle, tendon, and ligament problems; hindlimb pain and weakness; correlates with trigger point
Gall bladder (GB) 41	In the depression distal to the junction of MT 4 and 5, on the lateral side of the tendon of the extensor digitorum longus muscle	Local point for pain in the MTP area, urinary incontinence
Liver (LIV) 3	On the medial aspect of the second toe proximal to the MTP joint	Soreness in joints, especially medial tibiotarsal joint; liver and gallbladder problems
Governing vessel (GV) 14	On the midline, between the dorsal SPs of the seventh cervical and first thoracic vertebrae	Local cervical and back pain
Governing vessel (GV) 16	On the dorsal midline at the atlanto-occipital joint	Cervical hyperpathia
Bai-hui	In the depression on the dorsal midline just caudal to the wings of the ileum in the L7-S1 space	Hip, lumbar, or pelvic limb disorders
Bafeng	In the web between the toes of the hindlimbs	MTP pain, contracture of hindlimb toes
Baxie	In the web between the toes of the forelimbs	MC phalangeal pain, contracture of forelimb toes
Shen-shu	2 cun lateral to *bai-hui*	Similar to *bai-hui*
Shen-peng	2 cun cranial to *shen-shu*	Similar to *bai-hui*
Shen-jiao	2 cun caudal to *shen-shu*	Similar to *bai-hui*
Jian-jiao	Dorsolateral aspect of the hip, in the depression just ventral to the craniodorsal aspect of the iliac wing	Coxofemoral pain Aquapuncture at this point can provide lasting relief for hip pain
Xi-yan (eye of the knee)	In the depression below the patella, two points—one medial and one lateral to the patellar ligament	Stifle problems, rear limb weakness

*Cun, Unit of measure. In the dog, 8 cun = the distance from umbilicus to xiphoid.

CHAPTER 19

Physical Therapy and Rehabilitation in Dogs

Darryl L. Millis

The use of physical modalities in the treatment of acute and chronic pain has received little attention. The focus of pain management has largely relied on pharmacologic methods, with application of these agents in a number of ways. However, there are other modalities that appear to be efficacious in treating pain, alone or in combination with pharmaceuticals. Commonly used physical modalities include cryotherapy, thermotherapy, massage, physical rehabilitation and therapeutic exercises, transcutaneous electrical nerve stimulation (TENS), low-level laser therapy, extracorporeal shock wave treatment (ESWT), therapeutic ultrasound (US), and pulsed electromagnetic field (PEMF) therapy. Although most of these have their greatest application in the management of chronic pain, such as that from osteoarthritis (OA), some modalities are also useful for adjunctive management of acute pain. This chapter reviews the use of these modalities, potential mechanisms of action, indications, contraindications, and application.

In humans, there is limited but positive evidence that some physical modalities are effective in managing chronic pain associated with specific conditions, with the most support for the modality of therapeutic exercise. Different physical modalities have similar magnitudes of effects on chronic pain. The effect of various modalities on pain is generally strongest in the short term immediately after the intervention, but effects can last as long as 1 year after treatment. Veterinarians applying physical modalities should obtain training that includes the risks of and precautions for these modalities. If practitioners lack training in the use of physical modalities, it is important to consult with other healthcare professionals who have specialized training. Physical therapists have been trained to treat animals with most of the physical modalities discussed in this chapter. Healthcare professionals must be knowledgeable about the strength of evidence underlying the use of physical modalities for the management of pain.

CRYOTHERAPY

Cryotherapy is used to reduce inflammation, pain, and edema, which facilitates improved mobility. Cryotherapy decreases tissue blood flow by causing vasoconstriction and reduces tissue metabolism, oxygen use, and muscle spasm. Treatment with ice provides short-term analgesia and minimizes hematoma formation. Cryotherapy after contusion reduces the number of leukocytes adhering to endothelial cells and should therefore reduce edema.

Cryotherapy

Cold aids pain relief. Cryotherapy has effects locally and at the level of the spinal cord via neurologic and vascular mechanisms.

- Cold temporarily numbs the affected area by constricting the blood vessels.
- Cold raises the activation threshold of tissue nociceptors.
- Nerve cooling also increases the duration of the refractory period, the time when a nerve cannot be stimulated by a second impulse.
- Cold reduces the nerve conduction velocity of pain nerves. This effect is thought to be linear until 10° C, when neural transmission is blocked.
- Cold receptors may be overstimulated by cryotherapy, resulting in pain control at the spinal level by preventing pain transmission to higher centers via the spinal gate-control theory of pain transmission.
- The result is a local anesthetic effect called *cold-induced neurapraxia.*
- Cryotherapy may reduce painful reflex muscle spasms.

Indications for Cryotherapy

Cryotherapy is best applied during the acute inflammatory phase of tissue healing and after exercise to minimize any inflammatory response. Cryotherapy is effective in reducing pain, particularly acute postoperative pain. In addition, cryotherapy is effective in reducing edema when combined with compression and elevation. Cold also decreases the metabolic rate of reactions involved in tissue injury and healing. At joint temperatures of 30° C (86° F) or lower, the activity of cartilage-degrading enzymes (including collagenase, elastase, hyaluronidase, and protease) is inhibited.

Precautions for and Contraindications to Cryotherapy

- If there is a history of frostbite to the area, further cold application is contraindicated. Observe for signs of frostbite during and after cryotherapy application.
- Caution should be exercised when applying cryotherapy around superficial peripheral nerves because cases of cold-induced nerve palsy of the ulnar and superficial peroneal nerves have been reported in humans.
- Cold should also not be used in animals with generalized or localized vascular compromise or who possess an impaired thermoregulatory capacity.
- Use caution in applying cold over open wounds, areas of poor sensation, or in very young or old dogs.

Application of Cryotherapy

Topical cold treatment decreases the temperature of the skin and underlying tissues to a depth of 2 to 4 cm. Techniques for cryotherapy include the application of cold or ice packs, ice bath immersion, and massage with ice over painful areas or acupoints. Cryokinetics combines cryotherapy with motion (passive, active-assisted, or active) to facilitate normal, pain-free movement and to reduce edema through muscle pump action to return lymphatic fluid to the vascular system. The primary benefit of cryokinetics is to facilitate the animal's ability to perform pain-free exercise as long as the level of exercise remains below levels that cause further injury.

To prevent frostbite or cold-induced injuries, it is critical to observe the skin for response to cold. Near the end of a 20-minute treatment, the skin may normally be erythematous, but pale or white skin is an indication that cold-induced tissue damage may be occurring. The range of expected sensations during cryotherapy includes an initial sensation of cold, followed by burn, sting, and ache, and finally a numb sensation. Because animals cannot describe these sensations, careful observation of the animal's behavioral responses and skin condition every few minutes during the treatment session is critical.

Ice Packs

The simplest method of ice application is to wrap a freezer bag containing crushed ice in a thin damp cloth (such as a pillowcase) and apply it directly over the affected area. Another ice pack may be made by combining one-third part isopropyl alcohol and two-thirds part water and placing it in a resealable plastic bag and then in a freezer. The resulting slush more easily conforms to irregular dog extremities (Figure 19-1). A compression wrap to secure the bag to the body results in more effective tissue cooling. Cold compression units are commercially available and combine compression with cryotherapy. Cold water circulates in a fabricated sleeve that is applied to provide compression to the area. To prevent skin damage, apply a towel or cloth to prevent direct contact of the ice pack with the animal's skin. Apply the cryotherapy treatment for 15 to 25 minutes at a time, inspecting the tissue for its response after the first 5 to 10 minutes. Monitor closely for signs of frostbite.

Cold Immersion Baths

Cold immersion results in the greatest decrease in tissue temperature because it exposes the greatest body surface area to cold. The body part is immersed in an ice "slush" bath as part of the immediate first aid after injury. The analgesia from the immersion allows the animal to perform cryokinetics with relative ease.

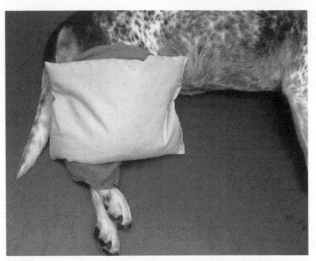

FIGURE 19-1   An ice pack may be wrapped in a thin towel before placement on a dog's limb.

Ice Massage

Ice massage is a quick and effective method of applying cryotherapy to the affected area with the muscle in a position of gentle stretch. Placing tongue depressors in paper cups filled with water and freezing them is a low-cost method to perform ice massage. Ice massage is applied parallel to the muscle fibers. The pressure from the ice massage stimulates mechanoreceptors more than other forms of cryotherapy. This technique is particularly useful for small, irregular areas. Treatment time is generally 5 to 10 minutes or until the affected area is erythematous and numb.

Treatment Duration and Frequency

The duration and frequency of cryotherapy depend on the severity of the injury, the area of injury, and the desired outcome. Treatment times may be cycled to 20 to 45 minutes on, followed by an equal amount of time off. Practically, cryotherapy is typically administered two to six times daily. Cryotherapy may be applied after an exercise session to minimize reactive swelling and pain.

THERMOTHERAPY

Heat therapy, which can be superficial or deep, is like cryotherapy in that it provides analgesia and decreased muscle tonicity. Unlike cryotherapy, thermotherapy increases tissue temperature, blood flow, metabolism, and connective tissue extensibility; aids muscle relaxation; and reduces stiffness. Because heat increases circulation to the affected area, there is some concern that this may worsen inflammation and edema.

Thermotherapy

Heat therapy may reduce pain.

- Heat causes vasodilation, which increases blood flow. This effect may reduce tissue ischemia by supplying oxygen and nutrients while simultaneously removing metabolites that accumulate during tissue damage or exercise.
- Thermoreceptor afferent input may act via the gate-control theory of pain control by acting on the dorsal horn of the spinal cord to block transmission of pain to higher pain centers.
- Heat causes general relaxation of painful muscle spasms.
- Heat may also act on muscle spindles and sensory nerve conduction. A decrease in neuronal activity of secondary nerve endings and an increase in activity of primary nerve endings and Golgi tendon organs have been measured after heat application to nerve endings and muscle spindles. This results in a net inhibition of motor neurons, which helps to break the pain-spasm-pain cycle.

Indications for Thermotherapy

Heat therapy is indicated for animals with chronic pain, especially pain from muscle spasm. Heat is also beneficial for animals in which stretching is indicated to help enhance collagen extensibility.

Contraindications to and Precautions for Superficial Heat Applications

- Superficial heat is contraindicated during acute inflammation (because it may exacerbate the inflammatory process), over an area of subcutaneous or cutaneous hemorrhage, if thrombophlebitis is present, or over malignant tissue.
- Superficial heat should be used with caution in animals with poor thermoregulatory capacity, edema, or impaired circulation or over open wounds.
- Dogs should be monitored closely because they cannot verbalize their intolerance.
- A tissue burn may result if the animal is not able to dissipate the heat load via vasodilation or if too much heat (too hot or too long) is applied. Burns can be avoided by using materials that cool as the treatment progresses, increasing the insulation layer between the animal and the hot pack, or limiting the initial temperature increase.
- Caution should be used with products generating high-intensity heat (greater than 45° C), such as hydrocollator packs or electric heating pads.
- Monitor the skin condition before, during, and after treatment for any adverse effects.

Application of Heat Therapy

Superficial thermal therapy may be applied using commercially available packs containing cornhusks, gel material that can be used for hot or cold application, or iron filings (activation of such packs produces heat for several hours after a chemical reaction results in oxidation). Commercially available wraps may also be used for heat application by placement of heat packs inside the wraps (Figure 19-2).

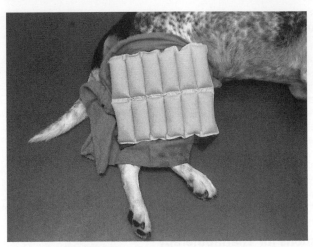

FIGURE 19-2   A hot pack applied to a dog.

Treatment Duration and Frequency

The duration and frequency of thermal treatment depends on the severity of the injury, the stage of tissue healing, the area of the injured part, and the desired outcome. Treatment times may be cycled to 30 to 45 minutes on, followed by an equal amount of time off. Thermal modalities should be applied to support the goal of pain-free function to obtain the best results in the shortest time.

CONTRAST THERMOTHERAPY

Contrast thermotherapy, in which the affected body part is immersed in cold water followed by immersion in hot water, is commonly used in rheumatic conditions and regional pain in humans. Contrast baths induce cyclic vasodilation and vasoconstriction to facilitate flushing debris and inflammatory mediators from the injured area. However, some authors do not agree with this proposed mechanism.

Few research studies have been performed regarding the efficacy of contrast thermotherapy for management of pain, but it is commonly used for sports injuries. Two well-controlled studies have shown that contrast thermotherapy has no effect on muscle tissue temperature.

Indications for and Contraindications to Contrast Thermotherapy

Contrast baths are most appropriate during the early phase of tissue healing or in cases of chronic edema. Clinically, it may be appropriate to use contrast baths during the transition from acute to subacute injury management. Contrast baths are not indicated in the immediate acute inflammatory phase.

Application of Contrast Baths

The body part is immersed in alternating cold and hot baths, in a ratio anywhere from 4 minutes cold–1 minute hot near the end of the acute phase of inflammation to 2 minutes hot–2 minutes cold in the chronic phase of injury. This cycle is repeated three to five times for a total of 15 to 30 minutes. If the injury is relatively acute, the final cycle should be in the cold bath to help reduce edema formation and the cold-hot ratio should be weighted toward longer times in cold. If contrast baths are used before exercise in subacute or chronic conditions, then the final cycle should be in the hot bath.

PHYSICAL REHABILITATION AND THERAPEUTIC EXERCISES

Active and passive exercise programs have been recommended for treatment of chronic pain, particularly OA. Reduced activity and deconditioning lead to decreased muscle mass and strength, loss of endurance, increased joint stiffness, and loss of cardiovascular fitness.

Exercise treatment in OA is useful to reduce pain and disability. This is achieved through improvement of muscle strength, stability of joints, range of motion (ROM), and aerobic fitness. These functions are often impaired in animals with OA, presumably contributing to pain and disability. Improving these functions is assumed to reduce pain and disability.

Application of Physical Rehabilitation

A specific exercise program must be developed for each animal that addresses the animal's impairments and functional needs. Therapeutic exercise should include stretching and ROM, aerobic conditioning, muscle strength and endurance training, and correction of gait abnormalities if possible. Baseline values should be established for exercise time and intensity. Exercise duration and intensity may then be increased in a stepwise fashion until aerobic activity is maintained for 20 to 30 minutes per session. Goals should also be set for any strengthening activities. Although the program should be monitored by the veterinary team, pet owners are encouraged to participate in a home exercise program with the animal. A log of the home exercise program should be maintained by the pet owner and reviewed by the veterinary team at regular intervals.

Massage

Massage has been reported to relieve pain, aid relaxation, and promote a feeling of well-being in humans. In addition to helping to improve lymphatic drainage, circulation, and tissue movement, soft tissue massage is also thought to provide symptomatic relief of pain.

Massage and Pain Relief

Suggested mechanisms of pain relief include the following:
- Relaxation
- Increase in the pain threshold through the release of endorphins and the gate-control theory of pain
- Increase in pain threshold

Massage causes traction at tissue interfaces. Horizontal plexuses lie at interfaces in the tissues, and gentle pulling on these vessels may stimulate the accompanying sympathetic nerves, which supply the mechanoreceptors. These receptors may be distorted by the massage, possibly lowering mechanoreceptor sensitivity and reducing pain and tenderness.

The flushing effect of massage on tissue fluids and removal of inflammatory mediators may increase the speed at which the inflammation resolves in humans with delayed-onset muscle pain after exercise.

Indications for Massage

Massage may be indicated for dogs having surgery to maintain mobility and ease pain, after exercise to reduce muscle soreness, in animals with edema, and in animals with chronic OA to help ease muscle tension.

Precautions for and Contraindications to Massage

- Massage is contraindicated in animals with open wounds, unstable fractures, severe pain, coagulation disorders, infections, or neoplasia.

Application of Massage

- Select a quiet area that is free of interruptions.
- Provide a soft, padded surface for the animal.
- Work in a systematic way.
- The therapist should relax and maintain proper body posture.
- Use larger muscles such as the shoulder muscles instead of the hands to minimize fatigue.
- Massage may be performed on isolated areas or on the entire limb and body. If the dog has a specific condition, local massage may be appropriate on a regular basis. General massage helps with treatment of compensatory conditions and biomechanical changes.

Massage Technique
Stroking

- Use good technique to start the treatment.
- Run hands over the dog from neck to tail and down the limbs with medium pressure.

- This aids in relaxation of the dog and allows assessment of tissues; note muscle tone and any swelling, masses, or temperature differences between body areas.

Effleurage

- Beginning at a distal area, such as the foot, the hands move proximally, using medium pressure.
- This helps to move fluids to the lymph nodes and aids drainage.

Petrissage

- Petrissage promotes muscle relaxation, decreases muscle stiffness, and increases blood flow.
- One rolls or kneads the soft tissues (Figure 19-3).
- Muscle bellies may be lifted and rolled.

Trigger Point Therapy

- Trigger point therapy is used for small areas of spasm felt within a muscle belly.
- Nodules are located, and ischemic compression is applied using one or two fingers.
- Compression is held for approximately 20 seconds and released for 10 seconds before reapplication of compression.
- In general, three or four repetitions may be required.

Joint Mobility

Normal ROM should be established as much as possible. Joint mobility, muscle tightness, and muscle weakness must be addressed for establishment of more normal ROM. OA often results in joint stiffness, and muscles secondarily become stiff and shortened. If this process continues, there is a cycle

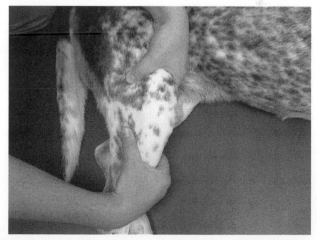

FIGURE 19-3   Applying petrissage massage technique to the caudal thigh muscles of a dog.

of continued weakness, tightness, abnormal movement, and pain. Treatment consists of ROM and stretching exercises.

Passive Range of Motion

- Treatment should be administered in a quiet and comfortable area, away from distractions, such as loud noises, other pets, and other persons who are not helping with the treatment.
- A muzzle should be applied for initial treatments or if the dog is in pain, resistant to treatment, or overly anxious.
- The animal is placed in lateral recumbency with the affected limb up. Help may be required to restrain the animal and to help keep it quiet and relaxed. In all forms of ROM activities, the therapist should be comfortable and use proper body mechanics to avoid injury to himself or herself.
- Place one hand on the limb above the joint. Place the other hand on the limb below the affected joint. Be certain that the entire limb is supported to avoid any undue stress to the involved joint (Figure 19-4).
- Begin by slowly and gently flexing the joint. The other joints of the limb should be allowed to remain in a neutral position (a position as if the animal were standing). Try not to move the other joints while working on the affected joint because some joints may be restricted by the position of the joints above or below the target joint. Slowly continue to flex the joint until the animal shows initial signs of discomfort, such as tensing the limb, moving, turning the head toward the therapist, or trying to pull away, but do not cause undue discomfort, such as causing the dog to vocalize.
- With the hands maintained in the same positions, slowly extend the joint. Again, try to keep the other joints in a neutral position and minimize any

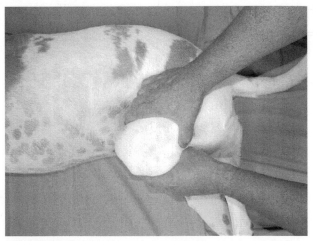

FIGURE 19-4 Placement of hands for passive range of motion to a dog's stifle.

movement of the other joints. Slowly continue to extend the joint until the animal shows initial signs of discomfort.

- Alternatively, a number of joints may be simultaneously placed through a ROM, a technique sometimes referred to as *ROM through functional patterns*. This form of ROM exercises may be appropriate as an animal nears active use of a limb. Flexing and extending all of the joints of a limb in a pattern that mimics a normal or exaggerated gait pattern may also be beneficial for neuromuscular reeducation.

- For most routine conditions, 15 to 20 repetitions performed two to four times per day are adequate. As the ROM returns to normal, the frequency may be reduced.

- Also important is to maintain normal ROM in the other joints of the affected limb.

Stretching

Stretching is often combined with ROM exercises to increase flexibility of tissues. Performance of some low-intensity active exercise is beneficial before stretching if possible. Application of superficial heat or therapeutic US before stretching may improve tissue extensibility. If the tissues are warmed first, less damage to the tissues may occur. The combination of muscles, tendons, skin, and joint capsule should be considered, and their relative contributions to restricted motion should be assessed. For example, the target tissue for lengthening a muscle that is contracted is the muscle belly, not the tendon.

- The animal should be in a comfortable position, which is generally in lateral recumbency, and should be on a padded surface. The animal should be as relaxed as possible, and in some cases, mild sedation or tranquilization may be beneficial.

- One hand should stabilize the bone proximal to the joint, and the other should stabilize the bone distal to the joint. The distal bone should be moved relative to the proximal bone.

- The affected joint should be slowly placed through one end of a ROM (usually beginning in flexion) until a restriction to motion is felt. Very gentle traction may be applied to the joint during slow stretching to the point of initial restriction.

- The animal may indicate that it feels mild discomfort, such as by turning the head or mildly tensing the muscles in the affected limb. Under no circumstances should more severe pain be inflicted, which might be indicated by vocalization or an attempt to bite.

- The stretch should be prolonged, ideally for at least 15 but no longer than 30 seconds. During the stretch, a conscious effort should be made to try to increase the joint excursion without increasing the level of discomfort. There should be no bouncing motions during the stretch.

- After the stretch at one end of the motion range, the pressure is slowly released and the opposite end of the ROM should be stretched.
- Each muscle group should be stretched three to five times in a session before other activities begin.
- The therapist should be patient and not try to achieve full ROM in one or two sessions. The ideal daily frequency of stretching is unknown for dogs. In general, two to four sessions per day may initially be required, with the frequency decreased as normal ROM and tissue extensibility improve. The process must be applied consistently and regularly for good results, and it may take 2 to 3 weeks to see noticeable improvement.

Active Range of Motion

More active ROM exercises may be initiated to encourage voluntary joint motion through a wider range than is typically achieved with only walking or trotting. Joint ROM is limited during normal walking and trotting, so the joints do not go through a complete normal ROM. If joint restriction is present, animals may benefit from performance of activities that encourage a more complete ROM.

- Swimming or walking in water results in greater flexion of joints and greater ROM. Decreased joint extension may occur with swimming, but walking in water maintains relatively normal active joint extension while increasing joint flexion, resulting in greater overall joint ROM.
- Other activities that may be performed include walking in snow, sand, or tall grass and crawling through a play tunnel.
- Climbing stairs may increase joint excursion while also increasing strength.
- Walking over cavaletti rails is an excellent method of achieving normal limb extension for walking while increasing joint flexion and overall ROM of the elbow, stifle, and tarsal joints as the dog negotiates the rails. In addition, the rails may be raised or lowered to encourage increased or decreased joint flexion, based on the needs of the individual animal.

Therapeutic Exercises

Strength and endurance improve if the level of exercise provides stress to tissues so that adaptation occurs with avoidance of excessive loading that may exacerbate structural weaknesses. In general, endurance, cardiovascular fitness, and obesity are initially addressed through endurance activities. It is critical to be certain that joints are stable before initiation of an exercise program. For example, performing weight-bearing exercises on a limb with a cranial cruciate ligament rupture hastens the development of OA.

- The level of activities is modified by *first increasing the frequency* of the activity, with adequate rest periods between sessions.

- Pet owners should be warned that animals may initially experience increased muscle soreness, discomfort, and fatigue for the first week or two, but care should be taken to be certain that joint inflammation is not exacerbated.
- After appropriate adaptation and conditioning have occurred at this level of activity, the *length of the activities* may be increased to provide further challenges.
- Finally, additional strength and conditioning may be achieved by *increasing the speed* of activities and *adding strengthening exercises.*

Daily exercise is preferable to exercise only once or twice a week. Caution should be used early in the exercise period to avoid overuse injuries and pain after exercise. In general, animals should begin with a conservative exercise program. Depending on the level of the disability and deconditioning, two exercise periods per day may be enough. If lameness and pain are not exacerbated at this level, exercise may be increased to three periods per day the next week, and four periods per day the following week, with care taken to ensure that lameness and pain are not increasing.

Chronic pain is not a static condition, and exercise periods must adapt to occasional "bad days." The level of activity should be decreased on days of worsened pain or lameness because forced exercise may exacerbate the inflammatory process in arthritic joints. When the degree of pain and lameness return to previous levels, the activity may be increased more gradually. The next step should be to increase the length of the walks.

A reasonable rule of thumb is to increase the length of activity by 10% to 15% per week, being vigilant for any exacerbation of pain or lameness; if pain or lameness is noted, the level of activity is decreased by 50% until the animal returns to baseline, and then the level of activity is increased more gradually.

Controlled leash walking, walking on a treadmill, jogging, swimming, and going up and down stairs or ramp inclines are excellent low-impact exercises. The length of the exercise should be titrated so there is no increased pain after activity. Also, it is better in the early phases of training to provide three 10-minute sessions rather than one 30-minute session. Avoiding sudden bursts of activity helps avoid acute inflammation of arthritic joints.

Slow Walks
- Slow leash walks are perhaps the most important therapeutic exercise for animals with debilitating chronic diseases. These walks are also frequently performed incorrectly.
- Leash walks must be performed very slowly to allow the dog to bear weight without undue stress on painful joints.
- Leash walks must be performed according to the speed of the dog, not the handler.

- Leash walks are performed for only 5 minutes, two or three times daily to begin. If the lameness or limb use is not worse after the first couple of days, the length and time of the walks may be gradually increased by 1 to 3 minutes per session every few days.
- Dogs may be walked up and down inclines, hills, or ramps to add more challenges and to encourage muscular and cardiovascular fitness.

Treadmill Walking

- Treadmill walking reduces stress and pain of limb movement in some conditions, such as the pain of hip extension in dogs with hip dysplasia or the pain of stifle extension after repair of a cranial cruciate ligament.
- Most dogs trained to leash readily take to treadmill walking.
- Many treadmills are available, and some models for humans may be adapted for canine use.
- A harness to provide support and prevent falls, side walls to prevent stepping off the treadmill, variable speed of the treadmill, a timer, and the ability to change the incline angle are useful features for canine treadmills.
- Do not face the treadmill toward a wall; have it face down a hallway or toward the middle of a room.
- One person may be in front of the dog to encourage it or provide treats.
- One person may stand over the dog to help keep it moving straight.
- A sling may be used to help support especially weak dogs.
- The treadmill may be angled up or down to reduce or increase stress on the forelimbs or rear limbs.
- Joint motion is similar between walking on a treadmill and normal walking over ground, but the treadmill provides some active assistance for movement of painful joints. In addition, the stance time of weight bearing is greater on a treadmill.

Ramp Walking and Stair Climbing

- Ramp walking and stair climbing are useful to improve power in rear limb extensors.
- The dog may begin ramp walking or stair climbing if the dog is consistently using the limb at a walk with decreasing lameness over time.
- Exercises must begin slowly to encourage proper use of rear limbs. The dog should step up with each limb rather than skipping up steps or jumping up steps by using both rear limbs ("bunny hopping") (Figure 19-5).
- This therapy is best started with ramp walking, then low, gradually rising steps, and progressing to increasingly steeper steps.
- Begin with ramp walking for 5 minutes, then five to seven steps, and increase to two to four flights once to three times daily.

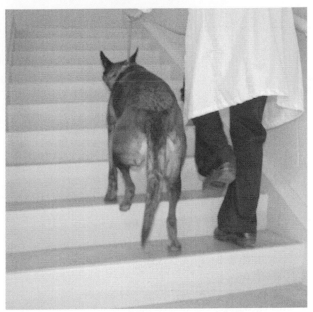

FIGURE 19-5   Dogs may begin slowly walking up stairs for strengthening and active range of motion if the surgical repair (if surgery has been performed) is stable and the dog is increasingly less lame with lower level rehabilitation activities such as leash walking.

Jogging

- Jogging may be initiated in many cases in dogs that are walking on the limb with minimal lameness and pain.
- Begin jogging slowly to improve muscle strength and cardiovascular fitness—2 to 3 minutes two or three times daily, increasing up to 20 minutes two to four times daily.
- Be certain that lameness is not worse after jogging. If so, the dog should rest for several days and receive anti-inflammatory medication; and when jogging is reinitiated, it should be at slower speeds and for less time.
- The dog may jog up hills for greater effect if there are no problems jogging on flat surfaces.

Sit-to-Stand Exercises

- Sit-to-stand exercises help to strengthen hip and stifle extensors without causing extension of the hip, stifle, and hock more than is achieved with walking. The exercises may be beneficial for dogs with hip dysplasia, in which full extension of the hips is painful.
- Sit-to-stand exercises should be combined with training, occasionally using a low-calorie treat.

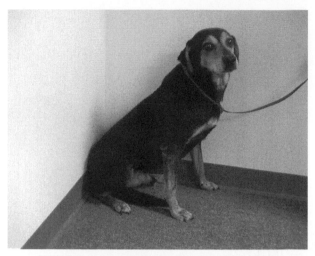

FIGURE 19-6 Proper positioning for sit-to-stand exercises.

- It may be easier to back the dog into a corner, with the affected leg against a wall. This encourages the dog to push up evenly with both rear limbs when rising, and not push up with a good leg while pushing the affected leg out away from the body (Figure 19-6).
- The handler should concentrate on having the dog sit and stand correctly, with both rear limbs flexing equally while sitting, and pushing off evenly with both rear limbs to stand.
- Start with 5 to 10 repetitions once or twice daily, and work up to 15 repetitions three or four times daily.

Wheelbarrowing

- Wheelbarrowing exercises are designed to improve use of the forelimbs and strengthen the weight-bearing muscles.
- The rear limbs are lifted off of the ground through support of the abdomen, and the dog is moved forward. Dogs with normal proprioception will move the forelimbs so that they do not fall (Figure 19-7).
- Some dogs with weakness of the forelimbs may require support to prevent them from collapsing.
- As dogs become stronger and endurance improves, they may be wheelbarrowed up and down inclines for greater effect.

Dancing Exercises

- Dancing exercises are designed to improve use and strength of the rear limbs.
- Because it may be difficult to encourage some dogs to exercise on an affected limb, it is recommended to apply a muzzle to the dog.

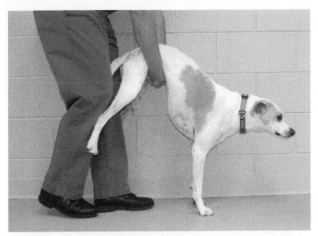

FIGURE 19-7   Wheelbarrowing for strengthening of forelimb muscles.

- The forelimbs are lifted off the ground, and the dog is moved forward or backward. Dogs with normal proprioception will move the limbs so that they do not fall.
- Most dogs dance forward, but others may stretch until they are nearly on the ground. In these situations, the handler should get behind dog and place the arms under the axillary region of the dog to support it and walk forward.
  - Forward dancing results in less extension of the hip joint and may be beneficial for dogs with painful hips. Backward dancing results in a more vertical position of the dog, and hip joint extension is much greater compared with forward dancing.
- As dogs become stronger and endurance improves, they may dance up and down inclines for greater effect.

Cavaletti Rails
- Cavaletti rails are raised rails or poles that are spaced apart on the ground. In some cases a ladder that is laying on the ground may act as cavaletti rails (Figure 19-8).
- Cavaletti rails are useful to help with increasing stride length, limb use, and active ROM of joints.
- The height of the rails may be raised to encourage greater active flexion and extension of the elbow, stifle, and tarsal joints, but care should be taken to prevent jumping over the rails.
- The rails are spaced equally or with varying widths. Initially it is a good idea to space the rails equally, somewhat less than the normal stride length of the animal. As the animal's condition improves, the rails may be spaced at varying distances to provide challenges to proprioception, or they may be spaced farther apart to encourage a longer stride length.

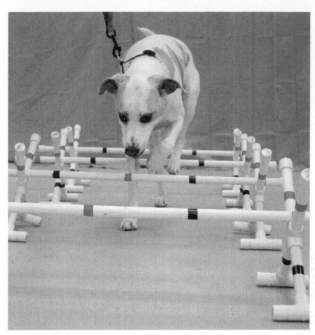

FIGURE 19-8   Walking over cavaletti rails increases active flexion of the elbow, stifle, and tarsal.

Pole Weaving

- Weaving back and forth between vertical poles is an exercise that is useful for encouraging lateral flexion of the spinal column, proprioceptive training, and weight shifting during gait to encourage use of limbs and strengthening of muscles in preparation for more challenging exercises, such as turning sharply while running.
- A series of vertical poles is placed in a straight line.
- The distance between the poles should be less than the length of the dog to encourage lateral bending of the spinal column and weight shifting.

Muscle-Strengthening Activities

Exercises that concentrate on strengthening muscles are designed to improve power and speed. These exercises include pulling or carrying weights, working against elastic bands, playing ball, and running for short distances at high speed.

Pulling or Carrying Weights

- Pulling or carrying weight is a method of increasing the force that muscles must use and encourages muscle strengthening. These exercises are similar to weight lifting in humans.

- Many harnesses are available to pull sleds or carts. The harnesses should be well designed and padded and should fit the animal very well to avoid problems with pressure sores. Dogs may pull various weights, depending on the stage of recovery and the dog's strength.
- The position of the dog's head and neck is important when the animal is pulling weight. If strengthening of the forelimb muscles is desired, the dog's head should be lower than the back to encourage transfer of weight to forelimbs to allow pulling; if strengthening of the rear limb muscles is desired, the dog's head should be higher than the back to encourage transfer of weight to the rear limbs to allow the animal to drive off the rear limbs for pulling weight.
- Backpacks are also available, and various weights may be placed in the backpack to allow strengthening of multiple muscle groups.
- Strap-on leg weights may be used to help strengthen flexor muscles during gait. Initially, the weights should be placed relatively proximally on the limb to reduce the muscle force and stress on joints during the early rehabilitation period. As strength and stamina improve, the weights may be moved further distally to provide more challenges. In general, 0.25-kg, 0.5-kg, 1-kg, and 2-kg weights may be used for small, medium, large, and very large dogs, respectively.

Elastic Bands
- Elastic bands of various stiffness are available and may be fastened to a dog's limb to provide resistance while it walks.
- It is important that the resistance not be so great that the normal gait is hindered; rather, the therapist should provide mild resistance to allow the dog to walk or jog normally.
- The band should be held parallel and close to the ground to allow normal joint flexion and extension.
- Elastic bands may also be used with treadmill walking (Figure 19-9).

Controlled Ball Playing
- Controlled ball playing is a fun activity for dogs and their owners and is an excellent method to establish strength and speed. However, control and gradual introduction of ball playing are essential to avoid reinjury.
- Begin ball playing on a relatively short leash or in an enclosed kennel or room to avoid overly explosive activity in the early postoperative period.
- Progress to ball playing in an enclosed area, such as a small dog run or room.
- As the animal nears full return to function, activity on a long leash is instituted, and if there are no problems, off-leash activity is introduced in a safe environment.

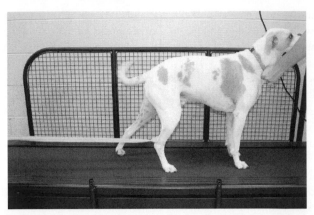

FIGURE 19-9   Elastic bands may be placed on a dog's limb while the dog walks on a treadmill to provide resistance during walking.

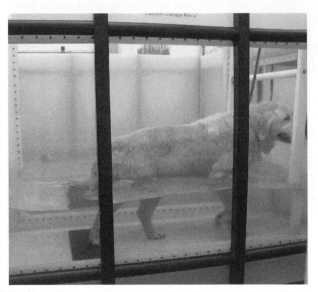

FIGURE 19-10   Walking on an underwater treadmill provides buoyancy for painful joints and results in increased active joint movement compared with walking over ground.

Swimming and walking in water are some of the best activities for dogs with chronic OA (Figure 19-10). The buoyancy of water is significant and limits the impact on the joint while the exercise promotes muscle strength and tone and joint motion. Training on an underwater treadmill may increase peak weight-bearing forces by 5% to 15% in a short period of training, which is comparable to achievements obtained using medication in many animals.

After exercise, a 10-minute warm-down period allows muscles to cool down. A slower-paced walk may be initiated for 5 minutes, followed by ROM and stretching exercises. A cool-down massage may help decrease pain, swelling, and muscle spasms. Finally, cryotherapy may be applied to painful areas for 15 to 20 minutes to control postexercise inflammation.

TRANSCUTANEOUS ELECTRICAL NERVE STIMULATION

TENS is an inexpensive, safe, noninvasive modality with few side effects that can be used to treat a variety of painful conditions. The clinical application of TENS involves the delivery of an electrical current, usually from a small battery-operated device, to the skin by surface electrodes. A variety of stimulators are available with a wide range of stimulation parameters to choose from, including frequency, intensity, pulse duration, and electrode placement sites.

Three important factors that determine the quality of TENS application include (1) the type of device (e.g., stimulators, electrode type, and design); (2) the wave form of the device, which is modified by adjusting the amplitude, rate, and width controls; and (3) the proper location of electrodes. Although four types of TENS device settings are currently used in human clinical practice, high-frequency (40- to 150-Hz, 50- to 100-microsecond pulse width, low to moderate intensity) or conventional TENS stimulators are most commonly used in animals because these stimulators are more comfortable and create less anxiety in small animals.

Transcutaneous Electrical Nerve Stimulation

- Transcutaneous electrical nerve stimulation (TENS) provides analgesia by several potential mechanisms of action.
- Conventional TENS provides peripheral stimulation with electrical impulses that activate non-noxious large myelinated afferent Aβ nerve fibers in the skin and inhibit small unmyelinated C fibers within the dorsal horn of the spinal cord.
- This gate theory is based on the principle that there is a gateway in the dorsal horn of the spinal cord that regulates the flow of pain signals that are ascending by small-diameter afferent nerve fibers and descending from higher levels of the brain for central processing, thus reducing the perception of pain.
- Most devices have a stimulation of approximately 100 Hz, which is thought to be comfortable to most persons. Individuals describe a "pins-and-needles" sensation under the electrodes, resulting in paresthesia.
- Some TENS units produce a more noxious high-intensity stimulus at 2 Hz. This stimulates small-diameter afferent fibers and results in the release of endogenous opiates and pain relief by stimulating the descending pain-inhibiting pathway.
- Different frequencies of TENS may act through different neurotransmitter systems.

Continued

Transcutaneous Electrical Nerve Stimulation—cont'd

- Low-frequency TENS analgesia may be mediated by activation of serotonin and µ opioid receptors, whereas conventional TENS activates δ opioid receptors. However, conclusive evidence regarding the more effective method of TENS is lacking. Five studies comparing conventional TENS and low-frequency TENS found no differences in pain-reducing effect.
- Pulse duration and stimulus intensity are also factors in providing analgesia. Greater analgesia has been achieved by increasing the stimulus intensity or pulse duration.
- Electrode placement may also influence the effectiveness of TENS. In general, electrodes are placed over the painful region.

Indications for Transcutaneous Electrical Nerve Stimulation

TENS is a form of neuromuscular electrical stimulation (NMES). TENS is used for pain control, primarily in chronic conditions but possibly also in acute conditions. Other forms of NMES are commonly used in the rehabilitation of animals that have had orthopedic or neurologic injury, such as fracture repair, cruciate ligament reconstruction, and meniscal debridement or repair. Animals that have neurologic conditions, such as cerebrovascular accidents, closed head injuries, spinal cord injuries, or other neurologic disease involving paralysis or paresis may also benefit from NMES. NMES has been used to increase joint mobility, decrease joint contracture, decrease edema, enhance circulation, minimize disuse atrophy, improve muscle strength, retard loss of volitional control, improve sensory awareness, decrease spasticity, diminish pain, and correct gait abnormalities.

Precautions for and Contraindications to Transcutaneous Electrical Nerve Stimulation

- Contraindications include high-intensity stimulation directly over the heart, animals with pacemakers, animals with seizure disorders, use over infected areas or neoplasms, use over the carotid sinus, or use over the trunk during pregnancy.
- Precautions include application over areas with impaired sensation; abdominal, lumbar, and pelvic regions during pregnancy; and areas of skin irritation or damage; and use in situations involving possible interference with electronic sensing devices such as electrocardiographic monitors.

Application of Transcutaneous Electrical Nerve Stimulation

In determining whether to use TENS in an animal, the use of other concurrent methods of pain control should be assessed. Some animals cannot tolerate medications, and in these animals TENS may provide an acceptable alternative. In other animals, the use of TENS may provide additional pain control.

The hair over the area to which electrical stimulation will be applied must be clipped to lower impedance. The skin may be cleaned with alcohol before treatment. Electrodes may be placed over the region to receive TENS. For TENS application, premodulated electrical stimulation (70 Hz) is applied to the affected area. In some situations, interferential current may be applied with four electrodes. If four electrodes are used, they are typically placed in a crossed fashion. Water-soluble electrode gel may be applied as a coupling agent, and the electrodes may be further secured with nonadhesive bandage material or Velcro straps.

Amperage (intensity) may be increased to the tolerance level of the animal and should be reduced if gross movement of the area is noted or if the animal displays any signs of distress or discomfort including turning its head in recognition of the stimulus or becoming agitated. Amperage may be reduced to a level just below that which produces these signs. Although the optimum time of treatment and the frequency of treatment are unknown, most clinicians believe that TENS should be applied to the desired area(s) for 30 minutes, three to seven times per week.

Precautions should be taken to avoid injury to the handler and animal. A muzzle should be applied, and the animal should be placed in lateral recumbency during the initial treatment. In some cases, tranquilization may be necessary if the animal is anxious. It is recommended that treatment be given only under the supervision of trained personnel.

THERAPEUTIC LASER TREATMENT

Therapeutic laser (TL) treatment involves a light source that consists of pure light of a single wavelength and has been recommended for managing chronic pain, especially in those with muscle injuries or chronic OA. The effect is not thermal but is related to photochemical reactions in the cells.

Until recently, TL devices were not widely used in the United States, but several have been approved by the Food and Drug Administration (FDA) in recent years. The effectiveness of laser therapy is still unclear, and the interpretation of studies regarding the efficacy of TL is hindered by specifics regarding the wavelengths and dosages of laser. But there is a growing body of evidence supporting the use of laser therapy in the multimodal management of pain.

The results of studies regarding pain management with lasers have been controversial. However, studies performed have resulted in FDA approval of low-level lasers for the management of chronic, minor pain, such as that from OA and muscle spasms, in people.

Therapeutic Laser Treatment

- Although the mechanisms of action of low-level laser therapy on pain are unclear, several mechanisms of action have been postulated.
- Laser therapy may have some analgesic effects by blocking pain transmission to the brain. Some studies have shown changes in the conduction of the radial and median nerve after low-level laser therapy, but others have shown no effect.
- Laser treatment may also increase the release of endorphins and enkephalins, which may further provide analgesic benefits.
- Laser therapy has been used to stimulate muscle trigger points and acupuncture points, which may provide pain relief.
- Nociceptive stimulation may be affected. The effects of diode laser irradiation (830 nm, 40 mW, 3 minutes, continuous wave) on peripheral nerves were examined by monitoring neuronal discharges elicited by application of various stimuli to the hindlimb skin of rats. Laser treatment of the saphenous nerve inhibited neuronal discharges elicited by pinch, cold, and heat stimulation. Injection of a chemical irritant into the hind paw skin elicited neuronal discharges in the ipsilateral dorsal root, and these discharges were significantly inhibited or abolished by laser irradiation. These results suggest that laser irradiation may selectively inhibit nociceptive neuronal activities.

Precautions for and Contraindications to Therapeutic Laser Use

- Protective eye gear should be worn to prevent damage to the retina if the laser shines into the area.
- Pregnant women should avoid laser treatment.
- Do not apply laser to open fontanels.
- To not apply laser over malignancies.
- Do not apply laser directly into the cornea.
- Avoid laser application over tattoos because of the high absorption of laser light by pigmented areas.
- Do not apply laser over growth plates of immature animals.
- Do not apply laser over photosensitive areas of the skin.

Application of Therapeutic Laser Treatment

The area should be clipped because the majority of the laser light is absorbed by hair. Little is known about the transmission of laser light to deeper tissues in darker dogs, but laser energy is likely to be absorbed because of the pigment. Any iodine or povidone-iodine should be washed off the area to allow greater transmission of light. Photosensitizing topical medications, such as cortisone, should be avoided. The therapist should wear protective eyewear specific to the laser used because serious damage may occur to the retina if the laser shines into the eyes.

The three variables for lasers used for TL are (1) the wavelength, (2) the number of watts or milliwatts, and (3) the number of seconds to deliver joules of energy. With these factors known, the length of time needed to hold the laser on a point to deliver the appropriate dose in joules must be calculated. For example, if a 904-nm laser with a maximum output power of 250 mW is used, it will take 4 seconds to deliver 1 J. Unfortunately, the optimal wavelengths, intensities, and doses have not been adequately studied in animals, and information in humans is difficult to interpret because of different conditions and treatment regimens.

Wavelengths of therapeutic lasers commonly used are in the infrared region of the light spectrum, such as 980 nm, because of their ability to penetrate tissues more deeply. The wavelength is the prime determinant of tissue penetration. Lasers that do not penetrate as deeply (630 to 740 nm) are suitable for acupuncture point stimulation and wound healing but have not proved their clinical efficacy with deep-seated musculoskeletal conditions. Infrared lasers (750 to 1000 nm) penetrate more deeply and are used to treat trigger points, ligaments, joint capsules, and intra-articular structures.

Power is measured in watts and is often expressed in milliwatts. One watt is equivalent to 1 J/sec. Power density is the power delivered under the area of the probe. Energy density is the amount of energy, or dose, per square centimeter of tissue. The greater the energy density and higher the wavelength, the deeper the penetration through tissues. A higher laser dose is not necessarily better, however, and it is possible that overdosage may retard the desired effect. Class IIIb lasers, commonly used in rehabilitation, are in the infrared region of the electromagnetic spectrum and have power up to 500 mW. Class IV therapeutic lasers are becoming more common because of the ability to deliver the dose of laser energy in a shorter period of time. The lasers are also typically in the infrared region of the electromagnetic spectrum and have 500 mW to 15 W of power. Class IV lasers heat tissues, and to avoid discomfort, it is important to keep the laser moving and monitor the animal for any discomfort, such as moving the limb or turning the head toward the area.

The following example illustrates how to calculate the number of seconds for which to apply the laser to a particular area to deliver a given dose of laser energy for a laser delivering 250 mW/sec, for a total dose of 1 J:

$$0.250\,W = 1\,J/X\,sec$$

$$(0.250\,W)(X\,sec) = 1\,J$$

$$X\,sec = 1\,J/0.250\,W$$

$$X = 4\,sec$$

With this particular laser, it is necessary to hold the laser at one point for 4 seconds to deliver 1 J of energy. The following doses have been suggested for treating pain.

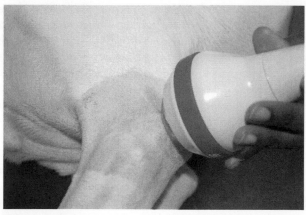

FIGURE 19-11   Application of a therapeutic laser. (From Millis D, Levine DL. Canine rehabilitation and physical therapy, ed 2, St. Louis, 2014, Saunders.)

- Analgesic effect:
  - Muscle pain: 4 to 6 J/cm^2
  - Joint pain: 8 to 10 J/cm^2
- Anti-inflammatory effect:
  - Acute and subacute: 1 to 6 J/cm^2
  - Chronic: 4 to 8 J/cm^2

TL treatment is generally administered with a handheld probe, with a small beam area that is useful to treat small surfaces. Laser energy may be applied with the laser probe in contact with the skin, which eliminates reflection from the skin and minimizes beam divergence, or with the probe not held in contact (Figure 19-11). With the noncontact method, it is necessary to hold the probe perpendicular to the treatment area to minimize wave reflection and beam divergence. The appropriate dose may be applied to larger areas by administering the calculated dose to each site in a grid fashion, or by slowly moving the probe over the entire surface, being certain to distribute the energy evenly to each site. In any case, the probe should be held perpendicular to the skin. A coupling medium is not necessary, as in US, because the laser beam is not attenuated by air.

EXTRACORPOREAL SHOCK WAVE TREATMENT

ESWT involves the application of high-energy, high-amplitude acoustic pressure waves to tissues. Shock waves are characterized by an extremely short buildup time of approximately 5 to 10 nanoseconds with an exponential decay to baseline. Shock waves behave like sound waves in tissue, in that the waves travel through soft tissue and fluid and release their energy into the tissues when a change in tissue density is encountered, such as the interface between bone and ligament. This energy release is thought to stimulate healing. Two primary methods are used to deliver the energy. Focused shock waves have the ability to focus the energy to different tissue depths. The shock waves are focused by means of a parabola to deliver an intense shock to a small area with a focused depth, up to 110 mm. Radial shock waves are delivered to the surface of the body. From there, the shock waves rapidly disperse through the tissues, releasing their energy to a wide area. Because of the energy dissipation, it is difficult to deliver energy to deeper tissues.

Orthopedic applications of ESWT in humans include delayed or nonunion fractures, plantar fasciitis, lateral epicondylitis, Achilles and patellar tendinitis, and, with limited experience, OA. Focal ESWT is currently FDA approved in the United States for use in chronic plantar fasciitis and lateral epicondylitis. Other potential applications include the use of ESWT to provide analgesia for humans with avascular necrosis of the femoral head, to treat calcified tendinitis of the shoulder, and to stabilize loose press-fit total hip replacements. Animals with humeral epicondylitis or plantar fasciitis tend to respond better to ESWT if the condition is chronic (>35 months) rather than more acute (3 to 12 months).

In veterinary medicine, ESWT has been used in horses for the treatment of suspensory ligament desmitis, tendinopathies, navicular disease, back pain, OA, and stress fractures. Although the treatment of dogs with shock wave therapy is relatively new, tendinitis, desmitis, spondylosis, nonunion fractures, and OA have been treated.

Extracorporeal Shock Wave Treatment

Pain may be modulated in animals receiving extracorporeal shock wave treatment, but the mechanisms of action are unclear. The following effects have been described and may contribute to analgesia:

- Reduced inflammation and swelling
- Short-term analgesia
- Production and release of growth factors
- Stimulation of nociceptors that may inhibit afferent pain signals

---

Indications for Extracorporeal Shock Wave Treatment

ESWT may be beneficial to animals with chronic OA of the major joints, especially if they cannot tolerate nonsteroidal anti-inflammatory drugs (NSAIDs) or other forms of treatment. In addition, ESWT may be useful as a nonpharmacologic form of adjunctive treatment along with medical management to obtain additional improvement. In addition, animals with OA of the vertebral column may benefit from ESWT, as well as animals with chronic nonunion fractures.

Precautions for and Contraindications to Extracorporeal Shock Wave Treatment

- Dogs with immune-mediated joint disease or neurologic deficits should not be treated with extracorporeal shock wave treatment (ESWT) because this treatment has no known effects on these conditions.
- Neoplastic joint disease, infectious arthritis, and diskospondylitis should not be treated with ESWT because of the risk of spreading the disease process with treatment.
- Acute unstable fractures and animals with unstable hardware are also not candidates for ESWT, even though this treatment has shown efficacy in treating nonunion fractures, because some stability of the fracture must be present to allow bone healing.
- Shock waves can have adverse effects if they are applied at excessively high energy levels, if a large number of shocks are used, or if they are focused on structures sensitive to their effects. Excessive and violent cavitation can lead to the production of free radicals, which can cause chemical or thermal damage to cells and tissues.
- Concurrent use of nonsteroidal anti-inflammatory drugs that affect platelet function is not recommended before ESWT because of the risk of petechiation and bruising.
- Shock waves should not be delivered over the lung field, brain, heart, major blood vessels, nerves, neoplasms, or a gravid uterus.

Application of Extracorporeal Shock Wave Treatment

Heavy sedation or anesthesia is required for focused ESWT. Because many animals requiring treatment are geriatric, adequate health screening should be performed before treatment, including a complete physical examination and appropriate ancillary tests such as radiographs, complete blood count, serum chemistry profile, and urinalysis.

A complete understanding of the anatomy of the treatment area and the spatial relationships of various anatomic landmarks is critical because ESWT is a localized treatment. Because shock waves may cause petechiation and bruising, aspirin and other non–cyclooxygenase-selective drugs should be discontinued before treatment because these drugs inhibit platelet function and may worsen the bruising.

The treatment area should be clipped, and the skin should be cleaned with alcohol if it is excessively oily. US gel is liberally applied to the area (Figure 19-12). Do not use other lotions or creams because these contain too much air, and this attenuates the sound waves.

At this time, the optimal energy level and the number of shocks for various conditions are not known. Based on the manufacturer's directions and the area(s) to be treated, the energy level and number of shocks to be delivered are selected. In general, treatments should not be repeated more frequently than every 2 weeks. Most conditions are treated two or three times, and the effects may last for several weeks to months.

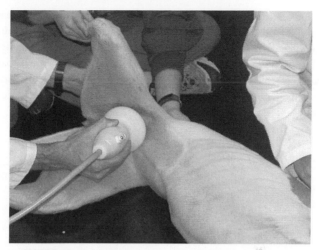

FIGURE 19-12 Application of extracorporeal shock wave treatment.

For treatment of joints, it is important to direct the probe at the insertion sites of the joint capsule, not the articular cartilage. If treating the supraspinatus or biceps tendons, direct the probe over these areas from proximal to distal. Do not direct the probe over the thorax or lungs if treating conditions of the forelimbs. Animals may be a bit sedate for the rest of the day after treatment and may develop some bruising, petechiation, or a hematoma over the treatment site. Some animals may be sore for several days after treatment and then have relative relief from pain. During this time, consider use of NSAIDs or other medications to provide analgesia. Continued improvement may be seen for up to several weeks after treatment. Some conditions seem to be more responsive to shock wave treatment than others. For example, the hips and back may respond well, whereas stifles may not respond to the same extent. Response rates of up to 80% may be seen, and the degree of improvement may be comparable to that seen with an NSAID.

THERAPEUTIC ULTRASOUND

Therapeutic US has been used for both thermal and microthermal biologic effects. Whereas superficial heating agents may penetrate to a depth of only 1 to 2 cm, US can heat tissues to a depth of up to 5 cm. Therapeutic US has been used for animals with restricted motion, joint contracture, pain, and muscle spasm and to enhance wound healing. Pain threshold is usually increased after US. Heating tissues may elevate the activation threshold of free nerve endings, produce counterirritation, or activate large-diameter nerve fibers. With intensities of 1 to 2 W/cm^2, US reduces the nerve conduction velocity of pain-carrying C fibers. This may help to reduce muscle spasm and reestablish circulation. US also has been used to treat pain associated with neuromas, low-back dysfunction, and skeletal muscle spasm. The mechanism of action for reduction of skeletal muscle spasm may be based on thermal effects that alter the skeletal muscle contractile process, reduce muscle spindle activity, or break the pain-spasm-pain cycle. Therapeutic US is also useful for wound healing.

Therapeutic Ultrasound

Several mechanisms of pain relief provided by therapeutic ultrasound have been suggested:
- Tissue heating.
- Decreased stiffness of tissues and joints.
- Increased local blood flow.
- Promotes resolution of inflammation.
- Promotes tissue repair.
- Pain threshold is usually increased after ultrasound.
- Heating may elevate the activation threshold of free nerve endings, produce counterirritation, or activate large-diameter nerve fibers.
- Peripheral nerve conduction velocities are either increased or decreased after ultrasound, partially depending on the intensity. Types A, B, and C nerve fibers have different sensitivities. Ultrasound reduces the nerve conduction velocity of pain-carrying C fibers. This may help to reduce muscle spasm and reestablish circulation.
- The mechanism of action for reduction of skeletal muscle spasm may be based on thermal effects that alter the skeletal muscle contractile process, reduce muscle spindle activity, or break the pain-spasm-pain cycle.

Indications for Therapeutic Ultrasound

Therapeutic US has recently shown efficacy for managing pain in OA in people, with one meta-analysis suggesting that US improved knee OA pain in people by 13%, and a similar effect with regard to functional improvements. A small study of people with hip OA indicated that the addition of therapeutic US to traditional physical therapy showed a longitudinal positive effect on pain, functional status, and physical quality of life.

Precautions for and Contraindications to Therapeutic Ultrasound Use

Avoid direct ultrasound (US) exposure to the following:
- Cardiac pacemakers
- Carotid sinus or cervical ganglia
- Eyes
- Gravid uterus
- Heart

Precautions for and Contraindications to Therapeutic Ultrasound Use—cont'd

- Injured areas immediately after exercise
- Areas over malignancies or tumors
- Spinal cord if a laminectomy has been performed; however, US applied to the tissues around the laminectomy site may be treated
- Testes
- Contaminated wounds
- Recent incision sites
  Exert precaution in the following situations:
- Bony prominences; treat around bony prominences rather than directly over them, to avoid overheating the periosteum
- Cold packs or ice before US could alter pain and temperature perception, limiting the animal's ability to respond if the US intensity is too high
- Decreased blood circulation
- Decreased pain and temperature sensation
- Animals that are overly sedated, restrained, or under local anesthesia
- Physeal areas in immature animals
- Injuries in the acute stage that should not receive heat therapy
- Acute inflammatory joint disease

Application of Therapeutic Ultrasound

The depth of the target tissue to treat should be determined. US frequency is the primary determinant of depth of tissue, and frequencies of common commercially available units are 1 and 3.3 MHz; 3.3-MHz US penetrates 1 to 3 cm of tissue depth, and 1-MHz US penetrates 2 to 5 cm of tissue depth.

It is necessary to clip the hair over the treatment site because US waves are attenuated by air. In addition, specific US gel should be used between the skin and sound head. Other gels or lotions may not be appropriate because they have not been degassed and the air trapped in them attenuates the transmission of US waves. A commercial gel pad may also be used, but US gel should be placed between the sound head and the gel pad, and between the gel pad and the skin (Figure 19-13). Alternatively, if small, irregular surfaces are to be treated, the clipped body part may be immersed in water and the US head may then be placed in water approximately 1 cm from the body surface for treatment administration. Air bubbles that form on the skin and transducer surfaces should be periodically wiped off.

Next, the duty cycle must be chosen. *Duty cycle* refers to the fraction of time that the US is emitted during one pulse period. With continuous mode the US intensity is constant, whereas pulsed US is interrupted so that energy is delivered in an on-off manner.

Duty cycle = Pulse duration (time on)/Pulse period (time on + time off)

Typical duty cycles for pulsed-mode US range from 0.05 (5%) to 0.5 (50%). Pulsed US decreases the pulse average intensity and decreases tissue

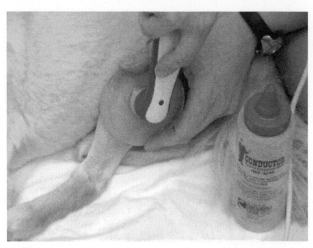

FIGURE 19-13   Application of therapeutic ultrasound treatment. (From Millis D, Levine DL. Canine rehabilitation and physical therapy, ed 2, St. Louis, 2014, Saunders.)

heating. Pulsed US may be used when the desired effect is based on biologic effects or when minimal heating is desired, such as treatment immediately postoperatively. Consideration should also be given to the tissue type to which the US is applied. Tissues with higher protein content absorb US to a greater extent, and therefore heating is expected to be greater in these tissues. Bone and cartilage absorb the most US, followed by tendon and ligament, skin, and muscle. Nervous tissue and fat absorb less US. Therefore, particular attention should be paid to US treatment over bones and joints. Normally dogs do not react to US treatment, but if the area becomes overheated, signs of discomfort may be noted, such as restlessness, moving of the limb, or vocalization. If such signs are noted, the treatment should be discontinued; tissue temperature will return to comfortable levels within a minute or so.

The intensity of US power must also be chosen. Intensity is the rate of energy delivery per unit area. Available intensities typically range from 0.25 to 3.0 W/cm^2. The greater the intensity, the more US is delivered to the tissues. For continuous US, this equates to a greater increase in tissue temperature. In general, small dogs with little soft tissue covering bones or joints are treated with 0.5 W/cm^2. Larger dogs with greater soft tissue mass, such as the thigh or shoulder muscles, are treated with intensities of 2 to 2.5 W/cm^2. Treatment time to achieve therapeutic heating is typically 5 to 10 minutes.

Although US units strive to produce even intensity throughout the sound head area, there are areas of greater intensity ("hot spots") and areas of lesser intensity. Measurement of the total output (W) of the transducer divided by the transducer surface area (cm^2) is referred to as the *spatial average intensity*. The greatest intensity anywhere within the sound head is termed the *spatial peak intensity*. The beam nonuniformity ratio (BNR) compares the maximal intensity from the transducer with the average intensity. This ratio should be low (between 2 and 6) to indicate that the energy distribution is relatively uniform. However, because there are areas of greater power emitted from the sound head, it is important to keep the sound head moving during treatment to avoid overheating.

The treatment area is generally two to four times the size of the sound head, with 4 minutes of treatment time per sound head area generally being necessary to achieve therapeutic effects. Increasing the total area beyond the recommended area or treating for shorter time periods decreases the dose and the heating effect. To avoid overheating of an area, the sound head is moved over the skin at approximately 4 cm/sec to achieve uniform distribution of energy to the target tissues. Moving the transducer too quickly may reduce heating and the therapist may have a tendency to cover too large an area. A back and forth grid or overlapping circular pattern may be used. Treatment may be administered daily initially, followed by less frequent sessions as the condition improves.

Typical treatment parameters in studies of human knee OA patients have used a 1-MHz frequency, with power ranging from 1 to 2.5 W/cm^2, with treatments administered two or three times weekly for 4 to 8 weeks. If US is used to heat tissues before ROM or stretching, stretching should begin near the end of the US treatment and immediately after because tissue temperature returns to normal within 5 to 10 minutes after US is discontinued.

PULSED ELECTROMAGNETIC FIELD THERAPY

PEMF therapy has been used for a variety of purposes, including pain control. In addition to other cellular and biochemical effects, PEMF therapy may help stabilize intracellular calcium stores that may reduce free radical production by mitochondria and subsequent inflammation. However, few clinical trials have demonstrated PEMF therapy to be an effective treatment for pain and tissue trauma, particularly in the early stages of inflammation. A randomized controlled clinical trial that evaluated the effect of PEMF therapy on postoperative pain in dogs after ovariohysterectomy found that although no clear benefit was seen, the results suggested that PEMF may augment morphine analgesia after ovariohysterectomy. PEMF therapy appears to have benefits for the treatment of certain conditions, and although many of the biophysical effects on cells and tissues have been confirmed, its use is still limited because of confusing and often conflicting results.

Indications for Pulsed Electromagnetic Fields

One of the most common uses for PEMF therapy is the treatment of OA. PEMF treatment has a number of physiologic effects on cells and tissues, including the upregulation of gene expression of members of the transforming growth factor-β (TGF-β) family, an increase in glycosaminoglycan levels, and perhaps an anti-inflammatory action. A review assessed the effectiveness of PEMF therapy compared with placebo for treating knee OA in people. Overall, no effect was demonstrated for pain or stiffness. However, there was an effect on activities of daily living. The authors concluded that PEMF treatment improves clinical scores and function as an adjuvant treatment in animals with knee OA, but there is no evidence for an effect on pain. A clinical trial in dogs with OA indicated some positive effects of PEMF therapy. Peak vertical force was significantly more improved in the treatment group from day 0 to day 11, but not from day 0 to day 42. The improvement in the Canine Brief Pain Inventory (CBPI) score and measured joint extension was significantly greater in the treatment group for both time points. This study suggested that pulsed-signal therapy, a form of tPEMF, was useful in treating dogs with OA.

Application of Pulsed Electromagnetic Fields

As with many modalities used in human and veterinary medicine, dose, frequency, and characteristics of the modality used in studies are inconsistent, making the meaningful interpretation of studies difficult. In addition, dogs must remain relatively quiet when in a PEMF unit. This can prove a challenge for many dogs. Although the modality may show promise for certain conditions, its common use in veterinary medicine is hampered by the lack of prospective, blinded, placebo-controlled studies, the expense of the equipment, and the need to maintain dogs in a relatively quiet state during treatment. Dogs treated in the OA study received PEMF therapy for 1 hour (on 9 consecutive days) of pulsed direct current at a frequency of 1 to 30 Hz and 12.5 G (Gauss) with greater than 50% duty cycle.

SUGGESTED READINGS

Alfano AP, Taylor AG, Foresman PA, et al. Static magnetic fields for treatment of fibromyalgia: A randomized controlled trial, J Altern Complement Med. 7:53–54, 2001.

Baker K, McAlindon T. Exercise for knee osteoarthritis, Curr Opin Rheumatol. 12:456–463, 2000.

Beckerman H, de Bie RA, Bouter LM, et al. The efficacy of laser therapy for musculoskeletal and skin disorders: A criteria-based meta-analysis of randomized clinical trials. Phys Ther. 72:483–491, 1992.

Bischoff HA, Roos EM. Effectiveness and safety of strengthening, aerobic, and coordination exercises for patients with osteoarthritis. Curr Opin Rheumatol. 15:141–144, 2003.

Bjordal JM, Couppè C, Chow R, et al. A systematic review of low level laser therapy with location-specific doses for pain from chronic joint disorders. Aust J Physiother. 49:107–116, 2003.

Bochstahler B, Levine D, Millis D: Essential facts of physiotherapy in dogs and cats: Rehabilitation and pain management. Babenhausen, Germany, 2004, BE VetVerlag.

Brosseau L, Robinson V, Wells G, et al. Low level laser therapy (classes I, II and III) for treating osteoarthritis. Cochrane Database Syst Rev. Issue 3, 2004, Art. No. CD002046.

Brosseau L, Robinson V, Wells G, et al. Low level laser therapy (classes I, II and III) for treating rheumatoid arthritis. Cochrane Database Syst Rev. Issue 4, 2005, Art. No. CD002049.

Brosseau L, Yonge KA, Robinson V, et al. Thermotherapy for treatment of osteoarthritis. Cochrane Database Syst Rev. Issue 4, 2003, Art. No. CD004522.

Brown CS, Ling FW, Wan JY, Pilla AA. Efficacy of static magnetic field therapy in chronic pelvic pain: a double-blind pilot study. Am J Obstet Gynecol. 187:1581–1587, 2002.

Buchbinder R, Green SE, Youd JM, et al. Shock wave therapy for lateral elbow pain. Cochrane Database Syst Rev. Issue 4, 2005, Art. No. CD003524.

Calderhead RG. Watts a joule: On the importance of accurate and correct reporting of laser parameters in low reactive level laser therapy and photoactivation research. Laser Ther. 3:177–182, 1991.

Carreck A. The effect of massage on pain perception threshold, Manipulative Physiotherapist 26 (2):10–16, 1994.

Carroll D, Moore RA, McQuay HJ, et al. Transcutaneous electrical nerve stimulation (TENS) for chronic pain. Cochrane Database Syst Rev. Issue 4, 2000, Art. No. CD003222.

Caselli MA, Clark N, Lazarus S, et al. Evaluation of magnetic foil and PPT insoles in the treatment of heel pain, J Am Podiatr Med Assoc. 87:11–16, 1997.

Cherkin DC, Eisenberg D, Sherman KJ, et al. Randomized trial comparing traditional Chinese medical acupuncture, therapeutic massage, and self-care education for chronic low back pain. Arch Intern Med. 161(8):1081–1088, 2001.

Cherkin DC, Sherman KJ, Deyo RA, Shekelle PG. A review of the evidence for the effectiveness, safety, and cost of acupuncture, massage therapy, and spinal manipulation for back pain. Ann Intern Med. 138:898–906, 2003.

Clarke GR, Willis LA, Stenner L, Nichols PJR. Evaluation of physiotherapy in the treatment of osteoarthrosis of the knee. Rheumatol Rehabil. 13:190–197, 1974.

Cochrane T, Davey RC, Matthes Edwards SM. Randomised controlled trial of the cost-effectiveness of water-based therapy for lower limb osteoarthritis, Health Technol Assess. 9(31):1–114, 2005.

Collacott EA, Zimmerman JT, White PT, Rindone JP. Bipolar permanent magnets for the treatment of chronic low back pain, J Am Med Assoc. 283:1322–1325, 2000.

Deal ND, Tipton J, Rosencrance E, et al. Ice reduces edema: A study of microvascular permeability in rats, J Bone Joint Surg Am. 84(9):1573–1578, 2002.

Enwemeka CS, Parker JC, Dowdy DS, et al. The efficacy of low-power lasers in tissue repair and pain control: A meta-analysis study, Photomed Laser Surg. 22(4):323–329, 2004.

Ernst E, Fialka V. Ice freezes pain? A review of the clinical effectiveness of analgesic cold therapy J Pain Symptom Manage. 9:56–59, 1994.

Ferretti M, Srinivasan A, Deschner J, et al. Anti-inflammatory effects of continuous passive motion on meniscal fibrocartilage, J Orthop Res. 23:1165–1171, 2005.

Franke A, Gebauer S, Franke K, Brockow T. Acupuncture massage vs Swedish massage and individual exercise vs group exercise in low back pain sufferers: A randomized controlled clinical trial in a 2×2 factorial design, Forsch Komplementarmed Klass Naturheilkd. 7(6):286–293, 2000.

Fransen M, McConnell S, Bell M. Exercise for osteoarthritis of the hip or knee, Cochrane Database Syst Rev. Issue 2, 2001, Art. No. CD004376.

French SD, Cameron M, Walker BF, et al. Superficial heat or cold for low back pain, Cochrane Database Syst Rev. Issue 1, 2006, Art. No. CD004750.

Furlan AD, Brosseau L, Imamura M, Irvin E. Massage for low-back pain, Cochrane Database Syst Rev. Issue 2, 2002, Art. No. CD001929.

Garrison DW, Foreman RD. Effects of transcutaneous electrical nerve stimulation (TENS) on spontaneous and noxiously evoked dorsal horn cell activity in cats with transected spinal cords, Neurosci Lett. 216:125–128, 1996.

Grana WA. Physical agents in musculoskeletal problems: Heat and cold therapy modalities, Instr Course Lect. 42:439–442, 1993.

Grimmer K. A controlled double-blind study comparing the effects of strong burst mode TENS and high rate TENS on painful osteoarthritic knees, Aust J Physiother. 38:49–56, 1992.

Gur A, Cosut A, Sarac AJ, et al. Efficacy of different therapy regimes of low-power laser in painful osteoarthritis of the knee: A double-blind and randomized-controlled trial, Lasers Surg Med. 33:330–338, 2003.

Harlow T, Greaves C, White A, et al. Randomised controlled trial of magnetic bracelets for relieving pain in osteoarthritis of the hip and knee, Br Med J. 329:1450–1454, 2004.

Hecht PJ, Backmann S, Booth RE, Rothman RH. Effects of thermal therapy on rehabilitation after total knee arthroplasty: A prospective randomized study, Clin Orthop Relat Res. 178:198–201, 1983.

Hinman R, Ford J, Heyl H. Effects of static magnets on chronic knee pain and physical function: A double-blind study, Altern Ther Health Med. 8(4):50–54, 2002.

Hseuh TC, Cheng PT, Kuan TS, Hong CZ. The immediate effectiveness of electrical nerve stimulation and electrical muscle stimulation on myofascial triggerpoints, Am J Phys Med Rehabil. 76:471–476, 1997.

Hulme J, Robinson V, DeBie R, et al. Electromagnetic fields for the treatment of osteoarthritis, Cochrane Database Syst Rev. Issue 1, 2002, Art. No. CD003523.

Hurley MV, Scott DL. Improvements in quadriceps sensorimotor function and disability of patients with knee osteoarthritis following a clinically practicable exercise regime, Br J Rheumatol. 37:1181–1187, 1998.

Jensen H, Zesler R, Christensen T. Transcutaneous electrical nerve stimulation (TNS) for painful osteoarthrosis of the knee, Int J Rehabil Res. 14:356–358, 1991.

Jette DU. Effect of different forms of TENS on experimental pain, Phys Ther. 66:187–192, 1986.

Johnson M. Transcutaneous electrical nerve stimulation (TENS). In: Kitchen S, editor: Electrotherapy, evidence-based practice, ed 11, Edinburgh, 2002, Churchill Livingstone.

Johnson MI. The analgesic effects and clinical use of acupuncture-like TENS (AL-TENS), Phys Ther Rev. 3:73–93, 1998.

Kalra A, Urban MO, Sluka KA. Blockade of opioid receptors in rostral ventral medulla prevents antihyperalgesia produced by transcutaneous electrical nerve stimulation (TENS), J Pharmacol Exp Ther. 298:257–263, 2001.

Köke AJ, Schouten JS, Lamerichs-Geelen MJ, et al. Pain reducing effect of three types of transcutaneous electrical nerve stimulation in patients with chronic pain: A randomized crossover trial, Pain. 108:36–42, 2004.

Lampe GN. Introduction to the use of transcutaneous electrical nerve stimulation devices, Phys Ther. 58(12):1450–1454, 1978.

Law PPW, Cheing GLY, Tsui AYY. Does transcutaneous electrical nerve stimulation improve the physical performance of people with knee osteoarthritis? J Clin Rheumatol. 10:295–299, 2004.

Man D, Man B, Plosker H. The influence of permanent magnetic field therapy on wound healing in suction lipectomy patients: A double-blind study, Plast Reconstr Surg. 104:2267–2268, 1999.

Mangione KK, McCully K, Gloviak A, et al. The effects of high-intensity and low-intensity cycle ergometry in older adults with knee osteoarthritis, J Gerontol A Biol Sci Med Sci. 54: M184–M190, 1999.

McMaster WC, Liddle S. Cryotherapy influence on posttraumatic limb edema, Clin Orthop Relat Res. 150:283–287, 1980.

Meeusen R, Lievens P. The use of cryotherapy in sports injuries, Sports Med. 3:398–414, 1986.

Melzack R, Wall PD. Pain mechanisms: A new theory, Science. 150:971–979, 1965.

Menth-Chiari WA, Curl WW, Paterson-Smith B, Smith TL. Microcirculation of striated muscle in closed soft tissue injury: Effect on tissue perfusion, inflammatory cellular response and mechanisms of cryotherapy—a study in rat by means of laser Doppler flow-measurements and intravital microscopy [German], Unfallchirurg. 102:691–699, 1999.

Messier SP, Loeser RF, Miller GD, et al. Exercise and dietary weight loss in overweight and obese older adults with knee osteoarthritis: The arthritis, diet, and activity promotion trial, Arthritis Rheum. 50:1501–1510, 2004.

Michlovitz SL, Erasala GN, Hengehold DA, et al. Continuous low-level heat therapy for wrist pain, Orthopedics. 25:S1467, 2002.

Millis D, Levine D. Canine rehabilitation and physical therapy, St Louis, 2013, Elsevier.

Myrer JW, Measom G, Fellingham GW. Temperature change in the human leg during and after two methods of cryotherapy, J Athletic Training. 33:25, 1998.

Nadler SF, Steiner DJ, Erasala GN, et al. Continuous low level heat wrap therapy provides more efficacy than ibuprofen and acetaminophen for acute low back pain, Spine. 27:1012–1014, 2002.

Nadler SF, Weingand K, Kruse RJ. The physiologic basis and clinical applications of cryotherapy and thermotherapy for the pain practitioner, Pain Physician. 7:395–399, 2004.

Nadler SF, Weingand KW, Stitik TP, et al. Pain relief runs hot and cold, Biomechanics. 8:1, 2001.

Nash TP, Williams JD, Machin D. TENS: Does the type of stimulus really matter? Pain Clinic. 3:161–168, 1990.

Newton RA. Contemporary views on pain and the role played by thermal agents in managing pain symptoms. In: Michlovitz SL, editor: Thermal agents in rehabilitation, ed 2, Philadelphia, 1990, FA Davis.

Oezdemir F, Birtane M, Kokino S. The clinical efficacy of low-power laser therapy on pain and function in cervical osteoarthritis, Clin Rheumatol. 20(3):181–184, 2001.

Olson JE, Stravino VD. A review of cryotherapy, Phys Ther. 52:840–853, 1972.

O'Reilly SC, Muir KR, Doherty M. Effectiveness of home exercise on pain and disability from osteoarthritis of the knee: A randomised controlled trial, Ann Rheum Dis. 58:15–19, 1999.

Osiri M, Welch V, Brosseau L, et al. Transcutaneous electrical nerve stimulation for knee osteoarthritis, Cochrane Database Syst Rev. Issue 4, 2000, Art. No. CD002823.

Philadelphia Panel. Philadelphia Panel evidence-based clinical practice guidelines on selected rehabilitation interventions for knee pain, Phys Ther. 81:1675–1700, 2001.

Radhakrishnan R, King EW, Dickman JK, et al. Spinal 5-HT(2) and 5-HT(3) receptors mediate low, but not high, frequency TENS-induced antihyperalgesia in rats, Pain. 105:205–213, 2003.

Rakel B, Barr JO. Physical modalities in chronic pain management, Nurs Clin North Am. 38(3):477–494, 2003.

Rogind H, Bibow-Nielsen B, Jensen B, et al. The effects of physical training program on patients with osteoarthritis of the knees, Arch Phys Med Rehabil. 79:1421–1427, 1998.

Seichert N. Controlled trials of laser treatment. In Schlapbach P, Gerber NJ, editors: Physiotherapy: Controlled trials and facts (rheumatology), Basel, Switzerland, 1991, Karger.

Sjölund B, Eriksson M, Loeser J. Transcutaneous and implanted electric stimulation of peripheral nerves. In Bonica JJ, editor: The management of pain, vol 2, Philadelphia, 1990, Lea & Febiger.

Sjölund BH. Peripheral nerve stimulation suppression of C-fiber-evoked flexion reflex in rats. 1. Parameters of continuous stimulation, J Neurosurg. 63:612–616, 1985.

Sluka KA, Deacon M, Stibal A, et al. Spinal blockade of opioid receptors prevents the analgesia produced by TENS in arthritic rats, J Pharmacol Exp Ther. 289:840–846, 1999.

Sluka KA, Walsh D. Transcutaneous electrical nerve stimulation: Basic science mechanisms and clinical effectiveness, J Pain. 4:109–121, 2003.

Stelian J, Gil I, Habot B, et al. Laser therapy is effective for degenerative osteoarthritis: Improvement of pain and disability in elderly patients with degenerative osteoarthritis of the knee treated with narrow-band light therapy, J Am Geriatr Soc. 40:23–26, 1992.

Stockle U, Hoffmann R, Schutz M, et al. Fastest reduction of posttraumatic edema: Continuous cryotherapy or intermittent impulse compression, Foot Ankle Int. 18:432–438, 1997.

Sutton A. Massage. In Millis DL, Levine D, Taylor RA, editors: Canine physical therapy and rehabilitation, Philadelphia, 2004, Saunders.

Thomson CE. Crawford, Murray GD. The effectiveness of extra corporeal shock wave therapy for plantar heel pain: A systematic review and meta-analysis, BMC Musculoskelet Disord. 6:19, 2005.

Tsuchiya K, Kawatani M, Takeshige C, Matsumoto I. Laser irradiation abates neuronal responses to nociceptive stimulation of rat-paw skin, Brain Res Bull. 34:369–374, 1994.

Tulgar M, McGlone F, Bowsher D, Miles JB. Comparative effectiveness of different stimulation modes in relieving pain, 1. A pilot study Pain. 47:151–155, 1991.

Ueda W, Katatoka Y, Sagara Y. Effect of gentle massage on regression of sensory analgesia during epidural block, Anesth Analg. 76(4):783–785, 1993.

van Baar ME, Dekker J, Oostendorp RAB, et al. Effectiveness of exercise in patients with osteoarthritis of hip or knee: Nine months' follow up, Ann Rheum Dis. 60:1123–1130, 2001.

Walsh DM, Baxter GD. Transcutaneous electrical nerve stimulation (TENS): A review of experimental studies, Eur J Phys Med Rehabil. 6:42–50, 1996.

Walsh DM, Foster NE, Baxter GD, Allen JM. Transcutaneous electrical nerve stimulation: relevance of stimulation parameters to neurophysiological and hypoalgesic effects, Am J Phys Med Rehabil. 74:199–206, 1995.

Walsh DM, Lowe AS, McCormack K, et al. Transcutaneous electrical nerve stimulation: effect on peripheral nerve conduction, mechanical pain threshold, and tactile threshold in humans, Arch Phys Med Rehabil. 79:1051–1058, 1998.

Walsh DM. TENS: Clinical applications and related theory, New York, 1997, Churchill Livingstone.

Wang B, Tang J, White PF, et al. Effect of the intensity of transcutaneous acupoint electrical stimulation on the postoperative analgesic requirement, Anesth Analg. 85:406–413, 1997.

Weintraub M. Magnetic bio-stimulation in painful diabetic peripheral neuropathy: A novel intervention—a randomized, double-placebo crossover study, Am J Pain Manage. 9:8–17, 1999.

Weintraub MI, Wolfe GI, Barohn RA, et al. Static magnetic field therapy for symptomatic diabetic neuropathy: A randomised, double blind, placebo-controlled trial, Arch Phys Med Rehabil. 5:736–746, 2003.

Winemiller MH, Billow RG, Laskowski ER, Harmsen WS. Effect of magnetic v sham-magnetic insoles on plantar heel pain: a randomized controlled trial, J Am Med Assoc. 290:45–56, 2003.

Wittink H, Cohen LJ, Michel TH. Pain rehabilitation: physical therapy treatment. In Wittink H, Michel TH, editors: Chronic pain management for physical therapists, ed 2, Boston, 2002, Butterworth and Heinemann.

Wolsko PM, Eisenberg DM, Simon LS, et al. Double-blind placebo-controlled trial of static magnets for the treatment of osteoarthritis of the knee: Results of a pilot study, Altern Ther Health Med. 10:36–43, 2004.

Woolf CJ. Transcutaneous electrical nerve stimulation and the reaction to experimental pain in human subjects, Pain. 7:115–127, 1979.

Yurtkuran M, Kocagil T. TENS, electroacupuncture and ice massage: Comparison of treatment for osteoarthritis of the knee, Am J Acupunct. 27:133–140, 1999.

Zemke JE, Andersen JC, Guion WK, et al. Intramuscular temperature responses in the human leg to two forms of cryotherapy: Ice massage and ice bag, J Orthop Sports Phys Ther. 27:301–307, 1998.

CHAPTER 20

Physical Examination With Emphasis on Isolating and Detecting Pain

James S. Gaynor

A complete physical examination is a critical component of any pain management program. The physical examination is made up of three or four parts: (1) interviewing the pet owner or handler, (2) conducting a visual examination, (3) performing a hands-on examination, and (4) optimally but optionally performing a computerized gait analysis. It cannot be emphasized enough that an initial complete examination is only the beginning. The animal needs to assessed and reassessed regularly. This is really the fact-finding mission, both verbally and physically (Box 20-1).

CLIENT INTERVIEW

The initial interview with the pet owner or handler is critical to setting the stage for background, assessment, goals, and likely outcomes.

VISUAL ANALYSIS

Visual analysis is an important portion of the examination. The ability to look for abnormal posture, positioning, and walking helps affirm or challenge preconceived ideas. Also, look for muscle atrophy, deformities, quality of conformation, bruising, licking, and scars. Visualization also helps the practitioner focus more intently during the hands-on portion of the examination.
1. Posture
2. Positioning
3. Walking

HANDS-ON EXAMINATION

It is important to move slowly to avoid startling the animal. Pain in a nervous, scared animal may appear greater because of fear guarding. It is critical to palpate for movement of joints, swelling, heat, and any sensitivities. The hands-on component should be methodical and repeated virtually in the same manner from animal to animal, typically from neck to tail. When

| BOX 20-1 | **Keys to Good Physical Examination for Pain** |

- Be methodical.
- Perform overall visual assessment.
- Palpate muscles and joints, neck to tail.
- Conduct computerized gait analysis for objective assessment.

abnormalities are found, appropriate diagnostic tests should be performed. These diagnostic tests may include radiographs, musculoskeletal ultrasound, computed tomography (CT) scan, and magnetic resonance imaging (MRI).

Neck

1. Assess the full range of motion slowly: dorsiflexion, ventriflexion, and side-to-side movement.
2. Carefully avoid hurting the animal that has limited range of motion.
3. Although limitations in range of motion are commonly muscular in origin, the possibility of vertebral and intervertebral abnormalities must always be kept in mind.
4. A sore neck is common in animals with a front limb gait abnormality.

Limbs

Although it is important to be systematic and perform the examination in a repeatable manner, if a particular limb is obviously more painful than others, it may be best to leave that portion of the examination for last so as not to sensitize the animal to further palpation and manipulation.

1. Palpate musculature for swelling, tenderness, atrophy, and asymmetry.
2. Flex and extend joints with emphasis on resistance caused by pain and/or structural limitations.
3. Measure joint flexion and extension (goniometry) if an abnormality is detected. Be sure to compare with the opposite limb. This is a good objective measure to follow over time (Figures 20-1 and 20-2).
4. Although it is not a limb, be sure to manipulate the tail in all four directions.
   - A tail that is sensitive to manipulation may be coupled with perispinal pain.
   - Dogs that have naturally curled tails may have a "down" tail when they have perispinal muscle pain.
   - Pain on dorsiflexion should be followed by rectal palpation. Additional pain during rectal palpation may indicate lumbosacral stenosis and should be followed by appropriate imaging.

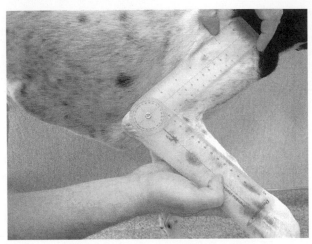

FIGURE 20-1 Goniometry of the right elbow in a dog. It is important to line up the goniometer with the pivot at the joint and the arms along the axis of the limb bones.

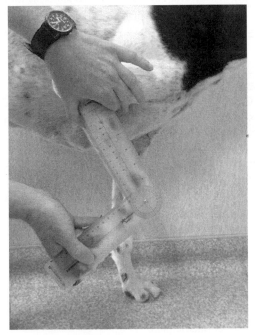

FIGURE 20-2 Goniometry of the right carpus in the dog. It is important to line up the goniometer with the pivot at the joint and the arms along the axis of the limb bones.

Spinal and Perispinal Muscles

1. Palpate muscles segmentally for swelling, tenderness, atrophy, and symmetry.
2. Be sure to include the iliopsoas muscles.
3. Painful perispinal and/or iliopsoas muscles are common in animals with rear limb gait abnormalities.

COMPUTERIZED GAIT ANALYSIS

Computerized gait analysis can be useful by providing an objective assessment of lameness. It should always be coupled with a complete hands-on examination.

Force Plate Analysis

1. Force plate analysis is the gold standard in research but has limited clinical value.
2. It involves measurement of ground reaction forces as a limb moves across the plate. Only one foot can be on the platform at a time, making it difficult to assess animals with potentially more than one limb involved.
3. The modality is not very portable.
4. Significant time is required to obtain and interpret data.
5. Velocity and acceleration must be monitored because they have opposite effects on peak vertical force and vertical impulse.

Pressure Analysis

1. Consists of platforms or walkways (Figure 20-3).
2. The modality is typically portable.
3. Typical ground reaction forces are nearly identical to measurements obtained via traditional force plates.
4. Provides detailed information on stance time, symmetry, stride length, peak pressure, and reach.
5. Helps determine lameness in one or more limbs.
6. Tends to be relatively simple for baseline and outcome assessment.
7. More sensitive than a visual assessment and can pick up lameness that is subclinical, allowing a more focused examination and early intervention.
8. Very useful for baseline and outcome assessments.

CAT SPECIFICS

1. The interview with the cat owner is focused much more on changes in household activity and behavior. Pet owners typically think that changes are age related and not pain related.

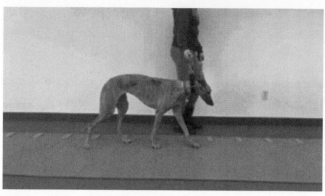

FIGURE 20-3   Walking a dog on a pressure mat. It is important for the dog to take several practice walks to get used to the surface and to not be too curious about its surroundings. The walker needs to keep a loose leash and avoid stepping on the mat.

- Limping is not usually detected, but when a pet owner identifies this, that particular limb should be examined in addition to the rest of the cat.
- Can the cat still jump onto furniture and countertops?
- Does the cat use the litter box appropriately?
- Similar to dogs, cats have a high incidence of muscular perispinal pain. Muscular back pain is commonly responsible for a cat's inability to jump. In addition, muscular back pain can lead a cat to get its front limbs into a litter box but then hesitate to arch and place the rear limbs in the litter box. Hence, the cat may urinate and/or defecate just outside the box as a result of pain, not behavioral issues.

2. The physical examination of a cat is similar except that the lameness examination and observation need to be well orchestrated.
- Because most cats will not walk on a leash and are often fearful, the opportunity for observation is limited. It is often useful to place the cat carrier in one corner of an examination room and then have the owner place the cat in the opposite corner. The practitioner must be ready to observe the cat as it runs to the carrier. Cats may not tolerate this more than once or twice.
- More than 90% of cats have radiographic evidence of osteoarthritis with a high incidence of spinal facet abnormalities.
- Assessment of joint movement with flexion and extension is important.
- As with dogs, it is critical to assess the neck and perispinal muscles by palpation. Movement away from gentle palpation is often more indicative of pain than vocalization.

Computerized Gait Analysis

1. Most gait analysis systems are not sensitive enough or do not have sensors concentrated enough to provide data from cats.
2. Systems that are appropriate for cats are not common and are costly but useful.
3. The technique to get a cat to walk across a gait system is similar to that for observation.
4. Training of cats may be necessary.

CHAPTER 21

Therapeutic Goals

Robin Downing; James S. Gaynor

One of our obligations as veterinary healthcare providers is to help pet owners understand what is happening to their animals during an illness or other medical issue. We have a responsibility to the animals and their owners to make a diagnostic plan, identify as complete a diagnosis as possible, create a treatment plan, translate that treatment plan into language understandable to the pet owner, set priorities among the treatment options, and articulate an expected illness trajectory, trajectory of treatments, and expected response to therapy. This cycle is repeated no matter whether we are dealing with an acute illness, a surgery, a chronic illness, chronic maladaptive pain, a lasting disability, or palliative care as the animal approaches the end of its life. Only by identifying expected outcomes and goals for the prescribed treatments can we accomplish several important things:

- We set the stage for the pet owner to be an active collaborator and participant in the treatment and healing process. Without owner engagement, we cannot achieve optimal outcomes for the animal.
- We create a "roadmap" for therapy that allows us to mark progress while adjusting treatment to meet the animal's changing needs.
- We provide ourselves and the pet owner with a reasonably objective way to measure the progress and success of our therapeutic choices.

Establishing therapeutic goals is a process no more exotic than creating expectations for ourselves and the pet owner. The pet owners need and deserve for us to be thoughtful about our treatment choices so that we make *rational* choices that maximize the animal's outcomes. It is critical to communicate clearly and openly with the pet owner to answer several key questions:

- *What have been the animal's routine activities of daily living (ADLs)?*

No one knows the animal better than their human family members. For that reason it is imperative that we engage those individuals in a dialogue to understand as best we can just what the animal's daily routine has been. It may be best to ask the family to write a log of those daily routines and activities to better understand what the family's expectations for treatment outcomes might be.

- *What outcome hopes and/or expectations does the family hold?*

No matter what the medical issue at hand, it is important to understand just what the human family hopes for. This is the starting place for articulating specific goals for therapy.

- *What incremental steps may be taken to move the animal toward the restoration of its ADLs?*

Once a desired outcome has been identified, then by working backward from that outcome it is possible to articulate specific incremental goals and specific therapies to achieve those goals.

- *How often will the animal be rechecked and reassessed, and the treatment plan revised?*

It is critical to create a reevaluation plan and schedule so the family can understand the steps to be taken and the timing of those steps. For many animals, the restoration of ADLs will be straightforward and will take little time. For others, the trajectory to anticipated or desired ADLs will be more convoluted and time-consuming. And for other animals, the ADLs themselves will have to be adjusted and adapted to more realistically reflect the future the animal faces with its existing medical issues.

- *How will the animal's ADLs be updated and modified to reflect its changing needs?*

Keeping an activity log at home will greatly facilitate any necessary adjustments of expectations. Sometimes an animal's improvement proceeds ahead of schedule. Sometimes it improves more slowly than expected. And sometimes permanent limitations emerge that require adjusting the expectations of the family as well as the veterinary healthcare team.

The process of establishing a diagnosis, creating a treatment plan, implementing that plan, and assessing progress is a logical sequence that lends itself to animals experiencing acute pain or chronic pain and those approaching the end of life. It will be useful to consider the application of this process to these three categories of animals.

THERAPEUTIC GOALS FOR ANIMALS WITH ACUTE PAIN

The arc of therapeutic goals and measured outcomes generally occupies a fairly short timeline for the animal with acute pain. The short time frame, however, does not lessen the need to articulate expectations for pain relief and healing. For the animal undergoing a fairly straightforward surgery such as castration, appropriate therapeutic goals might include the following:

- Appropriate perioperative analgesia to allow for restful sleep after surgery, and minimal reaction to palpation of the surgical site
- Appropriate postoperative analgesia that allows for normal eating and drinking.

- Appropriate analgesia after discharge from the hospital so that the animal does not traumatize the surgical site and returns to its normal ADLs once home

Contrast such an animal with a dog experiencing a forelimb amputation. In this case, therapeutic goals must be a bit more detailed and must occupy a slightly longer timeline. Appropriate therapeutic goals for a canine forelimb amputation might include:

- Appropriate perioperative analgesia to facilitate a smooth recovery from anesthesia and acceptance of palpation of the surgical wound.
- Appropriate postoperative analgesia to facilitate the dog's acceptance of assistance in rising and walking for the first time or two after anesthetic recovery.
- Appropriate postoperative multimodal analgesia to prevent the dog from developing a chronic maladaptive pain state (e.g., phantom limb phenomenon).
- Appropriate postoperative analgesia at discharge from the hospital to enable a comfortable transition to home and the ability to negotiate the home environment. This would include normal eating and drinking, the ability to go outside for elimination, and the ability to engage with human family members in the activities of the household.

Following an amputation, the therapeutic goals for postoperative activities must acknowledge and accommodate the animal's newly acquired limitations. For instance, a return to agility competition would be an inappropriate and unrealistic goal for this dog. Likewise, 5-mile walks should be off the agenda. That said, starting out with short walks of 10 minutes at a time two or three times per day is a reasonable initial goal. Walking has a cumulative effect, so three 10-minute walks translate to 30 minutes of walking for a dog who cannot walk 30 minutes all at once. The next therapeutic goal might be 20 minutes of walking two or three times per day, and so on, to a target of 30 to 45 minutes of walking all at once depending on the dog's age, comorbidities, and fitness level.

As is true for any animal being treated for pain, both the treatment plan and the goals of therapy for the animal with acute pain must be tailored to meet the needs of the individual and the expectations of the pet owner. Sometimes the expectations of the pet owner must be adjusted to reflect more accurately what the animal can and cannot do.

THERAPEUTIC GOALS FOR ANIMALS WITH CHRONIC PAIN

Establishing therapeutic goals for animals with chronic pain in some respects presents the most challenging scenario for this process. Among all animals with pain, the population of those with chronic pain is truly the most diverse for many reasons, including the following:

- The source of the pain may be elusive to uncover.
- There may be multiple origins for the pain phenomenon.
- Chronic pain from osteoarthritis (OA), for instance, may alter the animal's biomechanics, leading to secondary ergonomically induced pain.
- Older animals with chronic pain are likely to possess comorbidities that may influence or exacerbate their pain.
- Comorbidities in an animal with chronic pain may significantly influence or limit the treatment options available.
- Animals with chronic pain tend to be older when they are diagnosed, which means they are more likely than younger animals to have contributing comorbidities.
- Animals with chronic pain tend to have chronic degenerative conditions such as OA that progress over time. This means that successful management of these animals must also change over time.

When an animal with chronic pain is first evaluated, the pet owner may articulate ADLs that have been lost. These missing activities may, in fact, be the reason the pet owner has made the appointment. The owner may not yet appreciate that pain could explain the change in the animal's activity or activities. Even more important than limping, apparent stiffness, or difficulty rising, changes in everyday behavior provide important clues to the presence of pain. Because animals with chronic pain are generally older animals, it is easy for a pet owner to misinterpret behavior changes or lost ADLs as signs of aging. "She's just getting old" is a common refrain for veterinary healthcare providers to hear and it is critical that language about aging be "heard" as potentially about *pain* (Box 21-1).

Once an animal with chronic pain has been examined, its pain localized, the intensity of the pain identified, and appropriate diagnostics completed, it is time to engage the owner in a detailed dialogue about the pet. This is a conversation that must be repeated at regular intervals. It is important to mark the achievement of the therapeutic goals that have been set. Once goals have been achieved, it is logical to establish a new set of therapeutic goals. If, however, therapeutic goals have *not* been achieved in a timely fashion, it is appropriate to reassess the treatment plan as well as the goals themselves to answer the following important questions:

- *Does the treatment plan need to be modified?*

Should a medication dose be adjusted? Is there a medication missing that should be added?

- *Has enough time passed that the therapeutic goals could have been achieved?*

It is easy to be impatient when treating an animal with chronic pain because all parties desire a "quick fix." Unfortunately, it took time for the animal to develop chronic maladaptive pain, and it will take time to undo that process.

| BOX 21-1 | Barriers to Appropriate Pain Management |

There are many reasons why an animal may not receive the pain care it needs and deserves. Most of these reasons revolve around a lack of knowledge about pain, lack of understanding about how to evaluate an animal for pain, or a misinterpretation of animal behaviors, thinking that behavior changes reflect normal aging. Communication failures are equally common. Clearly, education and effective communication are the keys to excellent animal pain management—education of ourselves and our healthcare teams, and education of the pet owners—and a commitment to clear, two-way communication. Pain management barriers may take many forms, including the following:

- The pet owner's lack of understanding of what pain in the animal looks like.
- The pet owner's misinformation or misunderstanding about medications used for animal pain management.
- The pet owner's fear of the unknown.
- The pet owner's denial that the animal is experiencing pain.
- The pet owner's fears about the animal's suffering—that perhaps the animal's pain cannot be relieved.
- Difficulty giving medications. This may indicate a problem with the formulation, including the taste. It may be worth considering an alternative existing formulation or working with a compounding pharmacy if appropriate. Perhaps there is an injectable option.
- Dose timing that is problematic. It is always worth discussing openly with the pet owner whether a proposed administration schedule will be acceptable and achievable.
- Worry about costs. Transparency about short-term as well as long-term costs is critical to making the best choices for the animal in such a way that the pain management plan will be carried out.
- Discouragement. The pet owner does not perceive improvement with treatment and "gives up."
- The pet owner's reaction to an animal's adverse reaction to a medication.
- Poor communication from the pet owner about the animal's activities of daily living (ADLs).
- Unrealistic outcome expectations by either the veterinarian or the pet owner.
- Poor communication with the pet owner about chronic maladaptive pain—about "pain as disease."
- Lack of confidence by the veterinarian about assessing an animal's pain.
- Lack of appropriate and regular pain follow-up and reassessment independent of other preventive care procedures.
- Lack of clear, concise, and specific recommendations for animal pain management.
- Difficulty understanding how to juggle the multiple morbidities of an animal with pain.

Appropriate multimodal pain management clearly requires a team approach. It is critical for the veterinarian, the veterinary healthcare team, and the pet owner to work closely together on behalf of the animal with pain. The "Three Rs" of chronic pain management are "**R**eassess the animal. **R**eevaluate what is in place. **R**evise the pain management plan." By anticipating potential barriers to appropriate pain management, it may be possible to prevent lapses in the care of an animal in pain.

- *Were the therapeutic goals truly relevant and realistic for this animal at this time?*

Sometimes pet owners will set unrealistic goals for animals with chronic pain. These owners may desire to recapture times long gone. It is important to help these owners come to grips with any permanent limitations their animals are experiencing. It is fair to the animal *and* the owner to set *realistic* goals for therapy.

An animal with chronic pain needs to be reevaluated regularly to ensure that the overall pain management plan continues to meet the animal's needs. How often the animal is reevaluated and the therapeutic goals reviewed depends on the individual. Typically, it is appropriate to evaluate an animal with chronic pain every 2 to 3 weeks until a pain score on palpation of 1 or 2 of 10 is achieved. Once comfort is consistent, the focus can shift to activities that build strength and stamina to facilitate the reintroduction of desired ADLs. This is an important time for the veterinary healthcare provider to urge the pet owner not to push the animal for too much too soon, or to provide encouragement when things are not improving as quickly as desired. Therapeutic goals must be set incrementally, and this may be a challenging reality for some pet owners to face.

For instance, the therapeutic goal for an older dog with coxofemoral joint OA may be to walk 1 mile with the owner each day. For a young dog without OA, such a distance could be covered in 15 to 20 minutes if the owner walks briskly. For an older dog, a more realistic time goal would be 25 to 30 minutes. For the dog in this example, 25 to 30 minutes of walking all at once would be an unrealistic expectation. Once the dog's comfort level is acceptable, then it is appropriate to work on the walking goal. Create a conditioning plan to work up to the goal of 1 mile in 30 minutes of walking all at once. Start with 10 minutes of walking 2 to 3 times per day. After several weeks, if the dog acts as though 10 minutes is no longer challenging, move to 15 minutes at one time 2 to 3 times per day. Once that is no longer challenging, then it is time to extend a single walk to 20 minutes, and so on. The keys to success are incremental increases per walk, and building capacity over time (Box 21-2).

BOX 21-2 Pain Management Therapeutic Goals

Pain management therapeutic goals will vary dramatically with the animal and the family lifestyle. It is impossible to establish goals and to make a pain management plan without considering many things including the pet owner's outcome expectations as well as the veterinarian's outcome expectations.

It is important to understand the animal's activities of daily living (ADLs) early in its life, the ADLs before the current pain phenomenon, and the hoped-for ADLs once pain is controlled. Realistic therapeutic and outcome goals must be based on the animal's current condition and comorbidities.

Outcome goals for animals with pain will change over time as the response to therapy becomes apparent. Pet owners will see *behavior* changes, whereas veterinarians will see changes in the animal's pain score on palpation. On a 0 to 10 scale, a target pain score of 0 of 10 is unrealistic, a target pain score of 1 to 2 of 10 is both realistic and generally achievable, and a pain score of 3 or more of 10 is unacceptable and indicates a need to modify the pain management strategy.

Evaluating and adjusting therapeutic goals requires regular reassessment of the animal, open dialogue with the pet owner, and agreement on how to proceed. The pet owner should be encouraged to keep a daily log of the animal's activities, feeding, medications, behaviors, and family interactions. It is impossible to remember from day to day how things are going, so a written diary is invaluable. It may be appropriate to consider using a tool such as the Villalobos' Quality of Life Scale.

Let us consider two representative examples of animals with chronic maladaptive pain whose therapeutic goals changed over time—one dog and one cat.

CASE STUDY **Shiloh, FS, Labrador Retriever, 7 Years Old**

At 2 years of age, Shiloh was kicked by a horse and experienced a right cranial cruciate ligament (CCL) tear. Through misinformation, the owners simply confined Shiloh to crate rest for 8 weeks. She was neither evaluated nor treated for her CCL disorder. At 4 years of age, Shiloh had another equine encounter resulting in a rupture of her left CCL. Again acting on faulty information, the owners confined her to her crate for 2 months. She did not receive any formal treatment. Over time, through a combination of altered biomechanics and bilateral stifle OA with progressing degenerative joint disease (DJD), Shiloh developed multiple segments of bridging spondylosis in her spine and became less and less active. She lost interest in the outdoor activities of the family farm. She lost the ability to walk the perimeter of the property, then the ability to walk out to the barn to oversee chores. Finally, she lost the ability to walk across the living room of the house.

As her pain escalated, Shiloh's engagement with her family continued to diminish. At the time of her presentation for a pain assessment, Shiloh would not tolerate grooming, resulting in an unkempt, matted hair coat. She resented being asked to get up and move. She snapped at the other family dog if that dog approached her. She shied away and flinched anytime she was touched by a family member. Her family's perception was that she was experiencing an unacceptably low quality of life, and they were contemplating euthanasia. They thought they were witnessing behaviors borne of pain, but had not received either confirmation of those suspicions or any recommendations for how to make Shiloh's life bearable again.

On presentation, Shiloh's overall pain score on palpation was judged to be 8 of 10. Her pain was too generalized to allow for confident localization of its origin. She had to be muzzled during her initial evaluation. Her pain was so intense that she anticipated that any touch would be unacceptably painful, and she avoided escalation of her pain any way she could. Initial therapeutic goals for Shiloh were fairly conservative:

- Break the maladaptive pain cycle.
- Restore family interaction.
- Allow for grooming to clean up her unkempt appearance.
- Provide for more comfortable negotiation around the house.

Although these may seem to be incidental (perhaps insignificant) goals, these represented important milestones on Shiloh's therapeutic path. She was evaluated every 2 weeks initially to fine-tune her medication doses. By the 8-week reassessment, this first set of therapeutic goals had been achieved and it was time to articulate a new set of goals.

For Shiloh's family, reintegration of Shiloh into the activities of the family farm was an important overall therapeutic goal. The task was then to identify incremental goals of therapy leading to that end. Rebuilding strength and stamina were critical to success. Physical rehabilitation was initiated once Shiloh's pain was under control. The relief of her pain liberated her to reengage in her surroundings including her rehabilitation activities. A combination of joint mobilization, stretching, proprioceptive retraining, and hydrotherapy in an underwater treadmill was complemented by therapeutic exercise at home. At first, three or four repetitions of specific therapeutic exercises were all Shiloh could accomplish. Likewise, 5 minutes of walking on the underwater treadmill with the water just below the greater trochanter was her limit. The next incremental goal for her was five to seven repetitions of the exercises and 10 minutes of walking on the underwater treadmill. Once

---

| CASE STUDY | **Shiloh, FS, Labrador Retriever, 7 Years Old—cont'd** |

those benchmarks were met, the number of repetitions of her therapeutic exercises was increased, as was the walking time on the underwater treadmill. Each time she arrived for physiotherapy and the setting of new physiotherapy goals, Shiloh's pain was evaluated and her treatment plan was reassessed to guarantee that she remained comfortable with a pain score on palpation of 1 to 2 of 10.

By week 20 of treatment, Shiloh's owners reported that their goals for Shiloh had been met. She was able to walk the perimeter of their 100-acre farm comfortably. She once again engaged in play with the other family dog. She accepted grooming to keep her hair coat in good shape. She was once again fully integrated into the family and their daily routine. Shiloh was able to recapture ADLs not witnessed by her family for 3 or 4 years.

| CASE STUDY | **Boyd, MC, DSH, 14 Years Old** |

Boyd was presented for evaluation because over the course of the previous year, his interactions with his family had decreased dramatically. He was sleeping more and more, avoiding contact with the other animals in the household, and demonstrating intermittent inappetence. He no longer jumped up into the bay window to watch the birds outside at the feeder. Boyd was no longer grooming himself and had developed mats starting just behind his scapulae and extending to his tail base. He would not tolerate being combed by his family so his mats simply grew worse over time, putting constant tension over a large surface area of his torso. Radiographs revealed evidence of OA and DJD at the lumbosacral junction, as well as several bridging spondylosis lesions in the mid-thoracic area. Radiographic changes consistent with DJD take a very long time to accumulate, so that evidence demonstrated the chronic, and consequently maladaptive, nature of Boyd's pain. He could not bear to be petted because of the combined pain from his skin and from his OA.

Boyd's family recognized that he was in pain, but they had no idea how to make life better for him. On presentation, Boyd's overall pain score on palpation was judged to be 7 of 10. His pain was localized to be most intense in the paraspinal muscles from T10 to L/S, at the T/L junction, along the iliopsoas muscles, at the L/S junction, over the sacroiliac (SI) joints, and at the tail base. He had a normal body condition score—neither overweight nor underweight. A metabolic profile revealed chronic renal disease (CRD) but was otherwise within normal limits. He was euthyroid and normotensive.

The family's initial therapeutic goals for Boyd were straightforward:
- Break the maladaptive pain cycle.
- Relieve Boyd of his extensively matted hair coat in a way that was comfortable.
- Restore family relationships, including those with other animals.
- Restore Boyd's biomechanics to as normal a functional level as possible once his pain was under control.

The presence of CRD influenced medication, nutrition, and ancillary treatment choices. A non-steroidal anti-inflammatory drug (NSAID) was chosen for short-term use to bridge while a neuro-modulatory agent (gabapentin) targeted Boyd's chronic maladaptive pain. He began a therapeutic renal support diet to which was added supplemental eicosapentaenoic acid (EPA) for joint support. In addition, he began a long-term course of injectable polysulfated glycosaminoglycans administered at home. Boyd was reevaluated every 2 weeks, and his gabapentin dosage was adjusted up in response to ongoing pain. Boyd tolerated having his mats shaved by week 2, and his palpation pain score was 2 of 10 at week 6. Physical medicine modalities were added at that time. These

Continued

CASE STUDY **Boyd, MC, DSH, 14 Years Old—cont'd**

included chiropractic adjustment, medical acupuncture, as well as physiotherapy and rehabilitation techniques. Boyd participated in spinal stretching over a physioroll, proprioceptive retraining with a balance board, and hydrotherapy on the underwater treadmill.

By Boyd's 6-week assessment, his family reported that his progress had far exceeded their expectations. He was self-grooming as his hair grew back, he welcomed human handling, and he was even grooming the dogs in the household. Boyd was back to watching the birds and interacting with the family in ways they enjoyed and appreciated.

Starting at week 6, as physical medicine modalities were added, the NSAID dosage was titrated down, and ultimately that drug was discontinued in deference to his CRD. During the decreasing NSAID dosage titration, the gabapentin dosage was titrated up to sustain Boyd's comfort. By his eighth week of focused multimodal pain management he had achieved a pain score on palpation of 1 of 10. Boyd's physical medicine modalities were blended together to provide the broadest complementary effects. He received chiropractic adjustment every 2 weeks for 2 months, then monthly for 2 months, then every 6 weeks for two adjustments, and then every 8 to 12 weeks for maintenance. Boyd's physiotherapy sessions were scheduled twice per week for 4 weeks, and as he grew stronger, the interval between sessions was increased. Ultimately, Boyd received a physiotherapy "tune-up" every 6 to 8 weeks.

Throughout his treatments to get him comfortable and then to keep him comfortable, Boyd's family provided ongoing reports about his ADLs. They kept a detailed log of his medication administration, his interactions with the family and the other household pets, his eating habits, and even his time in the bay window watching the birds. Boyd's ongoing multimodal pain management including physical medicine modalities kept Boyd comfortable and mobile until he died at nearly 18 years of age (Box 21-3).

BOX 21-3 **Putting a Pain Plan in Place**

Pet owner expectations must be managed in dealing with an animal in pain, both for outcomes as well as for ongoing reassessments and pain management plan adjustments.

- Keep the focus on the animal. The animal needs to remain at the center of the caregiving circle.
- Prepare the pet owner for the fact that the initial evaluation of an animal in pain will take longer and be more involved than a regular examination.
- The initial evaluation should include:
  - Metabolic profile (do not overlook hypothyroidism, hyperthyroidism, or hypertension).
  - Demonstrate palpation pressure on the pet owner's forearm *before* palpating the animal.
  - Perform a careful pain palpation.
  - Create a "pain map." This is critical for future evaluations to determine and measure progress and success.
  - Careful and complete history:
    - What are the animal's ADLs?
    - What *were* the ADLs before pain took over?
    - What behaviors have changed?
    - How does the pet owner notice that the animal is in pain?
- Identify the pet owner's therapeutic goals for the animal:
  - Anticipated restoration of ADLs

BOX 21-3 **Putting a Pain Plan in Place—cont'd**

- Identify the veterinarian's therapeutic goals for the animal:
  - ADLs
  - Anticipated pain score changes over time
- Create expectations:
  - Short-term, middle-term, and long-term expectations
  - Medication usage
  - Dosage changes (increases and reductions)
  - Frequency of assessments
  - Adding physical medicine modalities (when available)
  - Keeping a log:
    - ADLs
    - Medications
    - Other parameters
  - Planned frequency of reassessment
- Schedule the next reassessment before the pet owner leaves.
- Be sure that all pet owner instructions are specific, detailed, and delivered with conviction. In addition, be sure to *write everything down* for the pet owner as well as for the medical record.
- Check in regularly with pet owners to ensure adequate understanding of the pain management plan.
- At each pain reassessment, conduct a medication, supplement, and feeding review. There is no better way to illuminate any discrepancies between the *prescribed* treatments and what is actually happening at home. This strategy, which should become second nature, is also an important way to prevent medical errors resulting in either harm to the animal or unnecessary suffering from inadequately treated pain.
- As the animal becomes more comfortable and functional, the interval between pain reassessments may be lengthened. It is inadvisable, however, to allow more than 3 to 4 months to pass between assessments. Chronic pain is the "gift that keeps on giving," and a part of our moral obligation to the animal is to be clear with the pet owner that managing chronic pain is an ongoing clinical process that will cease only at the end of the animal's life.

THERAPEUTIC GOALS FOR ANIMALS RECEIVING PALLIATIVE CARE

Establishing therapeutic goals and creating expectations for treatment options are important during any medical issue, but it is especially important as an animal approaches the end of its life. Palliative care is medical support provided to manage or treat *symptoms* without the intention of curing a disease process. Typically, animals receiving palliative care have multiple comorbidities. Our task as veterinary healthcare providers is to strike a balance among comorbidities to maximize the animal's quality of life. An in-depth discussion about quality-of-life measurement is found in

Chapter 6. The number one priority for working with animals receiving palliative care is managing their pain. All other therapeutic goals in palliative care are secondary to this one.

Establishing therapeutic goals for animals receiving palliative care is generally quite different from that for most other animals in pain. Most animals receiving palliative care experience diminished capacity that interferes with what were once considered its normal ADLs. One important task for the veterinary healthcare team is to work with the pet owner to establish and understand which ADLs to pursue at this stage of the animal's life. The concept of defining ADLs may be new for the pet owner. The owner may never before have thought through how the animal approaches and lives through its days. One effective first step in the process is to have the pet owner keep a log of the animal's day from start to finish over a period of a week. Have the owner document waking time, meal times, bathroom and elimination times and habits, walks (for dogs) including the length of time or distance, play (either with the owner or with other animals in the household), moving around the house, bed time, and so on. Be sure to have the owner include details of the animal's sleep habits as well.

Looking at such a log allows both the owner and the veterinarian to evaluate the *patterns* and *cycles* of the animal's activities. Reviewing the log together facilitates collaboration between the veterinarian and the owner to identify areas for improvement that help set and measure the goals of therapy. For instance, many animals receiving palliative care have pain and are too uncomfortable to sleep through the night. One therapeutic goal may be to achieve comfort that allows the pet (and the owner) to get a good night's sleep. Another example is the dog whose pain is so constant and distracting that it exhibits signs of canine cognitive dysfunction (CDS). CDS signs include aimless pacing, lost housetraining, decreased interactions with family members, and disrupted sleep cycles. These are also signs of chronic maladaptive pain. Only by relieving the chronic pain can we differentiate the signs of pain from the signs of CDS.

Therapeutic goals for animals receiving palliative care are most effective when they are as specific as possible, as realistic as possible, and as relevant as possible for the particular animal. It would be unrealistic and unfair to set a goal of walking 3 miles per day for a 15-year-old dog with cancer that also has multiple joint OA, even if that dog had been capable of taking a 3-mile walk at the age of 10. Because health, circumstances, and capacity change over time, the expectations for what the animal can accomplish must change as well. It is also important to remember that goals may be achieved by means other than medication. Let us review a specific palliative care case.

| CASE STUDY | Oreo, FS, DSH, 15 Years Old |

Comorbidities:

- Multiple joint OA
- Generalized chronic maladaptive pain
- Advancing CRD
- Chronic hypokalemia

Oreo's owners identified a host of lost ADLs:

- Oreo had stopped self-grooming and her hair coat had become matted because she was in pain and grooming hurt her.
- She had stopped jumping up into the window to watch the birds at the feeder outside.
- Oreo had stopped sleeping with the owners at night because she could no longer jump onto the bed.
- Oreo objected to being petted and handled by the owners.
- She experienced chronic low-level dehydration from CRD, causing her to, in the words of the owner, "feel bad."
- Oreo's hypokalemia caused generalized weakness, overall malaise, and decreased appetite.

Oreo's therapeutic goals included:

- Controlling chronic maladaptive pain to set the stage for reestablishing compensation of CRD and restoration of ADLs.

  Treatment: NSAIDs were not available as a treatment option because of Oreo's advanced renal disease. Gabapentin is an effective medication for chronic maladaptive pain. Oreo needed 300 mg orally (PO) per day in divided doses to achieve a pain score on palpation of 1 to 2 of 10. Once her pain was controlled, several important changes occurred. Oreo tolerated having her matted hair coat shaved, and she once again began self-grooming. She began interacting with her family again, seeking attention and sleeping with them. She became interested in sitting in the window again, thanks to the assistance of a strategically placed ottoman to give her an intermediate step up to the window sill. Oreo's conventional litter pan was replaced by one with lower sides to enhance appropriate bathroom behavior. Pain management was enhanced by raising her food and water dishes to mid-humeral level.

- Reestablishing and maintaining normal hydration to facilitate renal compensation to support Oreo's feeling as normal as possible.

  Treatment: Subcutaneous fluids were started at 120 mL bid. Renal serum chemistries were monitored regularly, and the fluid therapy was titrated down to 60 mL qd for maintenance. Fluid homeostasis facilitated the cat's feeling better overall, sustaining compensation of her CRD.

- Reestablishing normal serum potassium levels to facilitate normal muscle function, appetite, and a general sense of well-being.

  Treatment: Oral potassium gluconate was prescribed at 2 mEq PO bid initially, and titrated to 2 mEq PO qd.

Oreo's therapeutic goals were developed just for her. They reflected her specific medical and physical limitations, acknowledging those limitations yet maximizing her comfort and quality of life. Relieving her chronic maladaptive pain successfully opened the door for her to recapture and reclaim her lifestyle with just a few necessary environmental modifications. Dealing with her progressing CRD and her chronic hypokalemia helped her feel better in general and contributed both to enhanced quality of life and restored interest in her ADLs. Although Oreo ultimately needed an increased volume of subcutaneous fluids each day (60 mL subcutaneously [SC] bid) and a higher dose of gabapentin to control her OA pain (400 mg PO per day divided), her family's therapeutic goals for her were achieved and sustained over time. Oreo was euthanized in response to end-stage renal disease at the age of 18 years—3 years after her initial treatment plan using therapeutic goals was developed and implemented (Box 21-4).

BOX 21-4 | **Legal Considerations for an Animal in Pain**

Multimodal pain management for animals is a rapidly developing discipline in veterinary medicine. It means applying existing medications and modalities in new ways—specifically to animals—often based on extrapolation from the human pain management experience. The only U.S. Food and Drug Administration (FDA)–approved medications for pain in animals are the veterinary-licensed nonsteroidal anti-inflammatory drugs (NSAIDs), and then for chronic use only in dogs. This means that nearly every pharmaceutical agent we choose as a part of a multimodal pain management strategy is used in an "extra-label" or "off-label" fashion. This reality obligates the veterinary profession to consider the following:

- We must look to the evidence provided by clinical research for safety and efficacy data to abide by the Veterinarian's Oath to prevent and relieve animal suffering.
- We must take extra time to educate the pet owner about the medications we are using in an extra-label fashion to achieve *informed* consent. This includes:
  - Discussing the need for a specific medication
  - Articulating the intended and expected response to therapy
  - Communicating openly about any potential adverse events or other side effects (expected or unexpected)
  - Encouraging the pet owner to report *any* unusual behaviors or changes in the animal's demeanor
  - Educating the pet owner about any special medication handling techniques as well as offering guidance to keep the animal's medications (just like their own medications) well out of the reach of children
- We must maintain a thorough and accurate medical record. Extra-label use of medications opens the door for additional legal liability should anything untoward or unexpected occur. Anyone reviewing the medical record of the animal in pain should be able to understand:
  - What is the diagnosis (or diagnoses)?
  - What is the treatment plan?
  - Why are specific elements of the treatment plan in place?
  - What is the expected outcome or prognosis?
  - When will reassessments happen?
  - What is the schedule for medication refills?
- If we prescribe controlled drugs we must have a plan for:
  - Determining where these drugs will be dispensed—at the veterinary practice or at a human pharmacy
  - Monitoring refills and being alert for refills requested at too short an interval
  - Collection and disposal of controlled drugs in the event of a medication change, an adverse event, or the death of the animal
  - Educating the pet owner about handling these medications at home to reduce the risk for diversion by a family member or visitor
- A medication review at each and every visit is a "must-do" part of managing chronic pain in an animal. This is simply good due diligence. It allows clarification of dosing discrepancies, predicting refill intervals, as well as discussion of any medication concerns the pet owner may have.

We have an obligation to the animals, to the pet owners, and to our own veterinary healthcare teams to consider all elements of managing animal pain, and that means a consideration of the legal implications of our treatment decisions. Open communication, transparent decision making, detailed written instructions for the pet owners, and detailed medical records work together to protect all parties involved in the quest for comfort for animals with chronic pain.

CONCLUSION

Animals in pain need and deserve to have their pain adequately and appropriately managed, but more than that they and their families need to have a roadmap for care. We need to make as complete a diagnosis as possible, create a treatment plan, translate the treatment plan into terms the pet owner can understand, and articulate expected outcomes. Such a treatment plan is enhanced when the family and veterinary healthcare team work together to identify goals of therapy that reflect the individual nuances of the particular animal.

Establishing therapeutic goals is a process that helps us identify the animal's ADLs to make thoughtful treatment choices so that we may maximize the animal's outcome. It is critical to communicate clearly and openly with the pet owner throughout the treatment arc. It is important both to understand what the family desires for the animal as well as what is realistic to expect as treatment proceeds. A reevaluation plan and schedule must be created and maintained to measure the success of our efforts. For many animals, the restoration of ADLs will be straightforward and will take little time. For others, the anticipated or desired ADLs will take more time and effort to be restored. And for some animals, the ADLs will need to be adjusted to reflect limitations the animal now experiences. Working in partnership with the pet owner to establish and work toward therapeutic goals is a most rewarding aspect of veterinary pain medicine (Box 21-5).

BOX 21-5   **Building a Pain Management Pyramid**

The World Health Organization uses a stair-step model for escalating pain to communicate the idea that pain management strategies must "step up" to meet the needs of the animal in pain (Figure 21-1). For animals with chronic pain, it may be better to think of building a pain management pyramid with each layer added to the last as we strive to meet the animal's needs or as the animal's needs change over time. Recognize that there is no magic monotherapy, and that chronic pain is best addressed by a multimodal model. In a multimodal pain management plan, all the components complement one another, working better together than any single component can. It is also important to consider "targeted therapy" in which each component of the pain management pyramid has its specific target in the body (e.g., nonsteroidal anti-inflammatory drugs [NSAIDs] target inflammation and pain, opioids target the μ receptor in the central nervous system [CNS]).

The foundational layer of the pain management pyramid, on which the rest of the pain plan will be built, consists of several essential components:

- Weight normalization
- NSAIDs (when appropriate for a specific animal)
- Evidence-based nutrition and nutraceuticals for joint support
- Disease-modifying osteoarthritis agents (DMOAs)—for example, polysulfated glycosaminoglycans (PSGAGs)
- Neuromodulatory agent for the maladaptive component of chronic pain (e.g., gabapentin, amantadine)

Continued

BOX 21-5 **Building a Pain Management Pyramid—cont'd**

The next layer of the pain management pyramid would incorporate adjunctive physical medicine techniques:

- Medical acupuncture
- Chiropractic adjustment
- Physiotherapy or rehabilitation techniques
    - Therapeutic laser
    - Cryotherapy
    - Heat therapy
    - Hydrotherapy
    - Proprioceptive retraining
    - Stretching
    - Range of motion and joint mobilization
    - Therapeutic exercise

Next will come assistive devices for the animal in pain to make life at home easier to negotiate:

- Raised food and water dishes
- Nonskid floor surfaces
- Restricted access to stairs
- Areas of increased warmth and heated bedding
- Orthopedic foam for bedding
- Mobility devices such as slings, harnesses, and wheelchairs

Finally, as an animal's pain escalates and becomes more difficult to manage:

- Bisphosphonates for bone tumors
- Opioids
- Palliative radiation strategies for painful tumors
- Short-term hospitalization with IV intervention (continuous rate infusion)
- Palliative sedation and/or humane euthanasia

It is easy to see that most animals with chronic pain will benefit from the application of elements from all levels of the pain management pyramid; the top level is reserved for those animals facing exceptional pain. Our ethical obligation to animals in pain is to understand what tools are available for us to use, to understand how best to use those tools, to find access for those strategies we want to leverage on behalf of the animal but do not have available, and to engage in active reassessment and revision of the pain management pyramid as the animal's needs change over time. We have an obligation to look for and abide by the evidence to support the use of the various components of our pain management strategies, but we are truly limited only by our creativity in helping animals find their way out of the maze of relentless chronic pain.

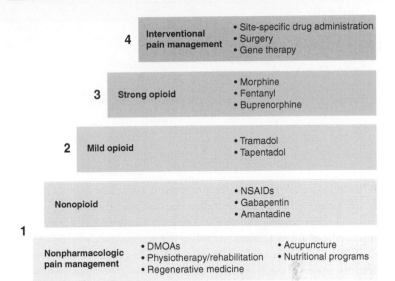

FIGURE 21-1   Modified World Health Organization pain management pyramid. Note that step 1 includes nonpharmacologic and nonopioid pain management. (Key: *DMOAs*, Disease-modifying osteoarthritis agents [e.g., chondroitin sulfate, polysulfated glycosaminoglycan (PSGAG), hyaluronic acid]).

SUGGESTED READING

American Animal Hospital Association (AAHA); American Association of Feline Practitioners (AAFP); AAHA/AAFP Pain Management Guidelines Task Force Members, et al. AAHA/AAFP pain management guidelines for dogs and cats. J Am Anim Hosp Assoc. 2007; 43(5):235–248.

Palliative medicine and hospice care. Vet Clin North Am Small Anim Pract. 2011; 41(3).

Villalobos A, Kaplan L. Quality of life scale. In: A Villalobos, L Kaplan (Eds.): Canine and feline geriatric oncology: Honoring the human-animal bond. Ames, Iowa, 2007, Blackwell Publishing.

CHAPTER 22

Acute Pain Management
A Case-Based Approach

James S. Gaynor; William W. Muir III

The following are specific cases of animals in pain. The cause of pain and the rationale for specific treatment are described. Each case presents a unique aspect or challenge as it relates to pain management. Various drugs and procedures are mentioned, including the analgesic techniques and dosages of drugs administered. Details on each drug and procedure are provided in earlier chapters of the *Handbook*. All animals should be considered healthy unless otherwise noted.

CASE 1 CANINE OVARIOHYSTERECTOMY

Analgesic management was for a dog scheduled for an ovariohysterectomy (OHE) in a veterinary practice that discharges animals the same day as surgery.

Signalment: A 6-month-old female mixed-breed dog weighing 20 kg.

Challenge: Most pet owners do not like to take their pet home sedated. The veterinarian is likely to be called if an animal remains sedated for hours after discharge. The challenge is to provide adequate analgesia without an extended period (>24 hr) of sedation.

Sources of Pain: The pain from OHE generally originates from the surgical incision and from manipulation of the abdominal viscera—uterus and ovaries—and from stretching of associated ligaments (Box 22-1).

BOX 22-1 CASE 1 Canine Ovariohysterectomy: Description of Pain

- Somatic and visceral pain
- Mild to moderate
- Inflammatory and surgically induced tissue trauma
- Acute onset, short duration

Treatment and Rationale

Many dogs exhibit minimal or no signs of pain in the presence of humans. Therefore, as with any other surgical procedure, it is best to treat pain preemptively and preventatively, with appropriate rescue analgesia and postoperative evaluation.

Preemptive-Preventative Analgesia

Appropriate preemptive analgesic therapy should include a full opioid agonist: morphine, oxymorphone, hydromorphone, or methadone. This dog received morphine 0.5 mg/kg subcutaneously (SC) combined with acepromazine 0.02 mg/kg and atropine 0.04 mg/kg. Acepromazine was added for tranquilization. Atropine was added to offset vagal-induced bradycardia associated with the morphine.

Immediate Postoperative Analgesia

Morphine produces analgesic effects for approximately 4 to 6 hours when administered at this dose SC. Most dogs do not require additional analgesic therapy on recovery from anesthesia, although the postoperative administration of a nonsteroidal anti-inflammatory drug (NSAID) or weak opioid (tramadol) may be appropriate for some dogs. If the OHE is performed in the morning, an additional dose of morphine at 0.5 mg/kg SC can be administered to provide analgesia for the rest of the day.

Analgesia at the End of the Day

Dogs are treated with tramadol at 2.0 mg/kg PO as the dog leaves the hospital to ensure several more hours of analgesia with minimal or no sedation.

24-Hour Analgesia

Mild to moderate pain can be treated with an NSAID (see Table 8-1) such as injectable carprofen (4 mg/kg SC) or robenacoxib 1 mg/kg SC. NSAIDs provide no clinically relevant analgesic advantage when administered preoperatively, but can be administered preoperatively if the animal has normal renal function, is undergoing a reasonably routine procedure, is receiving intravenous fluids, and is having blood pressure monitored. Postoperative administration of an NSAID helps to avoid NSAID-related renal toxicity in animals that were not given IV fluids or when arterial blood pressure monitoring is not available.

NOTE: The benefit of administering an NSAID before surgery is controversial at best and potentially dangerous at worst. Preoperative NSAID therapy has been linked to the development of postoperative acute renal failure in dogs and cats, mandating a thorough physical examination and appropriate evaluation of renal function before drug administration and comprehensive (arterial blood pressure) intraoperative monitoring. Furthermore, there are no evidence-based clinical trials that have demonstrated that the administration of an NSAID before surgery provides clinically relevant analgesia effects in otherwise normal healthy or ill dogs or cats.

FDA Announces Addition of Boxed Warning to Metacam (Meloxicam) Labels
Warning
Repeated use of meloxicam in cats has been associated with acute renal failure and death. Do not administer additional injectable or oral meloxicam to cats. See Contraindications, Warnings, and Precautions for detailed information.

4-Day Analgesia

Some practices like to provide approximately 3 days of analgesia after performing an OHE.

1. Carprofen 4.4 mg/kg orally (PO) qd. Carprofen should not be administered PO if another NSAID was originally administered parenterally. This particular dog received this protocol.
2. Robenacoxib 2.0 mg/kg PO qd. Robenacoxib should not be administered PO if another NSAID was originally administered parenterally.
3. Oral tramadol 2 to 3 mg/kg PO bid.
4. Transdermal fentanyl patch 2 to 3 µg/kg/hr. Caution should be used if depending on transdermal fentanyl patches because the plasma concentrations of fentanyl may vary over a 3-day period, with times when there may not be any detectable fentanyl in the blood.

BOX 22-2 | CASE 1 | **Canine Ovariohysterectomy: Therapeutic Options**

- Preemptive analgesia: Morphine 0.5 mg/kg SC
- Postoperative analgesia: Morphine at 0.5 to 1.0 mg/kg SC
- Analgesia at the end of the day: Tramadol 2.0 mg/kg PO
- 24-hour analgesia: Carprofen 4.4 mg/kg SC
- 3-day analgesia:
  - Carprofen 4.4 mg/kg PO qd and/*or*
  - Oral tramadol 2 to 3 mg/kg PO bid *or*
  - Transdermal fentanyl patch 2 to 3 µg/kg/hr

CASE 2 | **CANINE OVARIOHYSTERECTOMY 2**

This case is an example of an analgesic protocol used for dogs that stay overnight in the veterinary hospital after OHE.

Signalment: A 6-month-old female mixed-breed dog weighing 8 kg.

Challenge: The goal is to provide analgesia for 24 hours. The challenge is that the facility is not staffed in the evening to provide readministration of analgesic medications.

Sources of Pain: The pain from OHE generally originates from the surgical incision as well as from manipulation of the abdominal viscera—uterus and ovaries—and from stretching of associated ligaments.

Treatment and Rationale

See Box 22-3.

BOX 22-3 ■ CASE 2 ■ **Canine Ovariohysterectomy 2: Description of Pain**

- Somatic and visceral pain
- Mild to moderate
- Inflammatory and surgically induced tissue trauma
- Acute onset, short duration

Preemptive-Preventative Analgesia

The dog was administered morphine 7.5 mg SC (approximately 1 mg/kg) 30 minutes before induction to anesthesia. Morphine has a duration of action of approximately 4 to 6 hours when administered at this dosage SC. The dog was also given acepromazine 0.02 mg/kg SC and atropine 0.04 mg/kg combined with the morphine. The acepromazine was added to the premedication for tranquilization. Atropine was added to offset any potential for vagal-induced bradycardia associated with the morphine.

Immediate Postoperative Analgesia

Because most OHE surgical procedures are short (20 to 40 minutes) and relatively atraumatic when performed properly, most dogs do not require additional analgesic therapy. This OHE was performed in the morning, and an additional dose of morphine of 1.0 mg/kg SC was administered 4 hours after the first dose to provide analgesia for the rest of the day. Morphine is a full opioid agonist, is well tolerated by dogs, and provides excellent analgesia.

Analgesia at the End of the Day

Because no one is available to readminister morphine after 6 PM, this dog received buprenorphine 0.01 mg/kg SC. The advantage of buprenorphine is that it has a long duration of action, approximately 4 to 12 hours. The analgesia is not as good as that produced by morphine, but it should be adequate, especially when an NSAID is coadministered postoperatively.

24-Hour Analgesia

Analgesia can be supplemented by administering an NSAID such as meloxicam, carprofen, or robenacoxib. The NSAID should be given after the procedure during recovery to limit renal complications produced by anesthetic-associated hypotension if fluid therapy and blood pressure monitoring are not provided (Box 22-4).

BOX 22-4   CASE 2   Canine Ovariohysterectomy 2: Therapeutic Options

- Preemptive analgesia: Morphine 1 mg/kg SC
- Postoperative analgesia: Morphine 1.0 mg/kg SC
- Analgesia at the end of the day: Buprenorphine 0.01 mg/kg SC
- 24-hour analgesia: Carprofen 4.4 mg/kg SC

CASE 3   CANINE CASTRATION

Signalment: A 10-month-old male dog weighing 30 kg.

Challenge: To provide analgesia that will extend for 24 hours.

Source of Pain: Castration causes mild to moderate somatic and visceral pain (Box 22-5).

BOX 22-5   CASE 3   Canine Castration: Description of Pain

- Somatic and visceral pain
- Mild to moderate
- Inflammatory and surgically induced tissue trauma
- Acute onset, short duration

Treatment and Rationale

Castration, like other surgical procedures, is painful. Animals should receive preemptive and preventative analgesic therapy.

Preemptive-Preventative Analgesia

This dog was administered acepromazine 0.025 mg/kg for tranquilization, atropine 0.04 mg/kg to prevent vagal-induced bradycardia, and hydromorphone 0.1 mg/kg. All drugs were combined and administered SC. Lidocaine (2 mg/kg) can be administered intratesticularly after induction of anesthesia to enhance analgesic effects.

Immediate Postoperative and 24-Hour Analgesia

Because the pain from castration is believed to be mild to moderate, an NSAID (robenacoxib 1 to 2 mg/kg SC, or carprofen 4 mg/kg SC) should be administered during recovery from anesthesia (Box 22-6).

BOX 22-6   CASE 3   Canine Castration: Therapeutic Options

- Preemptive analgesia: Hydromorphone 0.1 mg/kg SC
- Intratesticular lidocaine, 2 mg/kg
- Immediate postoperative and 24-hour analgesia: Robenacoxib, 1 to 2 mg/kg SC

CASE 4   FELINE OVARIOHYSTERECTOMY

This case is an example of a cat that will go home the same day as surgery.

Signalment: A 6-month-old female domestic shorthair cat weighing 3 kg

Challenge: To provide analgesia for a 24-hour period.

Sources of Pain: The pain from OHE generally originates from the surgical incision and from manipulation of the abdominal viscera—uterus and ovaries—and from stretching of associated ligaments (Box 22-7).

BOX 22-7   CASE 4   **Feline Ovariohysterectomy: Description of Pain**

- Somatic and visceral pain
- Mild to moderate
- Inflammatory and surgically induced tissue trauma
- Acute onset, short duration

Treatment and Rationale

Preemptive-Preventative Analgesia

The cat was given buprenorphine 0.01 mg/kg SC and dexmedetomidine 0.01 mg/kg for analgesia and sedation. Atropine was administered to prevent bradycardia induced by the other two drugs. The effects of buprenorphine should last 4 to 8 hours in cats. Coadministration of anticholinergics (e.g., atropine, glycopyrrolate) may predispose to cardiac dysrhythmias. Pharmaceutical companies recommend that anticholinergics should be administered 20 minutes before α_2-agonists to avoid this problem, but this is often inconvenient and difficult to achieve.

Postoperative Analgesia

Robenacoxib 1 mg/kg PO can be administered after recovery from surgery, and its effects should persist for 24 hours. Alternatively, robenacoxib can be provided PO before the procedure and given PO for 2 additional days to provide 72 hours of analgesia (Box 22-8). Buccal buprenorphine 0.01 mg/kg can be administered as rescue analgesia if needed. Practitioners should be aware that the feline dosage of buprenorphine is likely to change by more than a factor of 10 based on new clinically derived data.

BOX 22-8   CASE 4   **Feline Ovariohysterectomy: Therapeutic Options**

- Preemptive analgesia: Buprenorphine 0.01 mg/kg and dexmedetomidine 0.01 mg/kg SC
- Postoperative analgesia: Robenacoxib 1 mg/kg SC or PO preoperatively
- Buccal buprenorphine 0.1 mg/kg: administered as rescue analgesia

---

CASE 5   FELINE CASTRATION

Signalment: An 8-month-old male Abyssinian cat weighing 3 kg.

Challenge: Providing analgesia without sedation so the pet owner can take the cat home the same day as surgery.

Source of Pain: Castration causes visceral pain related to spermatic cord and cremaster muscle tension. This pain is probably mild to moderate (Box 22-9).

BOX 22-9   CASE 5   **Feline Castration: Description of Pain**

- Somatic and visceral pain
- Mild to moderate
- Inflammatory and surgically induced tissue trauma
- Acute onset, short duration

Treatment and Rationale

Preemptive-Preventative Analgesia

This cat was given hydromorphone 0.10 mg/kg and dexmedetomidine 0.01 mg/kg for analgesia and sedation. Atropine was administered to prevent bradycardia induced by the other two drugs. Hydromorphone should produce analgesia for 3 to 4 hours in a cat.

Postoperative Analgesia

Robenacoxib 1 mg/kg SC on day one and 1 mg/kg PO for an additional 2 days. Alternatively, robenacoxib could be administered PO before surgery and continued for 2 additional days (Box 22-10).

BOX 22-10   CASE 5   **Feline Castration: Therapeutic Options**

- Preemptive analgesia: Hydromorphone 0.1 mg/kg and dexmedetomidine 0.01 mg/kg SC
- Robenacoxib 1 mg/kg SC on day 1 and 1 mg/kg PO for an additional 5 days

---

CASE 6   DECLAW—FRONT FEET

Signalment: A 1½-year-old castrated male domestic longhair cat weighing 5.5 kg.

Challenge: Pain from a declaw procedure is one of the most difficult sources of pain to treat. Anecdotally, some pet owners believe their cats are much meaner after being declawed, presumably from the intense pain experienced.

Source of Pain: Declawing produces severe pain originating from severed ligaments, tendons, and potentially traumatized bone and periosteum (Box 22-11).

BOX 22-11 | **CASE 6** | **Declaw—Front Feet: Description of Pain**

- Somatic pain (inflammatory and neuropathic)
- Severe
- Inflammatory and surgically induced tissue trauma
- Nerve damage
- Acute onset, short duration

Treatment and Rationale

Preemptive-Preventative Analgesia

1. This cat was coadministered methadone 0.25 mg/kg and dexmedetomidine 0.01 mg/kg SC for analgesia and sedation. Atropine was given to counteract bradycardia. Methadone was specifically chosen because of its μ receptor–induced analgesia and its potential to block N-methyl-D-aspartate (NMDA) receptors, ostensibly to help prevent tissue hypersensitization and the potential development of problem chronic pain. The dose of methadone was considerably higher than that used for most other procedures in cats because of procedure-related pain intensity. The effects of methadone last 3 to 5 hours in cats.

2. A local anesthetic nerve block was performed using bupivacaine (0.5%) 1.5 mg/kg plus lidocaine (2%) 1.5 mg/kg split between both front paws before surgery. A digital nerve block lasts approximately 3 to 6 hours. This combination allows rapid onset (lidocaine) plus long duration (bupivacaine). Bupivacaine without epinephrine should be administered for peripheral nerve blocks. The epinephrine component causes vasoconstriction and decreased perfusion, potentially causing tissue ischemia.

Postoperative Analgesia

A multimodal approach to analgesia is preferred because of the potential for severe pain.

1. Robenacoxib 1.0 mg/kg SC can be administered at the end of the procedure. This should provide analgesia for up to 24 hours. Alternatively, robenacoxib can be administered preoperatively 1 mg/kg PO.

2. Four hours after the initial dose of methadone, another dose of methadone 0.25 mg/kg SC was administered to ensure analgesia after bupivacaine effect subsided.

   Buprenorphine 0.01 mg/kg SC was administered 3½ hours after the last methadone dose. Buprenorphine has a longer duration of action than methadone, and when administered with robenacoxib should help keep the cat comfortable throughout the night. Practitioners should be aware that the feline dosage of buprenorphine is likely to change by more than a factor of 10 based on new clinically derived data.

3. Butorphanol was specifically not used in this case because of the intensity of pain. Butorphanol provides only mild to moderate analgesic effects (see Chapter 9). Methadone produces excellent analgesia in cats (Box 22-12).

BOX 22-12 ■ **CASE 6**   **Declaw—Front Feet: Therapeutic Options**

- Preemptive analgesia: Methadone 0.25 mg/kg and dexmedetomidine 0.01 mg/kg SC; bupivacaine declaw block
- Postoperative analgesia: Robenacoxib 1.0 mg/kg SC; methadone 0.25 mg/kg SC 4 hours after local anesthetic infiltration
- Overnight analgesia: Buprenorphine 0.01 mg/kg SC 3½ hours after the last morphine administration
- Analgesia to go home: Buprenorphine 0.01 mg/kg buccally bid for 2 days and robenacoxib 1 mg/kg PO once daily (range 1 to 2.5 mg/kg) for up to 6 days

---

Analgesia to Go Home

Onychectomy is a surgical procedure that requires an extended period of analgesia (4 to 7 days).

1. Robenacoxib, 1 mg/kg PO once daily (range 1 to 2.5 mg/kg) for up to 6 days.
2. Buprenorphine 0.01 mg/kg buccally bid for 2 days. Administration of buccal buprenorphine for longer periods is likely to induce inappetence and lethargy.
3. Transdermal fentanyl patch 25 μg/hr; leave on for 5 days.
4. As an alternative, methadone can be administered buccally at 0.1 mg/kg bid to tid for multiple days. This may provide more reliable analgesia than a fentanyl patch and will allow alterations in dosage depending on the individual's pain and behavioral responses.

CASE 7   **INCISOR EXTRACTION**

Signalment: A 12-year-old spayed female Miniature Poodle, weighing 9 kg, with periodontitis requiring extraction of two left lower incisors. This dog also has mitral regurgitation and a 2/6 systolic murmur. There are no apparent signs of heart failure, and the dog is not being given any medications.

Challenge: To provide analgesia during and for several days after tooth extraction.

Source of Pain: Mild to moderate pain arising from the tooth root and surrounding soft tissue (Box 22-13).

BOX 22-13   CASE 7   **Incisor Extraction: Description of Pain**

- Somatic pain
- Mild to moderate
- Inflammatory and surgically induced tissue trauma
- Acute onset, short duration

Treatment and Rationale

Preemptive-Preventative Analgesia

A multimodal therapeutic approach is preferred.

1. The dog was coadministered hydromorphone 0.1 mg/kg SC for analgesia, along with glycopyrrolate 0.01 mg/kg to prevent oxymorphone-induced bradycardia.
2. Carprofen 4.4 mg/kg SC was given to provide the initial 24 hours of analgesia.
3. A left mental nerve block was performed by administering 0.5 mL of bupivacaine (0.75%) (see Chapter 12). The dosage of bupivacaine was approximately 0.4 mg/kg to limit the total volume of local anesthetic administered.

Postoperative Analgesia

1. The procedure took approximately 30 minutes to complete. The dose of hydromorphone (0.1 mg/kg SC) was repeated postoperatively to extend the period of analgesia.
2. The dog was prescribed oral morphine elixir (4 mg/mL) 0.5 mg/kg PO tid to qid to provide analgesia for mild pain for several days (Box 22-14).
3. Carprofen 4.4 mg/kg PO qd for a minimum of 3 days. Carprofen should not be administered PO if another NSAID was originally administered parenterally.

BOX 22-14   CASE 7   **Incisor Extraction: Therapeutic Options**

- Preemptive analgesia: Hydromorphone 0.1 mg/kg SC; bupivacaine mental nerve block.
- Postoperative analgesia: Hydromorphone 0.1 mg/kg SC; oral morphine elixir (4 mg/mL) 0.5 mg/kg PO tid or qid.
- Carprofen 4.4 mg/kg PO qd. Carprofen should not be administered PO if another nonsteroidal anti-inflammatory drug (NSAID) was originally administered parenterally.

CASE 8   MAXILLECTOMY

Signalment: An 8-year-old spayed female terrier mix dog weighing 9 kg.
Challenge: Mass was present just behind right upper canine tooth, necessitating a partial maxillectomy.
Source of Pain: Bone and soft-tissue surgical trauma (Box 22-15).

BOX 22-15 █ CASE 8 █ **Maxillectomy: Description of Pain**

- Somatic pain
- Moderate to severe
- Inflammatory and surgically induced tissue trauma
- Acute onset, short duration

Treatment and Rationale

Preemptive-Preventative Analgesia

1. This dog was coadministered oxymorphone 0.1 mg/kg SC to provide preemptive analgesia and atropine 0.04 mg/kg SC to counteract vagal-induced bradycardia.
2. An infraorbital nerve block was performed using 2.5 mg of 0.5% (0.5 mL) bupivacaine (see Chapter 11) to provide regional anesthesia to the nose and associated structures.

Postoperative Analgesia

1. This dog was given a fentanyl bolus 2 μg/kg intravenously (IV) followed by a fentanyl infusion of 5 to 10 μg/kg/hr IV. Occasionally the dog appeared disoriented, and as a result, acepromazine 0.01 mg/kg IV was administered (Box 22-16).

BOX 22-16 █ CASE 8 █ **Maxillectomy: Therapeutic Options**

- Preemptive analgesia: Oxymorphone 0.1 mg/kg SC; bupivacaine infraorbital block.
- Postoperative analgesia: Fentanyl bolus 2 μg/kg IV followed by fentanyl infusion 3 to 6 μg/kg/hr IV.
- Carprofen 4.4 mg/kg PO qd. Carprofen should not be administered PO if another nonsteroidal anti-inflammatory drug (NSAID) was originally administered parenterally.

---

2. Carprofen 4.4 mg/kg PO qd. Carprofen should not be administered PO if another NSAID was originally administered parenterally.

█ CASE 9 █ **MANDIBULECTOMY**

Signalment: An 8-year-old female spayed Golden Retriever dog weighing 25 kg.

Challenge: A dog presented with a mass under the left lower canine tooth that was diagnosed as osteosarcoma on previous biopsy. The surgical procedure included a complete rostral mandibulectomy, resecting 2.5 cm of mandible. Extensive bone trauma results in significant pain.

Sources of Pain: The pain originates from cut bone and periosteum along with severed nerves. The potential for severe pain exists (Box 22-17).

BOX 22-17	CASE 9	Mandibulectomy: Description of Pain

- Somatic pain
- Moderate to severe intensity
- Inflammatory and surgically induced tissue trauma
- Neuropathic; nerve damage
- Acute onset, short duration

Treatment and Rationale

Preemptive-Preventative Analgesia

A mandibulectomy can be very painful and difficult to treat. This dog, like most animals with potential severe pain, warranted a multimodal approach to pain control.

1. Parenteral analgesia: This dog was administered morphine 1.0 mg/kg SC as premedication, along with acepromazine 0.025 mg/kg SC and atropine 0.01 mg/kg SC.
2. Local anesthesia: Local anesthetic blocks (see Chapter 12) are effective when administered in conjunction with opioids to help prevent tissue hypersensitization resulting from the surgical insult.
   a. Mental nerve blocks are useful for cranial mandibulectomies. This dog's mandibulectomy resected bone caudal to the mental nerve. As a result, a mental nerve block was not used.
   b. Mandibular nerve blocks are useful for providing local anesthesia to the ramus of the mandible. This dog received bilateral mandibular nerve blocks using 7.5 mg of (0.5%; 1.5 mL) bupivacaine at each site. This low dose of local anesthetic is possible because the local anesthetic is deposited directly over the nerve.
   c. Ketamine was administered as a bolus 0.5 mg/kg IV immediately before surgical stimulation, followed by a ketamine infusion 10 µg/kg/min to help prevent tissue hypersensitization and help prevent pain-induced dysphoria postoperatively.

Postoperative Analgesia

1. This dog was administered a fentanyl infusion 5 µg/kg/hr, following a fentanyl bolus of 2 µg/kg IV immediately after induction to anesthesia. The infusion was adjusted as needed throughout the night. The infusion was discontinued 24 hours after surgery.
2. The ketamine infusion was lowered to 2 µg/kg/min for the next 24 hours.
3. This dog became anxious 12 hours after surgery. Acepromazine 0.01 mg/kg IV was administered. This calmed the dog and presumably potentiated analgesic drug effects.

Multiday Analgesia

This dog was discharged from the hospital approximately 24 hours after surgery. Sustained-release morphine at approximately 1.0 mg/kg PO bid was prescribed for 4 days. The pet owners discontinued the morphine after 3 days and replaced it with carprofen 100 mg PO qd for another 3 days. The dog exhibited normal behavior at home (Box 22-18).

BOX 22-18   **CASE 9**   **Mandibulectomy: Therapeutic Options**

- Preemptive analgesia: Morphine 1.0 mg/kg SC; bupivacaine mandibular nerve block
- Ketamine bolus 0.5 mg/kg IV immediately before surgical stimulation followed by a ketamine infusion 10 μg/kg/min
- Immediate postoperative analgesia: Fentanyl bolus 2 μg/kg IV followed by fentanyl infusion 5 μg/kg/hr IV
- Carprofen 4 mg/kg once daily administered for the next 3 days

---

CASE 10   NASAL BIOPSY

Signalment: A 12-year-old spayed female mixed-breed dog weighing 7 kg.
Challenge: This dog had a 4-month history of epistaxis requiring rhinoscopy and potential biopsy.
Source of Pain: Stimulation of nasal mucosa produced moderate to severe pain (Box 22-19).

BOX 22-19   **CASE 10**   **Nasal Biopsy: Description of Pain**

- Somatic pain
- Moderate to severe
- Inflammatory and surgically induced tissue trauma
- Acute onset, short duration

Treatment and Rationale

Preemptive-Preventative Analgesia

The dog was very calm and required little premedication for restraint purposes. Nonetheless, the dog was administered hydromorphone 0.2 mg/kg SC for basal analgesia and to produce an anesthetic-sparing effect. Atropine 0.02 mg/kg SC was administered to counteract opioid-induced vagal bradycardia. This dog received 0.5 mg/kg of 0.5% bupivacaine into the nose 5 minutes before initiation of the procedure.

- This dose of hydromorphone may not be adequate analgesia to prevent a response to rhinoscopy as the rhinoscope approaches the back of the nasal passage. Increasing concentrations of isoflurane and dexmedetomidine 0.001 mg/kg IV were administered when the dog demonstrated signs of pain. α2-Agonists and opioids are synergistic (see Chapter 16). Dexmedetomidine administration decreased movement and allowed completion of the procedure.

Postoperative Analgesia

Postoperative pain is mild to moderate after rhinoscopy and nasal biopsy. Therefore analgesics are administered based on the dog's behavior and clinical signs (Box 22-20).

BOX 22-20   CASE 10   Nasal Biopsy: Therapeutic options

- Preemptive analgesia: Hydromorphone 0.2 mg/kg SC.
- Intraoperative analgesia: Dexmedetomidine 0.001 mg/kg IV.
- Postoperative analgesia: Nonsteroidal anti-inflammatory drugs (NSAIDs) or tramadol may be administered.

CASE 11   SHOULDER SURGERY

Signalment: A 2-year-old castrated male Labrador Retriever mixed-breed dog weighing 41 kg.

Challenge: Osteochondritis dissecans (OCD) of the left shoulder.

Sources of Pain: Articular cartilage defect and surgical trauma producing moderate to severe pain (Box 22-21).

BOX 22-21   CASE 11   Shoulder Surgery: Description of Pain

- Somatic pain
- Moderate
- Inflammatory and surgically induced tissue trauma
- Acute onset, 3 to 5 days' duration

Treatment and Rationale

Preemptive-Preventative Analgesia

This dog was coadministered buprenorphine 0.01 mg/kg SC and acepromazine 0.02 mg/kg SC for calming and analgesia. Atropine 0.02 mg/kg SC was administered to counteract vagal-induced bradycardia. All drugs were combined in one syringe. Buprenorphine was administered with the intent of providing a long duration of analgesia.

Postoperative Analgesia

The dog had a very rough recovery from anesthesia and surgery. Pain was thought to contribute to delirium during the recovery period. A test dose of IV fentanyl (2 µg/kg) was administered. Fentanyl administration did not improve the dog's demeanor, possibly because of buprenorphine antagonism of fentanyl effects. The dog was then administered dexmedetomidine 1 μg/kg IV, which calmed the dog considerably. Carprofen 4 mg/kg SC was also administered. Dexmedetomidine was repeated approximately every 2 hours for two treatments. Four hours after surgery, morphine 1.0 mg/kg was administered SC and then repeated every 5 to 6 hours until the next morning (Box 22-22).

BOX 22-22   **CASE 11**   **Shoulder Surgery: Therapeutic Options**

- Preemptive analgesia: Buprenorphine 0.01 mg/kg SC
- Postoperative analgesia: Dexmedetomidine 1 μg/kg IV; carprofen 4 mg/kg SC; morphine 1 mg/kg SC

CASE 12   ELBOW SURGERY

Signalment: A 24-month-old female Newfoundland dog weighing 56 kg

Challenge: This dog had OCD of the right elbow joint.

Sources of Pain: Articular cartilage defect and surgical trauma producing moderate to severe pain (Box 22-23).

BOX 22-23   **CASE 12**   **Elbow Surgery: Description of Pain**

- Somatic pain
- Moderate to severe
- Inflammatory and surgically induced tissue trauma
- Acute onset, 3 to 5 days' duration

Treatment and Rationale

Preemptive-Preventative Analgesia

The dog was administered hydromorphone 0.1 mg/kg and acepromazine 0.015 mg/kg for calming and analgesia. Glycopyrrolate 0.01 mg/kg was administered to counteract hydromorphone-induced bradycardia. All drugs were combined in one syringe and coadministered SC.

Postoperative Analgesia: Multimodal Approach

1. A dose of 2.5 mg morphine and 7.5 mg bupivacaine was injected into the joint at the termination of surgery.
   a. Morphine should activate articular opioid receptors and provide some degree of analgesia.
   b. Bupivacaine should block sodium channels and provide good analgesia for 4 to 8 hours.
2. This dog recovered uneventfully and was very comfortable. Oral tramadol 150 mg three times daily was initiated 6 hours after surgery. Carprofen

4 mg/kg PO qd was started the morning after surgery and continued for the next 5 days (Box 22-24).

BOX 22-24 | CASE 12 | **Elbow Surgery: Therapeutic Options**

* Preemptive analgesia: Hydromorphone 0.1 mg/kg SC.
* Postoperative analgesia: Morphine 2.5 mg and bupivacaine 7.5 mg intra-articular injection.
* Multiday analgesia: Tramadol 3 mg/kg PO tid. Carprofen 4 mg/kg PO qd was started the morning after surgery and continued for the next 5 days.

CASE 13   RADIAL AND ULNAR FRACTURE REPAIR

Signalment: A 10-year-old castrated male mixed-breed dog weighing 30 kg.

Challenge: This dog jumped from the back of a truck and fractured its left radius and ulna 3 days before presentation for anesthesia and surgery. The dog was hemodynamically stable.

Sources of Pain: Fractured bones and associated soft-tissue injury can produce severe pain (Box 22-25).

BOX 22-25 | CASE 13 | Radial and Ulnar Fracture Repair:
Description of Pain

* Somatic pain
* Moderate to severe pain
* Inflammation and damage from trauma to tissue
* Acute onset

Treatment and Rationale

Limb instability can exacerbate tissue injury and limit locomotion; pain may cause additional functional limitations.

Preemptive-Preventative Analgesia: Multimodal Approach

1. This dog was administered morphine 1.0 mg/kg for analgesia along with atropine 0.01 mg/kg SC to counteract bradycardia. No sedative or tranquilizer was used because this dog was very calm.
2. A brachial plexus block was performed using 5 mL of bupivacaine (0.75%), equivalent to approximately 1.3 mg/kg after surgical preparation of the left forelimb (see Chapter 12).

Postoperative Analgesia

1. This dog was administered morphine 1.0 mg/kg SC during recovery from anesthesia.

2. Two hours later this dog was administered another dose of morphine 1.0 mg/kg SC.
3. The dog was uncomfortable on palpation and was unable to rest comfortably. The administration of an NSAID and electroacupuncture treatment were considered. Electroacupuncture consisted of:
   a. Small intestine meridian 3 to 9
   b. Large intestine meridian 4 to 15
   c. Pericardium meridian 6 to 3
   d. 2.5-Hz alternating current continuous stimulation for 20 minutes
4. This dog was comfortable throughout the night and did not require additional analgesics or sedation (Box 22-26).

BOX 22-26 | **CASE 13** | **Radial and Ulnar Fracture Repair: Therapeutic Options**

- Preemptive analgesia: Morphine 1.0 mg/kg SC; bupivacaine brachial plexus block.
- Postoperative analgesia: Morphine 1.0 mg/kg SC; electroacupuncture.
- Robenacoxib 2.0 mg/kg PO qd was started the morning after surgery and continued for the next 5 days.

CASE 14 | **FORELIMB AMPUTATION**

Signalment: A 12-year-old male Golden Retriever dog weighing 38 kg.

Challenge: Osteosarcoma of the right forelimb.

Sources of Pain: Cancer and soft-tissue surgical trauma resulting from scapulectomy and forelimb removal producing moderate to severe pain (Box 22-27).

BOX 22-27 | **CASE 14** | **Forelimb Amputation: Description of Pain**

- Somatic pain
- Moderate to severe
- Inflammatory and surgically induced tissue trauma
- Acute onset

Treatment and Rationale

Preemptive-Preventative Analgesia

1. The dog was administered morphine 1.0 mg/kg SC to provide preemptive analgesia and atropine 0.04 mg/kg SC to counteract morphine-induced bradycardia.
2. Low-dose ketamine was administered as 0.5-mg/kg bolus followed by 10 μg/kg/min infusion. Ketamine was infused throughout surgery. Ketamine blocks NMDA receptors and should help decrease postoperative pain and dysphoria.

Postoperative Analgesia

1. Fentanyl 5 µg/kg/hr was infused IV.
2. The low ketamine infusion was decreased to 2 µg/kg/min for the first 24 hours after surgery.
3. The dog remained comfortable while in the hospital (Box 22-28).

BOX 22-28   **CASE 14**   **Forelimb Amputation: Therapeutic Options**

- Preemptive analgesia: Morphine 1.0 mg/kg SC; low-dose ketamine 0.5-mg/kg bolus followed by 10 µg/kg/min IV
- Postoperative analgesia: Fentanyl 5 µg/kg/hr IV; microdose 2 mg/kg intravenous ketamine

---

CASE 15   **THORACOTOMY—STERNOTOMY**

Signalment: An 11-year-old spayed female domestic shorthair cat weighing 3.2 kg.

Challenge: Lung tumor.

Sources of Pain: Sternotomy and stretching of associated tissues producing moderate to severe pain (Box 22-29).

BOX 22-29   **CASE 15**   **Thoracotomy—Sternotomy: Description of Pain**

- Visceral and somatic pain
- Severe
- Inflammatory and surgically induced tissue trauma
- Acute onset

Treatment and Rationale

Preemptive-Preventative Analgesia

The cat was very fractious. High doses of ketamine or a potent sedative were needed to achieve adequate sedation and pain control. Excessive physical restraint would have produced an excessive amount of stress. The cat was box-induced with sevoflurane.

Intraoperative Analgesia

The cat was administered fentanyl 2 µg/kg IV bolus followed by 10 µg/kg/hr IV infusion before and during surgery to provide analgesia.

Postoperative Analgesia

1. The cat was administered lidocaine 1.0 mg/kg followed by bupivacaine 1.0 mg/kg interpleurally through the chest tube before waking up. This drug combination was administered every 4 to 6 hours.
2. Fentanyl was infused, 5 µg/kg/hr (Box 22-30).

BOX 22-30   **CASE 15**   **Thoracotomy—Sternotomy: Therapeutic Options**

- Preemptive and intraoperative analgesia: Fentanyl 2 μg/kg IV followed by fentanyl 10 μg/kg/hr IV
- Postoperative analgesia: Lidocaine 1.5 mg/kg followed by bupivacaine 1.5 mg/kg interpleurally through the chest tube; fentanyl infusion 5 μg/kg/hr IV

CASE 16   **THORACOTOMY—INTERCOSTAL**

Signalment: A 5-month-old female Labrador Retriever dog weighing 15 kg.
Challenge: Patent ductus arteriosus.
Sources of Pain: Soft-tissue surgical trauma plus displacement and stretching of soft tissue, cartilage, and bone, producing moderate to severe pain (Box 22-31).

BOX 22-31   **CASE 16**   **Thoracotomy—Intercostal: Description of Pain**

- Visceral and somatic pain
- Moderate to severe
- Inflammatory and surgically induced tissue trauma
- Acute onset

Treatment and Rationale

Preemptive-Preventative Analgesia

This dog was coadministered methadone 1.0 mg/kg SC, atropine 0.02 mg/kg to counter increased vagal tone, and acepromazine 0.02 mg/kg for calming. Methadone provides excellent intraoperative analgesia in addition to blocking NMDA receptors, thereby helping to prevent tissue hypersensitization and central sensitization.

Bupivacaine 2 mg/kg was divided and injected two intercostal spaces cranial and caudal to the surgical site at the time of closure (see Chapter 12).

Postoperative Analgesia

The dog was administered methadone 0.05 mg/kg IV on recovery from anesthesia followed by methadone 0.1 mg/kg/hr. The combination of local anesthetic and opioid provided excellent analgesia (Box 22-32).

BOX 22-32   **CASE 16**   **Thoracotomy—Intercostal: Therapeutic Options**

- Preemptive analgesia: Methadone 1.0 mg/kg SC
- Postoperative analgesia: Bupivacaine intercostal nerve block; methadone bolus 0.05 mg/kg IV followed by methadone infusion 0.1 mg/kg/hr IV

CASE 17   LAPAROTOMY—INTESTINAL RESECTION AND ANASTOMOSIS

Signalment: A 6-year-old castrated male Labrador Retriever dog weighing 47 kg.

Challenge: Intestinal foreign body requiring resection and anastomosis.

Sources of Pain: Body wall incisional trauma and abdominal ligament stretching, producing moderate to severe somatic and visceral pain (Box 22-33).

BOX 22-33   CASE 17   **Laparotomy—Intestinal Resection and Anastomosis: Description of Pain**

- Somatic and visceral pain
- Moderate to severe
- Inflammatory and surgically induced tissue trauma
- Acute onset

Treatment and Rationale

Preemptive-Preventative Analgesia

The dog was coadministered morphine 1.0 mg/kg SC as preemptive analgesia and acepromazine 0.01 mg/kg SC for calming. Atropine 0.04 mg/kg SC was administered to counteract bradycardia.

- An epidural injection of morphine 0.1 mg/kg combined with bupivacaine 0.1 mg/kg was unsuccessfully attempted at the lumbosacral vertebral space before surgery. A subarachnoid injection was performed at the lumbar 6-7 intervertebral space (see Chapter 12). The low dose of bupivacaine permitted no alterations in dose, despite injection in the cerebrospinal fluid instead of epidurally.

  1. Epidural morphine administration provides analgesia, but not anesthesia, for 12 to 24 hours. Typically, no change in morphine (0.1 mg/kg) dose is necessary, regardless of epidural or subarachnoid injection. Epidural morphine administration may cause urinary retention. Bladder expression or a urinary catheterization postoperatively may be required.

  2. Epidural local anesthetic administration can produce dose-dependent effects. Larger doses produce motor and sensory blockade. The doses of bupivacaine administered in this dog were small with the intent of blocking sensory nerve transmission without motor blockade. Doses intended for epidural injection should be reduced to one half or one third for subarachnoid injection.

Postoperative Analgesia

The skin was desensitized using 40 mg of 0.5% bupivacaine in 1:200,000 epinephrine, diluted in half with sterile normal saline. The combination of subarachnoid drugs and the incisional block produced excellent analgesia. The dog did not experience urinary retention (Box 22-34).

BOX 22-34	CASE 17	Laparotomy—Intestinal Resection and Anastomosis: Therapeutic Options

- Preemptive analgesia: Morphine 1.0 mg/kg SC; epidural morphine 0.1 mg/kg and bupivacaine 0.1 mg/kg
- Postoperative analgesia: Bupivacaine incisional block—40 mg of 0.5% in 1:200,000 epinephrine

---

CASE 18 LAPAROTOMY—CYSTOTOMY

Signalment: A 4-year-old male Cocker Spaniel mixed-breed dog weighing 12 kg.

Challenge: Urinary calculi requiring laparotomy and cystotomy.

Sources of Pain: Body wall incisional trauma and abdominal ligament stretching, producing moderate to severe pain (Box 22-35).

BOX 22-35	CASE 18	Laparotomy—Cystotomy: Description of Pain

- Somatic and visceral pain
- Moderate to severe
- Inflammatory and surgically induced tissue trauma
- Acute onset

Preemptive-Preventative Analgesia

Premedication

This dog had a history of idiopathic epilepsy and was extremely nervous and hyperactive. The dog was administered morphine 1.0 mg/kg SC for preemptive analgesia. Dexmedetomidine 5 µg/kg SC was administered with the morphine. Dexmedetomidine has synergistic effects with opioids and produced superior sedation and analgesia. Atropine 0.04 mg/kg SC was added to the mixture because both drugs increase vagal tone and can induce bradycardia.

Postoperative Analgesia

1. This dog was not administered epidural morphine or local anesthetic even though this would likely produce good postoperative analgesia. The dog's behavior made it extremely difficult to maintain a urinary catheter. Because epidural morphine administration can cause urinary retention and this dog was undergoing bladder surgery, it was believed best to not subject the cystotomy incision to excess intraluminal pressure.

2. An incisional block was performed before skin closure by administering 15 mg of 0.5% bupivacaine with 1:200,000 epinephrine diluted in half with 0.9% saline (see Chapter 12).

3. Fentanyl 5 to 10 μg/kg/hr was administered to provide somatic and visceral analgesia.
4. The dog became dysphoric and was administered dexmedetomidine 2 μg/kg IV as needed.
5. Robenacoxib 1 mg/kg once daily (range 1 to 2.5 mg/kg) was administered for the next 5 days (Box 22-36).

BOX 22-36   CASE 18   Laparotomy—Cystotomy: Therapeutic Options

- Preemptive analgesia: Morphine 1.0 mg/kg and dexmedetomidine 5 μg/kg SC.
- Postoperative analgesia: Bupivacaine incisional block; fentanyl bolus 2 μg/kg IV followed by fentanyl infusion 10 to 15 μg/kg/hr.
- Robenacoxib 1 mg/kg once daily (range 1 to 2.5 mg/kg) was administered for the next 5 days.

CASE 19   PANCREATITIS

Signalment: A 12-year-old spayed female Miniature Schnauzer dog.
Challenge: History of vomiting and lethargy for 3 days; abdominal pain; no abdominal obstruction; blood work consistent with pancreatitis.
Source of Pain: Severe visceral pain associated with pancreatitis (Box 22-37).

BOX 22-37   CASE 19   Pancreatitis: Description of Pain

- Visceral pain
- Moderate to severe
- Inflammatory
- Acute onset

Treatment and Rationale

- This dog was initially unsuccessfully treated with a continuous infusion of fentanyl 5 to 6 μg/kg/hr after a bolus of 2 μg/kg. The dog was still unable to rest comfortably.
- Interpleural local anesthetic administration can provide analgesia for thoracic and cranial abdominal pain. The nerves from the cranial abdomen enter the spinal cord in the thorax.
  1. Lidocaine 1.5 mg/kg was injected in the sixth intercostal space through a 22-gauge butterfly catheter. Lidocaine was injected initially to produce an immediate block.
  2. Bupivacaine 1.5 mg/kg was injected after lidocaine. Bupivacaine has a 15- to 20-minute duration until the onset of analgesia and can cause stinging. Lidocaine prevents the bupivacaine from stinging.
  3. This technique produced comfort, allowing this dog to sleep. The local anesthetic technique was repeated every 4 hours. The fentanyl was continued at 2 μg/kg/hr (Box 22-38).

BOX 22-38 CASE 19 **Pancreatitis: Therapeutic Options**

- Analgesia: Lidocaine 1.5 mg/kg followed by bupivacaine 1.5 mg/kg interpleural block every 3 to 6 hours as needed
- Fentanyl 2 µg/kg IV bolus followed by 2 µg/kg/hr

CASE 20 **LUMBOSACRAL DISK SURGERY**

Signalment: A 7-year-old spayed female miniature Dachshund dog weighing 8 kg.

Challenge: Lumbosacral disk protrusion.

Sources of Pain: Spinal cord swelling and disk entrapment of nerve roots cause severe pain (Box 22-39).

BOX 22-39 CASE 20 **Lumbosacral Disk Surgery: Description of Pain**

- Somatic and visceral pain
- Moderate to severe
- Inflammatory and surgically induced tissue trauma and underlying disease
- Acute onset

Treatment and Rationale

Preemptive-Preventative Analgesia

This dog was administered morphine 0.75 mg/kg SC to provide analgesia, along with glycopyrrolate 0.01 mg/kg to help counteract bradycardia.

Intraoperative Analgesia

This dog was administered fentanyl 2 µg/kg IV followed by fentanyl 20 µg/kg/hr to provide intraoperative analgesia and decrease the concentration of inhalant anesthetic, thereby helping to maintain cardiac output and arterial blood pressure. The fentanyl infusion was discontinued 30 minutes before the anticipated completion of surgery to facilitate recovery and extubation.

Postoperative Analgesia

Recovery was uneventful but the dog remained sedated. The fentanyl infusion was restarted at 5 µg/kg/hr. This dog remained comfortable for the next 36 hours before and was discharged from the critical care unit (Box 22-40).

BOX 22-40 CASE 20 **Lumbosacral Disk Surgery: Therapeutic Options**

- Preemptive analgesia: Morphine 0.75 mg/kg SC
- Intraoperative analgesia: Fentanyl bolus 2 µg/kg IV followed by fentanyl infusion 20 µg/kg/hr IV
- Postoperative analgesia: Fentanyl infusion 5 µg/kg/hr IV

CASE 21   TAIL AMPUTATION

Signalment: A 2-year-old castrated male domestic shorthair cat.

Challenge: The cat's tail got caught in a radiator fan, causing a degloving injury and a fracture distal to coccygeal bone 5.

Sources of Pain: Bone fracture and soft-tissue trauma, producing severe localized pain (Box 22-41).

BOX 22-41   CASE 21   **Tail Amputation: Description of Pain**

- Somatic pain
- Moderate
- Inflammatory and surgically induced tissue trauma and underlying disease
- Acute onset

Treatment and Rationale

Preemptive-Preventative Analgesia

1. This cat was coadministered dexmedetomidine 0.01 mg/kg and hydromorphone 0.1 mg/kg SC for analgesia and sedation. Atropine 0.02 mg/kg SC was also administered to counteract bradycardia.
2. Bupivacaine 0.75 mg/kg was injected epidurally between coccygeal bones 1 and 2 after induction of anesthesia
3. Robenacoxib 1.0 mg/kg PO was administered before anesthesia to provide analgesia and to reduce inflammation for 24 hours.

Postoperative Analgesia

1. The cat was administered hydromorphone 0.1 mg/kg SC 4 hours after the initial hydromorphone injections.
2. Robenacoxib 1.0 mg/kg PO was administered 24 hours after the initial dose to provide analgesia and to reduce inflammation (Box 22-42).

BOX 22-42   CASE 21   **Tail Amputation: Therapeutic Options**

- Preemptive analgesia: Hydromorphone 0.1 mg/kg SC and dexmedetomidine 0.01 mg/kg SC; bupivacaine epidural; robenacoxib 1 mg/kg PO
- Postoperative analgesia: Robenacoxib 1.0 mg/kg PO and hydromorphone 0.1 mg/kg SC

CASE 22   REAR LIMB AMPUTATION

Signalment: A 7-year-old spayed female Rottweiler dog weighing 42 kg.

Challenge: Osteosarcoma of the left rear limb, requiring amputation.

Source of Pain: Cancer surgical trauma producing severe pain (Box 22-43).

BOX 22-43 | **CASE 22** | **Rear Limb Amputation: Description of Pain**
- Somatic pain
- Moderate to severe
- Inflammatory and surgically induced tissue trauma
- Acute onset

Treatment and Rationale

Preemptive-Preventative Analgesia

1. The dog was administered morphine 1.0 mg/kg SC for preemptive analgesia and atropine 0.05 mg/kg SC. No other tranquilizer or sedative was administered.
2. Morphine 0.1 mg/kg and bupivacaine 0.3 mg/kg were combined and administered epidurally to provide supplemental intraoperative and postoperative analgesia of 12 to 24 hours' duration (see Chapter 12).

Postoperative Analgesia

The dog was administered fentanyl 3 to 10 μg/kg/hr IV over the next 24 hours to maintain analgesia. This was administered in conjunction with deracoxib 50 mg PO, which was continued for the next 5 days (Box 22-44).

BOX 22-44 | **CASE 22** | **Rear Limb Amputation: Therapeutic Options**
- Preemptive analgesia: Morphine 1.0 mg/kg SC; morphine and bupivacaine epidural
- Postoperative analgesia: Fentanyl bolus 2 μg/kg IV followed by fentanyl infusion 3 to 10 mg/kg/hr IV
- Deracoxib 50 mg PO qd continued for the next 5 days

CASE 23   BILATERAL FEMORAL FRACTURE REPAIR

Signalment: A 6-year-old spayed female Australian Shepherd mixed-breed dog weighing 26 kg.

Challenge: This dog slipped off an icy deck under construction and fell 25 feet; radiographs revealed bilateral comminuted femoral fractures.

Sources of Pain: Broken bones and soft-tissue trauma producing severe pain (Box 22-45).

BOX 22-45 | **CASE 23** | **Bilateral Femoral Fracture Repair: Description of Pain**
- Somatic pain
- Severe
- Inflammatory, surgically, and traumatically induced tissue trauma
- Acute onset

Treatment and Rationale

Preemptive-Preventative Analgesia

Femoral fracture repairs can be very painful and difficult to treat.

- This dog received morphine 1.0 mg/kg SC as premedication, along with acepromazine 0.025 mg/kg SC and atropine 0.01 mg/kg SC.
- An epidural catheter was inserted in the lumbosacral space and advanced three disk spaces cranially after induction of anesthesia (see Chapter 12). Preservative-free morphine 0.1 mg/kg along with bupivacaine 0.1 mg/kg was injected through the catheter before surgery. This catheter facilitated readministration of epidural analgesics for several days. Placing morphine in the epidural space provided good analgesia for 12 to 24 hours with minimal central nervous system side effects. The low dose of bupivacaine blocked sensory nerve transmission with minimal effect on motor nerve transmission. This technique allowed the dog to feel its legs in recovery, preventing self-trauma and mutilation, which sometimes occur with epidural regional anesthesia.
- This dog underwent uneventful anesthesia and surgery.

Postoperative Analgesia

The dog recovered from anesthesia but was in considerable pain and agitated.

- Morphine 0.1 mg/kg was administered IV and infused at 0.1 mg/kg/hr to provide analgesia. The infusion was continued for 18 hours.
- Dexmedetomidine 2 µg/kg IV was administered in recovery because of agitation. It was readministered 5 hours later.
- Epidural preservative-free morphine 0.1 mg/kg was readministered 12 hours after the initial dose and then at 24-hour intervals for 3 days, at which time the epidural catheter was removed (Box 22-46).

BOX 22-46   **CASE 23**   **Bilateral Femoral Fracture Repair: Therapeutic Options**

- Preemptive analgesia: Morphine 1.0 mg/kg SC; preservative-free morphine 0.1 mg/kg and bupivacaine 0.1 mg/kg via epidural catheter.
- Postoperative analgesia: Morphine bolus 0.1 mg/kg IV followed by morphine infusion 0.1 mg/kg/hr IV; epidural morphine administration.
- Dexmedetomidine 2 µg/kg IV was administered to quiet recovery from anesthesia.

CASE 24   **GENERAL TRAUMA**

Signalment: A 7-year-old castrated male domestic shorthair cat weighing 3 kg

Challenge: The cat was recently hit by a car and sustained head trauma, a broken left humerus, and general soft-tissue trauma.

Sources of Pain: General soft-tissue trauma and fractured bone, producing severe pain (Box 22-47).

BOX 22-47 | CASE 24 | **General Trauma: Description of Pain**

- Somatic pain
- Moderate to severe
- Inflammatory and trauma-induced tissue trauma
- Acute onset

Treatment and Rationale

Preemptive-Preventative Analgesia

- The immediate goal was to provide good analgesia overnight but to be able to assess mentation periodically to determine the effects of head trauma.

- Remifentanil does not require liver metabolism but is cleared via nonspecific esterases throughout the body. Remifentanil has a duration of action of 8 to 10 minutes regardless of infusion time. Remifentanil was administered at 7 µg/kg/hr, which kept the cat very comfortable. The remifentanil infusion was periodically discontinued when neurologic assessment was desired. Neurologic assessment was performed 10 minutes later. Analgesia was reestablished by administering a bolus of remifentanil 4 µg/kg and restarting the infusion (Box 22-48).

BOX 22-48 | CASE 24 | **General Trauma: Therapeutic Options**

- Continuous analgesia: Remifentanil 7 µg/kg/hr

CASE 25 | **EXERCISE-INDUCED TRAUMA**

Signalment: A 4-year-old spayed female mixed-breed dog weighing 25 kg.
Challenge: Limping on right rear limb after a long hike in the mountains.
Sources of Pain: The dog had mild hip dysplasia of the right coxofemoral joint resulting in moderate osteoarthritic pain. There was also evidence of periarticular muscle soreness (Box 22-49).

BOX 22-49 | CASE 25 | **Exercise-Induced Trauma: Description of Pain**

- Somatic pain
- Mild to moderate
- Inflammatory and exercise-induced tissue trauma
- Acute onset

Treatment and Rationale

The dog was successfully treated with carprofen 100 mg PO once daily for 7 days (Box 22-50).

BOX 22-50	CASE 25	**Exercise-Induced Trauma: Therapeutic Options**

- Analgesia: Carprofen 4.4 mg/kg PO qd

CHAPTER 23

Chronic Pain Cases

Robin Downing; James S. Gaynor

$\mathbf{T}$he following are actual cases of animals in chronic pain. These cases were chosen because they represent the diversity of chronic pain presentations veterinarians are likely to encounter. Although there are commonalities across the population, each animal in pain is unique and will provide its own challenges in both diagnosis and treatment. Human pain scientist and specialist Dr. James Giordano has affirmed that "Pain management is an ongoing clinical experiment with an *n* of 1" (Personal communication, RD). It is important to keep an open mind when approaching an animal with chronic pain, and to take as systematic an approach as possible so as not to overlook any aspect of the animal's presentation or condition that could influence therapeutic decisions.

Keeping an open mind means evaluating the entire animal, resisting the temptation to home in too quickly on the apparent lameness or the lack of cervical mobility. It means making as thorough and complete a diagnosis as possible, both for the presenting pain issue and for any other relevant conditions. For instance, hypothyroidism interferes with metabolism of nutrients and medications as well as undermining stamina. Physiotherapy and therapeutic exercise will not be as effective if hypothyroidism is not managed. Another example is the dog with lameness that persists despite treatment, that actually has osteosarcoma rather than osteoarthritis (OA).

Keeping an open mind during the treatment of chronic pain means understanding that there is no single "silver bullet" that meets the needs of all animals in pain. Chronic pain is complex and generally provides several targets on which treatments should focus. Recognizing this reality is at the heart of multimodal pain management, in which we leverage multiple approaches to pain, each focused on a specific target in the body. In a multimodal pain management treatment plan, all the components work together synergistically, providing better results than any of them could work on its own. Keeping an open mind during pain treatment also means understanding what options are available to treat animals in pain (pharmacologic and nonpharmacologic), what treatment options have scientific evidence to support their use versus pure speculation or anecdote, and how to weave together various treatment options to create a targeted multimodal pain management plan. It means listening carefully to pet owners as treatment unfolds to understand from *their* perspective how the treatment is going. Most pet owners are completely oblivious to the fact that their cat or their dog is in pain. They misinterpret changes in behaviors and habits as signs of aging or mere quirks. They do not understand how important behavioral cues are in communicating an animal's comfort status.

Keeping an open mind when treating animals with chronic pain means recognizing that a treatment plan or specific modality is not working and revising the pain management strategy. A definition of insanity, after all, is doing the same thing over and over and expecting a different outcome. If the animal is not achieving the anticipated or desired results, it means the treatment plan needs to change. The three Rs of chronic pain management are Review, Reassess, and Revise. *Review* the current treatment plan. *Reassess* the animal. *Revise* the treatment plan as needed.

Finally, keeping an open mind when treating animals in chronic pain means recognizing when the animal is out of options and humane euthanasia is the most appropriate recommendation. The underlying reason for choosing euthanasia may be end-stage organ system failure, but the most relevant detail is compromised quality of life. Intractable or badly controlled pain is a relevant and important reason for choosing humane euthanasia. If an animal in pain reaches a point at which comfort cannot be restored or sustained, then euthanasia is a viable option.

Among the following representative cases, various drugs and drug dosages, nutraceuticals, procedures, and modalities are described. The details of these cases, the treatment options used, and responses to therapy should be considered examples of possible outcomes because animals were subjectively assessed through a combination of pain palpation and observation by the veterinarian as well as quality-of-life evaluations by the pet owners. More detailed information on specific drugs and procedures can be found in various chapters of this *Handbook*. These animals should be considered systemically healthy unless otherwise noted.

Please note the abbreviations for frequency of administration as recognized within the pharmacy profession:

qd = once daily (every 24 hours)
bid = twice daily (every 12 hours)
tid = three times daily (every 8 hours)
qid = four times daily (every 6 hours)
qod = every other day (every 48 hours)

For pain scoring in these cases a 0 to 10 scale was chosen in which 0 represents no pain and 10 represents the worst possible pain. Scoring pain in another being is a highly subjective activity, but one must begin somewhere to attempt to objectify the subjective experience of pain to advocate on behalf of beings who cannot advocate for themselves. A realistic target pain score for animals with pain is 1 or 2 of 10.

CASE 1 CHRONIC CRANIAL CRUCIATE LIGAMENT DISEASE

Pain control for a dog with bilateral chronic cranial cruciate ligament (CCL) disease.

Signalment: A 4½-year-old spayed female Great Dane dog weighing 45.5 kg presents with a torn right CCL and a partially torn left CCL. The dog has developed OA in both stifles and back pain secondary to altered biomechanics.

Challenge: The right CCL tear occurred 2½ years earlier; it is unknown when the left CCL partial tear occurred. The dog has been persistently lame and has had pain in the right rear for 2½ years with no diagnosis of back pain and no management of her CCL disease, either surgical or medical. Unmitigated chronic pain causes pathologic changes in the nervous system resulting in maladaptive pain, or maldynia. This is "pain as disease" with both central and peripheral sensitization. The dog's initial overall pain score on palpation was 7 of 10.

Sources of Pain: The dog had OA and degenerative joint disease (DJD) in the stifle joints, and altered biomechanics with secondary maladaptive back pain (Box 23-1).

BOX 23-1 CASE 1 **Chronic Cranial Cruciate Ligament Disease: Description of Pain**

- Stifle osteoarthritis
- Moderate to severe intensity
- Inflammatory and maladaptive
- Long term to lifelong

Treatment and Rationale

- The dog began receiving 100 mg of carprofen orally (PO) bid.
  - Nonsteroidal anti-inflammatory drugs (NSAIDs) remain the cornerstone for controlling the inflammatory pain associated with OA.
  - NSAIDs alone cannot manage chronic maladaptive pain, so many animals with chronic OA cannot achieve the realistic target pain score of 1 or 2 of 10.

- After 6 months of a multimodal pain management strategy including nonpharmacologic management of inflammation, the carprofen was gradually reduced and then discontinued.
- One advantage of reducing or eliminating the NSAID from daily use (*only* if the animal's pain score and activities of daily living remain stable) is that in the case of an acute inflammatory event (e.g., injury or surgery), the therapeutic dose is available for use.
- Several times in previous years, this dog either sustained an acute injury (sprained carpus) or needed a surgical intervention (extraction of a fractured premolar), recovery from which was greatly facilitated by a therapeutic dose of an NSAID.
- The dog's initial dosage of gabapentin was 300 mg PO bid.
  - Gabapentin acts at the $\alpha_2\delta$ ligand of the calcium channel in the neurons of the dorsal horn of the spinal cord, modulating calcium permeability.
  - Gabapentin's neuromodulatory effects achieve the result of normalizing the threshold for neuronal depolarization.
  - Gabapentin *complements* the other components of a chronic pain management protocol without enhancing toxicity so it can be used *with* other agents.
  - Gabapentin will elicit *some* response within 24 hours and *maximal response* within 7 to 10 days.
  - Gabapentin dosage should be escalated at 2- to 4-week intervals until the target comfort level is achieved or sedation occurs.
  - Sedation or altered mentation is the relevant dose-limiting side effect in both the cat and the dog. If sedation occurs, lower the dosage by 20% to 50% for 1 to 2 weeks, then reassess; if the animal is still in pain, attempt a dosage escalation using a smaller increment.
  - Long-term or even lifetime administration of gabapentin is common because OA is a progressive disease.
  - This dog ultimately needed 900 mg PO bid to achieve a pain score of 1 of 10.
- The dog was transitioned to a therapeutic nutrient profile with demonstrated efficacy for improving comfort and function in dogs with OA.
  - Remember the fundamentals when constructing a pain management plan. Dogs must eat every day. Science has brought forward a nutrient profile that improves outcomes in most animals with OA. In these dogs, every meal contributes to better pain control.
- Based on a total daily dosage of 50 to 60 mg/kg, eicosapentaenoic acid (EPA) to supplement the amount in the therapeutic nutrition was initiated.
  - Omega-3 fatty acids, and specifically EPA, have been demonstrated to decrease inflammation and support joint integrity.

- It is important to choose a source of EPA that is both bioavailable and produced in accordance with pharmaceutical standards.
- Polysulfated glycosaminoglycans (PSGAGs) at a dosage of 4.4 mg/kg were provided by subcutaneous injection twice weekly for 4 weeks, once weekly for 4 weeks, then twice monthly for maintenance.
  - PSGAGs interrupt the enzymatic degradation of cartilage in joints with OA.
  - PSGAGs increase the viscosity of synovial fluid, improving joint lubrication.
- Therapeutic laser was applied to the painful soft tissues of the lumbar torso (980 nm, 12 W, class IV).
  - Light energy at a wavelength of 980 nm and a dose of 10 J/cm^2 at the surface penetrates to a depth of 1.5 to 2 cm.
  - Therapeutic laser decreases inflammation, increases microcirculation, and decreases nerve conduction velocities, all contributing to pain relief.
- Microlactin, a milk-based protein with anti-inflammatory and pain relieving effects, was given at a dosage of 50 mg/kg PO bid. Microlactin is a nutraceutical, not a drug. A brand with documented efficacy was chosen because nutraceutical production is not regulated by the U.S. Food and Drug Administration.
- Once the dog was more comfortable (pain score 2 of 10), physiotherapy was initiated to improve function and build strength and stamina.
  - The dog engaged in proprioceptive retraining involving a physioroll, balance board, and wobble board.
  - Hydrotherapy on an underwater treadmill allowed the dog to improve stifle range of motion (ROM), rear limb coordination and strength, and core strength.
- Once a pain score of 1 of 10 was achieved, therapeutic exercise was assigned as "homework" to complement physiotherapy.
  - Sit to stand strengthens core and rear limb function.
  - Backward walking enhances proprioception and hip extensor function.
  - Curb walking enhances proprioception and strengthens lateral and medial stifle stabilizers.

Outcomes

- Once a pain score of 1 of 10 was achieved, the dog was cleared to begin conditioning for longer walks. She ultimately achieved walking 25 to 30 miles per week.
- Approximately 18 months after beginning treatment, only nutrition, nutraceuticals, and PSGAGs were in place for long-term joint support (Box 23-2).

BOX 23-2 | CASE 1 | **Chronic Cranial Cruciate Ligament Disease: Therapeutic Options**

- *First therapy:* Carprofen 100 mg PO bid
- *Concurrent therapy:* Gabapentin 900 mg PO bid, therapeutic nutrition, EPA, PSGAGs, therapeutic laser, microlactin, physiotherapy, therapeutic exercise
- *Long-term management:* Therapeutic nutrition, EPA, PSGAGs, microlactin

Key: *EPA,* Eicosapentaenoic acid; *PSGAGs,* polysulfated glycosaminoglycans.

| CASE 2 | **GENERALIZED MALADAPTIVE PAIN** |

Pain control for an elderly cat with OA and chronic maladaptive back pain.

Signalment: A 12-year-old spayed female Ragdoll cat weighing 3 kg presented with inflammatory bowel disease (IBD), lumbosacral bridging spondylosis, and facet OA.

Challenge: The cat had become increasingly reclusive, hiding under beds and furniture to avoid visitors to the home, the other cats in the household, and the pet owner. She could not be handled at the veterinarian's office except under general anesthesia. The pet owner believed the cat was in pain; however, the primary care veterinarian denied the presence of pain. Trial treatment with an NSAID (at the pet owner's insistence) failed to change the cat's behavior. Pain score on palpation was 7 of 10.

Sources of Pain: The cat had concomitant lymphocytic, plasmacytic enteritis with signs of lower gastrointestinal (GI) IBD. Lateral spine radiographs revealed a bridging spondylosis lesion at the L-S junction as well as facet joint changes consistent with spinal OA. The long duration of the cat's pain coupled with the diffuse distribution, and the apparent failure of an NSAID to effect any improvement supported a diagnosis of generalized maladaptive pain (Box 23-3).

BOX 23-3 | CASE 2 | Spine Osteoarthritis: Description of Pain

- Generalized back pain
- Severe intensity
- Inflammatory and maladaptive
- Long term to lifelong

Treatment and Rationale

- IBD can make cats miserable with nausea, increased intestinal gas, and increased stool urgency.

- A hydrolyzed protein nutrient profile was introduced to limit antigenic stimulation from food.
- Prednisolone at 5 mg PO qd was introduced to mitigate the inflammation from IBD. This also addressed the inflammation from the cat's spinal OA.
- Chronic maladaptive pain typically responds well to the neuromodulatory effects of gabapentin (see Case 1).
  - Gabapentin was started at 50 mg PO qd in the evening for 3 days, then 50 mg PO bid.
  - Starting with a single dose in the evening for three or four doses minimizes the risk of sedation. If sedation occurs, it will happen at night when the household will be asleep.
  - After 3 weeks the cat was still quite reactive, although her pain score on palpation was now 3 of 10. Gabapentin was increased to a total daily dosage of 150 mg PO per day in divided doses.
- Chiropractic adjustment was initiated to restore movement to areas of the spine experiencing restricted movement that contributed to the animal's back pain.
  - Back pain is a common reason cited by humans seeking chiropractic adjustment.
  - Empirically the cat showed an immediate decrease in reactivity after chiropractic adjustment.
  - The cat was adjusted every 2 weeks for three adjustments, then every 4 weeks for three adjustments.

Outcomes

- The hypoallergenic diet and prednisolone improved the cat's signs of IBD.
- The pet owner reported that within 3 weeks of initiation of multimodal pain management the cat was more interactive with her and with the other cats in the household.
- After 4 months of multimodal pain management, the pet owner reported that the cat had begun interacting with visitors to the home. She accepted grooming by both the pet owner and the other cats in the household (Box 23-4).

BOX 23-4   **CASE 2**   **Spine Osteoarthritis: Therapeutic Options**

- *First therapy:* Prednisolone 5 mg PO qd
- *Concurrent therapy:* Gabapentin 50 mg PO tid, chiropractic adjustment

CASE 3 INTERVERTEBRAL DISK DISEASE

Pain control for a dog with intervertebral disk disease (IVDD), OA, and chronic maladaptive back pain.

Signalment: A 14-year-old neutered male Dachshund dog weighing 6.5 kg presented with multilevel chronic IVDD, facet and peripheral joint OA, and generalized back pain.

Challenge: The dog was so weak in the rear legs that he was to be fitted for a dog wheelchair. He demonstrated reduced proprioception in both rear limbs. His pain score on palpation was 8 of 10. It was impossible to determine if he was weak as a result of pain or because of a neurologic deficit. The family was close to deciding on euthanasia because of his diminished quality of life.

Sources of Pain: The dog had multilevel chronic IVDD, facet and peripheral joint OA, and altered biomechanics with secondary maladaptive back pain (Box 23-5).

BOX 23-5   CASE 3   **Intervertebral Disk Disease and Osteoarthritis: Description of Pain**

- Rare limb paresis caused by pain
- Severe intensity
- Generalized distribution
- Inflammatory and maladaptive
- Long term to lifetime

Treatment and Rationale

- The dog was already receiving 5 mg prednisone PO qd.
- Once the dog's pain score was reduced to 2 of 10, the dosage of prednisone was modified to 5 mg PO qod.
- After 2 months of multimodal pain management, the prednisone was discontinued.
- Gabapentin was added at 100 mg PO bid for its neuromodulatory effects (see Case 1).
- After 1 year, the gabapentin dosage was increased to 100 mg PO tid.
- Four months later the gabapentin dosage was again increased, to 200 mg PO bid. This was the dosage for the rest of the dog's life.
- A daily glucosamine and low-molecular-weight (LMW) chondroitin with avocado and soybean unsaponifiables (ASU) nutraceutical was added.
- The omega-3 fatty acid EPA was added at 100 mg PO bid.
- After 10 days, the dog's pain score was 2 of 10 and the dog was walking more normally with improved proprioception.

- At this time twice weekly physiotherapy was initiated.
  - Dry-needle acupuncture
  - Therapeutic laser (980 nm, 10 W, class IV) at a dose of 10 J/cm^2 delivered at the surface
  - Stretching, traction, weight shifting using a physioroll
  - Hydrotherapy on the underwater treadmill
- The pet owners initiated 10-minute walks three or four times per day.
- The pet owners were taught several medical massage techniques to use at home between physiotherapy sessions to increase blood and lymph circulation as well as to provide gentle peripheral nervous system modulation.

Outcomes

- The dog was incapacitated by its pain, and the pet owners mistakenly believed it needed a canine wheelchair.
- Within 2 weeks of initiation of multimodal pain management, the dog was functioning dramatically better and it was clear that the dog did not need a wheelchair.
- With a combination of pharmacology, nutraceuticals, physiotherapy, and periodic medication modifications, the dog enjoyed 3 additional years of life (Box 23-6).

BOX 23-6   **CASE 3**   **Intervertebral Disk Disease and Osteoarthritis: Therapeutic Options**

- *First therapy:* Prednisone 5 mg qd (eventually discontinued)
- *Concurrent therapy:* Gabapentin 200 mg PO bid; glucosamine, low-molecular-weight chondroitin, ASU, EPA; physiotherapy, acupuncture, at-home massage

Key: *ASU,* Avocado and soybean unsaponifiables; *EPA,* eicosapentaenoic acid.

CASE 4   **HIP AND SPINE OSTEOARTHRITIS**

Pain control for a cat with hip and spine OA and back pain.

Signalment: A 19-year-old neutered male domestic shorthair cat weighing 5 kg presented with bilateral hip OA, spine and facet joint OA, and back pain.

Challenge: The cat could no longer jump or play as he had for his entire life. The pet owners perceived decreased quality of life. Preexisting chronic renal disease raised concerns about the use of NSAIDs. The cat's pain score on palpation was 6 of 10.

Sources of Pain: The cat had cartilage damage in coxofemoral and facet joints, and secondary lumbar pain from altered biomechanics (Box 23-7).

| BOX 23-7 | CASE 4 | **Hip and Spine Osteoarthritis: Description of Pain** |

- Lumbar and hip pain
- Moderate to severe intensity
- Inflammatory
- Long term to lifetime

Treatment and Rationale

- Because of the renal disease, microlactin at 250 mg PO bid was chosen as an alternative to NSAID therapy (see Case 1).
- Therapeutic laser (980 nm, 10 W, class IV) was applied at a dose of 10 J/cm^2 at the surface. The treatment area included the lumbar torso and the area over the coxofemoral joints. Therapeutic laser was chosen to decrease inflammation, increase circulation, and decrease pain.
- PSGAGs at a dosage of 4.4 mg/kg were administered by subcutaneous injection twice weekly for 4 weeks, once weekly for 4 weeks, then twice monthly for maintenance (see Case 1).
- Once the cat's pain score was reduced to 2 of 10, physiotherapy was initiated.
  - Torso stretching over a physioroll to provide mild traction.
  - Side-to-side weight shifting on a balance board to improve proprioception and strengthen intrinsic muscles.
  - Weekly hydrotherapy sessions on an underwater treadmill were initiated to increase strength and balance as well as improve mobility and ROM of the coxofemoral joints. The cat responded well and built up to 30-minute sessions.
  - The cat underwent weekly physiotherapy sessions for 8 weeks, then every-other-week physiotherapy sessions for four additional sessions.
- Chiropractic adjustment was provided at every other physiotherapy session to restore movement in spinal segments that were experiencing restricted motion. Back pain is a common reason cited by humans seeking chiropractic care.

Outcomes

The pet owner reported that the cat was restored to a robust activity level that included jumping up onto windowsills and playing with the other cats and dogs in the household (Box 23-8).

BOX 23-8 | CASE 4 | **Hip and Spine Osteoarthritis: Therapeutic Options**

- *First therapy:* Microlactin
- *Concurrent therapy:* PSGAGs, therapeutic laser, physiotherapy, chiropractic adjustment

Key: *PSGAGs,* polysulfated glycosaminoglycans.

CASE 5 | **BILATERAL HIP DYSPLASIA**

Pain control in a dog with bilateral canine hip dysplasia (CHD) and OA, coxofemoral joint denervation, a lumbosacral dorsal laminectomy, and degenerative myelopathy (DM).

Signalment: A 9-year-old spayed female German Shepherd Dog weighing 36 kg presented with bilateral CHD, a history of lumbosacral surgery, and signs consistent with DM.

Challenge: The dog was experiencing profound, generalized chronic maladaptive pain. The initial pain score on palpation was 7 of 10. Early signs of DM and muscle atrophy contributed to rear limb paresis. The dog had had a lumbosacral dorsal decompression and denervation of the coxofemoral joints 3 years before presentation. The dog also had profound atopy with self-trauma from pruritus and previously undiagnosed hypothyroidism (Box 23-9).

BOX 23-9 | CASE 5 | **Lumbosacral Dorsal Laminectomy, Canine Hip Dysplasia, Coxofemoral Joint Denervation, and Degenerative Myelopathy: Description of Pain**

- Generalized back and hip pain
- Severe intensity
- Inflammatory and maladaptive
- Long term to lifetime

Sources of Pain: The dog had CHD with resulting DJD and cartilage degradation, post-lumbosacral laminectomy pain, and altered biomechanics from OA and DM causing secondary back pain.

Treatment and Rationale

- Hypothyroidism was managed with 0.8 mg levothyroxine PO bid.
- Despite corticosteroid and antihistamine therapy, the dog's pruritus and self-trauma from inhalant allergies were uncontrolled.
  - A hydrolyzed protein nutrient profile was introduced to assist with allergy management.
  - Cyclosporine at 100 mg PO qd was prescribed to blunt the immune response to inhaled allergens. Over a 6-month period the dose frequency of cyclosporine was reduced and eventually the drug was discontinued.

- Antihistamines and prednisone were continued long term.
- Because of the maladaptive nature of this dog's chronic pain, gabapentin was introduced at 300 mg PO bid.
  - At the 2-week reassessment, the pain score was reduced only to 4 of 10, so the gabapentin dosage was increased to 300 mg PO in the morning and 600 mg PO in the evening.
  - Over a 2½-year period, the dog's gabapentin dosage was escalated as needed to meet its pain management need. At the time of death, this dog needed (and received) 1200 mg PO bid.
  - At no time did the dog experience any sedation from escalating doses of gabapentin.
- To enhance the effects of gabapentin in controlling this dog's maladaptive pain, amantadine was added at 100 mg PO qd.
  - Amantadine acts as an N-methyl-D-aspartate (NMDA) receptor antagonist. The NMDA receptor has been implicated in the perpetuation of maladaptive pain.
- The dog remained on amantadine for 6 months, at which time her pain was well enough controlled for discontinuation.
- PSGAGs at a dosage of 4.4 mg/kg were provided by subcutaneous injection twice weekly for 4 weeks, then once weekly for 4 weeks (see Case 1).
- To supplement the amount of EPA in the therapeutic nutrition, a total daily dosage of 50 to 100 mg/kg of EPA was initiated (see Case 1).

Outcomes

- Within 5 weeks of initiation of a comprehensive multimodal pain management strategy, this dog's pain score on palpation was reduced from 7 to 1 of 10.
- The owner reported a dramatic improvement and increase in the dog's overall activity, interaction, and ability to negotiate the environment.
- Over the nearly 3-year course of multimodal pain treatment, this dog also experienced a progression of signs of DM. The dog began using a canine wheelchair mobility device when the rear limb paresis prevented it from going on the walks it had enjoyed with the family (Box 23-10).

BOX 23-10	CASE 5	**Lumbosacral Dorsal Laminectomy, Canine Hip Dysplasia, Coxofemoral Joint Denervation, and Degenerative Myelopathy: Therapeutic Options**

- *First therapy:* Gabapentin 300 mg PO bid; eventually 1200 mg PO bid
- *Concurrent therapy:* Cyclosporine (atopy; eventually discontinued), levothyroxine (hypothyroidism), PSGAGs, EPA
- *Second therapy:* Amantadine 100 mg PO qd (discontinued after 6 months)

Key: *EPA*, Eicosapentaenoic acid; *PSGAGs*, polysulfated glycosaminoglycans.

CASE 6   BACK PAIN RESULTING FROM TRAUMA

Pain control in a cat with midback pain resulting from a fall.

Signalment: An 18-month-old spayed female domestic shorthair cat weighing 4.5 kg.

Challenge: The cat was witnessed falling from an 8-foot height, landing askew on the carpeted floor. Because she stood up, shook herself, and ran off, the pet owner did not think the cat was hurt. Over the next 2 months the cat became less and less interactive and more difficult to handle. Radiographs of the spine revealed no significant findings. The initial pain score on palpation was 6 of 10 (Box 23-11).

BOX 23-11   CASE 6   Midback Pain Resulting From a Fall: Description of Pain

- Midback pain
- Moderate to severe intensity
- Inflammatory and maladaptive
- Intermediate to long term

Source of Pain: The cat sustained a midback injury as the result of a fall.

Treatment and Rationale

- A course of meloxicam was administered.
  - 0.1 mg/kg PO qd for 3 days, then 0.05 mg/kg PO qd for 3 days, then 0.25 mg/kg PO qd for 3 days.
  - A decreasing dosage was chosen to reduce the risk of toxicity.
  - The NSAID did not provide significant relief.
- Gabapentin was introduced at 50 mg PO qd in the evening for 3 days, then 50 mg PO bid.
  - The NSAID was ineffective in relieving this cat's pain, which is suggestive that this was not inflammatory but rather maladaptive pain following injury to the spinal nerves.
  - At the 2-week reassessment, gabapentin was increased to 100 mg PO bid.
  - Two weeks later, gabapentin was increased to 100 mg PO tid. This dosage was adequate to decrease the cat's pain score to 0 to 1 of 10.
- Chiropractic adjustment was introduced to mobilize areas of the spine that were experiencing restricted motion and contributing to the animal's pain.
  - Back pain is a common reason cited by humans seeking chiropractic care.
  - Empirically, and according to the pet owner, the cat demonstrated increased athleticism and increased activity during the first week after chiropractic adjustment.

Outcomes

- The cat had become impossible to handle in the veterinary examination room. She resented the pet owner handling her at home. Once the pet owner reported the cat's fall, mapping the cat's journey to a chronic maladaptive pain state was straightforward.
- Once the pain was adequately managed, the cat exhibited a personality transformation. The pet owner reported that the family's interactions with the cat improved dramatically (Box 23-12).

BOX 23-12   CASE 6   Midback Pain Resulting from a Fall: Therapeutic Options

- *First therapy:* Meloxicam with decreasing dose
- *Second therapy:* Gabapentin 300 mg per day divided, chiropractic adjustment

---

CASE 7   BILATERAL CANINE HIP DYSPLASIA AND HIP REPLACEMENT

Pain control in a dog with bilateral CHD and bilateral total hip replacement (THR).

Signalment: An 18-month-old spayed female Mastiff weighing 35.5 kg presented with bilateral CHD preparing for bilateral THR.

Challenges: This dog was very young to have diffuse chronic maladaptive pain. The dog was scheduled to undergo bilateral THR (staged 8 to 10 months apart); however, relief from current pain was needed to achieve an appropriate comfort level before surgery. The dog exhibited fear aggression when handled by new people. Her generalized maladaptive pain caused her great anxiety because she anticipated any handling would be painful. The dog's initial pain score on palpation was 8 of 10 (Box 23-13).

BOX 23-13   CASE 7   Bilateral Canine Hip Dysplasia and Total Hip Replacement: Description of Pain

- Hip and back pain
- Severe intensity
- Inflammatory and maladaptive
- Intermediate term

Sources of Pain: The dog had CHD with resulting DJD and cartilage degradation, as well as generalized chronic maladaptive pain from altered biomechanics and amplification of hip pain.

Treatment and Rationale

- The dog was receiving 100 mg PO bid of carprofen (a very high dose based on her body weight).
  - Despite daily NSAID therapy, the dog's pain score revealed the inability of an NSAID alone to address maladaptive pain.
  - The dosage was decreased to an appropriate dosage of 150 PO qd.
- Gabapentin was introduced to address the dog's maladaptive pain (see Case 1).
  - The initial dosage was 300 mg PO qd in the evening for 3 days, then 300 mg PO bid.
  - The gabapentin dosage was escalated every 2 weeks by 300 mg PO per day to a dosage of 900 mg PO bid. This dosage provided a pain score of 1 of 10 before THR surgery.
  - Postoperatively the gabapentin dosage was escalated with the addition of 600 mg PO before bed for 2 weeks, then was returned to 900 mg PO bid.
  - Six weeks after THR, the gabapentin dosage was reduced to 600 mg PO bid until the second THR was performed.
  - Following the second THR, no increase in gabapentin was required. Three weeks after the second surgery, gabapentin was reduced to 300 mg PO bid for 6 weeks, then 300 mg PO qd for 3 weeks, then discontinued.
  - The dog did not have any rebound pain after the slow withdrawal of gabapentin.
- The dog was fed a nutrient profile for overall joint support.

Outcomes

- Once this dog's pain was appropriately controlled, the first THR went smoothly. With physiotherapy, the dog was ready for the second THR 4 months later—4 to 6 months ahead of schedule.
- After the second THR, the dog was successfully weaned off all pain medication within 3 months. The dog was then able to participate in a lifestyle typical of a healthy 2-year-old dog (Box 23-14).

BOX 23-14 | CASE 7 | **Bilateral Canine Hip Dysplasia and Total Hip Replacement: Therapeutic Options**

- *First therapy:* Carprofen 150 mg PO qd (eventually discontinued)
- *Second and concurrent therapy:* Gabapentin 900 mg PO bid (eventually discontinued), therapeutic nutrition for joint support

| CASE 8 | **DEGENERATIVE JOINT DISEASE OF THE HIPS** |

Pain control for a dog with DJD in both hips (Box 23-15).

Signalment: A 10-year-old female spayed German Shepherd Dog weighing 36 kg presented with bilateral hip dysplasia, left worse than right.

Challenge: This dog has had chronic OA pain for 8 years. The pain continues to worsen with age.

Source of Pain: The dog had OA of the coxofemoral joints.

BOX 23-15 | CASE 8 | **Bilateral Hip Osteoarthritis:**
Description of Pain

- Hip pain
- Severe intensity
- Inflammatory
- Long term

Treatment and Rationale

- This dog was initially receiving aspirin as needed on bad days for several years. The pet owner and the veterinarian became concerned with the possibility of GI side effects (i.e., ulcers, hemorrhage).
- The dog began receiving carprofen 50 mg PO qd. This dosage was low, but the dog was much more comfortable within 1 day.
- The hip-associated pain worsened, and the dosage of carprofen was increased to 125 mg PO qd. This made the dog more comfortable for approximately 6 months.
- The dog was in pain again after 6 months. Rather than increasing the dosage of carprofen and risking side effects, the veterinarian recommended switching from carprofen to deracoxib.
- It is reasonable to expect that if one drug does not work well for an individual, another might work better.
- Considerable risk is present when immediately switching from one NSAID to another. It is possible to get additive side effects, such as GI ulceration or renal toxicity.
- It is advisable to have a washout period between ending one NSAID and starting another. A period of 5 to 10 days, or at least five half-lives of the drug being discontinued, is considered safe.
- If a washout period is not possible, administering a GI protectant, such as misoprostol or omeprazole, for approximately 4 to 10 days is advisable. For example, end one NSAID on the evening of one day and start misoprostol 2 to 5 μg/kg PO bid. Start the new NSAID the following day.

- To keep a dog comfortable during the washout period, opioids can be administered orally.
- Carprofen was discontinued for 5 days, during which time this dog became very uncomfortable. Deracoxib 50 mg PO daily was then administered. The dog did not demonstrate a great improvement in quality of life compared with carprofen.
- The veterinarian and pet owner then discussed the potential of acupuncture for relief of pain.
- Electroacupuncture was instituted twice weekly for 3 weeks, alternating hips at each treatment using the following protocol.
  - GB 29 to GB 30
  - BL 40 to BL 54
  - GB 34
  - Bilateral BL 11
  - Alternating current, 2.5 Hz, continuous for 20 minutes
- The dog became much more comfortable. During the fourth week of acupuncture the dog received only one treatment.
- Acupuncture was spread out to one treatment every 4 to 6 weeks.

Outcome

This dog remained comfortable with a combination of an NSAID and periodic acupuncture for the long term (Box 23-16).

BOX 23-16 | **CASE 8** | **Bilateral Hip Osteoarthritis: Therapeutic Options**

- *First therapy:* Nonsteroidal anti-inflammatory drug (NSAID)
- *Second therapy:* Alternative NSAID
- *Third and final therapy:* NSAID with tapering frequency of acupuncture

---

CASE 9   DEGENERATIVE JOINT DISEASE

Pain control for a dog with long-term DJD in both hips (Box 23-17).

Signalment: A 5-year-old female spayed 40-kg Old English Sheepdog presented with bilateral DJD of the coxofemoral joints.

Challenge: This dog has had chronic OA pain for 3 years. She has been receiving deracoxib 50 mg PO qd for 3 years. The deracoxib recently became less effective for controlling pain. The dog was switched to carprofen 150 mg PO qd, which maintained her comfort for several months before its efficacy began to decrease.

Source of Pain: The dog had inflammatory disease of both hips.

BOX 23-17   **CASE 9**   **Bilateral Hip Osteoarthritis:**
Description of Pain

- Hip pain
- Severe intensity
- Inflammatory and maladaptive (central neuronal hyperexcitability, or wind-up)
- Long term

Treatment and Rationale

- Amantadine 3 mg/kg PO qd for 21 days to treat potential central neuronal hyperexcitability (wind-up). Wind-up occurs because of a prolonged low- to medium-grade constant noxious stimulus bombarding the spinal cord. This case typifies the clinical presentation. In treating animals with OA and wind-up, NSAID administration can be maintained.
- Carprofen 150 mg PO qd.

Outcome

This dog became comfortable on the third day of treatment and remained comfortable for months on carprofen alone (Box 23-18).

BOX 23-18   **CASE 9**   **Bilateral Hip Arthritis: Therapeutic Options**

- *First therapy:* NMDA antagonist
- *Second and concurrent therapy:* Nonsteroidal anti-inflammatory drug (NSAID)

Key: *NMDA*, N-methyl-ᴅ-aspartate.

CASE 10   PAIN RELATED TO RADIATION THERAPY

Signalment: A 9-year-old spayed female Labrador Retriever dog weighing 31 kg.

Challenges: This dog had a mast cell tumor removed from the lateral aspect of the mid-left thigh and was treated with radiation therapy for 14 treatments over a 3-week period. The dog progressively developed more pain than could be managed at home with oral morphine and would not stand up (Box 23-19).

Source of Pain: The dog had radiation-induced soft tissue damage and inflammation.

Treatment and Rationale

The dog developed severe pain that affected its quality of life and the pet owner's ability to cope with it. The initial goal of therapy for this dog was to gain control of the pain.

BOX 23-19   CASE 10   **Radiation-Induced Pain: Description of Pain**

- Left thigh
- Severe intensity
- Neuropathic, central neuronal hyperexcitability
- Short to intermediate term

- The dog was hospitalized and a peripheral catheter was placed in the cephalic vein. Ketamine was diluted and administered as a bolus of 0.5 mg/kg IV, followed by 1 µg/kg/min. Ketamine was used as an NMDA receptor antagonist to decrease central neuronal hyperexcitability and reduce the chronic pain.

- Fentanyl was administered concurrently, initially as a 2-µg/kg bolus and followed by a 5 µg/kg/hr infusion. Within 1 hour, this dog was willing and able to stand and walk.

- Fentanyl and ketamine were administered for approximately 48 hours, with the fentanyl decreased to 2 µg/kg/hr during the last 12 hours.

- This dog was hospitalized for an additional 48 hours to make the transition to oral drug therapy before release back to the pet owner's care.

- Oral sustained-release morphine was started, 30 mg PO bid for 10 days. It was believed that this dosage of morphine would control the pain, based on the low dose of fentanyl that the dog had been maintained on during her initial therapy. This is the same dosage of morphine she was receiving before admission to the hospital. After 10 days, she was weaned to sustained-release morphine 30 mg PO qd for 5 days. Morphine was then discontinued completely.

- Amantadine was started, 100 mg PO qd for 5 days, to block the NMDA receptors and prevent central neuronal excitability.

Outcome

This dog was released from the hospital in a comfortable state and remained comfortable at home (Box 23-20).

BOX 23-20   CASE 10   **Radiation-Induced Pain: Therapeutic Options**

- *First therapy:* Ketamine and fentanyl
- *Second therapy:* Amantadine and oral morphine, then discontinued

---

CASE 11   PAIN RELATED TO FORELIMB AMPUTATION

Signalment: A 7-year-old spayed female Siberian Husky weighing 25 kg had osteosarcoma of the right front limb culminating in an uneventful forelimb amputation. The dog presented with the pet owner's complaint of intermittently crying out. The dog was receiving codeine 30 mg with acetaminophen 300 mg orally bid for 5 days. On physical examination, the dog was hypersensitive to touch and cried when lightly touched across her lateral thorax and abdomen. The dog had no neck or back pain. Allodynia was diagnosed.

Challenges: The dog had osteosarcoma of the right front limb culminating in an uneventful forelimb amputation and long-term complicated pain for which conventional approaches were not efficacious.

Source of Pain: The source of pain was unclear but was considered to be diffuse (Box 23-21).

BOX 23-21   CASE 11   **Forelimb Amputation Pain: Description of Pain**

- Diffuse pain
- Severe intensity
- Allodynia
- Short to intermediate term

Treatment and Rationale

- Current analgesic therapy was ineffective. Chronic refractory pain with allodynia is difficult to treat with a single drug (opioids) and generally requires a multimodal approach.
- Amantadine 100 mg PO qd for 5 days was initiated to block NMDA receptors and decrease central neuronal excitability, with the intent of decreasing allodynia.
- Oxycodone 5 mg PO qd was started for 10 days to provide analgesia from the chronic pain.
- The pet owner reported that the dog was comfortable within 2 days. The seventh day after the new analgesic protocol had started (2 days after discontinuation of the amantadine), the dog started developing allodynia again. Amantadine 100 mg PO qd was started for another 10 days, and sustained-release morphine was given for another 5 days (Box 23-22).

BOX 23-22   CASE 11   **Forelimb Amputation Pain: Therapeutic Options**

- *First and final therapy:* NMDA antagonist plus opioid

Key: *NMDA*, N-methyl-D-aspartate.

Outcome

The pet owner did not report that the dog had any more pain at the end of 10 days.

SUGGESTED READING

Giordano J, ed: Maldynia: Multidisciplinary perspectives on the illness of chronic pain, Boca Raton, 2011, CRC Press.

Woolf CJ: Pain: Moving from symptom control toward mechanism-specific pharmacologic management. Ann Intern Med. 2004; 140:441–451.

CHAPTER 24

Cat-Specific Considerations

Sheilah A. Robertson

Cats remain popular pets in many countries, with approximately 30% of households in the United States owning at least two cats. Most cats will undergo at least one surgery in their lifetime, usually elective neutering, that is associated with the potential for them to experience acute pain. There is a growing awareness and recognition of chronic pain in cats related to oral and dental disease, ocular diseases, idiopathic cystitis, various cancers, chronic wounds, and degenerative joint disease (DJD). Studies suggest that as many as 90% of cats have radiographic evidence of DJD, and although this is strongly associated with increasing age, young cats are also affected.[1]

Alleviation of pain in cats historically has lagged behind that in other companion animals, but this is rapidly changing; for example, in one survey the use of perioperative analgesics in cats increased fourfold over a span of 5 years.[2] The challenges of treating pain in cats are unique but not insurmountable, and methods of meeting them continue to improve (Box 24-1).

The drugs discussed elsewhere in this book can be used in a pain management plan for cats and include opioids (Chapter 9), nonsteroidal antiinflammatory drugs (NSAIDs) (Chapter 8), α2-adrenergic agonists (Chapter 10), local anesthetics (Chapter 11), and many of the drugs listed in the discussion of other drugs used to treat pain (Chapter 14). In addition, complementary therapies, physical rehabilitation, and exercise are applicable to cats (Chapters 17, 18, and 19). This chapter discusses the unique features of these drugs and modalities when used in cats and also provides practical information for managing common pain conditions in the feline patient.

BOX 24-1 Challenges of Treating Pain in Cats

- Difficulty in recognizing pain in cats
- Unique metabolism of drugs (e.g., low capacity for hepatic glucuronidation)
- Risk of unwanted or adverse side effects
- Paucity of drugs with market authorization
- Difficulty of administering medications to some cats

RECOGNITION OF PAIN IN CATS

There are no gold standard acute or chronic pain scoring systems for use in animals, but several scoring methods exist, and it is now recognized that validated methods will depend heavily on analyzing behaviors (Chapter 5). Studies that have tried to correlate easily measured objective physiologic data such as heart rate, blood pressure, respiratory rate, and rectal temperature with pain in cats have been unsuccessful because these are influenced by many factors other than pain, such as fear and stress.[3,4] Therefore, observation of behavior is the best means of assessing the presence and degree of pain experienced by a cat. The main things to consider are as follows (Box 24-2):

1. Does the cat maintain its normal behaviors before and after the procedure?
2. Does the cat stop displaying normal behaviors (e.g., a cat with abdominal pain may not perform a typical cat stretch, a cat with DJD may groom less and no longer jump up onto its favorite resting spots)?
3. Does the cat display new behaviors (e.g., the cat appears to be overgrooming; a previously friendly cat becomes aggressive; a social cat becomes reclusive)? Another example is a cat adopting a new posture when urinating, such as standing rather than squatting because of hip or spinal pain.

Knowing a cat's personality before onset of pain is important because changes in behavior may be specific for that patient, and often veterinarians must rely on information from the owner.

Acute Pain

Because even pain-free cats change their behavior in a veterinary clinic as a result of fear, this can make assessing pain very difficult. Cats that are stressed and/or in acute pain may be depressed, immobile, and tense, try to hide, and usually do not respond positively to human interaction such as stroking. The cat in pain that is immobile and hiding at the back of the cage is often overlooked and therefore goes untreated. Cats that are experiencing acute pain will often adopt specific postures and these can help to differentiate pain from fear or stress.

Brondani and colleagues[4] have identified specific domains that should be assessed when one is evaluating cats for pain related to ovariohysterectomy, and many of these also apply to other causes of acute pain (Box 24-3). Cats with abdominal pain frequently adopt a sternal posture, with the head down,

---

BOX **24-2** **Using Behavior to Assess Pain in Cats**

- Maintenance of normal behaviors
- Loss of normal behaviors
- Presence of new behaviors

BOX 24-3	Specific Domains to Consider in Assessing Pain in Cats

- Posture
- Comfort
- Activity
- Mental status
- Miscellaneous behaviors
  - Excessive tail activity
  - Contraction and extension of the hindlimbs
  - Partially closed eyes
  - Licking and chewing at the wound
- Reaction to palpation of the wound
- Reaction to palpation of the abdomen and flank
- Appetite
- Vocalization

elbows drawn back, stifles forward, abdominal muscles tensed, and back arched, and their eyes are often half-shut or squinting (Figure 24-1). An alternative posture that is adopted in the presence of abdominal pain is seen in Figure 24-2; the cat will hold its legs abducted and intermittently flex and extend them.

In some cats the response to pain is different and exhibited by manic and aggressive behavior, growling, hissing, and rolling around the cage, but this is less common. The latter behavior may be a response to restrictive bandages regardless of pain, but the two must be differentiated. Often if the bandage can be removed, the cat calms down; if it does not, then pain should be suspected and further investigated.

Limb pain prevents weight bearing; however, pain is often bilateral in cats (forelimb declaw) and therefore easily overlooked. One of the many commonly reported problems after onychectomy is excessive licking and chewing of the feet. If possible, one should assess the response to palpation on or around the source of pain; for example, a cat that has been given appropriate analgesic agents should tolerate gentle pressure around a surgical incision.

It is important that pain not go untreated just because one is unsure of its presence or severity. If in doubt, administer an analgesic agent and observe for a positive improvement in behavior or demeanor.

Pain should always be assessed and recorded in hospitalized individuals. A pain scoring system that suits the individual clinic should be adopted. This system must be user-friendly and not too time-consuming[4] (see Chapter 5).

Chronic Pain

The most common cause of chronic pain in cats is DJD, but cancer and oral, ocular, bladder, and long-standing skin diseases or wounds are also important causes.

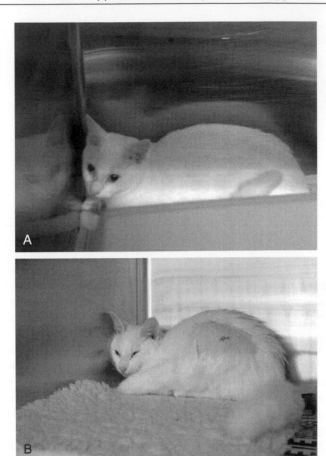

FIGURE 24-1   **A,** This image shows a cat before surgery that is fearful; note the posture and facial expression and position in the cage. **B,** This is the same cat after surgery (flank spay), with additional postures and expressions. The typical features suggestive of abdominal pain are a sternal posture with head down, elbows drawn back, and a tucked-up position or arched back with half-shut or squinting eyes.

Because of their small size and their innate agility, cats can often cope with orthopedic disease; and because of a pet cat's lifestyle, lameness and exercise intolerance are not common owner complaints. In addition, bilateral involvement—for example, both elbows or both hip joints—is common, and this makes lameness more difficult to detect. Eliciting pain on clinical examination of some cats is also notoriously difficult and not always correlated with joint pain. More work is needed to develop pain scoring instruments to detect DJD in cats.[5,6]

Clinical experience suggests that the behavioral changes that accompany DJD are insidious and easily missed or are assumed to be inevitable with

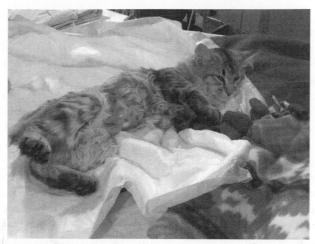

FIGURE 24-2   Abducted hind limbs that are alternately flexed and extended are suggestive of abdominal pain. Also note the facial expression in this cat.

advancing age; therefore the owner does not seek veterinary advice. Changes in behavior including decreased grooming, reluctance to jump up to favorite places, inability to jump as high as before, and soiling outside the litter box should prompt the veterinarian to look for sources of chronic pain. Other changes that owners may report are altered sleeping habits (increase or decrease), withdrawing from human interaction, hiding, and dislike of being stroked or brushed. Inactivity, which may result from chronic joint pain, is much more difficult to determine in cats because they naturally sleep a lot and are often solitary, and in many cases the owners are not home all day to monitor their cat's activity level. Although DJD affects mobility, nonactive activities are also important to a cat's overall quality of life.[7]

Analgesic trials may sometimes be the only way to confirm that chronic pain was present. For example, after intervention with an NSAID in cats with a presumptive diagnosis of DJD, the majority of owners believed that their cats made an improvement, and the most common clinical signs of improvement were a reduced unwillingness to jump, a higher jump, and a noticeably less stiff gait.[6,8,9]

METABOLISM OF DRUGS

Compared with other mammals, cats have a low capacity for hepatic glucuronidation of exogenously administered drugs.[10] Cats may lack these metabolic pathways because of their all-meat diet; they are not exposed to plants containing phytoalexins and therefore have not developed mechanisms to metabolize them.

These metabolic differences can lead to toxic side effects if doses and administration intervals are not adjusted. Alternatively, if the parent compound must be metabolized to an active component via this pathway, the drug may be less effective. The deficiency of the glucuronidation pathway in cats explains their susceptibility to the toxic side effects of phenolic drugs such as acetaminophen (paracetamol) and long half-lives of other drugs such as carprofen and aspirin. Only small amounts of morphine-6-glucuronide (M6G) are produced after administration of morphine in cats, and because this metabolite contributes to the overall analgesic profile of morphine in other species, morphine may be less effective in cats, especially if given in low doses.

Armed with a better understanding of feline drug metabolism, one can understand why the response to some drugs is unpredictable and different than in other species, and this allows clinicians to make more appropriate choices—for example, choosing a drug that relies more on oxidative pathways, such as meloxicam or robenacoxib, and using pharmacokinetic data such as half-life from research studies to devise administration intervals.

ANALGESIC DRUGS

Opioids

Opioids are the most versatile, reliable, and efficacious drugs for the treatment of pain and have an excellent safety record. In cats, opioids should be the foundation of most acute pain analgesic plans. As veterinarians study cats more, it is becoming clear that as in other species, there are genetic differences among individuals in their response to opioids. This may be correlated with individual differences in metabolism and with the number, type, and distribution of opioid receptors. For these reasons, one should not expect all cats to respond equally to a set dose of a specific opioid, emphasizing the need for careful pain assessment and individually tailored treatment protocols.

Timing of Administration

Opioids have distinct advantages when given before surgery; this is termed *preemptive* or *preventive analgesia*. Opioids can decrease but not fully prevent central sensitization, and animals that receive opioids before surgery have lower pain scores and higher pain thresholds for a longer period compared with those receiving them after surgery. When opioids are on board during a surgical procedure, heart rate and blood pressure tend to remain stable because they are less influenced by noxious stimuli.

Opioids decrease the need for inhalant agents less predictably and usually to a lesser extent in cats[11,12] compared with dogs, but having an opioid on board during surgery is still beneficial.

Side Effects

Many opioids can be used successfully in cats. The notion that cats are likely to become manic (so-called *morphine mania*) is a myth based on studies using doses far in excess of those needed to alleviate pain. Even at high doses undesirable behavior is uncommon,[13] and the opioids and doses suggested in this chapter usually result in sedation and euphoric behavior (rubbing against the cage or a person, purring, and kneading with the forepaws). Dysphoria is an unusual response to opioid administration in cats in pain or when an opioid is used in combination with drugs such as acetylpromazine or dexmedetomidine that provide sedation.

In contrast to many other species, opioids cause mydriasis in cats rather than miosis, but the analgesic effects can wear off before pupil size returns to normal, so pupil size should not be relied on as an indicator that analgesia is still present. Mydriasis, inability to focus, and poor depth perception may lead to cats becoming startled when approached quickly, bumping into objects, and showing aversion to bright light.

Nausea (licking of the lips, apprehension, and salivation) and vomiting are features of opioid administration in many species. In research and clinical settings the incidence of these side effects varies with the drug and the route of administration. Vomiting is most often associated with morphine and hydromorphone in cats, and vomiting is rarely seen after administration of butorphanol, buprenorphine, fentanyl, meperidine, methadone, or oxymorphone. Vomiting is most likely after subcutaneous injection and least likely after intravenous administration, with intramuscular administration lying between them.[14] These side effects are also more likely to be seen in a pain-free cat (e.g., when opioids are used before an elective procedure) and if opioids are not coadministered with acetylpromazine. Vomiting should be avoided in cats that are obtunded and may not have adequate airway protection and in those with a suspected increase in intracranial or intraocular pressure or with a corneal foreign body because the act of vomiting increases intracranial and intraocular pressure.

Long-term use of opioids is common in humans with chronic pain. However, in cats, inappetence is common after 2 to 3 days of opioid use and is likely associated with decreased gastrointestinal motility.

Route of administration also affects time to onset, intensity, and duration of action. It has been documented that the subcutaneous route is the least effective route for both hydromorphone and buprenorphine.[14,15] When an intravenous catheter is available, this is the recommended route of administration. This avoids repeated intramuscular injections, which can be painful and stressful for cats and more difficult for nursing personnel to perform.

Opioid-Related Hyperthermia. Hyperthermia can occur after opioid administration in cats. In a clinical setting with use of recommended doses (0.1 mg/kg) of hydromorphone, more than 60% of cats had temperatures greater than 40° C (104° F) at some time during recovery, with one cat reaching 42.5° C (108.5° F).[16] Moderately elevated temperatures have also been reported with morphine, buprenorphine, or butorphanol alone or with ketamine or isoflurane.[17] Depending on the severity of hyperthermia, cats can be treated with fans, bathed with cool water, or administered acepromazine to promote vasodilation; in severe cases naloxone has been successful after palliative measures failed. Mildly elevated rectal temperatures have been reported in association with transdermal fentanyl patches but rarely require treatment.

Cardiovascular depression, including bradycardia, is not a common side effect of opioids in clinical situations. If this does occur, it can be treated with atropine or glycopyrrolate (see Chapter 9). Respiratory depression is also uncommon, and during anesthesia it is often a result of other anesthetic agents and can easily be managed by providing manual ventilatory support. In conscious cats, hypoventilation after opioid use is rare and usually seen only after an overdose or if there is an underlying pathologic condition such as head trauma. In these situations, naloxone can be given *to effect* until respiratory rate increases; by doing this, respiratory depression can be selectively reversed while analgesia can be maintained. Naloxone (0.4 mg/mL) should be diluted in a 1:10 ratio with normal saline and given by slow intravenous injection until a response is seen. Alternatively, butorphanol (0.1 to 0.2 mg/kg) can be given to reverse μ opioid agonists and their respiratory depressive effects.

Clinical Use of Opioids

Buprenorphine. Buprenorphine is a partial μ-agonist that is widely used in cats. Buprenorphine is a popular choice in practice because it is versatile and is a less highly scheduled controlled drug than the pure μ-agonist agents. Onset of analgesia is faster than previously believed but dependent on route of administration; there is significant analgesia within 20 to 30 minutes after intravenous or transmucosal administration, and peak effect occurs 90 minutes after intravenous or transmucosal administration.

Transmucosal absorption through oral mucous membranes (oral transmucosal [OTM] administration) is effective in cats with almost 100% bioavailability by this route, likely a result of their alkaline saliva. Transmucosal administration has proved to be effective and acceptable in cats and can be used in the hospital if there is no easy intravenous access and mastered by owners for at-home treatment. The commercially available preparation for injection is used for transmucosal administration, and single dose formulations are better tolerated than multidose preparations.[18] The small volume (0.33 mL, at a dose of 0.02 mg/kg using a 0.3 mg/mL solution, in a 5-kg cat) can easily be placed on any oral mucous membrane such as under the tongue or in the cheek pouch. Buprenorphine (0.02 mg/kg) was equally effective when given by the intravenous and transmucosal routes and may provide analgesia for up to 6 hours.[19] Buprenorphine rarely causes vomiting or dysphoria in cats and is suitable for perioperative pain management because it is easily administered, highly effective, and long acting.

A sustained release preparation of buprenorphine for subcutaneous administration has been evaluated in cats undergoing ovariohysterectomy. A single sustained release dose of 120 μg/kg was as effective as 20 μg of buprenorphine per kilogram given by the OTM route every 12 hours until 60 hours after surgery.[20]

Butorphanol. Butorphanol is an agonist-antagonist opioid and exhibits a ceiling effect after which increasing the dose does not produce any further analgesia. In cats, this ceiling dose may be as low as 0.1 mg/kg.[21] Clinical and experimental investigations indicate that butorphanol is short acting in most cats (<2 hours) and requires frequent administration to be effective. It was found to be inferior to buprenorphine for control of pain after ovariohysterectomy.[22] Butorphanol appears to be an effective visceral but poor somatic analgesic and so may be a good choice for temporary relief of visceral pain syndromes such as interstitial cystitis.

Fentanyl. Fentanyl is a potent, short-acting pure μ-agonist that is used most commonly to supplement general anesthesia, during which it can be given as intermittent boluses or by infusion. Transdermal fentanyl patches that release fentanyl over several days have been used for alleviation of acute perioperative pain in cats. These patches enable a hands-off approach to pain management that is especially attractive for cats that are difficult to medicate. Plasma fentanyl concentrations are variable after patch placement in cats, and in some cats uptake is limited and does not reach an effective steady-state plasma concentration (>1 ng/mL); therefore, if patches are used, each cat must still be assessed carefully for comfort. The variability may be related to the size of the patch compared with the weight of the cat, skin permeability, placement site, skin perfusion, subcutaneous fat, and body temperature. When the patch is effective, cats achieve steady-state plasma concentration faster than dogs (6 to 12 hours compared with 18 to 24 hours), and plasma levels take longer to decline after patch removal in cats (up to 18 to 20 hours). Transdermal fentanyl patches have proved useful in a clinical setting for routine ovariohysterectomy and onychectomy. Significantly elevated temperatures (1.0° C above baseline) 4 to 12 hours after transdermal fentanyl patch application have been reported. Because a patch can be removed, there are liability issues related to accidental ingestion by children or deliberate diversion if cats are sent home with a patch in place.

Meperidine (Pethidine, Demerol). Meperidine (pethidine, Demerol), is a μ-agonist and should *be given only intramuscularly (IM)* because intravenous injection can produce excitement. Meperidine rarely causes vomiting in cats. The main drawback of meperidine is its short duration of action. In clinical practice, meperidine performs as predicted in experimental studies, producing good analgesia for little more than 1 to 2 hours. This drug is a reasonable choice for minor procedures of short duration but is not ideal for cats that require longer treatment because repeated intramuscular injections can be painful, and cats quickly become resentful of this. It can be a good choice of premedicant if sedatives and tranquilizers are contraindicated because it does produce reliable, but mild sedation.

Hydromorphone. Hydromorphone is a μ-agonist. Doses of less than 0.05 mg of hydromorphone per kilogram did not produce antinociception in a research model, whereas a dose of 0.1 mg/kg IV was effective for 3.5 to 7 hours, with considerable inter-cat variability on duration of effect. When combined with acepromazine (0.05 to 0.1 mg/kg), hydromorphone provides good analgesia and sedation. Hydromorphone can be associated with hyperthermia, and vomiting unless given by the intravenous route (see discussion of side effects).

Methadone. Methadone has been used in cats at doses ranging from 0.1 to 0.6 mg/kg, normally by the intramuscular or subcutaneous route, but intravenous administration is also commonly performed. Nausea and vomiting are rare after administration. In a clinical setting when used for ovariohysterectomy, methadone was effective and produced no undesirable behavioral, cardiovascular, or respiratory effects. In addition to its μ-agonist actions, methadone may also contribute to analgesia via antagonism of N-methyl-D-aspartate receptors. Methadone is a versatile analgesic agent for cats undergoing procedures likely to cause moderate to severe pain[23] and is also effective via the OTM route.[24]

Morphine. Morphine has been widely used in cats and does not produce excitation even when given in excess of the clinically recommended dose of 0.05 mg/kg IM.[13] No M6G, the active analgesic metabolite, was detected after intramuscular administration, but after intravenous administration M6G was detected in 50% of cats; therefore if intravenous access is available, this may be a more effective route of administration.

Oxymorphone. Oxymorphone has been a popular analgesic for many years in the United States, where it is licensed for use in the cat. Oxymorphone produces few undesirable side effects but is more expensive than other μ-opioid agonists.

Mixing of Opioids
It has been proposed that mixing of different classes of opioids may result in added benefits. However, the outcome seems variable; a combination of hydromorphone and butorphanol did not have additive effects but did produce a longer-lasting (up to 9 hours) but less intense effect than hydromorphone alone.[25] Combining butorphanol and buprenorphine provided no added benefits over either drug used alone and showed large inter-cat variation.[26]

Constant Rate Infusions

Fentanyl. Fentanyl is suitable for constant rate infusion in cats but should be titrated to effect to reduce accumulation. Fentanyl is most commonly used during anesthesia so that less inhalant agents are required, and it also allows the anesthetist to alter the level of analgesia rapidly. Fentanyl infusion can be continued into the postoperative period, when again it is easily titrated to individual needs. A loading dose of 5 to 10 µg/kg IV is suggested, followed by 10 to 45 µg/kg/hr during anesthesia, reducing the dose postoperatively to 2 to 5 µg/kg/hr, depending on the individual cat's needs.

Remifentanil. Remifentanil has an ideal pharmacokinetic profile for infusion, and reports of its intraoperative use in cats at doses of 0.1 to 1.0 µg/kg/min are promising. Elimination of remifentanil is independent of renal or hepatic function, so the drug is an ideal agent of choice when those body systems are compromised.

Epidural Opioid Administration

Morphine, fentanyl, pethidine, methadone, and buprenorphine have been given via the epidural route in cats. Epidural injection is technically more challenging in cats because of their small size, and because the spinal cord ends more caudally, entering the subarachnoid space is possible at the lumbosacral junction. Morphine has the greatest usefulness when given epidurally in cats.[27]

Each opioid drug is described in detail in Chapter 9, and recommended doses and routes of administration for cats are shown in Table 24-1.

Nonsteroidal Anti-inflammatory Drugs

Until recently, NSAIDs have not been widely used for long-term pain management in cats largely because of the fear of toxicity. For many NSAIDs, pharmacokinetic data are available only for single doses in cats, but there are now several studies that have examined the safety of chronic administration. The deficiency of glucuronidation pathways in cats results in slow metabolism of several NSAIDs, particularly the phenolic compounds. However, drug metabolism and excretion pathways other than glucuronidation, such as oxidation, sulfation, and active drug transport, do not appear to be deficient in cats. In recent years a number of newer NSAIDs have become licensed for use in cats in several countries. Robenacoxib is the most recently approved NSAID in the United States; it is used for the control of postoperative pain associated with inflammation related to orthopedic surgery, ovariohysterectomy, and castration, and can be given for a maximum of 3 days. This is the first coxib class of drug approved for cats. At clinical doses cyclooxygenase 1 (COX-1) inhibition is minimal and short lasting. Robenacoxib has a unique pharmacokinetic

TABLE 24-1 Commonly Used Opioid Drugs and Dosages for Cats

OPIOID	DOSE	ROUTE OF ADMINISTRATION	COMMENTS
Butorphanol	0.1-0.8 mg/kg	IV, IM	Little benefit to giving doses >0.2 mg/kg (ceiling effect). Short acting in some cats.
Buprenorphine	0.01-0.03 mg/kg	IV, IM Oral transmucosal	Not associated with vomiting or hyperthermia.
	35 μg/hr patch	Transdermal	Uptake occurs, but dosing regimens and efficacy in clinical settings not established.
Fentanyl			
Bolus	2-10 μg/kg	IV	
CRI intraoperative	10-45 μg/kg/hr	IV	All CRIs should be preceded by a bolus to achieve effective plasma concentration. Infusion rate can be adjusted to rapidly change degree of analgesia.
CRI postoperative	5-10 μg/kg/hr	IV	
TDF patch	25 μg/hr, 2.5 mg	Transdermal (over shaved skin)	May take up to 12 hours to reach effective plasma concentrations. Elevated body temperature reported in some cats.
Hydromorphone	0.05-0.1 mg/kg	IV, IM	Doses of 0.1 mg/kg regardless of route may be associated with hyperthermia.
Meperidine (pethidine, Demerol)	5-10 mg/kg	IM	Not to be given IV.
Methadone	0.1-0.6 mg/kg	IV, IM Oral transmucosal	Also has NMDA- antagonist properties. Not associated with vomiting or hyperthermia.
Morphine	0.2-0.5 mg/kg	IV, IM	Active metabolites reported only at low concentration; therefore may be less effective than in other species.
Oxymorphone	0.05-0.1 mg/kg	IV, IM	Hyperthermia not reported.
Tramadol	1-4 mg/kg	IV, IM	Has opioid actions.
Tramadol*	2 mg/kg	Oral (capsules, tablets, liquid)	

CRI, Constant rate infusion; NMDA, N-methyl-D-aspartate TDF, transdermal fentanyl.
*The human product Ultracet contains acetaminophen and must not be used in cats.

profile, with a short half-life but long residence time in target (inflamed) tissues.[28] NSAIDs have the advantage of being long acting, providing up to 24 hours of analgesia, and they are not subject to the purchase and storage restrictions of the opioids.

Side Effects

The adverse side effects of NSAIDs in cats are similar to those described for other species (see Chapter 8) and include renal, hepatic, and gastrointestinal toxicity. NSAIDs should not be used if there is preexisting renal or hepatic disease; if corticosteroids are being used; in the face of hypovolemia, dehydration, or hypotension; or if substantial blood loss is anticipated. A complete blood count and chemistry panel drawn before use may detect animals unsuitable for NSAID treatment (e.g., those with renal disease or significant liver disease) and provide baseline data if there is an unexpected complication after administration.

Clinically Useful Nonsteroidal Anti-inflammatory Drugs

Carprofen. Carprofen (2 to 4 mg/kg subcutaneously [SC] or IV) provides good postoperative analgesia for at least 24 hours in cats after soft-tissue surgery. Anecdotal reports of toxicity have been made, usually associated with concurrent disease and prolonged administration of the oral formulations. Carprofen undergoes glucuronidation, and problems with repeated administration may be a result of variable inter-cat pharmacokinetics; for example, in one study the half-life of carprofen after intravenous administration to healthy adult cats ranged from 9 to 49 hours. Repeat administration is not recommended.

Ketoprofen. Ketoprofen has proved to be an effective analgesic for use in cats; 2 mg/kg provided postoperative analgesia for at least 18 hours and was as effective as carprofen, meloxicam, and tolfenamic acid after neutering.[29] Ketoprofen can alter platelet function and increase bleeding; therefore it is usually given after surgery. Oral formulations (1 mg/kg once daily) have been used for longer periods to treat musculoskeletal disorders.

Meloxicam. Meloxicam is a COX-2 selective NSAID, and the injectable formulation is licensed for preoperative use in many countries (up to 0.3 mg/kg SC). Meloxicam is clinically effective for surgical procedures including ovariohysterectomy, castration, and orthopedic surgery.

The sweet-flavored oral formulation seems palatable to most cats, and in one study it was voted by owners as easier to administer than ketoprofen. The liquid formulation also allows for accurate dosage, which is important when this drug is used long term. Meloxicam has been used for long-term treatment of DJD in cats, with owners reporting considerable improvement.[8,9] Meloxicam does not have a prolonged half-life in cats because it is metabolized by hepatic oxidative pathways, and this may be why it has achieved success for long-term use. Meloxicam oral suspension has market authorization for the treatment of DJD in cats in several countries. The suggested dose is 0.1 mg/kg on day 1, followed by a maintenance dose of 0.05 mg/kg once daily. The daily dose can be given on food or directly into the mouth using the drop dispenser of the bottle or the measuring syringe provided. Some cats may respond to lower maintenance doses, and this can be decided by the owner depending on the cat's response.

If NSAIDs are used off-label (e.g., oral meloxicam suspension in the United States), the owner should be made aware of this. In all cases the owner should be informed of the possible side effects verbally and in writing. This should include what clinical signs to look for (e.g., vomiting, inappetence, and bloody stool) that would warrant calling the veterinarian and stopping treatment.

Although there are no standard guidelines for monitoring cats receiving NSAIDs over prolonged periods, the veterinarian should follow the cats carefully. It is suggested that the packed cell volume, total protein, blood urea nitrogen, creatinine, and liver enzymes be measured in addition to urine analysis before and after 1 week of treatment and then at 3-monthly intervals. Liver enzymes may rise with chronic drug administration but do not reflect hepatic function; an increase of more than 200% should prompt running liver function tests such as a bile acid assay. Excellent guidelines for long-term use of NSAIDs including information sheets for owners have been compiled by the International Society of Feline Medicine and the American Association of Feline Practitioners.[30]

Clinical Choices

There seems to be little difference in the efficacy of the various NSAIDs in the acute perioperative setting, and all provide good analgesia in the majority of cats for up to 24 hours.[29] More recently, robenacoxib was shown to perform better than meloxicam for the control of postoperative pain after a variety of surgical procedures.[31] Choice of agent depends on personal preference, convenience of administration, duration of use, and availability of licensed products. For long-term use, meloxicam is currently the best choice and the only NSAID labeled for treatment of chronic musculoskeletal disorders in cats, at least in some countries. Once an NSAID has been chosen, the cat should not be placed on a different one without a period of washout, which is arbitrarily said to be 5 to 7 days.

With the availability of newer NSAIDs the efficacy and safety of which are established, there appears to be little justification for use of the older NSAIDs such as aspirin, flunixin, and phenylbutazone to provide analgesia in cats. Paracetamol, ibuprofen, indomethacin, and naproxen are extremely toxic in cats and should never be used.

α₂-Adrenoceptor Agonists

The α_2-adrenoceptor agonists, which include medetomidine and dexmedetomidine, provide sedation, muscle relaxation, and analgesia in cats. These drugs are not commonly used for their analgesic effect alone because of the profound sedation and cardiovascular depression that accompany their use. It must be remembered that the dose required for analgesia is much higher than the dose required for sedation.[32] In cats with cardiovascular disease or preexisting hypovolemia, α_2-adrenoceptor agonists should be used with caution because of the vasoconstriction and decrease in cardiac output associated with their use.

Medetomidine and dexmedetomidine can be used alone for chemical restraint so that minor painful procedures (cleaning wounds, lancing abscesses) can be performed or fractious cats can be examined. These drugs can be used in combination with a variety of opioids to provide sedation and reliable analgesia.

Low-dose constant rate intravenous infusions can be used in cats; this is a good technique for fractious cats and facilitates nursing care, and the dose can be titrated up or down depending on what interventions are required. Suggested doses are 1 to 2 µg/kg/hr and 0.5 to 1 µg/kg/hr for medetomidine and dexmedetomidine, respectively.

Medetomidine and dexmedetomidine can be antagonized with atipamezole, but this will reverse analgesia in addition to sedation.

Local Anesthetics

The local anesthetic techniques described in Chapter 12 can be adapted for use in the cat. One of the most commonly used local anesthetic techniques in cats is a digital nerve block before onychectomy. Bupivacaine (total dose 2 to 3 mg/kg) *without* epinephrine is often used, but longer-acting agents would be more beneficial. Cats do not lose motor function with this technique but may have proprioceptive deficits. This technique offers good intraoperative analgesia, but the benefits are short-lived[33] and other analgesics (e.g., NSAIDs and opioids) are required for control of postoperative pain. Another useful technique is a coccygeal epidural with lidocaine for catheterization and pain management of cats with urethral obstruction.[34] These cats are often high-risk anesthesia cases, and use of this technique may reduce the doses of drugs, or avoid the need for general anesthesia.

Implantable wound catheters that can remain in situ for several days have been used in cats after major surgery including limb amputations and extensive fibrosarcoma resection. Injection of local anesthetic agents at 4- to 6-hour intervals or as an infusion maintains continuous analgesia, and in most cases the use of systemically administered opioids and NSAIDs can be reduced. When used as part of a multimodal approach, this technique resulted in cats returning to normal function (eating) and being discharged from the hospital sooner than cats not having a wound catheter placed.[35]

Topical liposome-encapsulated formulations of lidocaine is available, and a eutectic mixture of lidocaine and prilocaine can be applied to shaved skin to provide analgesia in advance of venipuncture, catheter placement, and skin biopsies. Transdermal absorption has been reported, but plasma concentrations were significantly below toxic values.[36]

Intravenous infusions of lidocaine decrease inhalant anesthetic requirements in dogs and may provide analgesia. At plasma concentrations that reduce isoflurane requirements in cats, significant cardiovascular depression and impaired tissue perfusion occur, and therefore *this technique is not recommended in cats.*[37]

Other Drugs

Tramadol

Although not classified as an opioid, tramadol has weak binding affinity at μ receptors and is also thought to act at adrenergic and serotonin receptors. Clinical experience shows that in cats, opioid-like effects such as dilated pupils and euphoria can be significant, depending on the dose. Tramadol (injectable formulation) has been used to treat acute pain in cats; in cats the effective injectable dose is greater than 1 mg/kg, and in the clinical setting, 2 to 5 mg/kg has provided analgesia for soft-tissue surgery.[38]

Oral bioavailability in cats is approximately 60%, and peak concentration is reached within 45 minutes, making oral administration potentially useful for postoperative pain control after hospital discharge and for treatment of chronic pain in cats. Reports on its use for chronic pain are anecdotal. Tramadol is bitter tasting and difficult to administer to cats, although some compounded formulations may be more palatable.[39]

Gabapentin

Gabapentin is most appropriate for neuropathic pain and therefore could play an important role in cats that undergo major surgery in which nerve damage is substantial, such as limb amputation, or in cats that are diagnosed with cauda equina syndrome or intervertebral disk disease. There are now several case reports on the use of gabapentin in cats that were challenging to treat with other analgesic drugs.[40,41] Recommended starting doses are 10 mg/kg PO two times daily; doses may be increased or decreased based on the response. At higher doses, some cats become sedated.

MULTIMODAL APPROACH

Nociception and pain involve many steps and pathways, so it seems unlikely that one analgesic agent could completely prevent or alleviate pain. Multimodal analgesia describes the combined use of drugs that have different modes of action and work at different receptors and at different places along the pain pathway with the assumption that this will provide superior analgesia or allow lower doses of each drug to be used, thereby lessening any adverse side effects. The most commonly used combinations of drugs are opioids and NSAIDs; use in combinations is superior to use of either drug used alone.[42]

DURATION OF TREATMENT

Clinically, there are two phases associated with surgery; the first is the sensory input arising directly from the surgery itself, and the second is from the resultant, more prolonged inflammatory response. It is now understood that unless an *effective* and *appropriate* level of analgesia is maintained into the postoperative period to include the duration of tissue injury associated with inflammation, reinitiation of pain is possible. To prevent prolonged or persistent postoperative pain, analgesic therapy should be started before surgery, be maintained during surgery, be robust in the immediate postoperative period, and not be withdrawn until the inflammatory response has subsided. Duration of treatment will depend on the degree of surgical trauma and resultant inflammatory response. The exact duration of the inflammatory response after different types of surgical procedures in cats is not well documented. Based on behavior evaluations, cats may experience pain for 3 days after ovariohysterectomy,[43] so a pain management plan must take this into consideration.

COMPLEMENTARY METHODS FOR TREATING FELINE PAIN

In recent years the popularity of more holistic approaches to medicine for humans and pets has increased. Complementary, alternative, or integrative veterinary medicine is challenging to define, but the American Veterinary Medical Association states that this approach to medicine includes aromatherapy; Bach flower remedy therapy; energy therapy; low-energy photon therapy; magnetic field therapy; orthomolecular therapy; veterinary acupuncture, acutherapy, and acupressure; veterinary homeopathy; veterinary manual or manipulative therapy (similar to osteopathy, chiropractic, or physical medicine and therapy); veterinary nutraceutical therapy; and veterinary phytotherapy.

Of these modalities, acupuncture is the best studied, with enough evidence for it to be endorsed by the National Institutes of Health for humans with chronic osteoarthritis. Contrary to popular belief, many cats are tolerant of acupuncture therapy (Figure 24-3), and it should be considered a viable

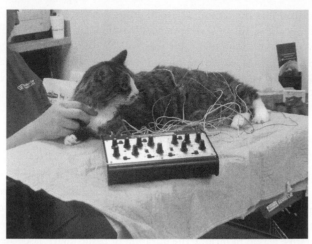

FIGURE 24-3   Many cats are tolerant of acupuncture and can benefit from the analgesia produced by this therapeutic modality.

choice for analgesic therapy, alone or in combination with drug therapy or other physical modalities. Some cats in pain will not eat, and acupuncture can be effective for appetite stimulation. The classic or traditional point that is often used is called *Shan-gen*, which is similar to GV 25 (GV means "governor vessel"), which is on the midline of the boundary between the hair and nonhair part of the nose.

ACUTE PAIN CASE STUDIES

See Boxes 24-4 to 24-6.

TREATMENT OF CHRONIC PAIN

Degenerative Joint Disease

As in dogs, weight control should be addressed in cats with DJD. If there are no contraindications to use, meloxicam is effective in many cats.[8,9,44] In some cats, this alone is not sufficient or preexisting disease precludes its use. In these cases, gabapentin can make many cats comfortable. Many veterinarians and owners report that chondroprotective agents, nutraceuticals, and acupuncture are beneficial.

Chondroprotective and Nutraceutical Agents

Animal nutritional supplements typically are not subject to premarketing evaluation by licensing authorities for purity, safety, or efficacy and may

---

BOX **24-4**	Ovariohysterectomy and Forelimb Declaw Pain

- Somatic and visceral pain
- Large inflammatory component to pain
- Moderate to severe intensity
- Potential to develop neuropathic pain (digits)
- Pain acute in onset
- Duration of several days or even weeks if complications arise

---

BOX **24-5**	Ovariohysterectomy and Forelimb Declaw—Anesthesia and Analgesia Plan

Premedication	Acetylpromazine 0.05 mg/kg IM
	Buprenorphine 0.02 mg/kg IM or methadone 0.5 mg/kg IM
	Robenacoxib 1-2 mg/kg PO* (30 min before induction)
Induction	Ketamine 5 mg/kg and diazepam 0.25 mg/kg IV
Local anesthetic block	Bupivacaine 2 mg/kg, digital nerve block
Postoperatively (in clinic)	Buprenorphine 0.01-0.02 mg/kg IV or IM q6-8h or methadone 0.3-0.5 mg/kg IV or IM
Postoperatively (at home)	Robenacoxib 1-2 mg/kg PO for 3 days

*If the injectable formulation is available, this is easier to use in the preoperative period.

BOX **24-6**	Hind Limb Amputation—Anesthesia and Analgesia Plan

Premedication	Dexmedetomidine 5 µg/kg IM
	Methadone 0.5 mg/kg IM
Induction	Ketamine 5 mg/kg and diazepam 2.5 mg/kg IV
Postoperatively	Methadone 0.3 mg/kg IV q4-6h for 24 hr
	Lidocaine 3 mg/kg infused into wound catheter, q4-6h (3 days); remove catheter on fourth postoperative day (send animal home)
	Gabapentin 10 mg/kg bid for 2 wk (start on day of surgery)
	Robenacoxib 1 to 3 mg/kg PO; duration of treatment will be based on evaluation of the cat

---

contain active pharmacologic agents or unknown substances. The mechanism of action of many of the proposed compounds is not known.

Chondroprotectants are available as oral nutraceuticals and as injectable (IM, IV, or intra-articular) pharmaceuticals, but their modes of action are poorly understood and their efficacy is controversial. Mixtures of chondroitin sulfate, glucosamine hydrochloride, and manganese are commercially available in flavored powders and capsules specifically aimed at cats. Polysulfated glycosaminoglycans can be given to cats but are licensed by the U.S. Food and

Drug Administration (FDA) for use only in dogs in the United States. Use of Adequan (polysulfated glycosaminoglycan) at 4.4 mg/kg IM or subcutaneously every 3 to 5 days for a total of eight injections has been reported in cats.[45] Commercially available joint diets containing various nutraceuticals can be beneficial.[46]

Cancer Pain

COX-2 has been identified in many human and dog carcinomas, and there is growing evidence from experimental, epidemiologic, and clinical trials that NSAIDs and in particular the COX-2–selective drugs may have a role in the prevention and treatment of some types of cancer. NSAIDs are thought to inhibit tumor growth by several different mechanisms including restoration of apoptosis (programmed cell death) and inhibition of angiogenesis.

Immunocytochemistry studies have been performed on a variety of feline neoplasms to determine COX-2 expression. There are species differences in COX-2 expression between canine and feline cancers; NSAIDs may have less of a role as anticancer agents in some feline cancers but may still be beneficial to alleviate cancer-related pain. Piroxicam is the most commonly used NSAID used in feline cancer patients and was well tolerated even in cats also receiving chemotherapy and/or radiation therapy.[47]

Oral Pain

Stomatitis, gingivitis, oral cancer, and dental disease are common medical conditions in cats and are accompanied by pain that can be severe and long-standing. In addition to specific surgical or medical intervention to treat the primary problem, pain must also be addressed. Cats with oral pain resent any attempts to administer pills by mouth, but buprenorphine can often be dropped into the corner of the mouth, and the liquid formulation of meloxicam can be mixed with soft food.

Administration of Drugs

Intravenous and intramuscular administration of drugs may be possible in a hospital setting; however, it is notoriously difficult for owners to medicate cats successfully in a home environment, resulting in poor compliance and thus failure of the treatment plan. Oral administration of pills, caplets, or capsules requires physical restraint, often by more than one person, and in most cats this quickly becomes an aversive procedure. Many drugs have an unpleasant taste; and because of their keen sense of smell, cats are suspicious of drugs placed in their food. It is important not to put medications in a prescription diet because there is a risk that the cat will refuse to eat it. Analgesics can be disguised or hidden in treats, pill pockets, or strongly flavored cat food or can be compounded in a liquid that the cat finds palatable.

Little data exist regarding the stability of individual drugs after compounding, and if done, one must adhere to all laws regarding compounding.

Transdermal fentanyl patches are a hands-off approach, but as noted previously, effective uptake is not achieved in all cats. Compounding of drugs in transdermal creams has become popular but is based on empirical information. Fentanyl compounded in pluronic lecithin organogel cream failed to be absorbed through the skin of the inner pinnae or dorsum of the shaved neck in cats even after a dose of 30 μg/kg.[48] There are no published scientific data to support the use of transdermal analgesics in cats.

Transmucosal administration of buprenorphine for short-term pain control at home is reported to be simple by most owners because it is a tasteless and odorless liquid. The oral formulation of meloxicam is accepted by most cats, and only very small volumes are required.

CONCLUSION

Great strides have been made in the field of feline analgesia. A better understanding of their unique metabolism has shown that extrapolation across species boundaries is unwise and has prompted valuable cat-specific studies. Opioids are now used more commonly in cats with good analgesic effect and few side effects. Excellent acute pain management is achievable in cats by using opioids, NSAIDs, α_2-adrenergic agonists, and local anesthetics. Although many studies use single drugs, a multimodal approach using agents that work at different parts of the pain pathway is commonly used in clinical settings with added benefit. Pain scoring tools for both acute and chronic pain are being developed for cats and will result in more objective assessment of pain.

Management of chronic pain in cats is a challenge because of the potential problems with long-term NSAID use; the success of long-term treatment with meloxicam is encouraging. As veterinarians gain experience with less traditional analgesics such as gabapentin and critically evaluate complementary therapies, the ability to provide comfort to cats will improve.

REFERENCES

1. Lascelles BD, Henry JB, Brown J, et al: Cross-sectional study of the prevalence of radiographic degenerative joint disease in domesticated cats. Vet Surg 39:535–544, 2010.
2. Joubert KE: Anaesthesia and analgesia for dogs and cats in South Africa undergoing sterilisation and with osteoarthritis—an update from 2000. J S Afr Vet Assoc 77:224–228, 2006.
3. Quimby JM, Smith ML, Lunn KF: Evaluation of the effects of hospital visit stress on physiologic parameters in the cat. J Feline Med Surg 13:733–737, 2011.
4. Brondani JT, Luna SP, Padovani CR: Refinement and initial validation of a multidimensional composite scale for use in assessing acute postoperative pain in cats. Am J Vet Res 72:174–183, 2011.

5. Benito J, Depuy V, Hardie E, et al: Reliability and discriminatory testing of a client-based metrology instrument, feline musculoskeletal pain index (FMPI) for the evaluation of degenerative joint disease-associated pain in cats. Vet J, 196:368–373, 2013.
6. Benito J, Hansen B, Depuy V, et al: Feline musculoskeletal pain index: responsiveness and testing of criterion validity. J Vet Intern Med 27:474–482, 2013.
7. Benito J, Gruen ME, Thomson A, et al: Owner-assessed indices of quality of life in cats and the relationship to the presence of degenerative joint disease. J Feline Med Surg 14:863–870, 2012.
8. Clarke SP, Bennett D: Feline osteoarthritis: a prospective study of 28 cases. J Small Anim Pract, 47:439–445, 2006.
9. Gunew MN, Menrath VH, Marshall RD: Long-term safety, efficacy and palatability of oral meloxicam at 0.01-0.03 mg/kg for treatment of osteoarthritic pain in cats. J Feline Med Surg 10:235–241, 2008.
10. Court MH, Greenblatt DJ: Molecular genetic basis for deficient acetaminophen glucuronidation by cats: UGT1A6 is a pseudogene, and evidence for reduced diversity of expressed hepatic UGT1A isoforms. Pharmacogenetics 10:355–369, 2000.
11. Ilkiw JE, Pascoe PJ, Tripp LD: Effects of morphine, butorphanol, buprenorphine, and U50488H on the minimum alveolar concentration of isoflurane in cats. Am J Vet Res 63:1198–1202, 2002.
12. Ferreira TH, Steffey EP, Mama KR, et al: Determination of the sevoflurane sparing effect of methadone in cats. Vet Anaesth Analg 38:310–319, 2011.
13. Kamata M, Nagahama S, Kakishima K, et al: Comparison of behavioral effects of morphine and fentanyl in dogs and cats. J Vet Med Sci 74:231–234, 2012.
14. Robertson SA, Wegner K, Lascelles BD: Antinociceptive and side-effects of hydromorphone after subcutaneous administration in cats. J Feline Med Surg 11:76–81, 2009.
15. Steagall PV, Pelligand L, Giordano T, et al: Pharmacokinetic and pharmacodynamic modelling of intravenous, intramuscular and subcutaneous buprenorphine in conscious cats. Vet Anaesth Analg 40:83–95, 2012.
16. Niedfeldt RL, Robertson SA: Postanesthetic hyperthermia in cats: a retrospective comparison between hydromorphone and buprenorphine. Vet Anaesth Analg 33:381–389, 2006.
17. Posner LP, Gleed RD, Erb HN, Ludders JW: Post-anesthetic hyperthermia in cats. Vet Anaesth Analg 34:40–47, 2007.
18. Bortolami E, Slingsby L, Love EJ: Comparison of two formulations of buprenorphine in cats administered by the oral transmucosal route. J Feline Med Surg 14:534–539, 2012.
19. Robertson SA, Lascelles BD, Taylor PM, Sear JW: PK-PD modeling of buprenorphine in cats: intravenous and oral transmucosal administration. J Vet Pharmacol Ther, 28:453–460, 2005.
20. Catbagan DL, Quimby JM, Mama KR, et al: Comparison of the efficacy and adverse effects of sustained-release buprenorphine hydrochloride following subcutaneous administration and buprenorphine hydrochloride following oral transmucosal administration in cats undergoing ovariohysterectomy. Am J Vet Res 72:461–466, 2011.
21. Lascelles BD, Robertson SA: Use of thermal threshold response to evaluate the antinociceptive effects of butorphanol in cats. Am J Vet Res 65:1085–1089, 2004.
22. Taylor PM, Kirby JJ, Robinson C, et al: A prospective multi-centre clinical trial to compare buprenorphine and butorphanol for postoperative analgesia in cats. J Feline Med Surg 12:247–255, 2010.
23. Rohrer Bley C, Neiger-Aeschbacher G, Busato A, Schatzmann U: Comparison of perioperative racemic methadone, levo-methadone and dextromoramide in cats using indicators of post-operative pain. Vet Anaesth Analg 31:175–182, 2004.

24. Ferreira TH, Rezende ML, Mama KR, et al: Plasma concentrations and behavioral, antinociceptive, and physiologic effects of methadone after intravenous and oral transmucosal administration in cats. Am J Vet Res 72:764–771, 2011.

25. Lascelles BD, Robertson SA: Antinociceptive effects of hydromorphone, butorphanol, or the combination in cats. J Vet Intern Med 18:190–195, 2004.

26. Johnson JA, Robertson SA, Pypendop BH: Antinociceptive effects of butorphanol, buprenorphine, or both, administered intramuscularly in cats. Am J Vet Res 68 (7):699–703, 2007.

27. Pypendop BH, Siao KT, Pascoe PJ, Ilkiw JE: Effects of epidurally administered morphine or buprenorphine on the thermal threshold in cats. Am J Vet Res 69:983–987, 2008.

28. Giraudel JM, Toutain PL, King JN, Lees P: Differential inhibition of cyclooxygenase isoenzymes in the cat by the NSAID robenacoxib. J Vet Pharmacol Ther 32:31–40, 2009.

29. Slingsby LS, Waterman-Pearson AE: Postoperative analgesia in the cat after ovariohysterectomy by use of carprofen, ketoprofen, meloxicam or tolfenamic acid. J Small Anim Pract 41:447–450, 2000.

30. Sparkes AH, Heiene R, Lascelles BD, et al: ISFM and AAFP consensus guidelines: long-term use of NSAIDs in cats. J Feline Med Surg, 2010. 12:521–538, 2010.

31. Kamata M, King JN, Seewald W, et al: Comparison of injectable robenacoxib versus meloxicam for peri-operative use in cats: results of a randomised clinical trial. Vet J, 2012 193:114–118, 2012.

32. Slingsby LS, Taylor PM: Thermal antinociception after dexmedetomidine administration in cats: a dose-finding study. J Vet Pharmacol Ther, 2008. 31:135–142, 2008.

33. Curcio K, Bidwell LA, Bohart GV, Hauptman JG: Evaluation of signs of postoperative pain and complications after forelimb onychectomy in cats receiving buprenorphine alone or with bupivacaine administered as a four-point regional nerve block. J Am Vet Med Assoc 118.03=08, 2000.

34. O'Hearn AK, Wright BD: Coccygeal epidural with local anesthetic for catheterization and pain management in the treatment of feline urethral obstruction. J Vet Emerg Crit Care (San Antonio), 21:50–52, 2011.

35. Davis KM, Hardie EM, Martin FR, et al: Correlation between perioperative factors and successful outcome in fibrosarcoma resection in cats. Vet Rec 161:199–200, 2007.

36. Fransson BA, Peck KE, Smith JK, et al: Transdermal absorption of a liposome-encapsulated formulation of lidocaine following topical administration in cats. Am J Vet Res 63:1309–1312, 2002.

37. Pypendop BH, Ilkiw JE: Assessment of the hemodynamic effects of lidocaine administered IV in isoflurane-anesthetized cats. Am J Vet Res 66:661–668, 2005.

38. Brondani JT, Luna SP, Marcello GC, et al: Analgesic efficacy of perioperative use of vedaprofen, tramadol or their combination in cats undergoing ovariohysterectomy. J Feline Med Surg 11:420–429, 2009.

39. Ray J, Jordan D, Pinelli C, et al: Case studies of compounded Tramadol use in cats. Int J Pharm Compd, 216:44–49, 2012.

40. Lorenz ND, Comerford EJ, Iff I: Long-term use of gabapentin for musculoskeletal disease and trauma in three cats. J Feline Med Surg 15:507, 2012.

41. Steagall PV, Monteiro-Steagall BP: Multimodal analgesia for perioperative pain in three cats. J Feline Med Surg 2013, Aug; 15(8):737–43.

42. Steagall PV, Taylor PM, Rodrigues LC, et al: Analgesia for cats after ovariohysterectomy with either buprenorphine or carprofen alone or in combination. Vet Rec 164:359–363, 2009.

43. Väisänen MA, Tuomikoski SK, Vainio OM: Behavioral alterations and severity of pain in cats recovering at home following elective ovariohysterectomy or castration. J Am Vet Med Assoc 231:236–242, 2007.

44. Bennett D, Morton C: A study of owner observed behavioural and lifestyle changes in cats with musculoskeletal disease before and after analgesic therapy. J Feline Med Surg 11:997–1004, 2009.

45. Beale BS: Use of nutraceuticals and chondroprotectants in osteoarthritic dogs and cats. Vet Clin North Am Small Anim Pract 34:271–289, 2004.

46. Lascelles BD, DePuy V, Thomson A, et al: Evaluation of a therapeutic diet for feline degenerative joint disease. J Vet Intern Med 24:487–495, 2010.

47. Bulman-Fleming JC, Turner TR, Rosenberg MP: Evaluation of adverse events in cats receiving long-term piroxicam therapy for various neoplasms. J Feline Med Surg 12:262–268, 2010.

48. Robertson SA, Taylor PM, Sear JW, Keuhnel G: Relationship between plasma concentrations and analgesia after intravenous fentanyl and disposition after other routes of administration in cats. J Vet Pharmacol Ther 28:87–93, 2005.

SUGGESTED READINGS

Lascelles BD and Robertson SA: DJD-associated pain in cats: what can we do to promote patient comfort? J Feline Med Surg 12:200–2012, 2010.

Robertson SA: A Review of Opioids in Cats, in Recent Advances in Veterinary Anesthesia and Analgesia: Companion Animals, RD Gleed, Ludders JW, Editor. International Veterinary Information Service 2007. Access available at: www.ivis.org.

Robertson SA: Managing pain in feline patients. Vet Clin North Am Small Anim Pract, 38:1267–1290, 2008.

Robertson SA and Lascelles BD: Long-term pain in cats: how much do we know about this important welfare issue? J Feline Med Surg 12:188–199, 2010.

Robertson SA and Taylor PM: Pain management in cats—past, present and future. 2. Treatment of pain—clinical pharmacology. J Feline Med Surg 6:321–333, 2004.

Taylor PM and Robertson SA: Pain management in cats: past, present and future. 1. The cat is unique. J Feline Med Surg 6:313–320, 2004.

WEB RESOURCE

How to perform a coccygeal epidural in a cat: www.youtube.com/watch?v=_oruduRgYkU.

CHAPTER 25

Rabbit- and Ferret-Specific Considerations

Matthew Johnston

A s of 2011, there were estimated to be 3.2 million rabbits and 748,000 ferrets kept as pets in the United States.[1] There is a perception among veterinarians who treat these animals that the demand for more advanced veterinary procedures on these species is increasing. The recent creation of a recognized veterinary specialty in exotic companion mammals by the American Board of Veterinary Practitioners reinforces this perception. Over the past 20 years, there has been a growing surge of interest and research in the field of veterinary pain management. As these two burgeoning fields have intersected, it has led to some important research in pain and its management in rabbits and ferrets. Because of the popularity of rabbits in the laboratory world and as pets, this species is more represented in the pain literature, whereas ferrets still remain very underrepresented. Much of the literature dealing with pain in rabbits and ferrets relates to these animals as laboratory specimens,[2-4] and extrapolation of this information to pet animals can be problematic.

The goal of this chapter is to focus on a practical, clinical approach to pain management in ferrets and rabbits. It should be understood that because of the shortage of published studies relating to analgesia in these two species, the author is drawing from personal clinical experience and extrapolating from what is known in other species. Whenever possible, reference is made to published information.

RECOGNITION OF PAIN

In some circumstances it is not difficult to recognize when a rabbit or ferret is in pain. Stimuli that cause pain in other animals, such as surgery or tissue trauma, should be assumed also to cause pain in these species. Though this concept seems simple, in a survey of British veterinarians published in 1999, only 22% of veterinarians administered some form of analgesia perioperatively to small mammals. This survey also showed that veterinary surgeons were more likely to administer analgesics to rabbits than to ferrets.[5] In a similar survey of veterinarians in New Zealand, it was concluded that veterinarians' knowledge base with regard to pain and its management in rabbits was inadequate.[6] There is some evidence that at least in the laboratory world, there is increased adherence to recommendations for provision of analgesia after surgical procedures[7]; furthermore, formal guidelines for assessment and management of pain in rabbits have been produced by the American College of Laboratory Animal Medicine.[8] No such guidelines or surveys are available specifically with regard to ferrets. Although surgical pain should be easy to identify, some stimuli that cause pain in ferrets and rabbits are more difficult to recognize, and an understanding of these species' unique physiology and behaviors is important (Box 25-1).

Ferrets and rabbits could not be any more different from a physiologic and behavioral standpoint. Ferrets are strict carnivores and predators that generally have a boisterous and gregarious demeanor, even when in an unfamiliar environment such as a veterinary hospital. Rabbits, however, are strictly herbivorous prey animals that are generally quiet and reserved and can appear anxious when in unfamiliar territory. Observations of normal ferrets and rabbits help the practitioner gain insight into behaviors associated with pain. Some behaviors are not specific for pain but could be associated with an underlying disease process, so the animal's entire clinical picture should be taken into account when one is assessing pain.

One of the biggest challenges facing veterinarians who treat ferrets is the lack of refereed literature examining assessment of pain. No studies exist specifically looking at ethograms associated with pain behavior, and though numerous reviews have been written in which ferrets are mentioned, the statements from these reviews reflect the authors' opinions and perceptions

---

BOX 25-1 | **Signs of Acute Pain in Ferrets and Rabbits**

FERRETS	RABBITS
• Balled-up posture and immobility	• Hyporexia or anorexia
• Hyperactivity and pacing	• Bruxism
• Tooth-baring	• Immobility
• Uncharacteristic aggression	• Lack of grooming behavior
• Hyporexia or anorexia	• Pinned ears
• Bruxism	• Epiphora and serous nasal discharge
• Shivering despite euthermia	• Fits of hyperactivity
• Bristle tail	• Flank biting
• Hunched abdominal posturing	• High-pitched vocalization
• Half-closed eyelids	• Bradypnea with pronounced nasal flare
• Focal muscle fasciculations	
• Lameness	
• Grunting or whining when handled	
• Generalized malaise	
• Lack of grooming behavior	

and are often directly opposed to one another. For example, although it has been my experience that ferrets in pain after painful procedures tend to stay curled up in a ball, this is in direct opposition to statements made by other authorities who mention increased activity levels.[9-11] Ferrets in pain may prefer to stay curled into a ball and exhibit aggressive biting behavior or teeth baring when disturbed. In addition, ferrets with visceral pain may have a decreased appetite and exhibit bruxism when presented with food. A hunched abdominal posture as shown in Figure 25-1 is common in ferrets following laparotomy incisions when pain management is not adequate. Uncomfortable ferrets may shiver despite a normal body temperature. Other signs of pain in ferrets include a bristle tail, in which the fur on the tail stands on end, resembling a pipe cleaner (Figure 25-2); eyelids that are held half closed (see Figure 25-1); focal muscle fasciculations; high-pitched vocalization or grunting when handled; lameness; lack of grooming behavior; and general disinterest in the surroundings (Box 25-2).

In rabbits, the most easily identifiable sign of pain is hyporexia or anorexia.[2-4,12,13] Rabbits are normally grazing animals that eat continuously, and when they are in pain this grazing behavior is reduced or ceases altogether. Rabbits in pain also grind their teeth, especially when visceral or dental pain is present. Though most rabbits in pain choose to sit motionless in a far corner of a cage, some rabbits may have fits of rapid and uncontrolled locomotion when handled. Rabbits in pain may vocalize or exhibit a decreased respiratory rate characterized by a pronounced nasal flare and deep breathing pattern. Rabbits normally have a very rapid respiratory pattern

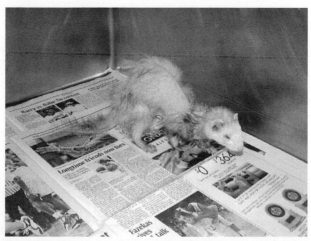

FIGURE 25-1   Appearance of a ferret approximately 6 hours after a laparotomy incision for a left adrenalectomy. Signs of uncontrolled pain are present, including a hunched abdominal posture, half-closed eyelids, and bristle tail.

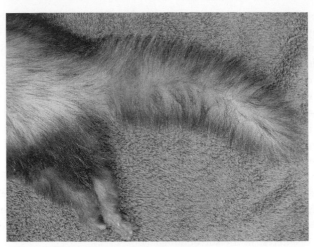

FIGURE 25-2 Example of a characteristic bristle tail appearance, one of the very common signs of pain in domestic ferrets.

BOX 25-2 Signs of Chronic Pain in Ferrets and Rabbits

FERRETS	RABBITS
• Weight loss	• Hyporexia
• Hyporexia	• Recurrent bouts of ileus
• Lameness	• Weight loss
• Bruxism	• Bruxism
• Lack of normal chewing behavior	• Ptyalism
• Unwillingness to grasp items with jaws	• Preferential selection of soft food items
• Generalized malaise	• Unkempt pelage
• Unkempt pelage	• Lameness
	• Fecal or urinary soiling of perineum

---

characterized by short, shallow breaths. The rabbit in pain may appear unkempt because of a lack of grooming and may avoid rearing on its hind legs to accept treat items. Epiphora and serous nasal discharge are sometimes present in rabbits that are in severe, acute pain.

ACUTE AND CHRONIC PAIN

As is true with most traditional companion animals, in general it is easier to recognize the signs of acute pain than chronic pain in ferrets and rabbits. However, in addition to surgical and traumatic pain, there are several medical conditions that lead to acute pain that are often overlooked. Analgesic management should be considered as part of the therapeutic plan for any medical condition that causes acute pain. For example, otitis media or otitis interna is an acute infectious or inflammatory medical condition that is common in rabbits. This condition is likely painful, based on the degree and extent of inflammation present within the ears, as well as the orthopedic postural abnormalities that result from the severe torticollis; furthermore, most rabbits with the condition are anorectic. However, it has been the experience at my referral hospital that many practitioners skip pain management in the treatment of this condition. At my hospital, rabbits with this condition seemingly benefit clinically from the administration of analgesic drugs, specifically nonsteroidal anti-inflammatory drugs (NSAIDs), in addition to nonpharmacologic methods of analgesia such as therapeutic massage, therapeutic laser therapy, and acupuncture. In rabbits, ileus leads to gastric and cecal dilation, which activates nociceptive fibers associated with the stretch receptors in the gastrointestinal (GI) tract. A similar pain pathophysiology occurs in ferrets with GI foreign bodies or trichobezoars. Both conditions lead to acute pain, but in many instances analgesia is not part of the initial treatment regimen. Experimentally in rabbits, several opioids have been shown to decrease pain behaviors after colorectal distention,[14] suggesting that this class of drugs may be useful for managing pain during these clinical presentations. Clinically, at my hospital, constant rate infusions (CRIs) of butorphanol (rabbits) or fentanyl (ferrets) can reduce the outward signs of pain associated with these GI problems.

Conditions that lead to chronic pain are often harder to recognize in ferrets and rabbits. A thorough history from the pet owner or caregiver that suggests changes in behavior may hint at chronically painful conditions. Neoplasia, arthritis, and dental problems are three common causes of chronic pain in ferrets and rabbits. Although some of these conditions cannot be cured, the quality of life of the animal can be greatly increased when analgesia is used to help manage these conditions. Often, simple changes in husbandry can lead to alleviation of the pain, and pharmacologic intervention may not be necessary. For example, geriatric rabbits with stifle and coxofemoral arthritis may benefit from a heavily bedded cage, whereas ferrets with chronic periodontitis may be kept comfortable by feeding them softened food.

PREVENTION OF PAIN

Several modalities may help prevent the cascade of factors that leads to pain. Gentle surgical technique leads to a reduction in inflammation and subsequent pain postoperatively. Crushing and pulling of tissues activates Aδ and C nociceptive fibers, which are not immediately recognized by the central nervous system when the animal is anesthetized. However, these noxious stimuli lead to central nervous system changes that are exhibited as pain behaviors on recovery from anesthesia (see Chapter 2).

Known in humans and assumed to be true in animals is that memory of a painful stimulus correlates strongly with the maximum intensity of pain. Therefore, if therapy can intervene and prevent central stimulation, the intensity of pain should be reduced. This concept is the basis for preemptive analgesia, or administration of antinociceptive drugs before the noxious stimulus to improve postoperative analgesia (see Chapter 2). Preemptive analgesia should be considered as a part of the anesthetic regimen for all rabbits and ferrets undergoing procedures that may lead to pain postoperatively.

NONPHARMACOLOGIC INTERVENTIONS FOR ANALGESIA

There have been some recent reviews written on physical modalities as well as acupuncture for the management of painful conditions in ferrets and rabbits, and at my hospital some of these modalities have become commonplace in the holistic pain management plans[15,16] (Box 25-3). It is beyond the scope of this chapter to cover all therapies in depth, so the reader is referred to other, more complete works on the subject.[15-17]

Cryotherapy—simply the application of ice packs to acute injuries, including surgical incisions—slows nociceptive transmission from the area.

BOX 25-3 Nonpharmacologic Interventions for Pain Management in Ferrets and Rabbits

- Cryotherapy (ice packs) of surgical wounds or acute tissue trauma
  - Useful in the first 48 hours after surgery or injury
  - 10- to 15-minute application two or three times daily
- Heat therapy
  - Animals with visceral abdominal pain
  - Use of a heating pad on the ventral abdomen for 15 minutes two or three times daily
  - Reduces sympathetic tone, promotes circulation, reduces muscle spasm
- Therapeutic laser therapy
  - 1 to 5 J/cm^2
  - Osteoarthritis
  - Myofascial restrictions
- Therapeutic massage
  - Usually performed at home by pet owners
  - Promotes human-animal bond
  - Reduces edema and sympathetic tone
  - Abdominal massage of rabbits with ileus
  - Osteoarthritis and myofascial restriction
- Acupuncture
  - Performed by certified veterinary acupuncturist
  - Chronic back pain
  - Osteoarthritis and myofascial restriction
  - Ileus

By causing local vasoconstriction, it can reduce edema and inflammation in the acute (first 48 hours) phase of the injury.[18] At my hospital, it is routine practice to use ice packs for surgical incisions or acute soft-tissue injuries, and I have observed a decrease in incisional complications such as overgrooming and dehiscence since the institution of this practice. Ice packs are easily available to pet owners, and if indicated, this modality can be continued once the animal has left the hospital.

There is evidence in humans that use of therapeutic lasers can ease pain in a focal treatment area.[19,20] This modality is gaining traction in veterinary medicine, although published analgesic efficacy studies are extremely limited in small animals[21] and nonexistent in pet ferrets and rabbits. However, there are numerous reports in the literature of use of various rabbit models and this modality, specifically with regard to wound healing. One of the more applicable studies of laboratory rabbits showed that low-level laser therapy is beneficial for the treatment of chemically induced stifle osteoarthropathy. Specifically, compared with a control group, treated animals had a reduction in inflammatory markers, less severe radiographic and computed tomography changes, and histologic evidence of reduction of inflammation and replacement with close to normal-appearing articular cartilage.[22] At my hospital this modality has demonstrated the most promise in chronically painful orthopedic conditions such as osteoarthritis and myofascial restriction secondary to torticollis. Although research is still needed to determine an optimum dosage regimen for specific conditions, clinically effective treatment seems to occur in the range of 1 to 5 J/cm^2.[15]

Heat therapy can be useful in the management of chronically painful conditions. The use of heating pads is an easy, practical way for many pet owners to implement this modality. Heat therapy can reduce sympathetic neurologic tone, promote circulation, and reduce muscle spasms. In pediatric human patients, a heating pad is placed across the abdomen to help modulate GI motility.[23] Because ileus is a common condition in rabbits, it is easy and practical to place a rabbit on a heating pad, if tolerated, thereby warming the ventral abdominal wall and potentially relieving the discomfort associated with ileus.

Therapeutic massage is generally not performed in the hospital environment, but is something that is commonly prescribed for pet owners to perform at home. Pet owners and companion animals seem to enjoy this activity, and massage may help reduce edema and sympathetic tone. In humans, massage can be used to regulate GI motility via stimulation of vagal afferent fibers in the visceral wall, and this technique is recommended for pet owners to use for rabbits with ileus.[24] Pet owners can be taught to gently massage the abdomen for 10 to 15 minutes several times daily. Studies in humans also describe additional benefits of myofascial massage, including increased range of motion, release of myofascial restriction, and reduced pain and anxiety.[25–27] In rabbits, myofascial massage can be used to reduce myofascial restriction associated with chronic torticollis as well as reduce pain and increase range of motion in muscles of limbs affected by osteoarthritis.

Acupuncture may be the most well studied and popular of all the non-pharmacologic interventions for analgesia, with entire textbooks written on its practice and principles in small animals. It is interesting that much of the basic research into acupuncture's mode of action, especially for analgesia, has been performed in rabbits. This topic is beyond the scope of this chapter, but a recent review provides further information specific to ferrets and rabbits.[16] At my hospital, acupuncture has been part of the analgesic plan for many rabbits and occasionally in ferrets. Like many physical therapies, it is rarely, if ever, used as a sole modality; therefore it has been challenging to formulate clinical opinions on its effectiveness. As part of a combined pharmacologic and physical modality analgesic plan, it seems to play an important role.

PHARMACOLOGIC ANALGESIC AGENTS

Table 25-1 gives dosage information on drugs discussed in the text.

Opioids

The use of opioid drugs remains a mainstay of analgesic therapy, especially when facing situations of moderate to severe acute postsurgical or traumatic pain. Opioids exert their effects via inhibition of pain transmission in the dorsal horn of the spinal cord, activation of inhibitory pathways from the brain, and inhibition of supraspinal afferent nerves and by causing a decrease in the release of neurotransmitters in the spinal cord (see Chapter 9). Some examples of opioids commonly used in ferrets and rabbits are butorphanol, buprenorphine, morphine, hydromorphone, oxymorphone, and fentanyl.

Some practitioners have been wary of using this class of drugs because of its potential for adverse side effects such as sedation, respiratory depression, and ileus. However, the beneficial analgesic properties of these drugs far outweigh the potential adverse effects in the majority of cases. Ferrets seem especially sensitive to the sedative and respiratory depressant effects of opioids, so lower dose ranges and careful monitoring should be used with this species. Preliminary work in my laboratory in a limited number of ferrets has demonstrated cardiorespiratory depression associated with morphine, hydromorphone, and butorphanol, but further work, including investigation into the pharmacokinetics, is needed before any conclusions can be drawn.[28] The ileus-inducing effects of opioids are a major concern for practitioners working on rabbits; however, pain-induced ileus is much more difficult to treat than that brought on by the administration of opioids, so this concern does not justify their exclusion from analgesia protocols. Usually the institution of forced feedings and adequate fluid therapy is enough to counteract the

TABLE 25-1	Dosages of Analgesic Drugs for Ferrets and Rabbits	
DRUG	**FERRET**	**RABBIT**
Butorphanol	0.1-0.5 mg/kg q2-4h IV, IM, SC 0.1-0.2 mg/kg/hr IV CRI	0.5 mg/kg q2-4h IV, SC 0.1-0.3 mg/kg/hr IV CRI
Buprenorphine	0.01-0.03 mg/kg q6-10h IV, SC, TM*	0.01-0.05 mg/kg q6-10h IV, SC
Morphine	0.2-2 mg/kg IM single dose preoperatively 0.1 mg/kg epidurally	0.5-5 mg/kg IM single dose preoperatively 0.1 mg/kg epidurally
Hydromorphone	0.1-0.2 mg/kg IV, IM, SC q6-8h 0.005-0.015 mg/kg/hr IV CRI	0.05-0.2 mg/kg IV, IM, SC q6-8h
Oxymorphone	0.05-0.2 mg/kg IV, IM, SC q6-8h	0.05-0.2 mg/kg IV, IM, SC q6-8h
Fentanyl	20-30 µg/kg/hr IV CRI during anesthesia to reduce volatile inhalant concentrations 1-4 µg/kg/hr IV CRI for analgesia	5-10 µg/kg IV loading dose followed by 10-40 µg/kg/hr IV CRI to reduce minimum alveolar concentration of isoflurane 1.25-5.0 µg/kg/hr IV CRI for analgesia[†]
Meloxicam	0.1-0.2 mg/kg SC, PO q24h	0.1-1.0 mg/kg SC, PO q12-24h
Lidocaine	<4 mg/kg SC 4.4 mg/kg epidurally	<4 mg/kg SC
Bupivacaine	<2 mg/kg SC 1.1 mg/kg epidurally	<2 mg/kg SC
Ketamine (analgesic)	0.5 mg/kg IV before surgery 10 µg/kg/min IV CRI during surgery 2 µg/kg/min IV CRI for 24 hours postoperatively[‡]	0.5 mg/kg IV before surgery 10 µg/kg/min IV CRI during surgery 2 µg/kg/min IV CRI for 24 hours postoperatively[‡]
Tramadol	5 mg/kg PO q12h	Further research is needed before dose recommendations can be made

NOTE: Many of these dosages are based on clinical experience and extrapolation from other species. It is the responsibility of the attending veterinarian to monitor for adverse effects associated with administration of these drugs.
Key: *CRI*, Constant rate infusion.
*Transmucosally—administer directly into space between molars and buccal mucosa.
[†]See text for cautionary statements regarding the use of fentanyl in rabbits.
[‡]Must be combined with an additional analgesic agent such as an opioid to provide adequate analgesia.

motility-slowing effects of opioids. In addition, because there are several different opioids available, in most cases a relatively safe drug can be found.

Opioids are classified as mixed agonist-antagonists, pure agonists, and pure antagonists. Pure antagonists are not discussed in this chapter because they are used primarily to reverse the effects of the other two classes and by themselves have no analgesic properties. Three different classes of opioid receptors are recognized: μ, κ, δ. The μ receptors are further broken down in to μ_1, μ_2, and μ_3 subgroups. In mammals, μ_1 and κ receptors are the primary receptors responsible for analgesia (see Chapter 9).

The most commonly used mixed agonist-antagonists are butorphanol and buprenorphine. Butorphanol has agonist effects mainly at κ receptors, with minimal to no μ effects, hence its classification as a μ-antagonist (see Chapter 9). Pharmacokinetic data are available for rabbits for this drug and suggest that a 0.5-mg/kg dose given intravenously (IV) results in a half-life of elimination of just over 1.5 hours. The same dose given subcutaneously (SC) resulted in an elimination half-life of just over 3 hours.[29] In one study looking at arterial blood gas effects in healthy rabbits breathing room air, it was found that statistically significant increases in blood pH and decreases in arterial oxygen tension (PaO_2) occurred in rabbits given butorphanol alone or butorphanol-midazolam combinations compared with controls. The clinical significance of these changes in healthy rabbits is probably negligible; however, use of butorphanol might require more intensive monitoring and oxygen supplementation in rabbits with respiratory compromise.[30] No pharmacologic studies are available for this drug in ferrets, and other than the preliminary work done in the laboratory that was previously mentioned,[28] no studies exist evaluating butorphanol alone. However, there is a series of papers published by Ko and colleagues assessing anesthetic, sedative, and cardiorespiratory effects of drug combinations that include butorphanol as one of the components.[31-34] In the tiletamine-zolazepam-xylazine-butorphanol study, butorphanol was shown to increase the duration of analgesia, ease endotracheal intubation, and increase time of dorsal recumbency, suggesting at least a synergistic analgesic and sedative effect. However, its addition to the cocktail also caused hypoxemia, prompting the author to conclude that supplemental oxygen should be given to ferrets if butorphanol is included in the cocktail with the other drugs.[31] In both the diazepam-acepromazine-xylazine-butorphanol and the diazepam-ketamine-acepromazine-xylazine-butorphanol experiments, statistically and clinically significant cardiorespiratory depression occurred in all the groups, but because of the presence of butorphanol in all of the cocktails and variance of other drugs, it is unclear how much the butorphanol had to do with this suppression.[32,33] In the medetomidine-ketamine-butorphanol study, the addition of butorphanol to the cocktail of drugs caused the greatest degree of respiratory depression and significantly increased the duration of sedation over the cocktails that did not contain butorphanol.[36] However, all four of these studies were done with a limited number of animals (9, 10, 10, and 10, respectively) and the combination of drugs used made evaluation of the effects of any single component very difficult.

Butorphanol is suitable for mild to moderate pain in rabbits because of its κ effects, but the frequency of administration makes it impractical for many situations. However, butorphanol can be given as an intravenous

CRI to counteract the need for frequent administration. As mentioned before, this method of administration is especially good at addressing visceral pain associated with GI disorders. In ferrets, butorphanol is mainly used for its sedative effects because the analgesic effects seem limited in this species, although further research is needed to answer this question.

Buprenorphine is classified as a partial μ-agonist and κ-antagonist. Buprenorphine binds strongly to the μ receptors, and because of this, buprenorphine can be difficult to reverse (see Chapter 9). Buprenorphine, like butorphanol, is suitable for management of mild to moderate pain. Unlike with butorphanol, the analgesic effects of buprenorphine seem to last longer, although no pharmacokinetic or dynamic data are available in either species. Unfortunately, there have been no studies relative to buprenorphine in ferrets. Clinically, analgesic effects seem to persist for 6 to 10 hours in both species after subcutaneous administration. However, one study demonstrated that behavior attributed to pain in rabbits was not diminished after administration of buprenorphine.[35] In a study in rabbits assessing the effect of buprenorphine on visceral pain, however, it was concluded that visceral pain may be attenuated by the preemptive administration of buprenorphine, but that buprenorphine administered after the noxious stimulus was in place was ineffective.[36] In this study, however, relatively low doses compared with what is recommended in Table 25-1 were used. Buprenorphine clinically appears to be safe in both species, and this is supported by research in rabbits showing that the addition of buprenorphine (0.03 mg/kg) to a cocktail of ketamine and medetomidine did not significantly change cardiorespiratory parameters other than a slight decrease in mean arterial blood pressure, although it did increase the duration of anesthesia.[37] However, a separate study evaluated buprenorphine alone in conscious, healthy rabbits at a dose of approximately 0.02 mg/kg. In this experiment, buprenorphine administration did cause a statistically significant decrease in respiratory rate and produced a mild hypoxemia, although the changes would not be considered clinically significant. The conclusion by the authors was that these changes would be well tolerated in healthy animals, but caution should be taken if buprenorphine is administered to rabbits with respiratory compromise.[38] In addition, buprenorphine has been shown to have transmucosal absorption in cats,[39] and this route is used with apparent clinical success in ferrets. Because transmucosal absorption of buprenorphine depends on the pH of the saliva, it would make sense that animals with similar digestive physiology (cats and ferrets) should respond similarly, although no studies have been done to back up this assumption. Consequently, until studies have been performed, this route of administration is not recommended in rabbits.

Morphine is considered the prototype opioid to which all other opioids are compared. Morphine has the added benefit of being inexpensive, hence its use as the primary opioid in most veterinary practices (see Chapter 9). Because of its rather large array of side effects, especially respiratory depression and emesis in ferrets and induction of ileus in rabbits, repeated systemic administration of morphine is rarely performed. Morphine is used commonly as a one-time premedication before noxious stimulus to provide preemptive analgesia. However, epidurally administered morphine can be an excellent analgesic technique for abdominal and hindlimb procedures in both species. In ferrets and rabbits, epidural or spinal morphine administration is known to attenuate postoperative pain responses.[40,41] For more complete analgesia, a local anesthetic such as lidocaine or bupivacaine may be combined with the morphine and administered epidurally. The analgesic effects of epidurally administered morphine last approximately 12 to 24 hours, and the adverse effects noted before are virtually eliminated.

The procedure for lumbosacral epidural puncture in ferrets and rabbits is similar to that described for dogs and cats[42] (see Chapter 12), except that there is rarely a definitive "popping" sensation when the epidural space is entered. Landmarks used for lumbosacral epidural puncture in both species are the wings of the ileum and the dorsal prominence of the first sacral vertebra. The three landmarks form a triangle, and the lumbosacral space is in the center of this triangle, directly on midline. Epidural puncture can be performed with the ferret or rabbit in ventral recumbency or in lateral recumbency. In both positions the coxofemoral and lumbosacral joints should be hyperflexed to help open up the space (Figure 25-3). It should be noted that in rabbits the spinal cord continues caudally into the sacral vertebrae, so the potential for accidental spinal puncture during lumbosacral epidural injection

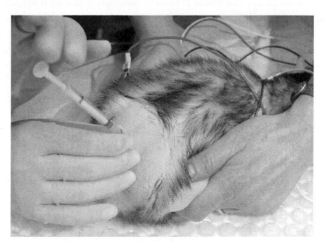

FIGURE 25-3 Lumbosacral epidural administration in a ferret. Landmarks are the wings of the ileum and the dorsal prominence of the first sacral vertebra. The three landmarks form a triangle, and the lumbosacral space is in the center of this triangle, directly on midline.

is higher.[43] If cerebrospinal fluid is seen in the hub of the needle during epidural puncture, half of the volume of drug should be administered because the drug will be confined to the subarachnoid space and may distribute further cranially.

Hydromorphone and oxymorphone are similar drugs and so are discussed together. Currently, hydromorphone is significantly less expensive than oxymorphone and so is used more frequently in veterinary practice. The analgesic effects of both drugs are similar to those of morphine, but both have the advantage of decreased adverse side effects (see Chapter 9). I have used both drugs extensively in ferrets and rabbits, with minimal adverse side effects. No data are available for either drug in either species except for anecdotal clinical reports. Hydromorphone and oxymorphone can be used as premedications to provide preemptive analgesia, postoperatively to manage moderate to severe pain, or as primary analgesics after trauma or for painful medical conditions. In ferrets, both drugs cause profound sedation, making assessment of their analgesic properties difficult. In ferrets and rabbits, subcutaneous injection seems to provide approximately 6 hours of analgesia. In ferrets the sedative effects of the hydromorphone seem attenuated when it is used as an intravenous CRI along with ketamine.

Fentanyl is a very short-acting pure μ-agonist with analgesic effects similar to those of morphine. The effects of fentanyl last less than 30 minutes after a single intravenous injection (see Chapter 9). Although no scientific publications are available on this drug's clinical use in ferrets, at my hospital fentanyl is used commonly in ferrets intraoperatively as a CRI to decrease volatile inhalant anesthetic concentrations and to provide analgesia for moderate to severe pain. A fentanyl CRI is the most commonly used analgesic modality for ferrets in the immediate postoperative period at my hospital. Fentanyl is also available as a transdermal patch, the use of which has been evaluated in rabbits. Although this study reported therapeutic blood concentration with use of a 25-μg/hr patch in rabbits, it also reported a loss in body weight of the fentanyl-treated rabbits.[44] This observation correlates with my experience with fentanyl in rabbits, whether administered transcutaneously or IV. Rabbits administered fentanyl at the currently recommended dosages seem to have a severely decreased appetite, and management of ileus associated with fentanyl can be difficult. For this reason, and until further clinical and pharmacokinetic data are available for this drug, fentanyl is used sparingly in rabbits at my hospital. However, some recent work in rabbits looked at targeted controlled intravenous infusions of fentanyl and its ability to reduce the minimum alveolar concentration of isoflurane. In this study the targeted infusions that significantly reduced MAC correlated to a clinical dose of 5 to 10 μg/kg as a loading dose followed by 10 to 40 μg/kg/hr during anesthesia. Apnea occurred throughout the dose range (which is expected with fentanyl in other species), and at the higher dose ranges, excessive spontaneous movement, extensor rigidity, and increased heart rate and respiratory rate occurred. However, the authors of this study believed that these side effects may have been caused by over-reduction in the isoflurane and consequent loss of anesthesia, and not necessarily caused by the fentanyl.[45] Rabbits were not evaluated long term after the study, so the GI effects of these doses could not be examined.

Nonsteroidal Anti-inflammatory Drugs

NSAIDs as a class share common therapeutic actions, including anti-inflammatory, analgesic, and antipyretic effects. This discussion focuses on the analgesic effects. NSAIDs are the most commonly used analgesic drugs in veterinary medicine because they are effective for acute and chronic pain and have few side effects. NSAIDs exert their analgesic effects via inhibition of the cyclooxygenase enzyme, which decreases tissue inflammation (see Chapter 8). NSAIDs are generally contraindicated in ferrets or rabbits that are pregnant, have hepatic or renal dysfunction, are in shock or have other conditions limiting perfusion, or have known GI ulceration.

Many NSAIDs have been used in rabbits and ferrets throughout the past 10 to 15 years, but by far the most commonly used NSAID today in these animals is meloxicam. The increased use of meloxicam in ferrets and rabbits is primarily a result of its apparent relative safety, ease of administration (it is commercially available as a palatable liquid suspension), and apparent effectiveness. Meloxicam is a cyclooxygenase-2–selective NSAID, which means that clinically its side effects are minimal (usually affecting the GI system when seen). Although caution should be used with long-term administration of NSAIDs in ferrets because of their apparent sensitivity to certain NSAIDs,[46] based on my clinical experience it appears that meloxicam is safe to use for short-term administration. No pharmacokinetic or clinical data regarding this drug in ferrets are available. Any ferret or rabbit receiving a long-term NSAID regimen should have plasma liver enzymes, blood urea nitrogen, and creatinine monitored periodically to ensure that toxicosis is not occurring. Rabbits seem to tolerate meloxicam especially and NSAIDs generally very well, with minimal adverse effects. At my hospital, meloxicam has been used in numerous rabbits with chronic painful conditions (dental root overgrowth, arthritis, neoplasia) for long periods at doses higher than those for dogs with apparent clinical efficacy and no changes in plasma biochemistry values or GI signs. It is always prudent to use the lowest possible clinically effective dose, however, until further studies on safety and efficacy are performed. One clinical study involving meloxicam in rabbits was performed to assess the isoflurane-sparing effects of meloxicam in rabbits, and the results of this study showed that when used alone, meloxicam was not successful in reducing the minimum alveolar concentration of isoflurane. However, a meloxicam-butorphanol combination had greater isoflurane-sparing effects than butorphanol alone, suggesting that meloxicam indeed has analgesic effects in rabbits.[47] Another effectiveness trial was conducted in Dutch belted rabbits, where the analgesic effects of meloxicam were compared with those of buprenorphine in a post-ovariohysterectomy group. The authors of this study concluded that meloxicam administered at 0.2 mg/kg SC q24h provided the same analgesic effects and lack of GI side effects as buprenorphine administered at 0.03 mg/kg intramuscularly (IM) q12h.[48] Single- and repeated-dose pharmacokinetics of oral meloxicam administration in rabbits were evaluated, and it was concluded that a dose of greater than 0.3 mg/kg given once daily was necessary to achieve optimal plasma levels over a 24-hour period.[49] A similar study by a different group suggested a dose of 0.2 to 0.3 mg/kg orally (PO) q24h; however, this group conceded that higher doses may be required for optimal effects and suggested that further safety studies are necessary to assess these higher-dose regimens.[50] In a study using behavioral variables to assess the effects of meloxicam after ovariohysterectomy, some degree of analgesia was obtained with doses of 1 mg/kg initially followed by 0.5 mg/kg daily, and a conclusion was made that either a higher dose or combination with another analgesic drug may be required for consistent, adequate analgesia after ovariohysterectomy.[51] These three studies provide some support for the higher dosage regimen recommended in Table 25-1.

Local Anesthetics

Local anesthetics such as lidocaine and bupivacaine are also commonly used in veterinary practice. Local anesthetics provide regional anesthesia by reversibly blocking the transmission of nociceptive stimulation from nerve endings or fibers. Local anesthetics can be used topically; via direct infiltration into soft tissue containing nerve endings; intra-articularly (not practical in ferrets or rabbits); IV; or epidurally (see Chapter 11). Care in calculation of appropriate volumes for administration must be taken when using these drugs in small animals such as rabbits or ferrets to avoid reaching toxic drug concentrations. When injecting SC, always aspirate back on the syringe to ensure that the drug is not being accidentally administered IV. Practically, for bupivacaine and lidocaine, use less than 2 and 4 mg/kg, respectively, of drug to avoid accidental toxicosis. When used epidurally, bupivacaine may lead to motor weakness in the hindlimbs for up to 12 hours after injection. This motor weakness can be agitating to rabbits and may lead to increased morbidity postoperatively. For this reason, my hospital uses bupivacaine epidurally in ferrets only. One of my most common uses of local anesthetics is as a line block before surgical incisions. For abdominal procedures, a 1½-inch, 22- or 25-gauge needle is used to infiltrate the subcutaneous tissue with lidocaine or bupivacaine before incision. Care should be taken not to puncture the abdominal wall and viscera accidentally when performing this technique. Other common uses include infraorbital and mandibular nerve blocks in animals undergoing dental work as well as subcutaneous infusion via infusion

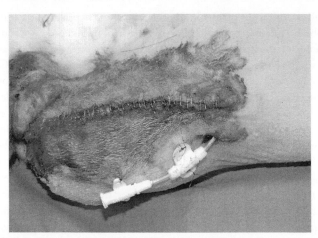

FIGURE 25-4 Example of a placement of a subcutaneous infusion catheter in a rabbit hind leg amputation incisional site. The catheter is fenestrated in multiple areas along its length and then tunneled into the subcutaneous tissue surrounding the incision to allow for distribution of local anesthetic into the entire incisional area.

catheters in animals with large surgical wounds. Commercially available subcutaneous infusion catheters are often too large for small ferrets or rabbits. My hospital fabricates these catheters from sterile 3.5- or 4-French infant feeding tubes or 18- or 20-gauge long intravenous catheters into which multiple holes have been cut to allow for infusion of the drug over a large surface area SC (Figure 25-4).

Ketamine

Ketamine is known primarily for its anesthetic properties. Ketamine is used frequently in ferrets and rabbits as a premedication and has recently been used to augment analgesia by administration of a microdose CRI intraoperatively and postoperatively. Ketamine has been shown to act as preemptive analgesic by inhibiting the N-methyl-D-aspartate (NMDA) receptor in the central nervous system. NMDA stimulation has been shown to increase central nervous system sensitization. Therefore, blockade of this receptor aids in prevention of pain perception (see Chapter 14). It should be noted that no studies confirm this effect in rabbits or ferrets and that ketamine alone is not an acceptable analgesic in most instances. However, a ketamine CRI may allow a lower dose of an opioid or other analgesic to be administered.

Tramadol

Tramadol has recently become popular in veterinary medicine as an analgesic agent for treatment of mild to severe acute and chronic pain. The popularity of tramadol stems from the fact that it is efficacious in certain circumstances, is not controlled, and is cost-effective. The mechanisms of action of tramadol are not completely understood, but it appears to have opioid-like properties and serotonin and norepinephrine reuptake inhibition (see Chapter 14). There are no published reports of pharmacokinetic data or clinical efficacy of this drug in ferrets, though it has been used occasionally at my hospital with apparent safety. More clinical experience is needed before efficacy can be commented on. Doses have been extrapolated for other mammals and applied to ferrets. At this time tramadol appears to have limited clinical usefulness in rabbits because of its short half-life and lack of clinical effect.[52,53] However, further studies are necessary to assess pharmacokinetics and pharmacodynamics as well as analgesic efficacy of higher dosage regimens before this drug is disregarded in rabbits. One important consideration when administering tramadol to ferrets and rabbits is its palatability. Tramadol is intensely bitter, and because rabbits and ferrets generally require medications to be compounded into a liquid formulation, a strong flavoring agent is necessary to mask this bitter taste.

REFERENCES

1. American Veterinary Medical Association. *U.S. Pet ownership & demographics sourcebook.* Schaumburg, Ill., 2012, Author.
2. Flecknell PA: Analgesia of small mammals. Vet Clin North Am Exot Anim Pract. 2001; 4:47–56.
3. Flecknell PA: Analgesia in small mammals. Semin Avian Exotic Pet Med. 1998; 7:41–47.
4. Flecknell PA: Pain relief in laboratory animals. Lab Anim. 1984; 18:147.
5. Lascelles BDX, Capner CA, Waterman-Pearson AE: Current British veterinary attitudes to perioperative analgesia for cats and small mammals. Vet Rec. 1999; 145:601–604.
6. Keown AJ, Farnworth MJ, Adams NJ: Attitudes towards perception and management of pain in rabbits and guinea pigs by a sample of veterinarians in New Zealand. N Z Vet J. 2011; 59:305–310.
7. Coulter CA, Flecknell PA, Leach MC, Richardson CA.: Reported analgesic administration to rabbits undergoing experimental surgical procedures. BMC Vet Res. 2011; 7:12.
8. ACLAM Task Force Members, Kohn DF, Martin TE, et al: Public statement: Guidelines for the assessment and management of pain in rodents and rabbits. J Am Assoc Lab Anim Sci. 2007; 46:97–108.
9. Oostrom HV, Schoemaker NJ, Uilenreef JJ: Pain management in ferrets. Vet Clin North Am Exotic Anim Pract. 2011; 14:105–116.
10. Brown SA: Clinical techniques in domestic ferrets. Semin Avian Exotic Pet Med 6:75–85, 1997.
11. Pollock C: Emergency medicine of the ferret. Vet Clin North Am Exotic Anim Pract. 2007; 10:463–500.
12. Weaver LA, Blaze CA, Linder DE: A model for clinical evaluation of perioperative analgesia in rabbits (*Oryctolagus cuniculus*). J Am Assoc Lab Anim Sci. 2010; 49:845–851.
13. Mayer J: Use of behavioral analysis to recognize pain in small mammals. Lab Anim. 2007; 36:43–48.
14. Borgbjerg FM, Frigast C, Madsen JB, Mikkelsen LF: The effect of intrathecal opioid-receptor agonists on visceral noxious stimulation in rabbits. Gastroenterol. 1996; 110:139–146.

15. Rychel JK, Johnston MS, Robinson NG: Zoological companion animal rehabilitation and physical medicine. Vet Clin North Am Exotic Anim Pract. 2011; 14:131–140.

16. Koski MA: Acupuncture for zoological companion animals. Vet Clin North Am Exotic Anim Pract. 2011; 14:141–154.

17. McGowan C, Goff L, Stubbs N, eds: *Animal physiotherapy: Assessment, treatment, and rehabilitation of animals*. Ames, Iowa, 2007, Blackwell.

18. Heinrichs K: Superficial thermal modalities. In: Millis DL, Levine D, Taylor RA, eds: *Canine rehabilitation and physical therapy*. St. Louis, 2004, Saunders.

19. Hegedus B, Viharos L, Gervain M, Gálfi M: The effect of low-level laser in knee osteoarthritis: A double-blind, randomized, placebo-controlled trial. Photomed Laser Surg. 2009; 27:577–584.

20. Venezian GC, da Silva MA, Mazzetto RG, et al: Low level laser effects on pain to palpation and electromyographic activities in TMD patients: A double-blind, randomized, placebo-controlled study. Cranio. 2010; 28:84–91.

21. Draper WE, Schubert TA, Clemmons RM, et al: Low-level laser therapy reduces time to ambulation in dogs after hemilaminectomy: a preliminary study. J Small Anim Pract. 2012; 53:465–469.

22. Cho HJ, Lim SC, Kim SG, Miles SA: Effect of low-level laser therapy on osteoarthropathy in rabbit. In Vivo. 2004; 18:585–591.

23. Lane E, Latham T: Managing pain using heat and cold therapy. Paediatr Nurs. 2009; 21:14–18.

24. Diego MA, Field T, Hernandez-Reif M et al: Preterm infant massage elicits consistent increases in vagal activity and gastric motility that are associated with greater weight gain. Acta Paediatr. 2007; 96:1588–1591.

25. Huang SY, Santo MD, Wadden KP et al: Short-duration massage at the hamstrings musculotendinous junction induces greater range of motion. J Strength Cond Res. 2010; 24:1917–1924.

26. Donoyama N, Shibaski M: Differences in practitioners' proficiency affect the effectiveness of massage therapy on physical and psychological states. J Bodyw Mov Ther. 2010; 14:239–244.

27. Albertin A, Kerppers II, Amorim CF, et al: The effect of manual therapy on masseter muscle pain and spasm. Electromyogr Clin Neurophysiol. 2010; 50:107–112.

28. Johnston MS, Allweiler S, Smeak D: Cardiorespiratory effect of morphine, butorphanol, and hydromorphone in conscious ferrets. *Proceedingsof the Association of Exotic Mammal Veterinarians Annual Conference*, 2011, 137.

29. Portnoy LG, Hustead DR: Pharmacokinetics of butorphanol tartrate in rabbits. Am J Vet Res. 1992; 53:541–543.

30. Schroeder CA, Smith LJ: Respiratory rates and arterial blood-gas tensions in healthy rabbits given buprenorphine, butorphanol, midazolam, or their combinations. J Am Assoc Lab Anim Sci. 2011; 50:205–211.

31. Ko JC, Nicklin CF, Montgomery T, Kuo WC: Comparison of anesthetic and cardiorespiratory effects of tiletamine-zolazepam-xylazine and tiletamine-zolazepam-xylazine-butorphanol in ferrets. J Am Anim Hosp Assoc. 1998; 34:164–174.

32. Ko JC, Nicklin CF, Montgomery T, Kuo WC: Evaluation of sedative and cardiorespiratory effects of diazepam-butorphanol, acepromazine-butorphanol, and xylazine-butorphanol in ferrets. J Am Anim Hosp Assoc. 1998; 34:242–250.

33. Ko JC, Smith TA, Kuo WC, Nicklin CF: Comparison of anesthetic and cardiorespiratory effects of diazepam-butorphanol-ketamine, acepromazine-butorphanol-ketamine, and xylazine-butorphanol-ketamine in ferrets. J Am Anim Hosp Assoc. 1998; 34:407–416.

34. Ko JC, Heaton-James TG, Nicklin CF. Evaluation of sedative and cardiorespiratory effects of medetomidine, medetomidine-butorphanol, medetomidine-ketamine, and medetomidine-butorphanol-ketamine in ferrets. J Am Anim Hosp Assoc. 1997; 33:438–448.

35. Robinson AJ, Muller WJ, Braid AL, Kerr PJ: The effect of buprenorphine on the course of disease in laboratory rabbits infected with myxoma virus. Lab Anim. 1999; 33:252–257.
36. Shafford HL, Schadt JC: Effect of buprenorphine on the cardiovascular and respiratory response to visceral pain in conscious rabbits. Vet Anaesth Analg. 2008; 35:333–340.
37. Murphy KL, Roughan JV, Baxter MG, Flecknell PA: Anaesthesia with a combination of ketamine and medetomidine in the rabbit: Effect of premedication with buprenorphine. Vet Anaesth Analg. 2010; 37:222–229.
38. Shafford HL, Schadt JC: Respiratory and cardiovascular effects of buprenorphine in conscious rabbits. Vet Anaesth Analg. 2008; 35:326–332.
39. Robertson SA, Taylor PM, Sear JW: Systemic uptake of buprenorphine by cats after oral mucosal administration. Vet Rec. 2003; 152:675–678.
40. Sladky KK, Horne WA, Goodrowe KL, et al: Evaluation of epidural morphine for postoperative analgesia in ferrets (*Mustela putorius furo*). Contemp Top Lab Anim Sci. 2000; 39:33–38.
41. Kero P, Thomasson B, Soppi AM: Spinal anaesthesia in the rabbit. Lab Anim. 1981; 15:347.
42. Eshar D, Wilson J: Epidural anesthesia and analgesia in ferrets. Lab Anim. 2010; 39:339–340.
43. Greenaway JB, Partlow GD, Gonsholt NL, Fisher KR: Anatomy of the lumbosacral spinal cord of rabbits. J Am Anim Hosp Assoc. 2001; 37:27–34.
44. Foley PL, Henderson AL, Bissonette EA, et al: Evaluation of fentanyl transdermal patches in rabbits: blood concentrations and physiologic response. Comp Med. 2001; 51:239–244.
45. Hawkins MG, DiMaio Knych HK, Pypendop BH et al: Reduction of minimum alveolar concentration of isoflurane by fentanyl citrate in rabbits. In: *Proceedings of the Association of Avian Veterinarians, 33rd Annual Conference and Expo.* Louisville, Ky. 23; 2012.
46. Richardson JA, Balabuzsko RA: Ibuprofen ingestion in ferrets. 43 cases. J Vet Emerg Crit Care. 2001; 11:53–58.
47. Turner PV, Kerr CL, Healy AJ, Taylor WM: Effect of meloxicam and butorphanol on minimum alveolar concentration of isoflurane in rabbits. Am J Vet Res. 2006; 67:770–774.
48. Cooper CS, Metcalf-Pate KA, Barat CE, et al: Comparison of side effects between buprenorphine and meloxicam used postoperatively in Dutch belted rabbits (*Oryctolagus cuniculus*). J Am Assoc Lab Anim Sci. 2009; 48:279–285.
49. Turner PV, Chen HC, Taylor WM: Pharmacokinetics of meloxicam in rabbits after single and repeat oral dosing. Comp Med. 2006; 56:63–67.
50. Carpenter JW, Pollock CG, Koch DE, Hunter RP: Single and multiple-dose pharmacokinetics of meloxicam after oral administration to the rabbit (*Oryctolagus cuniculus*). J Zoo Wildl Med. 2009; 40:601–606.
51. Leach MC, Allweiler S, Richardson C et al: Behavioural effects of ovariohysterectomy and oral administration of meloxicam in laboratory housed rabbits. Res Vet Sci. 2009; 87:336–347.
52. Souza MJ, Greenacre CB, Cox SK: Pharmacokinetics or orally administered tramadol in domestic rabbits (*Oryctolagus cuniculus*). Am J Vet Res. 2008; 69:979–982.
53. Egger CM, Souza MJ, Greenacre CB et al: Effect of intravenous administration of tramadol hydrochloride on the minimum alveolar concentration of isoflurane in rabbits. Am J Vet Res. 2009; 70:945–949.

CHAPTER 26

Bird-Specific Considerations
Recognizing Pain Behavior in Pet Birds

Joanne Paul-Murphy; Michelle G. Hawkins

All animals possess the neuroanatomic and neuropharmacologic components necessary for nociception and detection of, transmission of, and response to noxious stimuli. It stands to reason, therefore, that all animals can experience pain even if they cannot give verbal expression to the emotional component of pain. Although humans are challenged to assess emotion in birds, emotional behaviors have been preserved in evolution so that there is little survival advantage for emotional display for some avian species, whereas for another there may be benefit. For the purposes of this chapter, it is accepted that birds perceive and respond to noxious stimuli and that birds feel pain.

Birds are often undertreated for pain. Poor understanding of avian behaviors makes it difficult to identify when birds are in pain and the severity of their pain (Box 26-1). The difficulty is compounded when birds are isolated in a hospital setting because social isolation can alter the bird's response to pain.[1]

Assessment of pain must take into consideration the species, gender, age, environment, and concurrent disease. When a bird is in pain, there is a change in or absence of one or more normal behaviors (Table 26-1). Social interactions decrease in species of birds that have complex social systems. This may be an obvious change, such as perching away from the flock, or might be more subtle, such as a reduction in social grooming. When birds are housed as single pets, their social interactions with the owner may be reduced. Birds in pain may display guarding behavior, which may manifest as antisocial behaviors, to protect a painful area. Some forms of aggression have been linked to painful conditions in birds whereby aggressive behaviors are reduced or dissipate after treatment of the painful condition. A change in feather-grooming behavior is common to both solitary and social birds with

---

BOX 26-1

Birds are often undertreated for pain. Poor understanding of avian behaviors makes it difficult to identify when birds are in pain and the severity of the pain.

TABLE 26-1	Effect of Chronic Pain on Pet Bird Behavior
BEHAVIORAL CHANGES	**EXAMPLES**
Decreased social interactions	Perching away from other birds
	Decreased grooming of self and/or conspecifics
	Decreased interactions with pet owner
Guarding behavior	Change in posture to protect a painful area
	Decreased activity
Increased aggression	Toward conspecifics
	Toward pet owner
Grooming behavior: at painful site or generalized	Feather-destructive behaviors
	Self-mutilation

The effect of chronic pain on a bird's behavior can be subtle. When a pet owner reports changes in the bird's behavior such as those listed above, consider the possibility of a painful condition.

painful conditions. Decreased self-grooming is a withdrawal behavior that can occur when a bird's focus is on pain; however, increased self-grooming or overgrooming of cagemates has also been reported when birds are stressed or in pain. Grooming and feather damaging behavior may increase over an area of the body associated with the region of discomfort. Studies of chickens with induced sodium urate arthritis demonstrated that shifting the bird's attention reduced the severity of pain and may potentially reduce peripheral inflammation.[2]

Behavioral change does not manifest uniformly among different species of birds, and observers must become familiar with the full range of normal behaviors for the species as well as the individual. It is important to observe birds at appropriate times for each species—for example, observing nocturnal species at night. Without knowing the range of normal behavior, an observer will find it extremely difficult to detect abnormal behavior, especially in prey species, which often demonstrate only cryptic and subtle changes.

Treating avian pain is limited by the reliability of pain assessment, which remains highly subjective, and clinicians often need to rely on indirect measures of pain. Having an identified set of behaviors that correlate with pain provides a response that can be used to monitor analgesic therapy. It is difficult to state when a bird's condition has been effectively treated if it cannot be measured before and after therapy. Nonetheless, having an identified behavior or set of behaviors that correlates with pain provides a means to monitor response to pain treatment. Pain scales and score sheets are tools that are increasingly being used to assess pain in animals, especially when specifically designed for a given species under well-defined conditions. Pain score sheets can help maximize the efficacy of pain scoring using behavioral analysis. Score-sheet descriptions of behavior must be refined, and terms must be clearly defined to reduce observer bias and interobserver variability.

Once such a system is implemented, well-trained staff can perform scoring. These pain scales take time and effort to design.

Pain is not just a "yes-or-no" condition; it occurs along a gradient. In lieu of species-specific pain score sheets for birds, there is tremendous value in using a generic pain scale of 1 to 10 to evaluate a bird's pain and the response to treatment and recovery from a painful condition. In a study completed by one of the authors (JPM), pigeons that had undergone orthopedic surgery were evaluated with use of a detailed numeric rating scale plus a simple 1-to-10 pain scale, and there was significant correlation between the outcome using both scales. In a recent evaluation of a fracture pain model using pigeons, two of four tested pain scales ("Fractured limb's position in the presence of the observer" and "Subjective observer evaluation of the level of pain") showed good to excellent sensitivities and specificities and were found to be reliable in a research setting.[3] Effective analgesia is expected to show a marked, easily discernable change in posture or behaviors that will effect a reliable change in the subjective pain score. If no change in pain score occurs, then the drug, dosage, or frequency of administration needs to be reevaluated for that individual animal.

PHYSIOLOGY OF AVIAN PAIN

The physiology of pain in all animals involves detection of a noxious stimulus in the periphery (mechanical, thermal, or chemical) and transmission of the impulses to the spinal cord, where they are modulated and projected to the brain for central processing of the information, which then determines the perception of the noxious stimulus. Taxonomic differences in central nervous system (CNS) anatomy and complexity are apparent, but anatomic, physiologic, and biochemical studies in nonmammalian vertebrates have found that pain perception is expected to be analogous to mammals. Genetic variability with response to pain has been demonstrated at the individual level and in different strains of chickens.[4,5]

Peripheral nociceptors have been studied in birds and include high-threshold mechanothermal, mechanochemical, mechanical, and thermal types. Mechanothermal nociceptors are multifunctional and respond to mechanical stimulation and temperatures higher than 40° C. These nociceptors are similar to cutaneous free nerve endings in mammals with slow conducting unmyelinated C-fiber components. Compared with mammals, the receptive fields of some of the polymodal fibers are greater in birds. As stimulus intensity increases, the number of responses increases. Some fibers have continuous response up to 56° C, whereas other fibers peak at lower temperatures, and increasing the thermal stimulus above this peak results in a reduction of impulses.[6]

Thermal and mechanical nociceptors are polymodal and can be Aδ or C fibers with discharge patterns and receptor field size similar to those in mammals.[7] The avian counterpart may be less sensitive to low temperatures and have a greater threshold to high temperatures, perhaps related to the higher body temperatures of birds. Recent studies have demonstrated polymodal nociceptors (mechanochemical) in the nasal and oral mucosa of chickens similar to those in mammals, with chemical sensitivity to a range of compounds.[8] Birds have multiple ascending pathways in the dorsal horn laminae of the spinal cord transmitting pain signals to the midbrain and forebrain. The distribution of neurons in the nociceptive spinothalamic tract cells is similar between birds and mammals.[9]

Peripheral sensitization occurs when inflammation at the site of injury creates an increased response to a normally painful stimulus. Cell damage and leakage lead to a series of responses resulting in increased sensitivity of the peripheral receptors. Central sensitization is an increase in the excitability of spinal cord neurons and a recruitment of neurons not involved in pain perception under normal circumstances. When stimulation from the peripheral nociceptors to the spinal cord continues for an extended period, a wide range of spinal neurons becomes sensitized and hyperresponsive.[10] Although sensitization has not been experimentally demonstrated in birds, mammalian studies have demonstrated that when analgesics are given before a painful event rather than after the start of the stimulation, the spinal excitability can be dampened.[11,12] The earlier the pain is treated, the less total drug required to maintain analgesia during and after surgery (Box 26-2). Preemptive analgesia with opiates, nonsteroidal anti-inflammatory drugs (NSAIDs), and local anesthetics can block sensory noxious stimuli from onward transmission to the CNS, thus reducing the overall potential for pain and inflammation and potentially improving short-term and long-term recovery.

TREATMENT OF PAIN

Diagnosing the cause of pain can be challenging in birds, and identification of the disease process or site of tissue damage affects the choice of analgesic drugs and supportive care. Therapy should be directed at resolving the injury or disease in addition to using analgesics to decrease peripheral pain signals and their effect on the central neural processing of the pain. Conversely, the

---

BOX 26-2

Treat for pain before and during surgery so that less total drug will be required to maintain analgesia during and after the procedure.

BOX **26-3**

A bird's signs of pain may be recognized before a diagnosis is reached. In these cases, treatment of the pain becomes a critical component of the symptomatic therapy.

animal's signs of pain may be recognized before a diagnosis is reached, and in these cases, treatment of the pain becomes a critical component of the symptomatic therapy (Box 26-3).

Combining analgesics that act by different mechanisms can augment pain relief and is termed *balanced analgesia*. Administration of two or more analgesics frequently produces a synergistic effect. Surgical analgesia commonly includes a local anesthetic at the incision site, an opioid administered directly before and after surgery, and an NSAID given postoperatively and for several days after the procedure (Box 26-4). Balanced analgesic protocols usually allow the dose of each drug and the concentration of inhalation anesthetic to be reduced, thereby reducing the adverse effects of each drug. Adjunctive drugs, such as tranquilizers, used in conjunction with analgesic drugs can enhance the analgesia by reducing anxiety through relaxation. The most common sedatives used in avian medicine are the benzodiazepines, which calm birds before handling for anesthesia.

Supportive care is important to the management of pain. This includes keeping the bird warm, dry, and clean. Keep perches low in the cage and close to the food and water if the bird has difficulty moving about the cage. Hospital environment stressors such as barking dogs or strong smells of cats, ferrets, or other "predators" can be minimized by having a separate area for avian critical care. Gentle human contact and use of a soothing voice are beneficial for the pet bird.

REGIONAL ANESTHESIA AND ANALGESIA

Local anesthetics such as lidocaine and bupivacaine block sodium channels in the nerve axon, which interferes with the conduction of action potentials along the nerve. When local anesthetics are used preoperatively, the number and frequency of impulses are reduced, thereby reducing nociceptor sensitization, which has the beneficial effect of minimizing central sensitization.

BOX **26-4** **Multimodal or Balanced Surgical Analgesia**

1. Local anesthetic at incision site
2. Opioid immediately before and after surgery
3. Nonsteroidal anti-inflammatory drug (NSAID) given intramuscularly after surgery
4. Oral NSAID and tramadol administration for 3 to 5 days after the procedure
5. Continue oral tramadol and NSAID as needed, often with discontinuation of tramadol before discontinuation of NSAID

Regional infiltration using a local line or splash block is the most common method used in birds. A 25- or 27-gauge needle is used to make several subcutaneous injections of small volumes into the operative area. The subcutaneous space in birds is very thin. A line block follows the course of the intended incision; a small bleb of local anesthetic is injected subcutaneously (SC) then the needle is withdrawn and reinserted at the edge of the bleb. Another bleb is made under the skin, and the process is repeated until the length of the incision has been blocked.

Local anesthetic dosage recommendations for birds are lower than for mammals because birds may be more sensitive to the effects (Box 26-5). Systemic uptake of the drug can be rapid in birds, and metabolism may be prolonged, increasing the potential for toxic reactions. Toxic side effects include fine tremors, ataxia, recumbency, seizures, stupor, cardiovascular effects, and death. Toxic effects can be acute in the case of accidental intravenous injection. Chickens given intra-articular injections of high doses of bupivacaine (4 to 5 mg/kg) showed immediate signs of toxicity such as drowsiness and recumbency.[13] The duration of action of local anesthetics depends on the molecular properties and lipid solubility of the drug. Neither the time to effect nor duration of action has been determined for these drugs in birds. In a study of bupivacaine using mallard ducks, the absorption rate was slower than the elimination rate.[14]

Dose recommendations for lidocaine are 2 to 3 mg/kg; thus the commercial preparation of 20 mg/kg often needs to be diluted 1:10 with sterile water to achieve adequate volume for perfusion. Diluting to a 2-mg/kg concentration of lidocaine increases accuracy of dosing and provides the volume needed for blocking a surgical site (Box 26-6). The commercial preparation of bupivacaine is a 0.5% solution (5 mg/mL), and doses of 1 mg/kg have been safely administered to large birds. Dilution of bupivacaine is also recommended to increase the volume for administration. Intra-articular administration of bupivacaine (3 mg in 0.3 mL saline) was studied for its analgesic effects in chickens with experimentally produced acute arthritis. Chickens given bupivacaine were able to feed, peck, and stand on the affected limb similar to birds without arthritis.[13] Topical benzocaine has been used for minor wound repair in small birds.[15] A topical bupivacaine–dimethyl sulfoxide mixture applied to the amputation site of beak-trimmed chickens provided 4 hours of analgesia.[16]

Lidocaine and bupivacaine have been used for brachial plexus blockade in a variety of avian species using palpation, ultrasound, or nerve locator techniques; however, most studies have concluded that these techniques do not always produce an effective block and further study is necessary to develop a useful block for surgical analgesia.[17–19] Local anesthetics in the form of transdermal patches and transdermal creams have not been studied for use in birds. In addition, epidural infusions, spinal blocks, intravenous blocks are difficult to perform in birds; therefore the use of local anesthesia through these applications has not been reported.

OPIOIDS AND OPIOID-LIKE DRUGS

Opioids are used for moderate to severe pain, such as traumatic or surgical pain. These drugs reversibly bind to specific receptors in the central and peripheral nervous system. Opioids vary in their receptor specificity and efficacy in mammals, which results in a wide variety of clinical effects in different species. Clinical effects are also influenced by the commercial preparation of the opioid and the dose and route of administration to the species receiving the drug. It stands to reason that the type of opioid and the dosage also have a wide range of clinical effects in different avian species. The distribution, number, and type of opioid receptors are conserved across vertebrate species in the brainstem and spinal cord but vary substantially in the forebrain. Autoradiography was used to identify μ, κ, and δ opioid receptors in the forebrain of rats, mice, and humans, and κ receptors represented 9%, 13%, and 37% of the total opioid receptor population, respectively.[20] In contrast, the pigeon forebrain has a relatively high proportion (76%) of κ receptors,[20] although opioid receptor distribution may be highly variable amongst avian species not yet studied. The κ receptors have multiple physiologic functions in the bird, and the analgesic function of these receptors needs further investigation.

Physiologic and analgesic effects of butorphanol have been studied in parrots with use of the isoflurane-sparing technique. With this method, healthy birds are anesthetized with isoflurane with determination of the minimum anesthetic concentration (MAC) by use of a noxious stimulus (toe pinch or electrical stimulus) and observation of a withdrawal response with a cognitive movement. Each bird is then treated with the opioid and the MAC redetermined. If the concentration of isoflurane can be lowered, then this sparing effect is considered to be a result of the analgesic effects of butorphanol. Butorphanol (1 mg/kg) was administered to three species of parrots, and the isoflurane MAC was significantly lowered in cockatoos and African grey parrots but not Amazon parrots.[21,22] A higher dose of butorphanol may be necessary to achieve a sparing effect in Amazon parrots. When turkeys were given a low dose of butorphanol (0.1 mg/kg) in a similar anesthesia-sparing model, the halothane MAC was not changed.[23] A MAC-sparing study using chickens compared three doses of morphine (0.1, 1.0, and 3.0 mg/kg) and an experimental κ opioid, and found that both μ and κ opioids had isoflurane-sparing effects.[24]

The effect of opioids on conscious parrots has been evaluated by studying the change in withdrawal threshold from noxious electrical and thermal stimuli before and after receipt of an opioid and by evaluating the pharmacokinetics of the drug. When African grey parrots were given butorphanol (1 mg/kg intramuscularly [IM]), 50% of the birds had significant increases in withdrawal thresholds; and when given 2 mg/kg, a greater percentage of birds demonstrated significant analgesia. Butorphanol doses of 3 and 6 mg/kg had similar analgesic effects on Hispaniolan Amazon parrots with use of this same thermal withdrawal evaluation. Doses of 3 mg/kg demonstrated significant analgesia, but increasing the dose to 6 mg/kg did not increase the effect.[25,26] In evaluation of the pharmacokinetics of butorphanol, the bioavailability of 5 mg/kg administered orally (PO) in Hispaniolan Amazon parrots was less than 10%, making this route ineffective[27] (Table 26-2).

Currently butorphanol at 1 to 3 mg/kg IM is recommended for parrots but needs to be administered every 2 to 3 hours (Box 26-7). Butorphanol (1, 3, and 6 mg/kg IM) was recently evaluated in the American kestrel with use of the same thermal threshold testing modality, and there was no evidence that it had any effect on thermal antinociception in this species.[28]

Nalbuphine exerts its agonistic activity at the κ receptors and is a partial antagonist at the μ receptor, similar to butorphanol. In mammals it has a lower incidence of respiratory depression that does not increase with additional dosage administration. Nalbuphine was rapidly cleared after both intravenous and intramuscular administration of 12.5 mg/kg to Amazon parrots and had excellent bioavailability after intramuscular administration, with little sedation and no adverse effects. The same dose increased thermal foot withdrawal threshold values in this species for up to 3 hours; higher doses (25 and 50 mg/kg IM) did not significantly increase thermal foot withdrawal threshold values above those of the 12.5-mg/kg dose.[29]

Buprenorphine at 0.1 mg/kg IM in African grey parrots did not show an analgesic effect on evaluation by thermal nociception,[25] but pharmacokinetic analysis suggests that this dose may not achieve effective plasma concentration.[30] Pigeons given 0.25 and 0.5 mg of buprenorphine per kilogram showed an increased latency period for withdrawal from a noxious electrical stimulus of 2 and 5 hours, respectively.[31]

TABLE 26-2	Opioid and Opioid-like Analgesics Evaluated in Avian Species by Either Pharmacokinetic (PK) or Pharmacodynamic (PD) Studies					
DRUG	**DOSAGE (mg/kg UNLESS OTHERWISE INDICATED)**	**ROUTE**	**STUDY DESIGN**	**SPECIES**	**COMMENTS**	**REFERENCES**
Butorphanol	5.00	PO, IM, IV	Single dose	Hispaniolan Amazon parrots	Intravenous dose q2h, intramuscular dose q3h	27
	1.00-3.00	IM, IV	Single injection	Psittacines	Oral bioavailability <10%; oral administration not recommended	21,22,25,73
Buprenorphine	0.10	IM	Single injection	African grey parrots	May not achieve effective plasma concentrations at this dose; no change in withdrawal response to noxious stimuli	30
	0.25 0.50	IM	Single injection	Domestic pigeons	Increased withdrawal latency from noxious stimulus for 2 hr at 0.25 mg/kg and for 5 hr at 0.5 mg/kg	31
Fentanyl	0.15-0.50 µg/kg/min	IV	Constant rate infusion	Red-tailed hawks	Reduced isoflurane MAC 31%-55% in a dose-related manner, without significant effects on heart rate, blood pressure, $Paco_2$, or Pao_2	34
Nalbuphine	12.50 25.00 50.00	IM	Single injection	Hispaniolan Amazon parrots	PK: $t_{1/2}$ IM and IV less than 0.35 hr Excellent intramuscular bioavailability PD: 12.5 mg/kg produced 3 hr analgesia; higher doses did not increase effect	29,74
Tramadol	7.50	PO	Single dose	Peafowl	PK: Maintained plasma human therapeutic concentrations for 12-24 hr	38
	11.00	PO	Single dose	Red-tailed hawks	PK: Maintained human plasma therapeutic concentrations for approximately 4 hr	39
	5.00	PO	Single dose	American bald eagles	PK: Bioavailability high at 11 mg/kg; sedation with multiple doses; therefore 5 mg/kg q12h recommended	37
	30.00	PO	Single dose	Hispaniolan Amazon parrots	PK: Maintained human plasma therapeutic concentrations for approximately 6 hr PD: Reduced thermal withdrawal response for approximately 6 hr	42

MAC, Minimum anesthetic concentration.

Fentanyl 0.02 mg/kg was evaluated in cockatoos, and it did not affect the thermal withdrawal threshold; however, a 10-fold increase in the dose of fentanyl (0.2 mg/kg SC) did produce an analgesic response, but many birds were hyperactive for the first 15 to 30 minutes after receiving the high dose.[32] Recently hydromorphone (0.1, 0.3, and 0.6 mg/kg IM) was evaluated through similar thermal nociception techniques in the American kestrel, and there was a distinct dose-responsive thermal antinociception, suggesting that this drug will produce analgesia in this species.[33] Most opioids evaluated in birds have rapid absorption and rapid elimination, with mean residence times of less than 2 hours. Because of its short-acting properties, fentanyl delivered via constant-rate infusion (CRI) is an excellent analgesic adjunct to inhalant anesthesia in mammals; and when used in birds at low doses as a CRI, fentanyl may be effective in avian anesthetic protocols. Fentanyl administered as an intravenous CRI in red-tailed hawks (Buteo jamaicensis) to target plasma concentrations of 8 to 32 ng/mL reduced the MAC of isoflurane 31% to 55% in a dose-related manner, without statistically significant effects on heart rate, blood pressure, $PaCO_2$, or PaO_2.[34] Fentanyl may also be combined with ketamine as a CRI, thereby reducing the doses of each needed. Butorphanol has also been studied as an effective CRI component to provide analgesia and reduce MAC in cockatoos.

Tramadol is an analgesic that has become popular despite minimal evidence regarding its efficacy. It is active at opiate, α-adrenergic, and serotonergic receptors.[35] Tramadol is a weak μ agonist, but the O-desmethyl metabolite (M1) is a much more potent agonist in mammals. The conversion to the M1 metabolite is variable among species, but it has been present in the bird species studied thus far.[36-39] In humans, less respiratory depression and constipation are seen with tramadol than with μ-agonist opioids. Pharmacokinetic data have been reported for American bald eagles (Haliaeetus leucocephalus), Hispaniolan Amazon parrots, red-tailed hawks, and Indian peafowl (Pavo cristatus), and species differences exist with regard to pharmacokinetics.[36-38,40] Oral bioavailability of tramadol was higher for American bald eagles than for humans and dogs, suggesting this as a useful route of administration in this species.[37] Tramadol 11 mg/kg PO achieved plasma concentrations in the human analgesic range for 10 hours in five of six bald eagles; M1 plasma concentrations reached the human therapeutic range in only two eagles at much earlier time points.[37] The $t_{1/2}$ of tramadol in American bald eagles after oral administration was twice that reported in dogs, but half as long as in humans.[37] In Indian peafowl administered 7.5 mg/kg PO once, plasma M1 concentrations remained at or near the human therapeutic range for 12 to 24 hours.[38] Because specific analgesic plasma concentrations for tramadol and its metabolites are not known in birds, it is difficult to predict how these differences may affect appropriate administration frequency after repeated doses. For example, sedation was seen with repeated administration in the American bald eagles; therefore, careful monitoring with reduced doses or frequency may be necessary.[37] Tramadol has also been investigated in American kestrels and significantly increased the foot withdrawal threshold to noxious thermal stimulus at lower doses (5 mg/kg PO), whereas higher doses (15 and 30 mg/kg PO) resulted in a lower antinociceptive effect.[41] In a study evaluating 10 to 30 mg/kg tramadol PO in Hispaniolan Amazon parrots, plasma concentrations associated with analgesia in humans were reached for approximately 6 hours when 30 mg/kg was administered,[40] and a companion study found a reduction in thermal withdrawal response for approximately 6 hours after this same oral dose.[42] Thus the oral bioavailability of tramadol was much lower for Hispaniolan Amazon parrots then other species studied to date. Although this analgesic holds great promise for use in birds, much work is still needed to evaluate appropriate doses, efficacy and safety of this drug in different species.

NONSTEROIDAL ANTI-INFLAMMATORY DRUGS

NSAIDs inhibit cyclooxygenase (COX) enzymes, thereby disrupting eicosanoid synthesis and reducing inflammation at the site of injury. NSAIDs also decrease sensitization of nerve endings and have a modulating effect within the CNS. Based on limited studies, it is assumed that the chemistry and mechanism of action are similar with administration to birds.[43,44] A broad tissue distribution of COX has been demonstrated in chickens,[45] but more information is needed to differentiate the physiologic effects of NSAIDs in various avian species.

NSAIDs are used in birds to reduce visceral and musculoskeletal pain, acute pain associated with trauma, and inflammation and sensitization associated with surgery and to treat chronic pain such as that caused by arthritis. The most common NSAIDs used in current avian medicine are meloxicam, carprofen, ketoprofen, piroxicam, and celecoxib (Table 26-3). As new NSAID formulations appear on the human and veterinary pharmaceutical market, the extra-label use of these drugs in birds will emerge. In recent years, meloxicam has become the most widely used anti-inflammatory medication in exotic animal practice. A survey to investigate NSAID toxicity in captive birds treated in zoos reported zero fatalities associated with meloxicam, which was administered to over 700 birds from 60 species.[46]

TABLE 26-3 Nonsteroidal Anti-inflammatory Drugs Evaluated in Avian Species by Either Pharmacokinetic (PK) or Pharmacodynamic (PD) Studies

DRUG	DOSAGE (mg/kg)	ROUTE	FREQUENCY	SPECIES	COMMENTS	REFERENCES
Carprofen	3.0	IM	q12h	Hispaniolan Amazon parrots	PK: Arthritis pain partially reduced, effect less than 12 hr	66
	30.0	IM	Single injection	Chickens	PD: Arthritis pain behaviors reduced 1 hr after treatment	64
	1.0	IM	Single injection	Chickens	PD: Improved locomotion of lame birds 1 hr after treatment	66
Ketoprofen	2.0	IV, IM, PO	Single injection	Quail	PK: Low bioavailability IM, PO; short intravenous $t_{1/2}$	59
	12.0	IM	Single injection	Chickens	PD: Arthritis pain behaviors reduced 1 hr after treatment	64
	2.5	IM	q24h for 7 days	Budgerigars	TOX: Tubular necrosis	75
	5.0	IM	Single injection	Mallard ducks	PC: 12-hr activity	60
	2.0	PO	q12-24 h	Eiders	TCX: Mortality associated with male Eiders	54
	5.0	IM, IV				
Meloxicam	1.0	IM	q12h	Hispaniolan Amazon parrots	PD: Improved weight bearing on arthritic limb; lower doses did not	65
	1.0	IV, IM, PO	Single injection	PK: Hispaniolan Amazon parrots	IV and IM similar PK; PO low bioavailability	77
	2.0	IM	q12h for 14 days	TOX: Quail	Muscle necrosis at injection. No other chemistry or histopathology	67
	0.1	IM	q24h for 7 days	TOX: Budgerigars	Mild glomerular congestion	75
	0.5	IV	Single injection	PK: Chickens, ostrich, ducks, turkeys, pigeons	Variable distribution, slow clearance except ostrich	56,57,77
	2.0	IM, PO	Single treatment	PK: Cape Griffon vultures	Short $t_{1/2}$ (<45 min)	78
Piroxicam	0.5-0.8	PO	q12h	CS: Cranes	Used for acute myopathy and chronic arthritis	JPM (unpublished data)

TOX, toxicology.

Specific NSAIDs such as diclofenac and flunixin meglumine are not recommended for birds because of significant toxic effects reported in vultures and quail, respectively.[47–51] Diclofenac toxicity in vultures resulted from a combination of increased reactive oxygen species (chemically reactive molecules containing oxygen such as oxygen ions and peroxide) and interference with uric acid transport.[48] Alternatively, safety of meloxicam was studied in three vulture species at doses as high as 2 mg/kg, and serum uric acid concentrations were not increased.[52] In quail given meloxicam (2 mg/kg) for 14 days, no significant changes were identified in renal histopathology, complete blood cell (CBC) count, or biochemistry parameters; however, muscle necrosis at the injection site was severe, and therefore multiple intramuscular injections are discouraged.[53]

Renal prostaglandins have an important role in regulating water and mineral balances and modulating intravascular tone. COX-2 is constitutively expressed in the kidney in chickens, similar to mammalian species studied, and is highly regulated in response to alterations in intravascular volume.[45] Therefore, in conditions of relative intravascular volume depletion and/or renal hypoperfusion such as dehydration, hemorrhage, hemodynamic compromise, heart failure, and renal disease, interference with COX enzyme activity can have significant deleterious effects. A field anesthesia study using ketoprofen, propofol, and bupivacaine in Eider ducks associated ketoprofen administration with mortality of male birds with histopathologic renal lesions; however, a poor hydration status of these wild birds was suspected to be a contributing factor.[54] In birds, NSAIDs should not be used if there is any indication of renal impairment, moderate to severe dehydration, hepatic dysfunction, or gastric ulceration. A fecal occult blood test can detect gastrointestinal bleeding in birds not being fed meat products.[55] Increased monitoring is indicated with high-risk birds, establishing a baseline of plasma uric acid, phosphorous, and hepatic enzyme concentrations before NSAID administration and reevaluation of these parameters at fixed intervals.

The analgesic efficacy of NSAIDs related to dose and frequency of administration depends on pharmacodynamic evaluations as well as pharmacokinetic data and has not been well studied in any avian species. Pharmacokinetic trials in several species of birds have found NSAIDs to have rapid elimination. The half-life of 0.5 mg/kg meloxicam in chickens and pigeons was 3.2 hours and 2.4 hours, respectively, compared with 13.7 hours in humans.[56,57] Oral administration of meloxicam (1 mg/kg) to Amazon parrots had lower bioavailability than when the drug was administered parenterally, with maximum concentrations occurring at 6 hours after oral administration.[58] Pharmacokinetics of ketoprofen (2 mg/kg) given PO, IM, and intravenously (IV) to quail (*Coturnix japonica*) showed a very short half-life and low bioavailability with oral (24%) and intramuscular (54%) administration.[59]

Unfortunately, plasma concentrations may not have a direct correlation to physiologic activity of the NSAID, because NSAIDs tend to accumulate in tissue areas of inflammation. A few pharmacodynamic studies of NSAIDs in birds have been completed. In mallard ducks, 5 mg of flunixin per kilogram and 5 mg of ketoprofen per kilogram significantly suppressed thromboxane B_2 levels within 15 minutes of intramuscular administration and maintained this physiologic effect for 4 hours.[60] Ketoprofen 5 mg/kg IM administered to wild mallard ducks anesthetized with isoflurane had an analgesic effect 30 to 70 minutes after administration.[61] A carprofen dose of 1 mg/kg SC given to chickens raised their threshold to pressure-induced pain for at least 90 minutes.[62] Carprofen (1 mg/kg) given to chickens with chronic lameness improved their ability to walk and navigate a maze, with peak plasma levels occurring at 1 to 2 hours after subcutaneous administration.[63] However, another study using chickens concluded that 30 mg of carprofen per kilogram given IM was required to eliminate behaviors associated with experimental arthritis.[64] An experimental arthritis model in Hispaniolan Amazon parrots was used to evaluate NSAID analgesia by measuring return to normal weight bearing.[65] Carprofen (2 mg/kg IM) was effective for up to 6 hours but was less effective than butorphanol in improving weight bearing on the arthritic limb.[66] Alternatively, in a dose-response study using the same model of arthritis, meloxicam (1 mg/kg IM q12h) was effective at returning the parrots to normal weight bearing on the arthritic limb throughout 30 hours of observation, whereas lower doses of meloxicam were ineffective.

CHRONIC PAIN

Assessment of analgesia is challenging when the condition is progressive, such as chronic degenerative joint disease or neoplasia. Response to analgesia therapy is based on evaluation of a set of behaviors particular for each bird.

NSAIDs are the first course of therapy for chronic disorders because they have no sedative effect and have a longer duration of analgesic effect than most opioids. Carprofen and meloxicam are the current drugs of choice because of their widespread use and the low incidence of reported toxicities. Injectable forms of meloxicam and carprofen will cause myositis and muscle necrosis[67,68]; therefore oral formulations are recommended. However, oral bioavailability of NSAIDs varies greatly among avian species. Therefore it is critical to monitor response to dosage and frequency of NSAID treatment for each bird. The commercially prepared oral suspension of meloxicam has an advantage of being easily administered in small volumes for small birds; however, in larger birds, meloxicam or carprofen tablets may be selected based on dosage and cost. NSAIDs are often initiated at a high-end dosage, which can be decreased gradually over time while the bird is monitored for response to treatment. If pain gradually increases over time, the dosage can be increased. Monitoring the complete blood count, fecal occult blood, and renal (uric acid, blood urea nitrogen, and phosphorous) and hepatic (aspartate aminotransferase and bile acids) plasma values every 4 to 6 months is recommended, and more frequently in the older bird. If pain recurs after several months of treatment, the next set of options includes changing to another NSAID. If pain persists or increases, especially with neoplasia, adding tramadol or opioid therapy may be indicated. Butorphanol, although short-acting, was shown to reduce pain behaviors associated with chronic arthritis in turkeys.[69] Unfortunately, parenteral forms of recommended opioids are effective only for a few hours. Studies using an experimental long-acting liposome-encapsulated butorphanol in parrots with experimentally induced arthritis reported greater efficacy at reducing pain and lameness than NSAIDs.[70]

Piroxicam may have synergistic action with anticancer drugs and is also an effective NSAID for degenerative joint disease in birds. Piroxicam is noted for renal toxicity and gastric ulceration in mammals. In a study using chickens with ascites syndrome, a high dose of piroxicam (0.6 mg/kg) caused gastrointestinal ulceration.[71] However, long-term use of piroxicam (0.5 to 1.0 mg/kg once daily) has been administered and closely monitored for several consecutive months to captive cranes with chronic degenerative joint disease and has not caused clinical problems.[72]

CONCLUSION

Avian analgesia is recognized as a critical component of avian medicine and surgery. Further progress needs to be made to recognize pain, provide pain relief, and identify when treatments effectively reduce pain behaviors in the individual bird. Several published research investigations, using several species of birds, have begun to provide avian analgesia therapeutics with information for clinical application. The challenge is to continue pushing this research forward with appreciation that there are approximately 10,000 known species of birds, perhaps 200 species commonly kept as pets, and that each species has a range of behaviors as varied as their species-specific pharmacokinetics and pharmacodynamics to each analgesic drug.

REFERENCES

1. Jones RB, Harvey S. Behavioural and adrenocortical responses of domestic chicks to systematic reductions in group size and to sequential disturbance of companions by the experimenter. Behavioural Processes. 1987; 14:291–303.
2. Gentle MJ, Tilston VL. Reduction in peripheral inflammation by changes in attention. Physiol Behav. 1999; 66:289–292.

3. Desmarchelier M, Troncy E, Beauchamp G, et al. Evaluation of a fracture pain model in domestic pigeons (*Columba livia*). Am J Vet Res. 2012; 73:353–360.

4. Sufka KJ, Hoganson DA, Hughes RA. Central monoaminergic changes induced by morphine in hypoalgesic and hyperalgesic strains of domestic fowl. Pharmacol Biochem Behav. 1992; 42:781–785.

5. Hughes RA. Strain-dependent morphine-induced analgesic and hyperalgesic effects on thermal nociception in domestic fowl (*Gallus gallus*). Behav Neurosci. 1990; 104:619–624.

6. Gentle M. The acute effects of amputation on peripheral trigeminal afferents in *Gallus gallus var domesticus*. Pain. 1991; 46:97–103.

7. Gentle MJ. Sodium urate arthritis: Effects on the sensory properties of articular afferents in the chicken. Pain. 1997; 70:245–251.

8. McKeegan DE. Mechano-chemical nociceptors in the avian trigeminal mucosa. Brain Res Brain Res Rev. 2004; 46:146–154.

9. Zhai SY, Atsumi S. Large dorsal horn neurons which receive inputs from numerous substance P-like immunoreactive axon terminals in the laminae I and II of the chicken spinal cord. Neurosci Res. 1997; 28:147–154.

10. Roughan JV, Flecknell PA. Effects of surgery and analgesic administration on spontaneous behaviour in singly housed rats. Res Vet Sci. 2000; 69:283–288.

11. Woolf CJ. A new strategy for the treatment of inflammatory pain. Prevention or elimination of central sensitization Drugs. 1994; 47(Suppl 5):1–9; discussion 46–47.

12. Woolf CJ, Chong MS. Preemptive analgesia—treating postoperative pain by preventing the establishment of central sensitization. Anesth Analg. 1993; 77:362–379.

13. Hocking PM, Gentle MJ, Bernard R, et al. Evaluation of a protocol for determining the effectiveness of pretreatment with local analgesics for reducing experimentally induced articular pain in domestic fowl. Res Vet Sci. 1997; 63:263–267.

14. Machin KL, Livingston A. Plasma bupivacaine levels in mallard ducks (*Anas platyrhynchos*) following a single subcutaneous dose. Proc Am Assoc Zoo Vet. 2001; 159–163.

15. Clubb SL. Round table discussion: Pain management in clinical practice. J Avian Med Surg. 1998; 12:276–278.

16. Glatz PC, Murphy LB, Preston AP. Analgesic therapy of beak-trimmed chickens. Aust Vet J. 1992; 69:18.

17. Brenner DJ, Larsen RS, Dickinson PJ, et al. Development of an avian brachial plexus nerve block technique for perioperative analgesia in mallard ducks (*Anas platyrhynchos*). J Avian Med Surg. 2010; 24:24–34.

18. Figueiredo JP, Cruz ML, Mendes GM, et al. Assessment of brachial plexus blockade in chickens by an axillary approach. Vet Anaesth Analg. 2008; 35:511–518.

19. da Cunha AF, Strain GM, Rademacher N, et al. Palpation- and ultrasound-guided brachial plexus blockade in Hispaniolan Amazon parrots (*Amazona ventralis*). Vet Anaesth Analg. 2013; 40:96–102.

20. Mansour A, Khachaturian H, Lewis ME, et al. Anatomy of CNS opioid receptors. Trends Neurosci. 1988; 11:308–314.

21. Curro TG, Brunson DB, Paul-Murphy J. Determination of the ED50 of isoflurane and evaluation of the isoflurane-sparing effect of butorphanol in cockatoos (*Cacatua* spp.). Vet Surg. 1994; 23:429–433.

22. Curro TG. Evaluation of the isoflurane-sparing effects of butorphanol and flunixin in psittaciformes. Proc Assoc Avian Vet. 1994; 17–19.

23. Reim DA, Middleton CC. Use of butorphanol as an anesthetic adjunct in turkeys. Lab Anim Sci. 1995; 45:696–698.

24. Concannon KT, Dodam JR, Hellyer PW. Influence of a mu- and kappa-opioid agonist on isoflurane minimal anesthetic concentration in chickens. Am J Vet Res. 1995; 56:806–811.

25. Paul-Murphy J, Brunson DB, Miletic V. Analgesic effects of butorphanol and buprenorphine in conscious African grey parrots (*Psittacus erithacus erithacus* and *Psittacus erithacus timneh*). Am J Vet Res. 1999; 60:1218–1221.

26. Paul-Murphy J, Ludders JW. Avian analgesia. Vet Clin North Am Exot Anim Pract. 2001; 4:35–45.

27. Guzman DS, Flammer K, Paul-Murphy JR, et al. Pharmacokinetics of butorphanol after intravenous, intramuscular, and oral administration in Hispaniolan Amazon parrots (*Amazona ventralis*). J Avian Med Surg. 2011; 25:185–191.

28. Sanchez-Migallon Guzman D, Drazenovich T, Olsen G, et al. Evaluation of the thermal antinociceptive effects and pharmacodynamics after intramuscular administration of butorphanol tartrate in American kestrels (*Falco sparverius*). Am J Vet Res. 2014; 75:11–18.

29. Sanchez-Migallon Guzman D, KuKanich B, Keuler N, et al. Antinociceptive effects of nalbuphine hydrochloride in Hispaniolan Amazon parrots (*Amazona ventralis*). Am J Vet Res. 2011; 72:736–740.

30. Paul-Murphy J, Hess J, Fialkowski JP. Pharmacokinetic properties of a single intramuscular dose of buprenorphine in African grey parrots (*Psittacus erithacus erithacus*). J Avian Med Surg. 2004; 18:224–228.

31. Gaggermeier B, Henke J, Schatzmann U. Investigations on analgesia in domestic pigeons using buprenorphine and butorphanol. Proc Eur Chap Assoc Avian Vet. 2001; 70–74.

32. Hoppes S, Flammer K, Hoersch K, et al. Disposition and analgesic effects of fentanyl in white cockatoos (*Cacatua alba*). J Avian Med Surg. 2003; 17:124–130.

33. Sanchez-Migallon Guzman D, Drazenovich T, Olsen G, et al. Evaluation of the thermal antinociceptive effects after intramuscular administration of hydromorphone hydrochloride to American kestrels (*Falco sparverius*). Am J Vet Res. 2013; 74:736–740.

34. Pavez JC, Hawkins MG, Pascoe PJ, et al. Effect of fentanyl target-controlled infusions on isoflurane minimum anaesthetic concentration and cardiovascular function in red-tailed hawks (*Buteo jamaicensis*). Vet Anaesth Analg. 2011; 38:344–351.

35. Scott LJ, Perry CM. Tramadol: A review of its use in perioperative pain. Drugs 2000; 60:139–176.

36. Souza MJ, Sanchez-Migallon GD, Paul-Murphy J, et al. Tramadol in Hispaniolan Amazon parrots (*Amazona ventralis*). Proc Assoc Avian Vet. 2010; 293–294.

37. Souza MJ, Martin-Jimenez T, Jones MP, et al. Pharmacokinetics of intravenous and oral tramadol in the bald eagle (*Haliaeetus leucocephalus*). J Avian Med Surg. 2009; 23:247–252.

38. Black PA, Cox SK, Macek M, et al. Pharmacokinetics of tramadol hydrochloride and its metabolite O-desmethyltramadol in peafowl (*Pavo cristatus*). J Zoo Wildl Med. 2010; 41:671–676.

39. Souza MJ, Martin-Jimenez T, Jones MP, et al. Pharmacokinetics of oral tramadol in red-tailed hawks (*Buteo jamaicensis*). J Vet Pharmacol Ther. 2011; 34:86–88.

40. Souza MJ, Sanchez-Migallon Guzman D, Paul-Murphy JR, et al. Pharmacokinetics after oral and intravenous administration of a single dose of tramadol hydrochloride to Hispaniolan Amazon parrots (*Amazona ventralis*). Am J Vet Res. 2012; 73:1142–1147.

41. Sanchez-Migallon Guzman D, KuKanich B, Drazenovich T, et al. Evaluation of thermal antinociceptive effects of oral tramadol hydrochloride to American kestrels (*Falco sparverius*). Am J Vet Res. 2014; 75:117–123.

42. Sanchez-Migallon Guzman D, Souza MJ, Braun JM, et al. Antinociceptive effects after oral administration of tramadol hydrochloride in Hispaniolan Amazon parrots (*Amazona ventralis*). Am J Vet Res. 2012; 73:1148–1152.

43. Papich MG. An update on nonsteroidal anti-inflammatory drugs (NSAIDs) in small animals. Vet Clin North Am Small Anim Pract. 2008; 38:1243–1266, vi.

44. Bergh MS, Budsberg SC. The coxib NSAIDs: Potential clinical and pharmacologic importance in veterinary medicine. J Vet Intern Med. 2005; 19:633–643.

45. Mathonnet M, Lalloue F, Danty E, et al. Cyclo-oxygenase 2 tissue distribution and developmental pattern of expression in the chicken. Clin Exp Pharmacol Physiol. 2001; 28:425–432.

46. Cuthbert R, Parry-Jones J, Green RE, et al. NSAIDs and scavenging birds: Potential impacts beyond Asia's critically endangered vultures. Biol Lett. 2007; 3:90–93.

47. Oaks JL, Gilbert M, Virani MZ, et al. Diclofenac residues as the cause of vulture population decline in Pakistan. Nature. 2004; 427:630–633.

48. Naidoo V, Swan GE. Diclofenac toxicity in Gyps vulture is associated with decreased uric acid excretion and not renal portal vasoconstriction. Comp Biochem Physiol C Toxicol Pharmacol. 2008.

49. Meteyer CU, Rideout BA, Gilbert M, et al. Pathology and proposed pathophysiology of diclofenac poisoning in free-living and experimentally exposed oriental white-backed vultures (Gyps bengalensis). J Wildl Dis. 2005; 41:707–716.

50. Swan GE, Cuthbert R, Quevedo M, et al. Toxicity of diclofenac to Gyps vultures. Biol Lett. 2006; 2:279–282.

51. Klein PN, Charmatz K, Langenberg J. The effect of flunixin meglumine (banamine) on the renal function of northern bobwhite quail (Colinus virginianus): an avian model. Proc Am Assoc Zoo Vet. 1994; 128–131.

52. Swan G, Naidoo V, Cuthbert R, et al. Removing the threat of diclofenac to critically endangered Asian vultures. PLoS Biol. 2006; 4:e66.

53. Sinclair K, Paul-Murphy J, Church M, et al. Effects of meloxicam on hematologic and plasma biochemical analysis variables and results of histologic examination of tissue specimens of Japanese quail (Coturnix japonica). Am J Vet Res. 2012; 73:1720–1727.

54. Mulcahy DM, Tuomi P, Larsen RS. Differential mortality of male spectacled Eiders (Somateria fischeri) and King Eiders (Somateria spectabilis) subsequent to anesthesia with propofol, bupivacaine, and ketoprofen. J Avian Med Surg. 2003; 17:117–123.

55. Gibbons PM, Tell LA, Kass PH, et al. Evaluation of the sensitivity and specificity of four laboratory tests for detection of occult blood in cockatiel (Nymphicus hollandicus) excrement. Am J Vet Res. 2006; 67:1326–1332.

56. Baert K, De Backer P. Disposition of sodium salicylate, flunixin and meloxicam after intravenous administration in broiler chickens. J Vet Pharmacol Ther. 2002; 25:449–453.

57. Baert K, De Backer P. Comparative pharmacokinetics of three non-steroidal anti-inflammatory drugs in five bird species. Comp Biochem Physiol C Toxicol Pharmacol. 2003; 134:25–33.

58. Molter C, Court M, Cole GA, et al. Pharmacokinetics of parenteral and oral meloxicam in Hispaniolan parrots (Amazona ventralis). Assoc Avian Vet. 2009; 375–380.

59. Graham JE, Kollias-Baker C, Craigmill AL, et al. Pharmacokinetics of ketoprofen in Japanese quail (Coturnix japonica). J Vet Pharmacol Ther. 2005; 28:399–402.

60. Machin KL, Tellier LA, Lair S, et al. Pharmacodynamics of flunixin and ketoprofen in mallard ducks (Anas platyrhynchos). J Zoo Wildl Med. 2001; 32:222–229.

61. Machin KL, Livingston A. Assessment of the analgesic effects of ketoprofen in ducks anesthetized with isoflurane. Am J Vet Res. 2002; 63:821–826.

62. Danbury TC, Weeks CA, Chambers JP, et al. Self-selection of the analgesic drug carprofen by lame broiler chickens. Vet Rec. 2000; 146:307–311.

63. McGeown D, Danbury TC, Waterman-Pearson AE, et al. Effect of carprofen on lameness in broiler chickens. Vet Rec. 1999; 144:668–671.

64. Hocking PM, Robertson GW, Gentle MJ. Effects of non-steroidal anti-inflammatory drugs on pain-related behaviour in a model of articular pain in the domestic fowl. Res Vet Sci. 2005; 78:69–75.

65. Cole GA, Paul-Murphy J, Krugner-Higby L, et al. Analgesic effects of intramuscular administration of meloxicam in Hispaniolan parrots (*Amazona ventralis*) with experimentally induced arthritis. Am J Vet Res. 2009; 70:1471–1476.

66. Paul-Murphy JR, Sladky KK, Krugner-Higby LA, et al. Analgesic effects of carprofen and liposome-encapsulated butorphanol tartrate in Hispaniolan parrots (*Amazona ventralis*) with experimentally induced arthritis. Am J Vet Res. 2009; 70:1201–1210.

67. Sinclair KM, Church ME, Farver TB, et al. Effects of meloxicam on hematologic and plasma biochemical analysis variables and results of histologic examination of tissue specimens of Japanese quail (*Coturnix japonica*). Am J Vet Res. 2012; 73:1720–1727.

68. Zollinger TJ, Hoover JP, Payton ME, et al. Clinicopathologic, gross necropsy, and histologic findings after intramuscular injection of carprofen in a pigeon (*Columba livia*) model. J Avian Med Surg. 2011; 25:173–184.

69. Buchwalder T, Huber-Eicher B. Effect of the analgesic butorphanol on activity behaviour in turkeys (*Meleagris gallopavo*). Res Vet Sci. 2005; 79:239–244.

70. Sladky KK, Krugner-Higby L, Meek-Walker E, et al. Serum concentrations and analgesic effects of liposome-encapsulated and standard butorphanol tartrate in parrots. Am J Vet Res. 2006; 67:775–781.

71. Valle K, Diaz-Cruz A, Avila E, et al. Antioxidant action of piroxicam on liver, heart and lung in broiler chicks. J Vet Pharmacol Ther. 2001; 24:291–293.

72. Paul-Murphy J, Sladky K, Krugner-Higby L. Analgesic effects of carprofen and liposome-encapsulated butorphanol tartrate in Hispaniolan parrots (*Amazona ventralis*) with experimentally induced arthritis. Am J Vet Res. 2009; 1201–1210.

73. Klaphake E, Schumacher J, Greenacre C, et al. Comparative anesthetic and cardiopulmonary effects of pre- versus postoperative butorphanol administration in Hispaniolan Amazon parrots (*Amazona ventralis*) anesthetized with sevoflurane. J Avian Med Surg. 2006; 20:2–7.

74. Keller D, Sanchez-Migallon Guzman D, KuKanich B, et al. Pharmacokinetics of nalbuphine hydrochloride in Hispaniolan Amazon parrots (*Amazona ventralis*). Am J Vet Res. 2011; 741–745.

75. Pereira ME, Werther K. Evaluation of the renal effects of flunixin meglumine, ketoprofen and meloxicam in budgerigars (*Melopsittacus undulatus*). Vet Rec. 2007; 160:844–846.

76. Molter CM, Court MH, Cole GA, et al. Pharmacokinetics of meloxicam after intravenous, intramuscular, and oral administration of a single dose to Hispaniolan Amazon parrots (*Amazona ventralis*). Am J Vet Res. 2013; 74:375–380.

77. Baert K, De Backer P. Disposition of sodium salicylate, flunixin, and meloxicam after intravenous administration in ostriches (*Struthio camelus*). J Avian Med Surg. 2002; 16:123–128.

78. Naidoo V, Wolter K, Cromarty AD, et al. The pharmacokinetics of meloxicam in vultures. J Vet Pharmacol Ther. 2008; 31:128–134.

CHAPTER 27

Reptile-Specific Considerations

Craig Mosley

Analgesic management of pain in reptiles is challenging because of their unique physiologic, anatomic, and behavioral adaptations. In addition, pain and nociception in reptiles have not been extensively studied, although there is compelling evidence that reptiles are capable of nociception. However the sensory *significance* of nociception, the emotional experience of pain, to the individual is poorly understood. Pain is often described as "an unpleasant sensory and *emotional experience* associated with actual or potential tissue damage, or described in terms of such damage." Pain is essentially an emotional experience. It is not possible to quantitatively or qualitatively describe this experience in reptiles given our current level of understanding and technology. However, it is certain that reptiles experience noxious insults as some sort of negative event and modify their behavior to escape such insults. Perhaps a more robust and inclusive definition of pain in animals would be "a sensory experience representing awareness of damage or the potential for tissue damage that results in a behavioral and physiologic response to minimize/prevent the recurrence and promote healing of damage"[1] (modified from Molony). This definition suggests that the experience in nonhuman animals may be similar to the experience in humans but recognizes that human and animal pain may not be the same and that they are perhaps quantitatively and qualitatively different. The evidence for animal pain in reptiles is briefly presented here, allowing the reader to more fully appreciate the balance of evidence.

EVIDENCE FOR ANIMAL PAIN IN REPTILES

Presence of Nociceptors

- Primarily nociceptive neurons (slowly adapting polymodal C fibers) have not been identified in reptiles.
- High-threshold $A\delta$ mechanical nociceptors and C-fiber mechanical nociceptors have been identified in one species of snake.

Ascending Transmission Pathways to the Brain

- Spinothalamic projections analogous to the neospinothalamic (fast pain) and paleospinothalamic (slow pain) tracts have been identified in reptiles.

- Trigeminal tracts have also been identified.
- No functional studies have examined the role of these pathways in nociceptive processing.

Suitable Brain Structures

- Reptiles posses brain structures necessary for experiencing pain (neocortex), and morphologically there are direct spinal connections to the brainstem and dorsal thalamus in the midbrain.
- Functional studies are lacking.
- Differences in reptiles' brain systems compared with those of birds and mammals may be a matter of degrees of elaboration rather than presence or absence of structures. It is possible (and even likely) that the response to a noxious stimulus (pain) in reptiles is one associated with less fidelity and range compared with mammals. "Emotions" and the experience of pain may be an all-or-nothing phenomenon (rage or no rage, pain or no pain) rather than the graded experiences of human emotions (e.g., rage, anger, irritation, discontent, neutrality, happiness). Humans describe a range of painful experiences from those that are mildly irritating to those that are intolerable.

Opioid and Other Nociceptive Receptors and Substances

- Presence of opioid receptors and endogenous opioids has been described.
- Their exact role, the receptor subtype present, and their anatomic locations are somewhat less clear.
- Good behavioral evidence supports an antinociceptive role (i.e., decreasing the intensity of neural trafficking associated with noxious stimuli) of the opioid system in reptiles.
- Several nociceptive related neuropeptides (e.g., glutamate, substance P, calcitonin gene–related peptide) have been identified in reptiles, but their functions are not well elucidated.

Evidence That Known Analgesics Reduce Nociceptive or Nocifensive Behaviors

- Several experimental models have examined the response of reptiles to substances known to be analgesic in mammals, primarily the opioids.[2]
- Studies suggest that some opioids reduce response to some stimuli, although there is inconsistency among different experimental nociceptive models used and the response of different reptile species to similar testing situations and individual drugs.
- Models have not been extensively validated for efficacy (i.e., discriminatory abilities) in reptiles.
- Thermal testing in ectothermic animals raises some concern; reptiles are prone to thermal burns if unprotected from heat sources capable of

inducing tissue trauma, suggesting that in some circumstances heat may not be perceived as sufficiently noxious to prevent thermally induced tissue damage.

- Nociceptive testing is also typically applied to a specific part of the body, and because of the wide anatomic variation and specific thermoregulatory adaptations of each reptile species, the locations and density of various nociceptors may vary among areas of the body.

Avoidance Learning

- No known studies have examined avoidance learning in response to a noxious stimulus in reptiles.

Suspension of Normal Behavior

- No specific studies in reptiles
- Reasonable anecdotal information from clinicians and reptile owners; may be influenced by preconceived biases and beliefs
- Some suggestions that a reptile's normal behaviors (eating, basking, social interaction) are altered by animal pain and that provision of appropriate analgesics will hasten resumption of normal behaviors. Evidence is largely circumstantial.

> Reptiles are capable of nociception, and evidence suggests they are capable of experiencing animal pain; however, the significance of this experience is not clear. Analgesic techniques to minimize the negative effects of nociception should be used in these animals.

ASSESSING PAIN IN REPTILES

- Pain assessment in reptiles is challenging and requires a good understanding of normal reptile behavior, physiology, and unique species-specific adaptations. An approach similar to pain assessment in other veterinary species can be adapted for use in reptiles. Remote observation may be required to evaluate pain in reptiles accurately (Box 27-1).

ANALGESIC THERAPY IN REPTILES

- Plan should include analgesic drugs, route of drug administration, and also steps to monitor individual response to therapy and the provision of ongoing supportive care.
- Recognize that there are few studies examining the pharmacokinetics and pharmacodynamics of analgesic drugs in reptiles, and significant species variation.

BOX 27-1 **An Approach to Pain Assessment in Reptiles**

Behavior

Species Considerations

Requires proper species identification and familiarity with species-specific behaviors. Basic species differences affect behavioral patterns, and these are important when one attempts to differentiate normal from abnormal behaviors.
- Predominant activity pattern (diurnal, nocturnal)
- Predated or predator species
- Habitat (arboreal, aquatic, terrestrial, fossorial)

Individual Considerations
- Stage of ecdysis
  - Some may become more aggressive during this time.
- Hibernation status
  - Hibernating animals or those inclined to hibernate may be more docile and less responsive than normal.
- Socialization
  - Altered response to human interaction (normally docile animal to biting) occurs; poor response to caregiver occurs.
- Concurrent illness
  - Animal may be incapable of exhibiting behaviors associated with pain, or behaviors associated with disease may be mistaken for pain behaviors.
- Owner assessment
  - Owners are often more familiar with their animal's normal behavior; however, owners may also be biased based on their own understanding and belief regarding their animal's conditions.

Environmental Considerations
- Enclosure
  - Home enclosures are often more "interesting" than hospital enclosures, providing animal with plenty of opportunity to exhibit normal behaviors.
- Preferred optimal body temperature
  - Ambient environmental temperature is one of the main determinants of metabolic rate in resting reptiles, and consequently normal behavior may be influenced by alterations in metabolic rate.
- Observer
  - Good evidence suggests that reptiles may suppress behaviors and activity that may be associated with pain in the presence of an observer (i.e., they may not withdraw from a painful stimulus).

Locomotor Activity
- Posture
  - Hunched, guarding of affected body area, not resting in normal posture
- Gait
  - Must differentiate neurologic and mechanical dysfunction from pain-induced lameness
- Other
  - Excessive scratching or flicking foot, tail, or affected area
  - Unwillingness to perform normal movements (look up, step up, thrash with tail)
  - Exaggerated flight response

BOX **27-1** **An Approach to Pain Assessment in Reptiles—cont'd**

Miscellaneous
- Appetite
  - Reduced appetite may be related to underlying disease but may also be related to pain.
- Eyes
  - Eyelids may be held closed when animal is in pain or ill.
- Color change
  - Species capable of color change may do so in response to stress and/or pain.
- Abnormal respiratory movements
  - Respirations may be associated with primary respiratory disease but also pain affecting the muscles and tissues involved in respiration.

Anticipated Level of Pain
The anticipated level of pain is commonly used to evaluate pain in reptiles and is based on the likelihood and severity of tissue trauma associated with a particular procedure or condition. This is a well-accepted approach in veterinary medicine, particularly when dealing with less familiar species.[37,38] However, in addition to significant species differences, significant individual differences in response to therapy and response to tissue trauma can be seen.

Physiologic Data
Most physiologic parameters have been shown to be poor indicators of pain in most species. Physiologic parameters can be influenced by disease and excitement. In addition, the physiologic parameters of reptiles may be influenced by a number of metabolic processes, such as activity level, temperature alterations, and feeding.

Response to Palpation
In some species a negative response to palpation can be a useful indicator of pain. However, in reptiles this may be less sensitive because most reptiles withdraw from touch regardless of whether the animal is experiencing pain.

ROUTE OF DRUG ADMINISTRATION

Considerations for route of drug administration include ease of administration, unique anatomic or physiologic structures, and variable bioavailability and uptake among various routes.
- Intravenous drug administration not always feasible.
  - Good technique, practice, appropriate patient selection, and skilled physical restraint can facilitate predictable venous access.
  - Intravascular injection ensures complete bioavailability of drug and may avoid tissue irritation associated with intramuscular or subcutaneous administration
- Intramuscular administration is commonly used.
  - Hindlimb and tail injection are normally avoided because of concerns related to first-pass and toxic effects associated with passage of administered drug through kidneys via renal portal system; clinical significance is highly species dependent.

- Bioavailability and time to effect (peak plasma drug concentrations) of intramuscularly administered drugs may be reduced and prolonged, respectively.
- Subcutaneous route is practical and easy in many species.
  - Evidence shows good absorption in some species.
  - Tissue irritation (rare with analgesic drugs) and required volume may be limitations.
- Oral drug administration may be desirable for animals that require chronic analgesic therapy.
  - Feeding tubes can greatly simplify and facilitate this process.
  - Consider gastrointestinal differences among reptiles; strict carnivores (snakes) may fast for days to weeks between meals, versus primarily herbivores (turtles, tortoises, and some lizards), which feed continuously, and this may affect bioavailability and pharmacokinetics of drugs given orally.
  - Evidence suggests that this may be a viable route in some reptile species, with bioavailability and pharmacokinetic profiles similar to intravenous administration.
- Transcutaneous.
  - Fentanyl levels have been detected after patch application; there are no current analgesic studies for directing clinical use.

Significant pharmacokinetic and pharmacodynamic differences exist between reptiles and mammals, making extrapolation of drug doses and intervals difficult. When available, species-specific analgesic drug studies in reptiles can provide valuable insight to help guide analgesic therapy. However, critical evaluation is required to interpret the results of these studies accurately.

DRUGS: CLASSES OF ANALGESIC DRUGS COMMONLY USED IN REPTILES

See Table 27-1.

Classes of Analgesic Drugs Commonly Used in Reptiles
- Opioids and opioid-like drugs
- Nonsteroidal anti-inflammatory drugs
- Local anesthetics
- Others (ketamine, α_2-agonists)

TABLE 27-1	Doses of Drugs with Potential Analgesic Effects in Reptiles			
DRUG	ROUTE	DOSAGE	COMMENTS	REFERENCES
Opioids				
Buprenorphine	IM, IV, SC	0.4–1.0 mg/kg	No evidence of analgesic efficacy in reptiles	3–5
Butorphanol	IM, SC	1.0–8.0 mg/kg	Very questionable analgesic efficacy in reptiles	3, 6–12
Fentanyl	Transdermal	12.5 mcg/hr 2.5 mcg/hr	No analgesic efficacy studies, plasma concentrations obtained	13, 14
Hydromorphone	SC, IM	0.5 mg/kg	Evidence for analgesic efficacy in red-eared sliders, likely similar efficacy to morphine	5
Meperidine	SC, IM	1.0–5.0 mg/kg 20.0–50.0 mg/kg	Analgesic effect short in red-eared sliders, wide range of doses reported	15, 16
Morphine	SC, IM	1.0–40.0 mg/kg	Very good evidence for analgesic efficacy, wide range of doses reported, respiratory depression can be seen	3, 6–8, 15–18
Tramadol	PO	5–10 mg/kg	Evidence of analgesic efficacy in red-eared sliders, long duration, less respiratory depression compared with morphine	19, 20
Nonsteroidal Anti-inflammatory Drugs (NSAIDs)				
Carprofen	IM, IV, SC	1.0–4.0 mg/kg	No evidence of analgesic efficacy in reptiles, extrapolated from mammals	21
Flunixin meglumine	IM	0.1–0.5 mg/kg	No evidence of analgesic efficacy in reptiles, extrapolated from mammals	21
Ketoprofen	IM, SC	2.0 mg/kg	No evidence of analgesic efficacy in reptiles, extrapolated from mammals	21, 22
Meloxicam	IM, IV, PO	0.1–0.3 mg/kg	No evidence of analgesic efficacy in reptiles, extrapolated from mammals	12, 21, 23, 24

Continued

TABLE 27-1 Doses of Drugs with Potential Analgesic Effects in Reptiles—cont'd

DRUG	ROUTE	DOSAGE	COMMENTS	REFERENCES
Local Anesthetics				
Bupivacaine (0.5%)	Local infiltration, intrathecal	Toxic dose unknown; recommend <2 mg/kg	Dilute to 0.25% to increase volume	21, 25
Lidocaine (2%)	Local infiltration, intrathecal	Toxic dose unknown; recommend <5 mg/kg	Dilute to 1.0% to increase volume	21, 25–27
Mepivacaine (2%)	Local infiltration	Toxic dose unknown; recommend <5 mg/kg	Dilute to 1.0% to increase volume	28
Other Analgesics				
Ketamine	IM, IV, SC	10-100 mg/kg	No evidence of analgesic efficacy in reptiles, high doses are associated with anesthesia, lower doses <10 mg/kg possibly associated with analgesia without sedation, extrapolated from mammals	29–32
Medetomidine	IM, IV, IO	50-300 mcg/kg	No evidence of analgesic efficacy in reptiles, lower doses may be effective for analgesia	31, 33–35
Xylazine	IM	1.0-1.25 mg/kg	No evidence of analgesic efficacy in reptiles, lower doses may be effective for analgesia	36

Repeat administration pharmacokinetics have not been fully studied for any of the analgesic drugs; variability in duration of clinical effects should be expected among species and individuals. Clinical effects of those opioids demonstrating analgesic efficacy are variable; morphine, and hydromorphone may persist for 24 hours, meperidine may be present for only 2 to 4 hours, and tramadol may have effects for 48 to 72 hours.

Opioids and Opioid-like Drugs

- Butorphanol (κ-agonist, μ-antagonist): Despite frequent use, does not appear to produce significant analgesic effects in most studies.
- Morphine (μ-agonist): Good evidence as an effective analgesic in many reptile species.
- Hydromorphone (μ-agonist): Only a single study showing evidence for analgesia in red-eared sliders, but probably very similar profile to morphine in others species.
- Fentanyl (μ-agonist): Plasma concentrations have been obtained using fentanyl patches, but no studies evaluating efficacy.
- Buprenorphine (partial μ-agonist): No evidence for analgesic efficacy in reptiles.
- Tramadol (μ-agonist, serotonergic and adrenergic effects): Not a classic opioid; evidence for long-acting analgesic effect in reptiles with good oral bioavailability.
- Time for onset of action may be variable among opioids (minutes to hours); evidence of respiratory depression (less with tramadol).
- Opioids appear to be safe for use in reptiles with minimal side effects at clinically recommended doses.

Nonsteroidal Anti-inflammatory Drugs

- Role of cyclooxygenase in pain and inflammation physiology of reptiles not studied; very limited efficacy (no evidence of analgesic efficacy) and safety information, although clinical use common.
- Limited pharmacokinetic data. Note that plasma levels of nonsteroidal anti-inflammatory drugs (NSAIDs) do not always correspond to their clinical effect.
- Based on available data, very difficult to recommend appropriate doses and administration intervals; extended administration intervals compared with mammals probably most appropriate.
- Consider possibility of side effects similar to those seen in mammals (gastrointestinal irritation, renal compromise, platelet inhibition).
- Hydration status, concurrent medications (steroids), presence of coagulopathy, gastrointestinal disease, and renal disease should be addressed before administration.

Local Anesthetics

- Local anesthetics often used to facilitate minor surgical interventions.
- Limited duration of analgesic effect (2 to 6 hours) and accompanying motor paralysis limit use to the immediate perioperative period or hospitalized animals.

- Few specific locoregional techniques described (mandibular and intrathecal).
- Careful attention to total dose (do not exceed mammalian toxic doses) required to avoid toxicity; many animals are very small.
- Excessive dilution of local anesthetics may decrease efficacy; probably best not exceed 50% on a per-volume basis.

Other Drugs

- Ketamine administered at subanesthetic dosages is used as an analgesic in many mammalian species, but its analgesic potential in reptiles has not been studied.
- The α_2-agonists produce analgesia, sedation, and muscle relaxation in mammals; the analgesic effects of α_2-agonists have not been evaluated in reptiles.
- The effects of other analgesic drugs and adjuncts such as gabapentin, amantadine, tricyclic antidepressants, and various forms of nutraceutical and physical therapy have not been explored in reptiles, but may have a role to play as our understanding of nociception, pain, and analgesic treatments in reptiles increases.

CONCLUSION

Reptiles are a unique and diverse class of animals that have distinctive mechanisms for managing alterations in their body temperature and metabolic rate that are not seen in most other animals. Because of the limitations in our current understanding of reptile physiology, nociception, pain, and analgesia, an indiscriminate and generalized approach is often used to manage pain in reptiles. As our knowledge and understanding increase, our approach to pain management in these animals will become modified and refined to more specifically address their pain. New information should be evaluated objectively and without the influence of personal bias or beliefs. The unique mechanisms reptiles have developed for managing pain and avoiding the negative consequences associated with pain are yet to be completely understood.

REFERENCES

1. Molony V. Comments on Anand and Craig, PAIN, 67 (1996) 3-6. Pain. 1997; 70 (2–3):293.
2. Sladky KK, Mans C. Clinical analgesia in reptiles. J Exotic Pet Med. 2012; 21:158–167.
3. Greenacre CB, Takle G, Schumacher J, et al: Comparative antinociception of morphine, butorphanol, and buprenorphine versus saline in the green iguana, *Iguana iguana*, using electrostimulation. J Herp Med Surg. 2006; 16(3):88–92.
4. Kummrow MS, Tseng F, Hesse L, et al: Pharmacokinetics of buprenorphine after single-dose subcutaneous administration in red-eared sliders (*Trachemys scripta elegans*). J Zoo Wildl Med. 2008; 39(4):590–5.

5. Mans C, Lahner LL, Baker BB, et al: Antinociceptive efficacy of buprenorphine and hydromorphone in red-eared slider turtles (*Trachemys scripta elegans*). J Zoo Wildl Med. 2012; 43(3):662–665.

6. Sladky KK, Miletic V, Paul-Murphy J, et al: Analgesic efficacy and respiratory effects of butorphanol and morphine in turtles. J Am Vet Med Assoc. 2007; 230(9):1356–1362.

7. Sladky KK, Kinney ME, Johnson SM. Analgesic efficacy of butorphanol and morphine in bearded dragons and corn snakes. J Am Vet Med Assoc. 2008; 233(2):267–273.

8. Sladky KK, Kinney ME, Johnson SM. Effects of opioid receptor activation on thermal antinociception in red-eared slider turtles (*Trachemys scripta*). Am J Vet Res. 2009; 70 (9):1072–1078.

9. Fleming GJ, Robertson SA. Assessments of thermal antinociceptive effects of butorphanol and human observer effect on quantitative evaluation of analgesia in green iguanas (*Iguana iguana*). Am J Vet Res. 2012; 73(10):1507–1511.

10. Fleming GJ, Robertson S. Use of thermal threshold test response to evaluate the antinociceptive effects of butorphanol in juvenile green iguanas (*Iguana iguana*). Proceedings. Annu Meet Am Assoc Zoo Vet. 2006; 279–280.

11. Mosley CA, Dyson D, Smith DA. The cardiac anesthetic index of isoflurane in green iguanas. J Am Vet Med Assoc. 2003; 222(11):1565–1568.

12. Olesen MG, Bertelsen MF, Perry SF, et al: Effects of preoperative administration of butorphanol or meloxicam on physiologic responses to surgery in ball pythons. J Am Vet Med Assoc. 2008; 233(12):1883–1888.

13. Darrow BG, Meyers GE, Kukanich B. Fentanyl transdermal therapeutic system pharmacokinetics in ball pythons (*Python regius*). Proceedings. Annu Meet Am Assoc Zoo Vet. 2010; 238–239.

14. Gamble KC. Plasma fentanyl concentrations achieved after transdermal fentanyl patch application in prehensile-tailed skinks, Corucia zebrata. J Herp Med Surg. 2008; 18:81–85.

15. Wambugu SN, Towett PK, Kiama SG, et al: Effects of opioids in the formalin test in the Speke's hinged tortoise (*Kinixy's spekii*). J Vet Pharmacol Ther. 2010; 33 (4):347–351.

16. Kanui TI, Hole K. Morphine and pethidine antinociception in the crocodile. J Vet Pharmacol Ther. 1992; 15(1):101–103.

17. Kanui TI, Hole K, Miaron JO. Nociception in crocodiles: Capsaicin instillation, formalin and hot plate tests. Zool Sci. 1990; 7:537–540.

18. Mauk MD, Olson RD, LaHoste GJ, et al: Tonic immobility produces hyperalgesia and antagonizes morphine analgesia. Science. 1981; 213(4505):353–354.

19. Baker BB, Sladky KK, Johnson SM. Evaluation of the analgesic effects of oral and subcutaneous tramadol administration in red-eared slider turtles. J Am Vet Med Assoc. 2011; 238(2):220–227.

20. Cummings BB, Sladky KK, Johnson SM. Tramadol analgesic and respiratory effects in red-eared slider turtles (*Trachemys scripta*). Proceedings. Annu Meet Am Assoc Zoo Vet Am Assoc Wildl Vet Joint Conf. 2009; 115–116.

21. Funk RS, Diethelm G. Reptile formulary. In Mader DR, ed. *Reptile medicine and surgery.* ed 2, St. Louis, 2005, Elsevier.

22. Tuttle AD, Papich M, Lewbart GA, et al: Pharmacokinetics of ketoprofen in the green iguana (*Iguana iguana*) following single intravenous and intramuscular injections. J Zoo Wildl Med. 2006; 37(4):567–570.

23. Divers SJ, Papich M, McBride M, et al: Pharmacokinetics of meloxicam following intravenous and oral administration in green iguanas (*Iguana iguana*). Am J Vet Res. 2010; 71(11):1277–1283.

24. Trnkova S, Knotkova Z, Hrda A, et al: Effect of non-steroidal anti-inflammatory drugs on the blood profile in the green iguana (*Iguana iguana*). Vet Med. 2007; 52(11):507–511.

25. Mans C, Steagall PVM, Lahner LL. Efficacy of intrathecal lidocaine, bupivacaine, and morphine for spinal anesthesia and analgesia in red-eared slider turtles (*Trachemys scripta elegans*). 2011 Proceedings. Annu Conf Am Assoc Zoo Vet Proc Annu Conf Am Assoc Zoo Vet.

26. Hernandez-Divers SJ, Stahl SJ, Farrell R. An endoscopic method for identifying sex of hatchling Chinese box turtles and comparison of general versus local anesthesia for coelioscopy. J Am Vet Med Assoc. 2009; 234(6):800–804.

27. Rivera S, Divers SJ, Knafo SE, et al: Sterilisation of hybrid Galapagos tortoises (*Geochelone nigra*) for island restoration. Part 2: phallectomy of males under intrathecal anaesthesia with lidocaine. Vet Rec. 2011; 168(3):78.

28. Wellehan JF, Gunkel CI, Kledzik D, et al: Use of a nerve locator to facilitate administration of mandibular nerve blocks in crocodilians. J Zoo Wildl Med. 2006; 37(3):405–8.

29. Custer RS, Bush M. Physiologic and acid-base measures of gopher snakes during ketamine or halothane-nitrous oxide anesthesia. J Am Vet Med Assoc. 1980; 177(9):870–874.

30. Schumacher J, Lillywhite HB, Norman WM, et al: Effects of ketamine HCl on cardiopulmonary function in snakes. Copeia. 1997; 1997(2):395–400.

31. Greer LL, Jenne KJ, Diggs HE. Medetomidine-ketamine anesthesia in red-eared slider turtles (*Trachemys scripta elegans*). Contemp Top Lab Anim Sci. 2001; 40(3):9–11.

32. Bienzle D, Boyd CJ. Sedative effects of ketamine and midazolam in snapping turtles (*Chelydra serpentina*). J Zoo Wildl Med. 1992; 23(2):201–204.

33. Sleeman JM, Gaynor J. Sedative and cardiopulmonary effects of medetomidine and reversal with atipamezole in desert tortoises (*Gopherus agassizii*). J Zoo Wildl Med. 2000; 31 (1):28–35.

34. Dennis PM, Heard DJ. Cardiopulmonary effects of a medetomidine-ketamine combination administered intravenously in gopher tortoises. J Am Vet Med Assoc. 2002; 220 (10):1516–1519.

35. Lock BA, Heard DJ, Dennis P. Preliminary evaluation of medetomidine/ketamine combinations for immobilization and reversal with atipamezole in three tortoise species. Bull Assoc Reptil Amphib Vet. 1998; 8(4):6–9.

36. Bennett RA. Reptile anesthesia. Semin Avian Exot Pet Med. 1998; 7(1):30–40.

37. Flecknell PA. The relief of pain in laboratory animals. Lab Anim. 1984; 18:147–160.

38. Morton DB. Assessment of pain. Vet Rec. 1986; 119:435.

CHAPTER 28

Regulations Regarding Pain and Distress in Laboratory Animals

Andrea R. Slate

The assessment and treatment of pain in animals used for research, testing, and teaching are complicated by the fact that these animals do not have owners in the same sense as companion animals or livestock. In the United States, legal and ethical obligations require laboratory animal veterinarians to adequately assess and treat pain. The specific laws that each institution must follow depend on the species of animal used and the sponsor of the work. There is overlap among some of the regulations. Most of the regulations do not prescribe specific treatments but do require that animals receive standard veterinary care. Professional organizations offer textbooks, peer-reviewed literature, guidelines, and position statements to aid veterinarians and institutions in developing and updating programs of animal care.

PUBLIC HEALTH SERVICE POLICY ON HUMANE CARE AND USE OF LABORATORY ANIMALS

- The 1985 Health Research Extension Act mandated that the Secretary of Health and Human Services, acting through the Director of the National Institutes of Health (NIH), establish guidelines for the proper treatment of animals used in research. This law directs the development of guidelines (the Public Health Service [PHS] Policy) that require the appropriate use of "tranquilizers, analgesics, anesthetics, paralytics and euthanasia as well as appropriate pre-surgical and post-surgical veterinary medical and nursing care."[1]
- The NIH Office of Laboratory Animal Welfare (OLAW) is responsible for the general administration and coordination of the Policy.

Public Health Service Policy

- The PHS Policy applies to all work that is conducted or supported by the PHS involving live vertebrate animals. The PHS includes the Agency for Healthcare Research and Quality, the Centers for Disease Control and Prevention, the Food and Drug Administration, the Health Resources and Services Administration, the Indian Health Service, the NIH, and the Substance Abuse and Mental Health Services Administration.

- The PHS follows the *U.S. Government Principles for the Utilization and Care of Vertebrate Animals Used in Testing, Research and Training* (the U.S. Government Principles).
- The PHS Policy requires institutions to use the *Guide for the Care and Use of Laboratory Animals* (the Guide) as a basis for developing and implementing an institutional program for activities involving animals. The Policy also requires compliance with applicable regulations issued by the U.S. Department of Agriculture (USDA).
- Institutions with PHS-supported projects must have an Institutional Animal Care and Use Committee (IACUC) and an institutional veterinarian. The IACUC reviews proposed animal use protocols to ensure the following:
  1. Pain, distress, and discomfort to animals will be minimized.
  2. Procedures that may cause more than momentary or slight pain or distress to the animals will be performed with appropriate anesthesia, analgesia, or sedation. Exceptions to this may be approved when a scientific justification is provided and approved by the IACUC.
  3. Animals that would otherwise experience severe or chronic pain or distress that cannot be relieved will be euthanized during or at the end of the procedure.
  4. The living conditions and other nonmedical care will be directed by a veterinarian or scientist trained and experienced with the species.
  5. Medical care for animals will be available and provided as necessary by a qualified veterinarian.
  6. Personnel will be qualified and undergo training in the procedures they will be conducting with animals.
  7. Methods of euthanasia will be consistent with the American Veterinary Medical Association (AVMA) Guidelines on Euthanasia. Exceptions to this may be approved when a scientific justification is provided and approved by the IACUC.

The U.S. Government Principles

The U.S. Government Principles were written by the Interagency Research Animal Committee in 1985. These nine principles have been adopted by the PHS and the USDA.[2] The following principles relate to pain or distress in research animals:

- *Principle IV:* "Proper use of animals, including the avoidance or minimization of discomfort, distress and pain when consistent with sound scientific practices, is imperative. Unless the contrary is established, investigators should consider that procedures that cause pain or distress in human beings may cause pain or distress in other animals."
- *Principle V:* "Procedures with animals that may cause more than momentary or slight pain or distress should be performed with appropriate sedation,

analgesia, or anesthesia. Surgical or other painful procedures should not be performed on anaesthetized animals paralyzed by chemical agents."

- *Principle VI:* "Animals that would otherwise suffer severe or chronic pain or distress that cannot be relieved should be painlessly killed at the end of the procedure or, if appropriate, during the procedure."[3]

GUIDE FOR THE CARE AND USE OF LABORATORY ANIMALS, EIGHTH EDITION

- The Guide defines animals as all vertebrates produced for or used in research, teaching, or testing.
- The Guide supports the U.S. Government Principles and reiterates that it should be assumed that procedures that cause pain in humans may also cause pain in animals.
- The Guide describes pain as "a complex experience that typically results from stimuli that damage or have the potential to damage tissue; such stimuli prompt withdrawal and evasive action." Distress is described as "an aversive state in which an animal fails to cope or adjust to various stressors with which it is presented."[4]
- The recommendations of the Guide regarding treatment of pain in animals rely on the professional judgment of veterinarians rather than over arching prescriptive rules.

Development of Research Protocols

- A veterinarian should be consulted regarding the selection, dose, and use of anesthetic and analgesic medications. The recommendations should reflect professional veterinary judgment and consider clinical, humane, and research needs. Guidelines for the appropriate use of anesthetics and analgesics should be developed. These guidelines should be reviewed and modified as standards and techniques are refined.
- The research protocol should describe the plan for postsurgical monitoring and care, record keeping, and specific duties of the personnel involved in caring for the animals.
- If possible, humane end points (in contrast to experimental end points that are based on research needs) should be described before the start of the study. Pilot studies may be indicated for novel experiments to identify animal welfare issues and define appropriate humane end points. Humane end points and monitoring schemes should be determined through collaboration between the Principal Investigator (PI), the veterinarian, and the IACUC.

- The use of neuromuscular blocking agents should be carefully reviewed by the IACUC and the veterinarian. A pilot study conducting a similar procedure without the use of neuromuscular blocking agents is suggested for verification of the adequacy of the proposed anesthetic regimen.

Postoperative and Postprocedural Monitoring and Care

- Proper use of anesthetics and analgesics is required. Personnel working with and caring for animals should be trained to recognize pain in the specific species with which they are working. Some species may be stoic and will not show outward signs of pain until it is severe (e.g., prey species).
- Preemptive analgesia is recommended to improve patient stability during surgery and to reduce postoperative pain.
- Postsurgical observation and intervention by trained personnel is required to ensure animal well-being during recovery from anesthesia and surgery. During this time, animals should be housed in a clean, dry, and comfortable area that facilitates monitoring. Attention should be paid to maintenance of body temperature, cardiovascular and pulmonary function, electrolyte and fluid balance, and behavioral signs of postoperative pain or discomfort.
- Animals should be monitored during and after painful procedures. Individual animals may respond differently to analgesics. If pain or distress is beyond that anticipated, or interventional control is not possible, a veterinarian must be consulted. Animals should receive additional analgesic medications as needed.
- Routes of administration of analgesic drugs include enteral, parenteral, and local. Nonpharmacologic strategies may also be effective, including appropriate nursing support; a comfortable, warm, quiet environment; fluid administration; and supplemental feeding.

Drugs

- Anesthetic and analgesic agents as well as euthanasia drugs must be used before their expiration date. All use of medications should be in concordance with applicable federal and local laws.
- When available, pharmaceutical-grade substances should be used in laboratory animals to prevent toxic or unwanted side effects. When non–pharmaceutical grade chemicals are to be used in live animals, their use should be described and justified in the animal use protocol. Suggestions for parameters to be evaluated in these substances include "grade, purity, sterility, pH, pyrogenicity, osmolality, stability, site and route of administration, formulation, compatibility, and pharmacokinetics, as well as animal welfare and scientific issues relating to its use."[5]

Chronic Pain

Assessment and alleviation of chronic pain may be more difficult than for acute postprocedural pain. The Guide suggests considering the use of chronic administration of analgesics by alternate routes such as transdermal patches or osmotic mini-pumps.

Emergency Intervention

Emergency veterinary care must be provided for research animals. The veterinarian or his or her designee must be available to evaluate and treat or euthanize the animal. If the PI is not available or the PI and the veterinarian are in disagreement, the veterinarian must be provided with the authority to ensure animal welfare by providing appropriate medical care, removing the animal from the study, or euthanizing the animal when necessary.

Euthanasia

Methods of euthanasia must be consistent with the *AVMA Guidelines on Euthanasia*. Exceptions should be justified scientifically and approved by the IACUC.

Recommended Resources

Animal users are directed to additional sources such as: *Recognition and Alleviation of Pain in Laboratory Animals* and *Recognition and Alleviation of Distress in Laboratory Animals*.

ANIMAL WELFARE ACT, ANIMAL WELFARE ACT REGULATIONS, AND USDA ANIMAL CARE POLICY MANUAL

Animal Welfare Act

- The Animal Welfare Act (AWA) (initially the Laboratory Animal Welfare Act of 1966) authorizes the USDA to regulate the "transportation, purchase, sale, housing, care, handling, and treatment of animals by carriers or by persons or organizations engaged in using them for research or experimental purposes."[6]
- The USDA is also authorized to promulgate standards for research facilities that require that animal care and treatment minimize pain and distress. Veterinary care must be provided in the form of appropriate use of medications (anesthetics, analgesic, or tranquilizing drugs) or euthanasia.
- For any procedures that could cause pain to animals, the AWA requires the following:
  1. The PI considers alternatives to those procedures that could cause pain.

2. A veterinarian is consulted during the planning stages of those procedures to provide recommendations on the use of anesthetic, analgesic, and tranquilizing medications as well as recommendations on the observation and care to be provided to those animals by the laboratory staff. These recommendations should be based on current established veterinary standards.
3. Paralytic agents should not be used without anesthesia.
4. When there is a scientific need to withhold anesthetic, analgesic, or tranquilizing medications or euthanasia, those agents or euthanasia should be withheld only as long as necessary.

Animal Welfare Information Center

The AWA mandated the establishment of an information service at the National Agricultural Library (NAL). The NAL established the Animal Welfare Information Center (AWIC) to provide information to researchers with the goal of improving animal care in research and teaching.

Animal Welfare Regulations

- Animal Welfare Regulations (AWRs) apply to "any live or dead dog, cat, nonhuman primate, guinea pig, hamster, rabbit, or any other warm-blooded animal, which is being used, or is intended for use for research, teaching, testing, experimentation, or exhibition purposes, or as a pet."
- Animals excluded from these regulations are "birds, rats of the genus *Rattus*, and mice of the genus *Mus*, bred for use in research; horses not used for research purposes; and other farm animals, such as, but not limited to, livestock or poultry used or intended for use as food or fiber, or livestock or poultry used or intended for use for improving animal nutrition, breeding, management, or production efficiency, or for improving the quality of food or fiber."[7] The majority of mice and rats used in research are *not* covered by the AWRs.
- The AWRs require each research facility to have an IACUC.
- The AWRs require adequate veterinary care. Each research facility must have an attending veterinarian. This veterinarian should provide periprocedural care to animals in accordance with current established veterinary medical and nursing standards.

USDA Animal Care Policy Manual

- The USDA Animal Care Policy Manual is put forth by the USDA to clarify the AWRs. Policy 3 and policy 11, discussed later, relate to pain or distress in research animals.
- Specific details of veterinary care should be written in the animal use proposal. This includes the manner in which relief of pain and distress will be

provided to animals before, during, and after potentially painful procedures. The specific medications to be used should be noted and should
be available for use. The veterinarian maintains authority to alter the care
if unexpected pain or distress occurs. If the veterinarian recommends
changes to the care of subsequent animals, the IACUC should review this
change to the animal use protocol. Finally, if care to relieve pain or distress
will be withheld, a scientific justification must be provided in the animal
use protocol and approved by the IACUC.

* A painful procedure is defined as "any procedure that would reasonably
  be expected to cause more than slight or momentary pain or distress in a
  human being to which that procedure is applied—that is, pain in excess of
  that caused by injections or other minor procedures."[5] Animals experiencing pain are expected to receive standard veterinary care unless a scientific
  justification is provided to and approved by the IACUC.

AMERICAN VETERINARY MEDICAL ASSOCIATION

* The AVMA is a nonprofit organization of more than 82,000 veterinarians in the United States.[6] In 2000 the group published the Report of the
  AVMA Panel on Euthanasia. This document has since been revised and
  in 2007 was renamed the AVMA Guidelines on Euthanasia. The document gives recommendations for methods of euthanasia for various species and classifies them into acceptable, conditionally acceptable (used
  only under certain circumstances), and unacceptable. Multiple regulatory
  documents require adherence to these guidelines including the PHS Policy and the USDA Animal Care Policies.

ASSOCIATION FOR ASSESSMENT AND ACCREDITATION OF LABORATORY ANIMAL CARE INTERNATIONAL

* The Association for Assessment and Accreditation of Laboratory Animal
  Care International (AAALAC) is a nonprofit organization that offers a
  voluntary accreditation program with the mission of promoting the
  humane treatment of animals in science. This accreditation program is
  recognized by the PHS. AAALAC assessment of animal care and use
  programs takes a performance-based approach. Institutions are expected
  to adhere to local, state, and federal laws and specific primary standards,
  depending on the facility location and type of research conducted. The
  primary standards are the Guide; the Guide for the Care and Use of Agricultural Animals in Research and Teaching; and the European Convention for the Protection of Vertebrate Animals Used for Experimental and
  Other Scientific Purposes Council of Europe (ETS 123). Additional reference resources are available on the AAALAC website.

INSTITUTE FOR LABORATORY ANIMAL RESEARCH

- The Institute for Laboratory Animal Research (ILAR) is a component of the National Academies of Science with the mission to "evaluate and disseminate information on issues related to the scientific, technologic, and ethical use of animals and related biologic resources in research, testing, and education."[7]
- Useful references are available through ILAR including *ILAR Journal, Guide for the Care and Use of Laboratory Animals, Recognition and Alleviation of Pain in Laboratory Animals,* and *Recognition and Alleviation of Distress in Laboratory Animals,* among others.

AMERICAN ASSOCIATION FOR LABORATORY ANIMAL SCIENCE

- The American Association for Laboratory Animal Science (AALAS) is a professional organization with the goal to "advance responsible animal care and use to benefit people and animals."[8] There are also local branches of this national organization.
- AALAS organizes an annual meeting and supports training and certification programs. Two peer-reviewed journals are published: *Journal of the American Association for Laboratory Animal Science* (JAALAS) and *Comparative Medicine.*

GUIDE FOR THE CARE AND USE OF AGRICULTURAL ANIMALS IN RESEARCH AND TEACHING

- The Federation of Animal Science Societies (FASS) has published the Guide for the Care and Use of Agricultural Animals in Research and Teaching (the Ag Guide; initially published as the Guide for the Care and Use of Agricultural Animals in Agricultural Research and Teaching). This is a useful guide, especially for the use of animals that do not fall under the authority of the AWA and AWARs.
- The Ag Guide echoes the regulatory documents regarding animal pain and distress, but also suggests that certain potentially painful animal husbandry procedures, so-called "standard agricultural practices," may be conducted in very young animals without anesthesia if in accordance with accepted veterinary practice and approved by the facility IACUC.[1] It subsequently gives details on when these practices may be appropriate.
- FASS also publishes a number of peer-reviewed journals in the field of agricultural animal sciences.

AMERICAN COLLEGE OF LABORATORY ANIMAL MEDICINE

- The American College of Laboratory Animal Medicine (ACLAM) is an AVMA-recognized specialty board that serves to certify laboratory animal veterinarians. ACLAM was founded with the goals "to encourage education, training and research in laboratory animal medicine; to establish standards of training and experience for qualification of specialists in laboratory animal medicine; and to further the recognition of such qualified specialists by suitable certification and other means."[1] There are ACLAM-approved formal laboratory animal medicine training programs and a specialty board examination. ACLAM holds an annual conference.
- The ACLAM series of books, published by Academic Press, are valuable resources for those working with research animals. *Laboratory Animal Medicine, Anesthesia and Analgesia of Laboratory Animals*, and species-specific texts are available.
- ACLAM also publishes position statements on pain and distress that are available on the organization's website.
  - *Pain and Distress in Laboratory Animals.* This document reiterates the concepts adopted by the PHS and the USDA.
  - *Guidelines for the Assessment and Management of Pain in Rodents and Rabbits.* This document provides species-specific clinical assessment tools and information regarding treatment modalities, both pharmacologic and nonpharmacologic. It also discusses possible side effects of classes of analgesic drugs, including some that may confound research.

REFERENCES

1. Health Research Extension Act of 1985, PL 99-158, Anim Res. (Section 495 a.2.A, a.2.B) Retrieved from http://grants.nih.gov/grants/olaw/references/phspol.htm#HealthResearchExtensionActof1985.
2. Office of Laboratory Animal Welfare, National Institutes of Health: Public health service policy on humane care and use of laboratory animals. Bethesda, 2002, Author. Retrieved from http://grants.nih.gov/grants/olaw/references/phspol.htm#PublicHealthServicePolicyonHumaneCareandUseofLaboratory
3. National Institutes of Health. U.S Government principles for the utilization and care of vertebrate animals used in testing, research, and training. Retrieved from http://grants.nih.gov/grants/olaw/references/phspol.htm#USGovPrinciples.
4. National Research Council: The guide for the care and use of laboratory animals. Washington, D.C., 2011, National Academies Press. Retrieved from www.nap.edu/catalog.php?record_id=12910.
5. American Veterinary Medical Association: AVMA guidelines on euthanasia. 2007. Retrieved from www.avma.org/KB/Policies/Documents/euthanasia.pdf.
6. National Research Council: Recognition and alleviation of pain in laboratory animals. Washington, D.C., 2009, National Academies Press.

7. National Research Council: Recognition and alleviation of distress in laboratory animals. Washington, D.C., 2008, National Academies Press.

8. Animal Welfare Act. United States Code Title 7, Chapter 54, Sections 2131-2159. 2005.

9. Animal Welfare Information Center. www.awic.nal.usda.gov.

10. Animal Welfare Regulations. Code of federal regulations, Title 9, Chapter 1, Subchapter A, Parts 1-4. 2005.

11. Animal Care Policy Manual. www.aalas.org/association/about.aspx.

12. American Veterinary Medicine Association (AVMA). www.avma.org.

13. Association for Assessment and Accreditation of Laboratory Animal Care (AAALAC). www.aaalac.org.

14. Federation of Animal Science Societies: Guide for the care and use of agricultural animals in research and teaching, ed 3. Champlain, 2010, Author.

15. The European Convention for the Protection of Vertebrate Animals used for Experimental and Other Scientific Purposes, Strasbourg, 1986. Retrieved from http://conventions.coe.int/treaty/en/treaties/html/123.htm.

16. Institute for Laboratory Animal Research (ILAR). http://dels.nas.edu/ilar.

17. American Association for Laboratory Animal Science (AALAS). www.aalas.org.

18. Federation of Animal Science Societies (FASS). www.fass.org.

19. American College of Laboratory Medicine (ACLAM). www.aclam.org.

20. Fox JG, Anderson LC, Loew FM, Quimby FW, eds.: Laboratory animal medicine, ed 2. San Diego, 2002, Academic Press.

21. Fish RE, Brown MJ, Danneman PJ, Karas AZ: Anesthesia and analgesia of laboratory animals, ed 2. London, 2008, Academic Press.

Drugs Used to Treat Pain, Pain-Related Anxiety, and Anesthesia-Related Side Effects as Described in This Handbook

GENERIC NAME	TRADE NAME	DOG DOSAGE (mg/kg)	CAT DOSAGE (mg/kg)	OTHER SPECIES DOSAGES (mg/kg)
Acepromazine	Acepromazine	0.025-0.1 max 3 mg IV, SC, IM 0.5-2 PO	0.05-0.1 max 1 mg IV 0.1-2.25 PO	Swine: 0.1-0.2 (adult) IM q12h
Acetaminophen	Tylenol	10-15 PO q8-12h Use with caution	Not recommended	Not recommended for birds
Alendronate	Fosamax	0.5-1.0 PO daily	Unknown	
Amantadine	Symmetrel	3-5 PO q24h	3-5 PO q24h	
Amitriptyline	Elavil	1-2 PO q12-24h	5-10 PO q24h	
Aspirin	Aspirin	10-25 PO q8-12h	10-25 PO q48h	Av: 1.0-5.0 PO q12h Swine: 10 PO q6-8h
Atenolol	Tenormin	0.25-1.0 PO q12-24h	2-3 PO q24h	
Atipamezole	Antisedan	50-100 µg/kg IM	50-100 µg/kg IM	
Atropine		0.02-0.04 IV, SC, IM PRN	0.02-0.04 IV, SC, IM PRN	Av: 0.02-0.04 SC, IM
Bupivacaine	Marcaine	1-2 SC, interpleurally 1-1.5 epidurally	1-2 SC, interpleurally 1-1.5 epidurally	F: <1.5 SC, 1.1 epidurally Ra: <1.5 SC Av: <1.0 SC Ck: Toxic at 2.7 intra-articularly Re: Toxic dose unknown; recommend <2 mg/kg; dilute to 0.25% to increase volume

Continued

Buprenorphine	Buprenex, Carpuject	0.005-0.02 SC, IM, IV q4-8h	0.005-0.02 SC, IM, IV q4-8h 0.01-0.02 PO q6-12h	Re 0.4-1.0 IM, SC, IV F: 0.01-0.03 q6-10h IV, SC Ra: 0.01-0.05 q6-10h IV, SC *African Grey parrots: 0.1 IM *Domestic pigeons: 0.25-0.5 IM
Butorphanol	Torbugesic	0.4-1.2 SC, IM q2-6h 0.1-0.5 IV q0.5-2h 0.5-2 PO q6-8h	0.1-0.4 SC, IM q2-6h 0.1-0.2 IV q1-2h 0.5-2 PO q6-8h	Re: 10-8.0 IM, SC F: 0.1-0.4 q2-4h IV, IM, SC 0.1-0.2 mg/kg/hr IV CRI Ra: 0.5 q2-4h IV, SC 0.1-0.3 mg/kg/hr IV CRI; *Hispaniolan, Amazon parrots: 5 IV q2h, 5 IM q3h Psitaccines: 1-3 IV, IM
Cannabis, cannibinoids (THC)	Cesamet, Marinol, Sativex	0.05 PO extrapolated from human dosage; no investigational data	Unknown	
Carprofen	Rimadyl, Zenecarp	4.4 SC single dose 2.2 PO q12h 4.4 PO q24h	1-4 SC single dose Not recommended for oral use	Re: 1.0-4.0 IV, IM, SC *Hispaniolan, Amazon parrots: 3.0 IM q12h *Chickens 1.0 IM once
Chlorpromazine	Thorazine	0.05-0.50 SC, IM, IV q6-24h 0.8-4.4 PO q24h	0.5 IM, IV q6-8h 2-4 PO q24h	Swine: 0.5 IM once
Clomipramine	Clomicalm	1-3 PO q12-24h	1-5 PO q12-24h	
Clonidine	Catapres	0.01 IV 0.1/15-20 kg transdermal patch 20-30 µg/kg/hr epidural	0.01 IV 20-30 µg/kg/hr epidural	

GENERIC NAME	TRADE NAME	DOG DOSAGE (mg/kg)	CAT DOSAGE (mg/kg)	OTHER SPECIES DOSAGES (mg/kg)
Codeine		0.5-1 PO q4-6h	0.5 PO q6h	
Deracoxib	Deramaxx	1-2 PO q24h 3-4 PO q24h 7-day limit		
Detomidine	Dormosedan	Approx. 0.4-0.6 mg/kg on buccal mucosa	Approx. 0.4-0.6 mg/kg on buccal mucosa	
Dexamethasone		0.10-0.15 SC, PO, IV	0.10-0.15 SC, PO, IV	
Dexmedetomidine	Dexdomitor	0.002-0.005 IM, IV (sedation, analgesia) 0.0005-0.001 mg/kg/hr IV (supplemental CRI during inhalant anesthesia) 0.001-0.003 IV bolus (short-term sedation/analgesia) 0.0005-0.002 mg/kg/hr IV (extended sedation or analgesia CRI)	0.002-0.010 IM, SC, IV 0.0005-0.001 mg/kg/hr intraoperative or postoperative	
Dextromethorphan	Benylin	0.5-2 PO, SC, IV q6-8h	0.5-2.0 PO q6-8h	
Diazepam	Valium	0.1-0.5 IV, IM 0.5-2.2 PO	0.05-0.4 IV, IM 0.5-2.2 PO	Av: 0.5-1.0 mg/kg IM, IV
Diltiazem	Cardizem, Dilacor	0.5-1.5 PO 0.125-0.035 IV	1.75-2.5 PO 0.125-0.35 IV	
Dipyrone	Metamizole	25-100 IM, IV, SC, PO q8h	25 IM, IV, PO q12-24h	

Doxapram	Dopram	1-5 IV	1-5 IV	
Fentanyl	Sublimaze	0.01-0.04 SC, IM 0.002-0.005 IV 2-20 µg/kg/hr IV	0.005-0.04 SC, IM 0.002-0.005 IV 2-20 µg/kg/hr IV	F: 20-30 µg/kg/hr IV CRI during anesthesia to reduce volatile inhalant concentrations 1-4 µg/kg/hr IV CRI for analgesia Ra: 5-10 µg/kg IV loading dose followed by 10-40 µg/kg/hr IV CRI during anesthesia to reduce volatile inhalant concentrations 1.25-5.0 µg/kg/hr IV CRI for analgesia 25 g/hr transcutaneous patch Red-tailed hawks: 0.15-0.5 µg/kg/hr IV Re: 2.5-12.5 µg/hr
Fentanyl: transdermal patch	Duragesic	Loading: 2-5 g/kg CRI: 2-5 µg/kg/hr (pain management) 10-45 µg/kg/hr (surgical analgesia and MAC reduction) <5 kg 12 µg/kg/hr 5-10 kg: 25 µg/kg/hr 10-25 kg: 50 µg/kg/hr >25 kg: 75 µg/kg/hr	Loading: 1-3 µg/kg CRI: 1-4 µg/kg/hr (pain management) 0-30 µg/kg/hr (surgical analgesia) 5 µg/kg/hr	
Fentanyl: transdermal solution	Recuvyra	2.6 (0.052 mL/kg)	Not approved or recommended	
Firocoxib	Previcox	5 PO q8-12h		

Continued

GENERIC NAME	TRADE NAME	DOG DOSAGE (mg/kg)	CAT DOSAGE (mg/kg)	OTHER SPECIES DOSAGES (mg/kg)
Flumazenil	Romazicon	0.2 mg/dog IV PRN	0.2 mg/cat IV PRN	
Flunixin meglumine	Banamine	1.0 PO single dose 0.5-2.2 IV 1 IV, IM SC once	1.0 PO single dose 0.5-2.2 IV 1 IV, IM, SC once	Re: 0.1-0.5 IM
Gabapentin	Neurontin	2.5-40 PO bid-tid	5-10 PO bid	
Glycopyrrolate	Robinul-V	5-10 µg/kg IV, IM, SC	5-10 µg/kg IV, IM, SC	Swine: 3.3 µg/kg
Hydrocortisone	Cortef	2.5-5 PO q12h	2.5-5 PO q12h	
Hydromorphone	Dilaudid Hydrostat	0.05-0.2 SC, IM 0.05-0.1 IV q2-6h 0.05-0.1 mg/kg/hr	0.05-0.1 SC, IM q2-6h 0.03-0.05 IV q1h 0.01-0.05 mg/kg/hr	F: 0.1-0.2 IV, IM, SC q6-8h 0.005-0.015 mg/kg/hr IV CRI Ra: 0.05-0.2 IV, IM, SC q6-8h Re: 0.5 IM, SC
Imipramine	Tofranil	0.5-1.0 PO q8h	2.5-5.0 PO q12h	
Ketamine (as NMDA receptor antagonist, not anesthetic)	Numerous: Ketalar, Vetalar, Ketaset, Ketaflo	0.5 IV, followed by 20 µg/kg/min during surgery, followed by 2 µg/kg/min for next 24hr	0.5 IV, followed by 20 µg/kg/min during surgery, followed by 2 µg/kg/min for next 24hr	Re: 10-100 IM, IV, SC F: 0.5 IV before surgery 10 µg/min IV CRI during surgery 2 µg/kg/min for 24hr postoperatively Ra: 0.5 IV before surgery 10 µg/kg/min IV CRI during surgery 2 µg/kg/min for 24hr postoperatively
Ketoprofen	Ketofen, Anafen	1-2 IV, IM, SC initial dose 1 PO q24h up to 5 days	0.5-2 IV, IM, SC initial dose 0.5-1 PO q24h up to 5 days	Re: 2 q24-48h IM, SC Av: 1-5 IM, IV q24h *Chickens: 12 IM *once* *Mallard ducks: 5 IM *once*

Ketorolac	Toradol	0.3-0.6 PO, IV, IM q8-12h	0.25 IM q12h	
Lidocaine		2-4 IV bolus then 25-75 µg/kg IV infusion 4.4 of 2% epidural	0.25-1.0 IV bolus then 10-40 µg/kg IV infusion 4.4 of 2% epidural	Re: toxic dose unknown, recommend <5; Dilute to 1% to increase volume F: <4 SC 4.4 epidurally Ra: < 4 SC Av: 1-3, toxic at 4
Magnesium salts		5-15 IV 0.75-1 mEq Mg^{2+}/kg IV	5-15 IV 0.75-1 mEq Mg^{2+}/kg IV	
Meloxicam	Metacam	0.2 IV, SC 0.2 initial loading dose, then 0.1 PO q24h	C.3 SC	Re: 0.1-0.3 IM, IV, PO q24-48h F: 0.1-0.2 SC, PO q24h Ra: 0.1-1.0 SC, PO q12-24h; *Parakeets: 0.5-1.0 PO q12h *Hispaniolan, Amazon parrots: 1.0 IM q12h *Hispaniolan, Amazon parrots: 1.0 IV, PO once *Ostrich 0.5 IV once
Meperidine	Demerol	3-10 IV, IM q2-3h or PRN 2.5-6.5 IM (preanesthetic)	1-5 IV, IM PRN 2.2-4.4 IM (preanesthetic)	Re: 1.0-50.0 IM, SC
Mepivacaine	Carbocaine-V	0.5 mL of 2% solution, q30sec, epidurally, until reflexes are absent	0.5 mL of 2% solution, q30sec, epidurally, until reflexes are absent	Re: Toxic dose unknown; recommend <5; dilute to 1% to increase volume
Methadone	Dolophine	0.1-0.5 IV, IM, SC q2-4h 0.5 PO b d-qid	0.1-0.25 IV, IM, SC q2-4h 0.1-0.3 Buccally tid-tid 00.25-0.5 PO bid-qid	Swine: 0.1-0.2 IV

Continued

GENERIC NAME	TRADE NAME	DOG DOSAGE (mg/kg)	CAT DOSAGE (mg/kg)	OTHER SPECIES DOSAGES (mg/kg)
Methylprednisolone	Medrol, Depo-Medrol, Solu-Medrol	0.5-1 PO q12h 0.22-0.44 PO q12-24h 30 IV followed by 5.4 mg/kg/hr for 24 to 48hr	0.5-1 PO q12h 0.22-0.44 PO q12-24h 30 IV followed by 5.4 mg/kg/hr for 24 to 48hr; 20-40 mg IA	
Mexiletine	Mexitil	5-8 PO bid-tid	NA	
Midazolam	Versed	0.1-0.25 IV, IM	0.05-0.5 IV, IM	Av: 0.5-1.0 IV, IM Swine: up to 0.5 IM
Misoprostol	Cytotec	0.002-0.005 PO q8h	0.002-0.005 PO q8h	
Morphine	Morphine	0.25-1.0 SC, IM q4-6h 0.05-0.1 IV q1-2h 0.05-0.1 mg/kg/hr 0.1 epidurally q12-24h	0.05-0.1 IM, SC q4-6h	Re: 0.5-4.0 (crocodiles) 1.5-6.5 (turtles) 1.0-40.0 (others) F: 0.2-2 IM single dose preoperatively 0.1 epidurally Ra: 0.5-5 IM single dose preoperatively 0.1 epidurally
Morphine sulfate: sustained release	MS Contin	2-5 q12h	Not recommended	
Morphine sulfate tablets and oral liquid	Morphine sulfate	1.0 PO q4-6h	Not recommended	
Nalbuphine	Nubain	0.5-1 IV, IM q1-4h 0.03-0.1 IV	0.2-0.4 IV, IM q1-4h	*Hispaniolan, Amazon parrots: 12.5 IM

Drug	Trade name			
Nalmefene	Revex	1-4 SC		
Naloxone	Narcan	0.002-0.04 IV, SC, IM as needed to reverse opiate	0.002-0.04 IV, SC, IM as needed to reverse opiate	
Naltrexone	Trexan	0.05-0.1 SC, 2.2 PO q12h (behavioral problems)	0.05-0.1 SC	
Nimodipine	Nimotop	Unknown	Unknown	
Oxymorphone	Numorphan	0.025-0.2 IV, IM, SC	0.02-0.2 IV, IM, SC	F: 0.05-0.2 IV, IM, SC q6-8h; Ra: 0.05-0.2 IV, IM, SC q6-8h
Pamidronate	Aredia	1-2 mg/kg diluted over 2-4hr IV, SC	1-1.5 mg/kg diluted over 2-4hr	
Pentazocine	Talwin	0.5-1.0 IM, IV, SC q4h	0.5-1.0 IM, IV, SC q4h	
Phenylbutazone	Butazolidin	10-22 PO, IV q8-12h (max 800 mg/dog)	6-8 IV, PO once	Swine: 4 IV q24h
Phenytoin	Dilantin	2-4 (max 10) IV in increments 20-35 PO	2-3 PO	
Piroxicam	Feldene	0.3 PO q48 h	0.3 PO q2-4days	Cranes: 0.5-0.8 q12h
Prednisolone	Delta-Cortef	0.5-1 PO, IV, IM q12-24h initially then taper to q48h	0.5-1 PO, IV, IM q12-24h initially then taper to q48h	
Prednisone	Deltasone Meticorten	0.5-1 PO, IV, IM q12-24h initially then taper to q48h	0.5-1 PO, IV, IM q12-24h initially then taper to q48h	
Pregabalin	Lyrica	1-3 PO bid-qid	1-3 PO bid-qid	

Continued

GENERIC NAME	TRADE NAME	DOG DOSAGE (mg/kg)	CAT DOSAGE (mg/kg)	OTHER SPECIES DOSAGES (mg/kg)
Propranolol	Inderal	0.02-0.06 IV over 5-10 min 0.2-1 PO q8h (titrate dose to effect) 0.125-1.10 PO	0.4-1.2 (2.5-5 mg/cat) PO q8h 0.4-1.2 PO	
Omeprazole	Prilosec	0.5-1.0 PO q24h	0.56-1.0 PO q24h	
Oxycodone	Percocet (with acetaminophen) Oxycontin (sustained release)	0.1-0.3 PO q8-12h	Not recommended	
Oxymorphone	Numorphan Opana (sustained release)	0.05-0.2 IV, IM, SC q2-4h 0.03-0.05 IV	0.05-0.2 IV, IM, SC 0.02-0.1 SC, IM q3-4h 0.01-0.03 IV	
Piroxicam	Feldene	0.3 PO q24h for 3 days then every other day	0.3 PO q48h 1 mg/cat PO q24h max 7 days	Av: 0.1-0.5 PO q12h
Prazosin	Minipress	1 mg/15 kg (0.5-2 mg/dog) PO q8-12h	1 mg/15 kg (0.5-2 mg/cat) PO q8-12h	
Remifentanil	Ultiva	Loading: 4-10 µg/kg CRI: 4-10 g/kg/hr (pain management) 20-60 g/kg/hr (surgical analgesia)	Loading: 4-10 µg/kg CRI: 4-10 g/kg/hr (pain management) 20-60 g/kg/hr (surgical analgesia)	
Robenacoxib	Onsior	1-2 PO q24h	1-2 PO q24 h	

Drug	Trade name	Dose	Dose
Romifidine	Sedivet	0.02-0.04 IM, IV 0.01-0.02 IV (sedation, analgesia) 0.01-0.08 IM 0.005-0.01 IV (preanesthetic)	0.09-0.18 IM, IV 0.03-0.06 IM 0.015-0.03 IV (sedation/analgesia) 0.02-0.03 IM 0.01-0.02 IV (pre-anesthetic)
Ropivacaine	Naropin	1 mL of 0.2% or 0.5% per site intercostal nerve block 1-2 mL of 0.2%/kg intrapleural regional block 0.5 epidural	mL of 0.2% or 0.5% per site intercostal nerve block -2 mL of 0.2%/kg intrapleural regional block total dose 1 SC for declaw .5 epidural
Sufentanil	Sufenta	Loading: 5 g/kg 0.1 g/kg/min	
Tapentadol	Nucynta	5-10 PO bid-qid	
Tolazoline	Tolazoline	0.5-5 IV slowly	0.5-5 IV slowly
Tramadol	Ultram	2-4 PO bid-qid 1-4 IV	2-4 PO bid 1-4 IV F: 5 PO q12h Ra: Further research needed *Peafowl 7.5 PO *once* *Red-tailed hawks 11 PO *once* *American bald eagle: 5 PO *once* *Hispaniolan, Amazon parrots: 30 PO *once* Re: 5-10 PO
Triamcinolone	Vetalog, Triamtabs, Aristocort	0.5-1 PO q12-24h then taper dose to 0.5-1 q48h 0.11-0.22 PO, IM SC 1-3 IA	0.5-1 PO q12-24h then taper dose to 0.5-1 q48h 0.11-0.22 PO, IM SC

Continued

GENERIC NAME	TRADE NAME	DOG DOSAGE (mg/kg)	CAT DOSAGE (mg/kg)	OTHER SPECIES DOSAGES (mg/kg)
Xylazine	Rompun, Tranquived	1.1 IV 1.1-2.2 IM, SC 0.05-0.1 IV prn 0.2 SC, IM q1-2h	1.1 IM, SC 0.05-0.1 IV prn 0.2-0.4 SC, IM q1-2h	Swine: 0.5-3 IM Sheep: 0.05-0.1 IV 0.1-0.3 IM Goats: 0.01-0.5 IV 0.05-0.5 IM Re: 1-1.25 IM
Yohimbine	Yobine	0.1-0.3 IV 0.25-0.5 SC, IM	0.1-0.3 IV 0.25-0.5 SC, IM	

Specific use of each drug and dose is described in greater detail in the appropriate chapter.

Av, avian; *CRI*, constant rate infusion; *F*, ferret; *IA*, intra-articularly; *max*, maximum; *NMDA*, *N*-methyl-D-aspartate; *prn*, as needed; *Ra*, rabbit; *Re*, reptile; *THC*, Δ9-tetrahydrocannabinol.

*Pharmacodynamics available. All other avian doses are anecdotal from clinical use.

INDEX

Note: Page numbers followed by b indicate boxes, f indicate figures and t indicate tables.